Advanced Animal Nutrition

D.V. Reddy, BVSc, MVSc, PhD.

Dean incharge and Professor & Head
Department of Animal Nutrition
Rajiv Gandhi College of Veterinary & Animal Sciences, Pondicherry

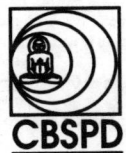

CBSPD

CBS Publishers & Distributors Pvt Ltd

New Delhi • Bengaluru • Chennai • Kochi • Kolkata • Lucknow • Mumbai
Hyderabad • Jharkhand • Nagpur • Patna • Pune • Uttarakhand

Advance Animal Nutrition

ISBN: 978-81-204-1756-4

OXFORD & IBH
New Delhi
(A Unit of CBS Publishers & Distributors Pvt Ltd)

Published by **Satish Kumar Jain** and produced by **Varun Jain** for

CBS Publishers & Distributors Pvt Ltd
4819/XI Prahlad Street, 24 Ansari Road, Daryaganj, New Delhi 110 002, India.
Ph: 011-23289259, 23266861, 23266867
Fax: 011-23243014

Website: www.cbspd.com
e-mail: delhi@cbspd.com;
cbspubs@airtelmail.in.

Corporate Office: 204 FIE, Industrial Area, Patparganj, Delhi 110 092
Ph: 011-4934 4934   Fax: 011-4934 4935
e-mail: publishing@cbspd.com; publicity@cbspd.com

Branches

- **Bengaluru:** Seema House 2975, 17th Cross, KR Road, Banasankari 2nd Stage, Bengaluru 560 070, Karnataka, India
  Ph: +91-80-26771678/79   Fax: +91-80-26771680   e-mail: bangalore@cbspd.com
- **Chennai:** 7, Subbaraya Street, Shenoy Nagar, Chennai 600 030, Tamil Nadu, India
  Ph: +91-44-26680620, 26681266   Fax: +91-44-42032115   e-mail: chennai@cbspd.com
- **Kochi:** 42/1325, 1326, Power House Road, Opp KSEB, Power House, Ernakulum Kochi 682 018, Kerala, India
  Ph: +91-484-4059061-65,67   Fax: +91-484-4059065   e-mail: kochi@cbspd.com
- **Kolkata:** 147, Hind Ceramics Compound, 1st Floor, Nilgunj Road, Belghoria, Kolkata-700056, West Bengal, India
  Ph: +033-25633055, 033-25633056   e-mail: kolkata@cbspd.com
- **Lucknow:** Basement, Khushnuma Complex, 7 Meerabai Marg (Behind Jawahar Bhawan),Lucknow-226001, UP, India
  Ph: +0522-4000032   e-mail: tiwari.lucknow@cbspd.com
- **Mumbai:** PWD Shed, Gala no 25/26, Ramchandra Bhatt Marg, Next to JJ Hospital Gate no. 2, Opp. Union Bank of India, Noorbaug, Mumbai-400009, Maharashtra, India
  Ph: 022-66661880/89   e-mail: mumbai@cbspd.com

Representatives

• Hyderabad	0-9885175004	• Jharkhand	0-9811541605	• Nagpur	0-9421945513
• Patna	0-9334159340	• Pune	0-9623451994	• Uttarakhand	0-9716462459

Printed at Chaman Enterprises, Daryaganj, New Delhi, India

Preface

Indian Council of Agricultural Research (ICAR), New Delhi constituted 18 Broad Subject Matter Area (BSMA) committees in January 2008 to revise the course curricula in respect of Post Graduate and Doctoral programme. BSMA committee on Livestock Production Technology & Production Management (Animal Science, Animal Husbandry, Animal Physiology, Animal Nutrition & AFT, LPM, APT, and Poultry Science) was headed by Dr. N.Balaraman, and the members were Dr.B.K.Joshi, Dr.S.K.Jindal, Dr.B.T.Deshmukh, Dr.Arjava Sharma, Dr.V.K.Tanwar, Dr.C.L.Marwah and Dr.R.S.Yadav. The new and restructured post-graduate curricula & syllabi had been published in January 2009 and are being implemented from 2009-2010 academic year for MVSc and PhD students' course work.

The implementation of the new restructured curricula is expected to build knowledge and skill portfolio of the students so as to enhance their employability and marketability as multi-service providers with practical skills and comprehensive knowledge of the entire subject area after masters.

The following courses are listed in Animal Nutrition Subject: Animal Nutrition: energy, protein, minerals, vitamins and feed additives; Feed Technology; Feed Conservation, Storage and Quality Control; Ruminant Nutrition and Non-ruminant Nutrition; Nutrition of Companion/ Laboratory, Wild and Zoo Animals; Nonconventional Feedstuffs and Toxic constituents/ Antimetabolites in Animal feedstuffs; Modern Concepts of Feeding Ruminants and Forage Utilization; Modern Concepts of Feeding Monogastric Animals; Nutrition and Rumen Fermentation; Advances in Micronutrients; Advances in Feed Technology; Clinical Nutrition; Nutrient and Drug interaction; New Feed resources and Toxicants in Animal Feeding.

My two companion textbooks on Animal Nutrition for BVSc & AH students - 'Principles of Animal Nutrition & Feed Technology 2nd edition 2010, and Applied Nutrition 2nd edition 2009' fairly covers the basic and applied aspects comprehensively.

The contents of the textbook Advanced Animal Nutrition have been carefully drawn to fill the gaps in information to meet the curriculum of MVSc and PhD students. Except 'Nutrient and Drug interaction' course, all the other courses are majorly covered in the above mentioned textbooks. "Complete information in a comprehensible way" is the watchword of the book. The book consists of IX sections as General Animal Nutrition, Ruminant Animal Nutrition, Monogastric Animal Nutrition, Toxins and Antinutritional Factors in Feedstuffs, Feed Technology, Feed Plant Management, Clinical Nutrition, Quality Control of Feed and Appendix, each with several chapters to delineate the contents in a straightforward and lucid style.

Being in the teaching line with a research bent of mind and with a passion for communication of experimental findings to the 'endusers', and being a life member of several professional bodies, I have had the great opportunity over the years to be associated with the happenings in the subject around the world. The goal of this publication is to bring "cutting-edge" nutrition information to students, teachers and researchers of Livestock and Poultry Production.

The textbook will be useful to all UG and PG students of Animal Production subjects & Research Scholars, teachers and research workers. These include Animal Nutrition, Animal Physiology, Livestock Production Management, Avian Production Management, Animal Husbandry Extension, Animal Genetics and Breeding, Livestock Products Technology. This textbook is an added resource to all students of Veterinary Science for their preparation to face competitive examinations. I take this opportunity to express my gratitude to the publishers for their meticulous planning and intelligent publishing of the textbook. The services of Thiru B.Kumaran are greatly appreciated for neat typing of manuscript meticulously. Above all, I thank God for His guidance and inspiration.

June 2011   DUVVURU VENKA REDDY

Acknowledgements

I would like to extend special thanks to Prof K.Pradhan, Vice Chancellor (Retired) and Prof N.Krishna, Associate Dean (Retired) for their valuable contribution to the textbook in the form of chapters "Utilization of fibrous feeds for dairy production" in Ruminant Animal Nutrition section and "Roughages and their processing" in Feed Technology section.

June 2011   DUVVURU VENKA REDDY

Content

SECTION III
Monogastric Animal Nutrition

SECTION IV
Plant Feedstuffs and the associated Toxic & Antinutritional Factors and Mycotoxins

SECTION V
Feed technology

SECTION VI
Feed Plant Management

SECTION VII
Clinical Nutrition

SECTION VIII
Quality Control of Feed

SECTION IX
Appendix

SECTION I
General Animal Nutrition

1

Discovery of Nutrients Briefly

INTRODUCTION

The knowledge that we have today on the amount and number of nutrients to use in animal feeding did not happen by chance alone. The changes in animal nutrition occurred during the last 125 years are even hard to believe. For the 1000 years before that, little seemed to change. The chemists of 1860 were knowledgeable and had developed very good analysis of the major grains. Observations by producers and some very observant University personnel began to make progress in the late part of the 1800's and during the first twenty years of the 1900's.

The early scientists were very dedicated individuals

The research workers of earlier years knew that they were there to help the people that employed them. The scientists were willing to come in at odd times of the week and at odd hours of the night if it would help get the experiment off and running. Their willingness to go the "extra mile", long hours, hard study and probably arguments with their superiors are responsible for much of what has happened.

Difference between compartmental stomach of ruminant animal and simple stomach of other animals was recognized in 400 B.C. Antoine Laurent de Lavoisier, a French scientist, established the chemical basis of nutrition in 1770, which led to understand that energy was derived from oxidation of food. German scientists, Wilhelm Henneberg and Friedrich Stohmann in 1860, developed the proximate analysis system of feed analysis. Around the turn of the 19th century, it was recognized that animals required proteins, fats and carbohydrates. Most progress until 1920 was made with regard to these nutrients as well as on energy utilisation, and less on minerals and vitamins.

The "Single Grain Experiments" from Wisconsin were a breakthrough. Babcock, the inventor of the "Babcock Test for butterfat" was a key person and the work was published in 1911. This stated that even though the so called chemical contents (those known at that time) of the diets were similar the results were quite different.

These results were reviewed by Casimar Funk in 1912 and proposed, "The vital amine theory" and later coined a term 'vitamine' for such substances. Around this time, McCollum began experiments with rats and in 1914, he reported that butter fat or egg yolk provided something ("fat soluble A") that lard or olive oil did not provide for animals. At this same time Osborne and Mendel (1914) reported that zein was very deficient in two amino acids called lysine and tryptophan.

After 1920 there was a rapid development in our knowledge in the field of vitamins, amino acids, essential fatty acids, macro and micro minerals, and energy metabolism. By late 1970's we knew that the body needs carbohydrates, fats and fatty acids, proteins and amino acids, vitamins and minerals, in contrast to the three recognized a century ago.

Nuclear Techniques for knowledge generation

Nuclear techniques had been employed since 1930s in solving problems of animal production and health. Isotope deuterium was used in the investigation of metabolism, stable isotope 15N and radio-isotopes ^{32}P and ^{35}S were used in assessing new diet formulations and feeding standards for livestock. Research work of Hansard (1964) favoured tritium (isotope) as the indicator of choice to measure total body water in farm animals because of its rapid equilibrium with body water, slow plasma protein binding and decreased metabolic breakdown. Later, Kay et al. (1966) reported tritiated water as superior to several diluents used to measure body water in living pigs, which attained a stable equilibrium in blood 2hr after intravenous injection in Large White Yorkshire pigs (Reddy and Prasad, 1983).

Knowledge of quantitative digestion and metabolism in ruminants was developed most rapidly when isotope dilution techniques become easy to apply, facilitated by improved instrumentation and mathematical approaches. The opportunity arose for the first time to examine ketone body metabolism in the whole animal (Leng and Anison, 1964) when radioactivity labeled β-hydroxybutyrate was first prepared by incubating ^{14}C-butyrate with sheep liver slices *in vitro*. Since then knowledge in this area has developed at an ever increasing rate.

Most of the earlier work focused on the contribution to new knowledge namely the elaboration of metabolic pathways, unraveling the complexity of disease transmission or understanding the endocrine system feedbacks in relation to reproductive and metabolic hormones. Hence the results obtained had more intellectual than economic / practical values. However, during the last 20-30 years nuclear techniques have been employed in reproduction, animal health/disease diagnosis to help resolve some of the difficult problems facing the third-world animal agriculture.

With the use of radio-tracers many reactions and turn over rates in the animal body can be estimated which otherwise is not possible with simple chemical determinations. Stable isotopes of nitrogen (^{15}N) helped to demonstrate that 25-50% of the microbial protein pool in the rumen may be turning over *in situ* and, therefore, unavailable to the host ruminant animal. The knowledge that developed has clearly shown that the way toward substantial increases in productivity of ruminants on forage based diets is through the balanced nutrient approach that considers the efficiency of rumen ecosystem and the availability of dietary nutrients post-ruminally.

Animal nutrition is an integral part of animal production

Animal nutrition is an integral part of animal production. It has changed drastically as a consequence of developments in the other disciplines of animal science and also because of changes in animal husbandry practices. Developments in disciplines have been so strongly related to one another that one discipline could not have developed in isolation without developments in the other. For instance, animals have been bred to have an increased production, but the expression of this enhanced genetic potential was only possible by continuous adjustment of nutrition to the genotype of the animal.

Solutions for problems in animal production can be at least partly achieved by developments in animal nutrition. In the past, this was done on one hand by determining requirements and on the other hand by determining composition of feedstuffs and diets. In recent years, mechanistic modelling is used increasingly. In addition, nutrition is used increasingly to determine biological reactions of animals.

Sustainable animal production

The word 'sustainability', according to a dictionary definition, refers to ' keeping an effort going continuously, the ability to last out and keep from falling'. In the context of agriculture, the technical advisory committee of the Consultative Group on International Agricultural Research (TAC/CGIAR 1992) states: "Sustainable agriculture should involve the successful management of resources for agriculture to satisfy changing human needs while maintaining or enhancing the quality of the environment and conserving natural resources". 'Sustainable' here simply means keeping something going for an indefinite period of time, with the emphasis on "indefinite".

More recently, the Millennium Ecosystem Assessment (2005) has given the following definition for sustainability: "A characteristic or state whereby the needs of the present and local population can be met without compromising the ability of future generation or population in other locations to meet their needs."

One of the biggest challenges of animal production is to have animals produced in a sustainable way. This also holds true for a selection of those animals that are robust enough to stay healthy and keep producing. Civil society increasingly gives signals to animal producers that it does demand animal production to be animal friendly and sustainable. The human food chain, including animal products has become an ethical issue. Food from animals should be safe, environmentally friendly and produced in a (animal) welfare friendly system. This means that emphasis is less on maximizing production but increasingly on optimizing production through optimum utilization of nutrients rather than maximum utilization of nutrients.

Nutrition can also become important for finding solutions for environmental pollution. Of course, nutritional improvements are continuously used for further improvements in production efficiency. Improvement in the ability of the animals to convert feed into products more efficiently are very significant and result in moderately priced, nutritious and healthful food for the public.

2

Feeding the Future

INTRODUCTION

Since the middle of the 20th century, global agricultural output has kept pace with a rapidly growing population, repeatedly defying Malthusian predictions of global food shortage. Between 1961 and 2005, the world's population increased by 111% (from 3.08 to 6.51 billion), whereas crop production rose by 162% (from 1.8 to 4.8 billion tons) (FAO, 2009 as reported by J.A.Burney et al., 2010). Although agricultural production has increased both by expanding the land area cultivated (extensification) and by improving crop yield from the land already under cultivation (intensification), the gains observed since 1961 were largely intensive.

"Men and women have the right to live their lives and raise their children in dignity, free from hunger and free from violence, oppression or injustice'.
—The United Nations Millennium Declaration 2000

From a humanitarian perspective, the agricultural intensification of the Green Revolution was a resounding success, but its environmental legacy is less clear. It has long been recognized that increased yields have spared forest and shrubland from conversion to cropland (N.E.Borlaug, 1983). The competition for feedstuffs and arable land at global level, including that for sugar cane, for the production of biofuel (biodiesel and ethanol), has recently destabilized the price of grains such that rice, the staple food of over two billion people soared recently. D.Farrell (2009) estimated the feed, food and land area that would be required to feed the people of the world by 2016-2018. He felt poverty and malnutrition would remain unchanged or would increase unless population growth is halted. Mother Earth can no longer cope with that and the brown footprint that accompanies it.

The aim of this chapter is to delineate the growth in livestock sector in India and its role in poverty alleviation, livestock population dynamics, enhanced demand for livestock products, feed resources to produce the needed animal products, integration of crop and livestock operations, efficiency of animal production and justification for raising livestock and poultry. It is stressed that optimal natural resources utilization is the need of the hour because the humanity's demand exceeds the regenerative capacity of the planet Earth. It is also emphasized the dire need for more investments in agriculture from both public sector and private sector to make our countrymen food secure.

Optimal Natural Resources utilisation

Two centuries ago, English clergyman and pioneer economist Thomas Malthus argued that population growth inevitably outpaces food output unless checked by moral restraint, disease or famine. His predictions were echoed in the mid 1960s. With just 2.4% of world's geographical area and 4% of world's fresh water resources, India has to meet the food and feed requirement of 17% of world's human population and 11% of livestock population.

All our Five Year Plans emphasized the need for efficient use of land, water and other natural resources for accelerated as well as sustainable economic development. Nevertheless, the problems of land degradation, ground water depletion and environmental pollution have assumed alarming proportions in many areas. Due to both population growth and urbanization, there is growing demand for conversion of agricultural lands to non-agricultural uses. The per capita availability of resources is about 4-6 times less as compared to the world average.

Population rich, but land hungry countries like India has no option except to produce more per units of land and water under conditions of diminishing per capita arable land and water availability, and expanding biotic and abiotic stresses. Stress is on evergreen revolution leading to the improvement of productivity in perpetuity without the associated ecological harm.

Scientific evidence today confirms that humanity's demand on the planet's living resources now exceeds its regenerative capacity by a wide margin. It now takes the Earth one year and four months to regenerate resources used in a single year. Thus it is clearly unsustainable.

Investment in agriculture and food security

Agriculture's share in total Official Development Assistance slumped from 17% in 1980 to a mere 3.8% in 2006. The share of agriculture in GDP has been a steady decline from 36.4% in 1982-83 to 18.5% in 2006-07. The agricultural sector is the primary source of livelihood for 52% of India's workforce. Yet, this sector contributed barely 17% of the country's gross domestic product (GDP) in 2007-08. The very fact that over a period the growth in agriculture has remained much lower than the growth in the non-agricultural sectors explains the unpleasant plight of the rural people. Underinvestment in agriculture over the past 30 years, high and volatile food prices and continuing economic turmoil increased the level of global food insecurity. Investment in sustainable agriculture is the key to ensuring the food security of present and future generations.

Food security refers to access by all people at all times to sufficient food for an active and healthy life. During the reform decade (1990-91 to 2000-01) in India, agricultural growth was at a mere 1.71%, and below the annual population growth of 1.87% per annum, signaling the advent of the "Malthusian" phenomenon of population growth outstripping food production. Prof M.S.Swaminathan emphasized "we need more science, both in public and private sectors, related to agriculture for falsifying the Neo Malthusian predictions of widespread food and drinking water insecurity".

Growth in livestock sector

It has been said that required growth rate in food grain production is only about 2.0-2.3%, while the growth in non-food grain output had to be about 6.0% so as to achieve the overall farm sector target of 4%. Non-food grain production would also include non-crop farming such as livestock and fisheries.

It is now well-accepted that the Animal Husbandry and Dairying sector play an important role in the national economy, significantly supplementing family income and generate gainful employment. Livestock rearing has remained the most effective employment generation and livelihood security enterprise for the uneducated and educated unemployed rural youth. Over the last three decades, livestock sector has consistently accounted for over 4% of the country's GDP, while its share in the GDP from agricultural sector steadily increased from 14 to 25%, while remaining greater than 20% over the last two decades. The gross domestic product (GDP) from livestock sector during 2004-05 is 24.72% share in agriculture and allied GDP, which increased to 29% in 2007-08. A target of 6-7% growth per annum for the livestock sector with milk production growing at a rate of 5% has been set during the 11th Five Year Plan (2007-2012).

Sustained growth in per capita income, fast increasing urban population and increasing awareness of nutrition-rich foods of animal origin among both urban and rural consumers suggest that livestock sector is sure to emerge as engine of growth of rural economy with potential to achieve higher growth rates of 6% per annum (V.K.Taneja, Agriculture Year Book, 2009 pp122). Further, the growth in livestock sector is poverty reducing. Livestock sector registered an overall growth rate of 3.6% during 1991/92-2005/06 (milk 3.9%, meat 3.2%, other livestock products 2.9%) against a growth rate 1.8% for crop sector.

All out efforts are required to boost up livestock sub sector where the 70 million people are directly involved to produce quality food for 70% or 882 million consumers (K.M.Bujarbaruah, Agriculture Year Book, 2009 pp112). Around 80% of livestock in India is owned by small and marginal farmers, which is also the livelihood option for 50% people below poverty line besides being the income source for around 30-50 percent of the household. Hence, the very basic issue of poverty alleviation agenda of the government could be meaningfully addressed through livestock centric growth and development agenda.

Animal production

The primary objective of raising livestock and poultry is to produce good quality animal products in the form of milk, meat and eggs to the consumers as a profitable enterprise with least contribution to climate change. Towards meeting this, livestock and poultry need to be fed with wholesome feed in 'environmentally-friendly' way and profitably and thus nutrition plays a major role.

Animal nutrition depends on the availability of feedstuffs to provide feed to animals in addition to the needs of the growing human population. With increasing prosperity of people and changing needs of the society, companion animals are increasing in numbers and the field of pet animal nutrition has been attracting much attention of the scientists as well as feed industry personnel.

Objective of animal nutrition

Traditionally, the objective of animal nutrition is to provide all essential nutrients in adequate amounts and in optimum proportions to the animal.

Now the objective moved to topics such as food safety and quality, animal health, welfare and ethical issues, feed resources, nutrient economy, environmental aspects. More efficient use of limited feed resources, lowered emissions of greenhouse gases (CO_2, CH_4 and N_2O) and other pollutants (N, P, trace elements) from animal farms, and inclusion of agro-industrial byproducts and non conventional feed resources are to be considered while doing ration formulation.

Livestock production is threatened by climate change, land degradation, water pollution and above all feed shortages. These factors have put forward challenges to produce more from less in a sustainable and eco-friendly manner following the balanced nutrition and proper supply of nutrients as per the physiological stage in a precision nutrition mode.

Precision animal nutrition

Precision animal nutrition (PAN) is defined as providing the animal with the feed that precisely meet its nutritional requirements for optimum productive efficiency to produce better quality animal products (milk, meat and eggs) and to contribute cleaner environment and thereby ensure profitability. Cleaner environment means reducing the enteric emission of methane, excretion of nitrogen (ammonia), phosphorus and other compounds into the environment. It is aimed at supplying the nutrients to the animals matching their requirements to improve not only the animal physiology and health but also the enrichment of their products for the well-being of the consumer (Reddy and Krishna, 2009). In other words PAN is to optimize the nutrition of animals to produce safe and healthy food for consumers, to assure animal health and welfare and to minimize negative effects on the environment.

Voices of concern

Objections have been raised over the use of hormones and antibiotics in food animal production since they leave their residues in meat, milk and eggs. There is some concern that feeding of low concentration of antibiotics may favour the proliferation of antibiotic-resistant microorganisms, which could have serious consequences for disease control in humans and domestic animals.

Proliferation of bovine spongiform encephalopthy (BSE) in the British cattle (in 1986) is thought to have emerged originally from initial interspecies transmission of the scrapie-agent into cattle by the feeding of scrapie-infected sheep and goat meat, plus bone meal products to cattle. In view of the possible link between BSE and human's Creutzfeldt-Jacob disease, meat and bone meal (MBM) was banned from using in ruminant feed while some countries most notably UK, have a complete MBM ban for all farm animal feed.

Dioxins are unintentional byproducts of many industrial processes and the byproducts such as fish meal, fish oil, recovered vegetable oil, and the byproducts of food industry have found their way into animal feeds as energy sources. Thereby the dioxins get concentrated in animal products and are highly toxic posing a real health hazard.

Challenges of modern animal nutrition

Food safety has become a major issue in light of global disasters of mad cow disease / BSE, dioxin contamination of feeds (in Belgium in May 1999), and lesser mishaps (drug, mycotoxin, pesticide, hormone residues in food products). Hence the tide of consumer trust in food safety is at its low ebb. The concept of 'quality in, quality out' has to be remembered and so quality and safe food can only be produced from quality and safe feed. The challenge for modern animal nutrition is to produce animal products that are acceptable to the consumer, to develop rations without antibiotics, meat and bone meal, or other objectionable feeds and to formulate rations that do not cause environmental pollution, and that maintain animal health and remain economically viable.

Tools to achieve precision animal nutrition

PAN is the best way to improve the productivity of animals in developing countries by effective utilization of available feed resources with the aim of maximizing the animals' response to nutrients. The tools to achieve PAN include improved feed processing techniques, precise ration formulation, implementing phase feeding and the use of feed additives. Supplementation of unsaturated fatty acids, ionophore antibiotics, organic acids, plant secondary metabolites, essential oils, probiotics and fibrolytic enzymes help to achieve precision animal nutrition.

It is generally agreed that the more feed an animal consumes each day, the greater will be the opportunity for increasing its daily production, which is dependent upon improving the nutrient digestibility. Towards this, urea-ammoniation treatment of straws has been promising. Strategic supplementation of nutrients enhance rumen fermentative digestibility, which stimulates intake of feed. Further, it also balances the end products of rumen fermentation in lowering enteric methane production from ruminants. Efficiency of ruminal fermentation and digestibility of the nutrients are key factors in improving the efficiency of feed use.

Nutrient partitioning is the major component of productive efficiency that differs among the individual cows and increase in productive efficiency can be achieved with exogenous recombinantly derived growth hormone (bGH) injections. Use of restricted protein levels and supplementation of rumen protected amino acids with matching ruminal energy and monitoring the milk urea nitrogen help assess efficiency of nitrogen use. Feed additives play a pivotal role in achieving increased efficiency and reduced environmental load per unit of the animal product.

Livestock population and annual growth rates

India is blessed with the most fabulous livestock wealth in the world. According to the 2003 Census data, the country had 185 million cattle, 98 million buffaloes, 124 million goats, 61 million sheep, 13.5 million pigs (485 million livestock population) and 489 million poultry. Population figures indicate that Indian cattle, buffalo, sheep and goats constitute to 14, 58, 6 and 16% of the world population, respectively (Table 1). All this livestock and poultry have to be supported with only 2.4% of the world's geographical area and 4% of world's fresh water resources.

Perusal of data on livestock population (annual growth rates) of 1997 & 2003 and its dynamics showed positive trend in the annual growth rates (Table 1) of buffaloes (1.43%), sheep (1.12%), goats (0.22%) and pigs (0.28%) while negative trend was seen in cattle (-1.18%). Buffaloes and goats are considered the 'animals of the future for the country' for poverty alleviation programmes, since the increase in the chicken population is mainly within the commercial sector. With regards to cattle, it has been observed that there is clear shift of preference towards high yielding animals; crossbred cattle population has increased by 22.8% and indigenous cattle population has decreased by 10.2%. Further, the increase in female crossbred cattle and female buffalo population was 34% and 12.3%, respectively. These changes were reflected in the production of milk at 97.1 million tonnes in 2005-06, which is 4.97% more than that in 2004-05. Now India is the largest milk producer in the world producing 105 million metric tons per annum.

Table 1. Livestock population in the year 2003 (in Million Numbers): India Vs World and the growth trends

Species	India*	Annual growth rates 1997-2003, %	World**	% of world of population
Cattle	185.18	-1.18	1350.9	13.7
Buffaloes	97.92	1.43	170.3	57.5
Yaks	0.06	1.52	–	–
Mithuns	0.28	–	–	–
Sheep	61.47	1.12	1038.7	5.9
Goats	124.36	0.22	771.5	16.1
Horse & ponies	0.75	–1.59	55.1	1.4
Mules	0.18	–3.74	12.9	1.4
Donkeys	0.65	–4.95	41.5	1.6
Camels	0.63	–5.92	19.2	3.3
Pigs	13.52	0.28	941.5	1.4
Total	485.00	–	4401.6	11.0

* Source: 17th Livestock Census, Department of Animal Husbandry, Dairying & Fisheries, M/O Agriculture; Directorate of Economics & Statistics. M/O Agriculture - various census reports and Animal Husbandry Statistics Division, ** FAOSTAT - Website year 2006

Livestock production and rural economy

Livestock production forms an integral part of the rural economy. In India, 70 to 80% of the total livestock produce is contributed by the underprivileged (*viz.* landless, marginal farmers and smallholder farmers) families (Kurup, 2004) and livestock are central to their livelihoods and culture. Thus livestock are important assets for rural people and play a critical role in building their livelihoods. Livestock rearing can provide a pathway out of poverty through improvements to household nutrition, cash income, asset building and employment. Almost 73% of rural households keep animals of one kind or another, and livestock play a special role in household security, particularly in smallholder farming systems. In areas with high livestock populations, income from livestock accounts for 30 to 50% of total farm income.

Low productivity of Indian livestock is a matter of concern and one of the contributing factors is the insufficient and poor quality feed and fodder resources. Nutritious, balanced and adequate feeding of animals is a major factor to improve the livestock production in the country. The impact of climate change is likely to aggravate the shortage of feed resources. It is therefore necessary to improve the efficiency of utilization of existing feed resources through field-tested technologies.

Land utilization pattern in India

The geographical extent of land in our country is finite and its optimal utilization is warranted. The total geographical area is 328.73 million hectares and 305.8 m ha is the reporting area for land utilization purpose. The Net Area Sown increased from 118.75 m ha in 1950-51 to 142.5 m ha in 1992-93. The area under non-agricultural use also increased to 8.0% from 3.3% and the area under barren and uncultivable land has been decreased to 5.8% from 13.4% during 1950-51 to 2003-04, respectively. However, forest area has increased to 22.8% from 14.2% during the same period.

The net irrigated area and gross irrigated areas were increased nearly by 2 and 3 folds, from 20.85 m ha to 55.10 m ha and 22.56 m ha to 76.82 m ha, respectively in the years from 1950-51 to 2003-04. Due to increase in irrigation, introduction of new crops and early maturing varieties, cropping intensity increased from 111% in 1950-51 to 137% at the moment. Consequently, gross cropped area also increased from 131.89% in 1950-51 to over 190% at present. The changes in land-use pattern for pasture production over the years are presented in Table 2. Per capita availability of land declined from 0.89 ha in the early 1950's to 0.37 ha in the mid 1990's and is expected to reduce further to 0.19 ha by 2020. Similarly land base for livestock has been shrinking (Table 3).

Animal products and efficiency of plant food conversion

Production of milk, meat, wool and eggs is a function of complex interactions between animal potential and the environmental conditions. Animal nutrition is the major factor that limits their production. Provision of nutrients in excess of maintenance allows the animal to become productive thus generating a return on the investment. Animals differ in their requirements according to their genetic potential and the desired level of production.

Table 2. Changes in Land-use pattern for pasture production (Area, million ha)

Item	1950-51	1990-91	2000-01
1. Total geographical area	305.8	305.8	305.8
2. Area under forest	40.48	67.80	68.75
3. Area not available for cultivation	47.52	40.48	41.54
a) Area under non-agricultural use	9.36	21.09	22.45
b) Barren and uncultivable land	38.16	19.39	19.09
4. Other uncultivable land (excluding fallow land)	49.45	30.22	28.48
i) Permanent pastures and other grazing land	6.68	11.40	11.04
ii) Land under misc. tree crops and groves not included in net area sown	19.83	3.82	3.50
iii) Cultivable wasteland	22.94	15.00	13.94
5. Fallow land	28.14	23.36	32.22
a) Fallow land other than current fallows	17.45	9.66	9.89
b) Current fallows	10.68	13.70	13.33

Agricultural statistics at a glance, Directorate of Economics & Stat. GOI, 2001

Table 3. Land base available for livestock (ha/head)

Particulars	1950	1980	2000
Land available for livestock excluding forest land	0.37	0.15	0.10
Land available for livestock including forest land	0.51	0.321	0.24

Soil conservation report, Ministry of Agriculture, GOI, 2001

Animal products are inevitably costlier compared to plant products. The reasons include double conversion of basic food constituents, apart from cost of processing of byproducts into feeds. Soil nutrients are firstly converted into plant products, which upon feeding to animals later, are converted into animal products. One example of this double conversion is that the average efficiency of conversion of fertilizer nitrogen into plant protein is 50%, while the average efficiencies of conversion of plant into animal protein are approximately 25, 26, 23, 14 and 4 % for milk, egg, broiler chicken meat, pork, and beef and mutton, respectively. The readers may refer the chapter "Efficiency of feed conversion to animal products in farm animals and poultry" in Applied Nutrition textbook by the author for more details (Chapter 11, pp 228-232).

What then are the justifications for raising any livestock?
Animal products enhance quality of human life

Animal production is not simply a matter of producing food, it is also relieving the ill-health of resource poor people resulting from essential nutrient deficiencies in mainly cereal based diets which animal products rectify. Animal products, even in tiny quantities, support physical and intellectual development of young people and pregnant mothers. Most humans demand a mixed diet as man is an omnivorous species and the majority are willing to pay higher prices for foods of animal origin than they are for foods of plant origin. The consumption of meat, fish, milk and eggs contributes to meet the human requirements in amino acids and trace nutrients (Wennemer et al., 2005), have a considerable enjoyment value and are considered as a parameter of living standard.

Raising of livestock facilitates recycling of nutrients

There are many plant foods such as forages, crop residues, byproducts from food production and processing industry, several unconventional feedstuffs and some of them may be inedible by man. All these are not used for human food and can not be digested by monogastric animals while the ruminant animals can efficiently convert them into valuable animal products. Use of such waste materials in animal feeding facilitates recycling of nutrients (soil-plant-animal-soil), reduces environmental pollution as well and furnishes additional profits from animal enterprise.

Mixed crop-livestock farming

There are complementarities between crops and livestock, with animals fed on crop byproducts producing manure to return nutrients to the soil. Of course, indigenous cattle and buffaloes also provide draught power. Mixed crop-livestock farming contributes stability and sustainability. Stability is promoted by keeping animals, which serve as a form of insurance, they can be raised in years of good harvests and animal products consumed or animals may be sold when crops fail. Sustainability is promoted because of mixed crop-livestock system. Crop-livestock farming is environmentally the most desirable system. The crop residues are utilized in animal feeding and animal excreta are added to crop lands, which ensures some nutrient recycling, and is less likely to result in nutrient deficits or surpluses. Especially, livestock proved to be a crucial link in nutrient cycling on small farms, maintaining viability and environmental sustainability of agricultural production.

Integration of crop and livestock operations

Greater efficiency of resource use is claimed for agricultural systems, which incorporate forages and livestock relative to those based on cropping alone (Chantalakhana, 1990). Plants and animals are complementary in mixed farming system and the utilization of both as sources of food may increase total food production per unit area of available land. The animal excreta can be effectively recycled as fertilizer for crops thereby reducing huge expenses incurred towards purchase of chemical fertilizers. This also encourages organic farming. Community wasteland and private wasteland have been reclaimed by adopting different agro-forestry models such as horti-pasture, horti-silvipasture, silvi-pasture, etc. Integration of livestock with agro-forestry model can enrich soil fertility and reclaim the problem-soil.

Intensive integrated farming system has a variety of agricultural, aquaculture and livestock enterprises. These diversified farming enterprises on the same farm help in generating year-round employment and returns. These provide scope for maximum use of family labour as well. The intensive integrated farming system involves intensive use of biological resources of the farm to optimize the farm productivity per unit of soil, water and air.

In India, ruminant production from small, integrated farming systems is the common and indeed the dominant form. But the productivity of livestock is low. Growth in livestock production has to come from improvements in animal productivity through greater animal nutrition and health, since feeding and nutrition is the principal determinant of performance of animals among the non-genetic factors. Of course, the genetic enhancements of local breeds do need attention.

Demand for animal products

The term 'Livestock Revolution' was first used by Delgado et al (1999) to describe the rapid increase in demand for food of animal origin (Table 4) with profound implications for human health, livelihoods and the environment. This phrase was coined by the IFPRI/ILRI/FAO study in the 2020 Vision publication *Livestock to 2020: The Next Food Revolution* of which Chris Delgado was the senior author (Delgado *et al.* 1999). Global production and annual growth rates of meat, milk and eggs in the developed and developing countries as predicted by Farrell (2009) is presented in Table 5. The word 'revolution' only indicates that there is a large and rapid change occurring in the dietary preferences of people, manifested particularly in developing countries. In the last 25 years (1978-2003) the proportion of dietary calories coming from livestock products (meat, milk and eggs) in developing countries has increased from 6% to 10%. In developed countries the proportion has remained constant at around 20%. Consequently, a lower proportion of dietary calories is being derived from cereals and other plant products in the people of developing countries.

Livestock revolution

Livestock revolution is different from the green revolution of 1970s and 1980s in the sense that the green revolution was primarily supply-led, driven by technological change and supported by massive investment in agricultural infrastructure and institutions, while the livestock revolution is demand-driven (consumer-driven) fuelled by sustained income growth and increasing urban population.

Feed requirements for livestock

No attempt has been made here to calculate the feed requirements for the livestock of India. Perusal of land utilization pattern over the years in India reveals the following: the net area sown increased (area under barren and uncultivable land decreased); net irrigated area and gross irrigated area increased; area under forest increased to 22.8%; cropping intensity is increased due to increase in irrigation. Forages, herbages, crop residues and byproducts available should be put to optimal use.

Table 4. Projected trends in meat and milk consumption, 1993-2020

Region/ Country	Projected annual growth (%) of total consumption (1993-2020)		Total consumption (million metric tons) in 2020		Per capita consumption (kg) in 2020	
	Meat	Milk	Meat	Milk	Meat	Milk
India	2.9	4.3	8	160	6	125
Other South Asia	3.2	3.4	5	41	10	82
China	3.0	2.8	85	17	60	12
Sub-Saharan Africa	3.5	3.8	12	31	11	30
Developing world	2.8	3.3	188	391	30	62
Developed world	0.6	0.2	115	263	83	189
World	1.8	1.7	303	654	39	85

Table 5. Global production of meat, milk and eggs (millions of metric tonnes) in the developed* and developing countries** and those predicted to 2016 and by Delgado for 2020 where available. Annual change is given as % per year from 2006 to 2016 (D. Farrell, 2009)

Commodity	Region	Change %	2016	2020
Bovine	Developed	0	24.3	34
	Developing	3.1	43.7	52
Pig	Developed	1.2	42.3	39
	Developing	3.7	92.9	81
Turkey meat	Developed	3.3	7.7	NA
	Developing	3.5	0.8	
Duck meat	Developed	3.5	0.7	NA
	Developing	4.6	4.5	
Sheep and goat	Developed	4.9	4.3	NA
	Developing	4.4	15.1	
Chicken meat	Developed	2.3	37.0	39
	Developing	4.0	60.1	70
Milk	Developed	0.4	347	286
	Developing	2.9	304	375
eggs	Developed	0.1	20.2	NA
	Developing	3.5	57.1	

Developed* countries include Australia, Canada, Eastern Europe, European Union, other Western European countries, Israel, former Soviet Union, Japan, New Zealand, South Africa, USA. Developing countries** include all countries in FAO Statistical Database. NA is not available

The unfortunate consequences of the extremely rapid and short-sighted thrust to produce biofuels at global level will affect the developing countries and particularly the very poor. Cost of inputs to sustain yield of grain crops have escalated and with them food costs. There is fear of social upheaval in many developing countries as food prices surge.

There is clearly conflict between land used for crops for feed and for biofuel production, and that needed for crops to feed humans. Biofuel (ethanol and biodiesel) is produced from oilseeds, grains and sugar cane. About 330 kg of distillers dried grains with solubles (DDGS) are produced per tonne of maize in ethanol production. They must be dried at some cost or fed wet to ruminant animals. DDGS can be used in poultry diets at a maximum inclusion of about 5% for broilers and 12% for layers; for pigs the inclusion is higher, as it is for ruminant animals. Similarly, byproducts of biodiesel industry - oilseed meals are available for animal feeding.

It is doubtful if there will be sufficient feed to satisfy the requirements of that needed to drive livestock production. However, this can be overcome by a relentless search for newer feed resources and effective utilization of available feed resources.

3

Feeds (Conventional and Non-conventional) for Livestock

INTRODUCTION

Quantitative and qualitative insufficiency of feeds and fodder in the country is one of the main impediments in the way of improvement of livestock production (NCA, 1976). The working efficiency of indigenous bullocks can be enhanced by 30% by better and scientific feeding (First five year plan. Planning Commission, Government of India, New Delhi, 1951). Final report of the 'ICAR scheme for introduction of balanced rations for Ryots cattle for the period 1951-1953' also concluded that the milk yield of indigenous cows can be enhanced by 50% by better and scientific feeding. The Famine Inquiry Commission, earlier in 1945, had rightly stressed that "feeding was of crucial importance, for no lasting improvement could be brought about by breeding alone, since improved breeds deteriorate rapidly if not fed adequately. The Report of the National Commission on Agriculture (1976) furnished the feed requirements and the availability of feeds to feed the livestock and poultry on scientific lines.

Feed supply position

Feed is an important input for milk and meat production from ruminants. The cost of feed constitutes 50 to 75% of production cost of livestock products. While milk production in the country is increasing fast, and India holding the prestigious position of largest milk producer with 84 million tonnes of milk production (FAO, 2002), the feed and fodder resources are depleting very fast due to increased population, urbanization and pressure on land for cereal and cash crops.This led to qualitative and quantitative insufficiency of feeds and fodders, which is one of the main impediments for orderly development of livestock industry in India.

As early as in 1970s, National Commission on Agriculture (1976) estimated the requirements of feed and fodder vis-à-vis availability to feed the country's livestock and poultry on scientific lines. It was reported that green fodder, concentrates and dry fodder were in short supply to the tune of 38%, 44% and 40%, respectively. The recent survey carried out by National Institute of Animal Nutrition and Physiology (NIANP), Bangalore indicated that there is a shortage of 45, 44 and 38 per cent of dry roughages, concentrates and green fodder, respectively (Anon, 2001-2002). Their latest database on availability and requirements of feeds and fodder indicates the deficit with regard to dry fodder, green fodder and concentrates as 11%, 28% and 35%, respectively (NIANP Disc, 2005). Hence, the imbalance existing between the animal numbers and the available feed resources associated with frequent exposure to drought or dry spells of 4-5 months in a year with virtually no green forage for grazing led to more dependence on crop residues, agro-industrial byproducts (AIBP) and non-conventional feed resources (NCFR) for feeding of ruminant livestock.

Common feeds and fodders for livestock and poultry feeding: their classification, composition and nutritive value

Feeds for livestock and poultry feeding composed of naturally occurring products from food crops and field crops and of many of the byproducts of the milling, oil seed processing, sugar industry, starch manufacturing, vegetable and fruit processing, dairy, meat, fish, prawn, etc. processing and other food processing industries. This shows that there are various types of feedstuffs available for the livestock and poultry feeding.

Though strictly speaking no two feedstuffs are alike in the composition and characteristic, substitution of one feedstuff is made with another depending upon the market price and availability in a particular region/season in practical feeding. Therefore, it is necessary to know the categories of the feeds within which substitutions are justified for the feeds with similar nutritional properties. The readers may refer Principles of Animal Nutrition and Feed Technology for detailed classification of feedstuffs.

Feedstuffs can be grouped into different classes on the basis of bulkiness (bulk density) and chemical composition. They are classified into roughages and concentrates based on the crude fibre (CF) content, which is primarily responsible for bulk density of the feeds. Broadly feeds and fodders can be classified into roughages, concentrates and additives (nutritive and non-nutritive). Please see chapter Feed Quality Control for the chemical composition of certain feed ingredients.

Forages and roughages

The term 'roughage' is usually used to designate feeds that are high in fibre and low in net energy. Technically forages mean hay, straw, silage and pasture while roughages include rice husk, groundnut (peanut) shells. However, the terms forage and roughage are used interchangeably. Products containing more than 18% crude fibre or more than 35% cell wall in their dry state are classified as forages and roughages. Feedstuffs with less than 18% CF or less than 35% cell wall are called as concentrates.

Concentrates

Concentrates are described as feeds or feed mixtures which supply primary nutrients (protein, carbohydrate and fat) at higher level but contain less than 18% crude fibre on dry matter basis or in air-dry feeds. In general concentrates are feeds that are high in nitrogen free extract and total digestible nutrients (TDN) and low in CF. Concentrates are classified into energy supplements and protein supplements based on their CP content.

Energy supplements

These are concentrate feedstuffs with less than 20% protein and less than 18% crude fibre or less than 35% cell walls on dry matter basis. In case of certain brans, chunies some samples may contain over 18% CF and more than 20% CP and still they are classified as energy feeds. Examples include cereal grains, mill byproducts, fruits, nuts and roots. Many of the fruits and some roots are excellent sources of vitamins and minerals for humans. These are also referred to as carbohydrate feed ingredients.

Protein Supplements

These are concentrate feedstuffs, which contain 20% or more protein and less than 18% crude fibre or less than 35% cell walls on dry matter basis.

Energy supplements: Energy supplements are by far the most important in the practical feeding of livestock from both a quantitative as well as an economic standpoint. These are categorized into grains and seeds, mill byproducts, molasses and roots.

Cereal grains

Grains are the seeds from cereal plants. Cereal grains are essentially carbohydrates, the main component being starch which is concentrated in the endosperm. Cereal grains contain relatively low percentage of CP and less than 18% CF. However, CF content of harvested grain is highest in oats and paddy and is lowest in the nacked grains, wheat and maize. The crude protein content of grains and seeds varies between 8-12% which is deficient in lysine and methionine. Cereal grains contribute about one third to one half of protein in the diet of chickens. The normal fat content is about 2-5%. The cereal oils are unsaturated, the main fatty acids being linoleic and oleic, and this is the reason feeding of cereal grains such as maize produces soft body fat (soft pork in swine) in nonruminants. Examples rice, wheat, maize, barley, oats, bajra, sorghum, etc.

All cereals are deficient in vitamin D and in calcium (less than 0.15%) but are moderately rich in phosphorus (0.3-0.5%) and vitamin E. Cereals and cereal byproducts are rich in phosphorus though more than 60% of it is phytate phosphorus. Calcium deficiency is not normally experienced in cattle feeding, except for high-producing cows or rapidly growing calves because cattle are kept mainly on roughages that are rich in calcium. Poultry and pigs, which cannot tolerate large quantities of fibrous feeds, should be given supplements of calcium salts when fed mostly on cereal grains.

Grains are costly for animal feeding. Only 2% of rice and wheat, 5% of sorghum, 10% of barley and maize and 50% of bajra and ragi are diverted towards livestock and poultry feeding, the major chunk of which is fed to poultry and swine. They must be processed before they can be fed. High grain feeding in ruminants may cause digestive disturbances such as acidosis and parakeratosis of the rumen. Feeding of wheat grain to cattle is conducive to acidosis because of the high solubility of its starch.

Maize

Maize is the most popular and palatable grain for all kinds of livestock. Ruminants are often fed ground ear corn (corn and cob meal). Ground ear corn consists of whole ears of corn (80% grain and 20% cobs) ground to varying degrees of fineness. Maize contains about 65% starch, 85-90% TDN, about 10% proteins. Maize protein is deficient in tryptophan and lysine. Two types of proteins are present: zein and glutelin. Zein, the predominant protein of corn, is a prolamine. The principal site of zein and other proteins is the endosperm. Glutelin occurs in both endosperm and germ and it is a better source of tryptophan and lysine.

Varieties of maize: Field corn or the dent type; sweet corn; pop corn; high lysine corn, opaque 2 (Opaque 2 is called as Shakti Ratna and Protina in India); waxy corn. Yellow maize is the only grain with appreciable amount of carotene. Opaque-2 maize contains higher amount of lysine while other variety Floury-2 has both increased methionine and lysine.

Sorghum

Crude protein content is 8.5–12.5% and sorghum protein has uniform essential amino acid composition. The use of less satisfactory sorghum results in mottled egg yolks. Tannins are also a problem.

Wheat grain

Broadly, wheat grain has four components: bran, aleurone layer, endosperm and germ (embryo). Bran accounts for 12%, germ 3% and endosperm 85%. The bran is the brown outer layer and this contains bulk-forming carbohydrates, B-vitamins and minerals (especially iron). The aleurone layer is located right under the bran and is rich in proteins and phosphorus mineral. The endosperm is the white center, which consists mainly of starches and sugars and proteins. This is the part present in highly refined flours. The germ is the heart of the wheat. It is this part that makes sprouts and makes a new plant. Wheat germ is rich in thiamin, good quality protein, vitamin E.

The nutritional value of wheat is affected by both variety and environment, but the intrinsic factors responsible for variation are not yet completely established. Soluble fibre in wheat is related to viscosity, which has also been shown to be related to AME value of wheat (Dusel et al., 1997). Choct and Annison, (1992) reported that the NSP content of wheat increases the digesta viscosity, which reduces intestinal passage time and availability of nutrients. These negative effects had been alleviated by enzyme addition. Of all cereal grains, wheat is most variable in protein content (10 to 17%). It is reported that low protein varieties contain more of lysine and tryptophan per gram of protein than high protein varieties.

Wheat byproducts

Wheat bran: The coarse outer covering of the wheat kernels as separated from cleaning and scoured in the usual process of commercial milling is called wheat bran.

Wheat germ meal: Wheat germ meal consists of chiefly wheat germ together with some bran and middlings or shorts. It must contain not less than 25% CP and 7% EE.

Wheat middlings: The Association of American Feed Control Officials (AAFCO) have specified that wheat middlings must consist of fine particles of wheat bran, wheat shorts, wheat germ, wheat flour, and some of the offal from the 'tail of the mill'. This product must be obtained in the usual process of flour milling. It must not contain more than 9.5% CF.

Wheat shorts: Wheat shorts must consist of fine particles of wheat bran, wheat germ, wheat flour, and the offal from the 'tail of the mill'. This product must be obtained in the usual process of commercial milling. It must not contain more than 7% CF.

Wheat red dog: It consists of the offal from the 'tail of the mill' together with some fine particles of wheat bran, wheat germ and wheat flour. This product must be obtained in the usual process of commercial milling and must contain not more than 4% crude fibre.

Bulgur: Debranned (polished) and cracked parboiled wheat is known as bulgur.

Barley

Barley is the preferred grain for cultivation in many areas in the world due to its resistance to drought and ability to mature in climates with a short growth season. However, its use for poultry has been limited by the considerable amounts of fibre present in the grain. The soluble fibre fraction, which mainly consists of mixed-linked (1-3) (1-4) - β-glucan, is associated with an increased gut viscosity, which in turn inhibits digestion and absorption of nutrients. The majority of the insoluble fibre fraction is present in the hull and it has no antinutritive effect, though it reduces the nutrient concentration of the grain. Hulless varieties of barley are successfully grown at a commercial scale in Canada and are suitable for use in poultry diets when used together with an enzyme.

Oats

Oats are higher in CF compared to that in maize (10-18% vs 2%) and accordingly are lower in TDN (68% vs. 77%, for ruminants). The high fibre content limits the use of oats in pig and poultry. Non-starch polysaccharides (NSP) may comprise 30% and consist of, in decreasing order, arabinoxylans, mixed-linked (1-3) (1-4)- β-glucans, and cellulose (Bach-Knudsen, 1997). More than two-thirds of the NSP are contained in the hulls fraction. Oats usually contain 5-9% fat, and the fat consists of a high amount oleic and linoleic acid. Oats are used extensively in rations for horses, young growing stock, show stock and breeding animals. Inclusion of oats in the ration in poultry reduces the incidence of cannibalism, feather picking because of fibre and manganese content in it. **Oat groats/oat kernel:** Oat groats are oats grain from which the hull has been removed

Triticale

Triticale is developed from crosses between wheat and rye. Triticale has agronomic advantages over wheat because it can be grown on more marginal land (arid, acidic, etc.) and requires less fertilizer, pesticides, etc. Wheat and triticale can be grown in the climate, soil and irrigation conditions that are unsuitable to maize cultivation. The main NSP constituent in the endosperm cell walls of triticale is pentosans with some β-glucan, such as in wheat and rye. Several studies (Petterson and Aman, 1988; Flores et al., 1994; Choct and Annison, 1990) indicated that the soluble NSP cell-wall components of wheat, rye and triticale depressed the performance of broiler chickens and inhibited nutrient digestion in the foregut due to high viscosity and water retention. These negative effects had been alleviated by enzyme addition.

Processing of Maize

Maize is processed by two methods: wet milling and dry milling. Wet milling provides starch, syrup, oil and power alcohol; 25-35% of the total wet-milled maize results in byproducts available for inclusion in livestock feeding. Dry milling is less complicated than wet milling with primary objective being to obtain as high a yield of grits with the least contamination with fat and black specks of tip cap.

Products of dry milling

Grits	40 kg per 100 kg of maize
Meal	30
Flour	05
Germ meal	14
Hominy feed	11

Products from wet milling

Maize starch/flour	67
Maize gluten meal	05.3
Maize gluten feed	12.2
Maize germ meal	03.8
Maize oil	03.6
Condensed fermented corn extractives	07.1

Mill byproducts for animal feed: Bran, flour, germ meal, gluten, grain screenings, groats, hulls, middlings, polishings, red dog and shorts.

Husks: Husks are leaves enveloping an ear of maize or the outer coverings of kernels or seeds, especially when dry and membranous. Husk consists of strongly lignified floral integuments.

Hulls: Hulls are outer covering of grain or other seed.

Flour: Soft, finely ground meal of the grains. It consists primarily of gluten and starch from endosperm.

Germ: Germ is the embryo of any seed. Wheat germ meal must contain at least 25% CP and 7% EE.

Gluten: When flour is washed to remove the starch, a tough, viscid, nitrogenous substance remains and this is known as gluten eg., corn gluten, sorghum gluten.

Maize gluten meal: It is a byproduct of corn starch and corn oil manufacture. It is satisfactory as a source of supplemental protein (40+%) for ruminants. It has a low essential amino acid supplemental value with most grains and it is very poor as a protein supplement for nonruminants. Corn gluten is one of the richest natural sources of xanthophylll and is an excellent source of yellow colouring in the shanks and body fat of broilers.

Maize gluten feed: It may contain high levels of sulphur that induce polioencephalomalcia (PEM) when fed in high proportions of the diet. The high sulphur content that results from chemicals added during the extraction procedure may decrease the availability of thiamine, which results in PEM. It is high in phosphorus.

Hominy feed: Hominy feed is a byproduct of the manufacture of hominy, hominy grits and corn meal for human consumption. Hominy feed consists of a mixture of the corn bran, corn germ and varying amounts of the finer siftings of the starchy portion of the corn grain.

Maize cake: Maize cake is a byproduct of starch industry. Its nutritive value is about similar to maize grain.

Brans

With the increased diversion of grains for human consumption, brans form an important source of concentrate feed in livestock feeding. Bran is outer coarse coat (pericarp) of grain separated during processing e.g, rice bran, wheat bran, maize bran. Brans are laxative in action. Wheat bran and rice bran have been traditionally used in feeding of livestock and poultry.

Maize bran: Maize bran is the poorest in nutritive value. It consists of the outer coating of maize seed including the hull and tip-cap with little or none of the germ or starchy part of the grain.

Wheat bran

Wheat bran consists of the outer coating of the wheat kernel. This is one of the most palatable and popular livestock feeds. It is poor in calcium content but is very rich in phosphorus. It is extremely rich in vitamins B-complex and vitamin E, but contains little or no vitamin A potency. It is a mild laxative and acts as a corrective when mainly dry roughages are fed.

Rice bran

Rice bran is obtained from the outer layers of the brown rice. Generally it consists of pericarp, aleurone layer, germ and a part of endosperm. Bran removal amounts to 4% to 9% of the weight of the paddy milled. True bran amounts to 4 to 5% only, rest is polish consisting of inner bran layers and portion of the starchy endosperm. Rice bran traditionally represents one of the world's most frustrating feedstuffs. Rice bran quickly becomes rancid because of contact with an endogenous lipase enzyme during the milling process.

Commercial bran is always contaminated with some amount of husk which varies widely with the type of rice mill used. A major portion of the paddy produced in the country is milled in huller/sheller/modern mills spread all over the country. The huller-bran contains a very high amount of husk where as sheller-bran contains small amount of husk and the bran produced by the modern rubber roll type mill is almost pure containing negligible amount of husk. S.K.Ranjhan (1990) mentioned that small-scale village plants in most of the Asian and African countries produce only huller-bran, which contains about 60% rice hulls, 30% bran and 10% polishings, germ and broken rice.

Rice bran is slightly inferior to wheat bran in protein content. The energy content is similar in both the brans of good quality. However, rice bran when adulterated with husk contains higher fibre. Oil extracted-rice bran, deoiled rice bran (DORB), has longer keeping quality but is poorer in energy content by about 10%. Rice bran is richer than wheat bran in phosphorus content, while the calcium content is similar in both.

Rice bran can be classified into 3 groups

1. Full fatted raw bran that contains 12 to 18% oil
2. Full fatted parboiled bran that contains 20-28% oil
3. Deoiled rice bran that contains 1 to 3% oil

The most important and crucial property of rice bran is the instability of its oil caused by an oil-splitting enzyme, lipase, inherently present in it. This enzyme acts as a catalyst. The fat and enzyme are spatially distributed in aleurone and testa layers respectively in intact rice grain. So long the bran surface is uninjured and protected by the husk, the enzyme remains dormant and the enzymatic activity is not perceptible. As soon as the bran surface is ruptured and separated from the brown rice in milling operations, the lipase comes in contact with the oil bearing layers and they are intimately mixed with each other causing a very rapid hydrolysis of fats into free fatty acids (FFA). As the reaction is hydrolytic in nature it may be called hydrolytic type of rancidification. It is apparent that the rate of hydrolysis will be further enhanced with the increase of moisture in bran. Immediately after milling, the FFA content in bran may be as high as 1% per hour under favourable conditions. The FFA content increase beyond 5% making it unfit for human consumption in as little as 12 hours and useless even as animal feed with in a few days.

Factors affecting rate of formation of FFA: Factors affecting rate of formation of FFA in bran during storage are as follows

(a) Storage temperature: Formation of FFA in raw bran occur even at a storage temperature of 3° C whereas parboiled rice bran was quite stable even at 25°C. The rates of degradation accelerate under tropical conditions.

(b) Moisture content of bran: The rate of hydrolysis of fats into FFA decreases as the storage moisture content of bran decreases.

(c) Storage relative humidity: Rate of FFA formation increases with the increase of the relative humidity of storage and the final moisture content of bran as well.

(d) Particle size of bran: Finer the particle size of the bran higher is the rate of formation of FFA.

(e) Insect infestation: Some of the insects and microflora can contribute lipase to the bran. Fumigation of the storage space is to be done for the control of insect infestation.

Stabilization of rice bran: Stabilization of rice bran extends the storage of bran without any appreciable change in FFA content. Heat treatment inactivates the lipase enzyme. Rice bran stabilizers are developed to stabilize the bran. The stabilized bran can be stored for 3 months at 25-30° C with FFA content below 5%.

CFTRI'S method consists of spraying mineral acid on the bran in a rotary drum. The equipment needed is simple and the process takes place less than 4 minutes a batch to inactivate the enzyme. The process required no steam and the power consumption is extremely low.

FCI designed a steam heated continuous 'inline stabilizer' for stabilizing rice bran. Ideally suited for modern rice mills of four tonnes an hour capacity, this composite stabilizer and polisher helps in bagging of stabilized bran in the mill itself. Simple in design and easy to operate, the stabilizer consists of three cylindrical jacketed vessels with a capacity to handle 150 to 200 kg bran an hour. The bran coming out of the polisher is to be fed to one end of the stabilizer and can be collected as stabilized bran at the discharge gate. Steam at 60 psi is passed through the vessels to heat the bran to 110° C which will inactivate the enzymes that caused increase in FFAs.

Stabilize the rice bran by forcing through an 'extruder'. This machine creates enough frictional heat to destroy powerful enzymes that would otherwise breakdown the oil. Clear, odourless high quality cooking oil can be obtained. In US one Californian company is making a crunchy rice bran-and-germ product. Stabilization by means of specialized extrusion technology has become the most popular process for creating high quality Stabilized Rice Bran. Heat produced (>115° C) deactivates the lipase enzyme fairly well, but heat-sensitive nutrients (vitamin E, B- vitamins, some amino acids) tend to suffer. The raw bran has to be stabilized through an extruder quickly. On-site stabilization can maintain most of the nutritional components inherent in the raw bran.

Advantages of stabilization of rice bran

1. It increases the bulk density and reduces the handling problem
2. It increases the particle sizes and reduces the problem of fines and filtration.
3. It imparts hardening effect to the bran for the better extractability.
4. Stabilised rice bran is a 'functional food' or nutraceutical ingredient, 'generally recognized as safe' GRAS under US FDA rules. It has tocotrienols as well as gamma oryzanol (potent antioxidants) in addition to protein, fat and fibre.

Parboiled rice bran

Parboiling of paddy is a hydrothermal treatment followed by drying before milling for the production of milled parboiled rice. Nearly 50% of the paddy produced in India at present is parboiled.

Physico-chemical changes: Certain physico-chemical changes takes place during parboiling process. The **endosperm** of the raw rice grain contains mainly polygonal starch granules. The voids or intergranular spaces are filled with air and moisture in parboiled rice and that is why it looks opaque. Moreover, there are fissures and or cracks in the grain, developed during maturity, which can cause breakage of rice during milling. The most important change during parboiling is the **gelatinization of starch and disintegration of protein bodies in the endosperm.** The starch and protein expand and fill the internal air spaces. The fissures and cracks in the endosperm are sealed making the grain translucent and hard as a result of which the breakage of grain during milling is minimized.

The colour of the rice changes to yellow or yellowish brown depending upon the paddy variety, soaking time and temperature, steaming time and temperature, drying time and temperature and many other post harvesting factors. Discolouration of rice during parboiling is mainly due to nonenzymatic Maillard type browning, that can be inhibited by bisulphate.

Parboiled rice bran contains higher oil content (25-30%) compared to raw rice bran (10-20%). During parboiling many nutrients are diffused inside the endosperm. This is relatively stabilized compared to raw rice.

Rice polish

Rice polish is a finely powdered material obtained in the operation of polishing rice kernels after husk and bran have been removed. The crude protein content of rice polish is about 12% and the fat is about 15%. The TDN value of good quality rice polish is about 70%. As the fibre content is just 2%, it is a good ingredient for pigs and poultry. It is high in thiamine content. But its keeping quality is poor because of its high fat content. Hence it should be fed as fresh as possible. Like rice bran, rice polish is often adulterated with paddy husk.

Milling of pulses and their byproducts

Pulses are seeds of leguminous plants. Pulses are rich in proteins and are mainly consumed in the form of dehusked split pulses. Milling of pulses means removal of the outer husk and splitting the grain into two equal halves. Generally, the husk is much more tightly held by the kernel of some pulses than most cereals. Green gram, red gram, bengal gram, black gram, lentils are some of the common types of pulses. Milling of pulses is done through wet milling and dry milling, though dry milling is popularly used in commercial mills. In case of red gram, the husk is of 15% and endosperm is the remaining 85%.

Chunies: Chunies are mixture of broken kernels (cotyledons), germ and broken seed coat (husk) of pulses. The nutritive value of *chuni* depends on the amount of husk present. Chuni is relished by animals and is useful in increasing the palatability of the mixtures. Pulse chunies accounts for 15-20% of total weight of pulses. *Urad (Phaseolus mungo) chuni* contained CP 15.5%, ash 12.3%, CF 24.2%, NFE 46.6%, cellulose 25.4%, hemicellulose 14%, lignin 8.8%, Ca 0.9% and P 0.4%. *Urad chuni* as a sole feed could provide all the nutrients for 25 kg sheep with a growth rate of 50 kg/day as per ICAR (1985).

Husks: The feeding value of husks of pulses is low. The DCP content is practically nil and the TDN content about is about 55%. They are liked by cattle and are mixed in small quantities with concentrate mixture.

Fats and oils

Fats and oils are the most concentrated sources of energy. Animal fats are available from the meat processing industry while vegetable oil products are available from refining of vegetable oils and soap manufacturing units. Vegetable oils themselves are added in feeds, some times. These are used to increase energy content of the diet, to control dust, to lessen the wear and tear of the equipment, to increase palatability and as a pellet binder. But the free fatty acid content and hydrolytic rancidity has to be kept in mind while using them in feeds.

By products of the brewing industry for animal feeding

Brewing Process: In brewing, barley is first soaked and allowed to germinate. During this germination (or malting) process of about 6 days, starch hydrolysation to dextrins, maltose and other sugars is initiated (and completed in 'mashing'). After germination the grain or malt is dried ensuring that enzymes do not get inactivated. The sprouts are removed and are sold as **malt culms or coombs**. The dried malt is crushed, and small amounts of other cereals such as maize or rice may be added. Water is sprayed on to the mixture and the temperature of the mash increased to about 65°C. (The object of mashing is to provide suitable conditions for the action of enzymes on the proteins and starch).

After completion of the mashing process the sugary liquid or 'wort' is drained off and the remaining are sold as **wet brewers' grains or dried brewers' grain** as feed for farm animals. Brewers' grains consist of the insoluble barley residue left after removable of the wort. This product also contains maize and rice residues and the composition, therefore, is highly variable. The chemical composition and nutritive value of wet brewers' grain is furnished in Table1.

The wort is next boiled with hops to get characteristic aroma and flavour and the hops are filtered off to dry and sold as **spent hops**. The wort is then fermented in an open vessel with yeast for a number of days, during which most of the sugars are converted to alcohol and carbon dioxide. The yeast is filtered off, dried and sold as **brewers' yeast**.

Malt sprouts: The radicle of the embryo of the grain removed from sprouted and steamed whole grain e.g., barley, wheat, rye malt sprouts.

Utilization of Brewers' grain

Brewers' grains have 20% crude protein on dry matter basis, making them a good protein source in addition to their energy value. The brewing process makes this protein less soluble and could be valuable in rations which contain large amounts of soluble protein such as urea-ammoniated straws, urea-supplemented concentrate mixtures. Brewers' grains are fed both in the wet and dry form. They are not as palatable in the dried form as the original grain and usually are included at 25% or less in the concentrate mixture. Transportation and storage of the wet grains is a problem because of their high moisture content. Hence it is better to utilize them as wet brewers' grain.

Roots and tubers

A root crop consists of the fleshy subterranean (underground) parts of a harvested plant, grown primarily for its sugar content. e.g., turnips, sugarbeet, carrots, Swedes, etc. Tubers are short, thickened, fleshy stems usually formed underground such as potatoes, cassava, sweetpotatoes, etc. Tubers differ from the root crops in containing either starch or fructan instead of sucrose as the main storage carbohydrate.

Table 3: Chemical Composition (%) and Nutritive Value of Wet Brewers' Grain on DMB (*McDonald et. al. 1995 P.496;**From our Lab Analysis.)

Nutrient	Mean*	Range*	Mean**	Range**
Chemical composition				
Dry matter	26.3	24.4-30.0	22.52	22.25-22.80
Crude protein	23.4	18.4-26.2	17.01	16.88-17.14
Crude fibre	17.6	16.5-20.4	20.29	19.38-21.20
Ether extract	7.7	6.1-9.9	1.65	1.44-1.85
Total ash	4.1	3.6-4.5	5.22	3.40-7.04
Acid insoluble ash	–	–	3.05	1.30-4.79
Calcium	–	–	0.57	–
Phosphorus	–	–	0.64	–
Nutritive Value (In sheep)				
Metabolizable energy, (MJ/kg DM)	11.2	10.5-12.0		
Digestible crude protein, %	18.5	13.9-21.3		

Tapioca and its byproducts

Tapioca (*Manihot esculenta crantz syn. utilissima*), also called cassava, is one of the most productive tuber crops in tropical areas in terms of dry matter yield per hectare. The main world producers are Brazil and Thailand. The ease of propagation and the economy production make tapioca an inexpensive and valuable source of carbohydrate. These tubers are used for the production of tapioca starch for human consumption although the tuber is also given to ruminants, pigs and poultry. At harvest time, the tuber is collected and the leaves (tops) are thrown away.

Tapioca tubers for animal feeding

Tapioca tubers compete with other carbohydrate sources, especially maize and sorghum grains, on the basis of price, nutritional value, quality and availability. Immediately after harvesting, tubers are to be chipped and sundried, otherwise tubers perish because of high moisture (65%) content and once perished moulds may grow and mycotoxins are liberated. The dried tapioca chips have low protein content compared to other carbohydrate feed sources such as cereal grains and millets. Later these chips are milled and incorporated in animal feeds. Tapioca flour can be mixed with soybean meal in a ratio of 4:1 to form a 'cereal replacer' and several European countries include tapioca in this way in place of maize grain. The chemical composition and nutritive value of tapioca tuber, tapioca starch waste and tapioca leaf meal are furnished in Table 2.

Table 2. Chemical composition and nutritive value of tapioca tuber, tapioca starch waste and tapioca leaf meal on DMB

Nutrient	Tapioca tuber/chips	Tapioca starch waste	Tapioca lead meal
Dry matter	66.8	100	100
Crude protein	2.2	4.9	15.4
Ether Extract	0.9	1.0	12.2
Crude fibre	5.2	19.2	22.8
Nitrogen Free Extract	88.8	69.3	41.2
Ash	2.9	5.6	8.4
Calcium	–	0.5	1.4
Phosphorus	–	0.2	0.3
Digestible Crude Protein	–	2.0	9.7
Total Digestible Nutrients	–	64.0	50.7
Digestible Energy (Kcal/kg dry matter)	–	2853	2235
Metabolizable energy (Kcal/kg dry matter)	–	2339	1833

Byproducts of tapioca

In manufacturing starch/sago from tapioca, fresh tubers of 1000kg yield starch/sago of 250/240 kg and byproducts such as peelings of 20kg, low grade starch of 20 kg and dried thippi of 70 kg.

Toxic factors

Tapioca plants and tubers, primarily skins of tubers, contain varying proportions of two cyanogenetic glycosides (linamarin (phaseolunatin) and lotaustralin), which readily breakdown to give hydrocyanic acid (HCN) by means of an enzyme which is usually present in the plant. Linamarin yields glucose, acetone and hydrogen cyanide on hydrolysis.

Simple sun-drying of leaves alone eliminates almost 90% of the initial cyanide content. When combined with chopping and wilting, cyanide in the dried meal was reduced to levels that are safer for monogastric animals. This reduction is due to the action of endogenous linamarase on glycosides following loss of cell integrity (wilting) or tissue damage (chopping). The free tannin contents of leaves are also considerably lowered during drying.

Part of the plant	HCN yield (mg/100g DM)
Tapioca tubers with skin	113
Tapioca tubers without skin	10-15
Tapioca leaves	80-320

Utilization of tapioca products in animal feeding
Tapioca leaf meal

Fresh tapioca forage including tender stems, could be utilized directly for ruminant feeding. The foliage, including tender stems, could be wilted, chopped and used directly for ruminant feeding. Alternatively, the leaves could be stripped, dried and ground into meal. When fed to growing calves, 2.3 kg of partially dried tapioca leaves can replace 0.7 kg of groundnut cake. About 50% of groundnut cake can be replaced by tapioca leaf meal in the ration of milch animals. At an intake level of 0.5 to 0.8% of body weight, it does not produce any adverse effect.

Although tapioca leaves are rich in protein, factors such as high crude fibre may limit its nutritive value for monogastric animals. Wide variability in chemical composition primarily protein and fibre content are related to differences in cultivars, stage of maturity, sampling procedure, soil fertility and climate. Cassava leaf protein is deficient in methionine, possibly marginal in tryptophan, but rich in lysine. Almost 85% of the crude protein fraction is true protein. However, presence of condensed tannins and high fibre content lower the protein utilization. Hence supplementation with methionine (0.15-0.20%) and corn oil (3%) make leaf meal good for poultry. Tapioca leaf meal has some yellow pigments that gave a good egg yolk pigmentation.

Tapioca meal (flour) and tapioca starch waste

Drying tapioca effectively reduces the danger of toxicity from the cyanogenic glycosides and proper supplementation with protein, minerals and vitamins can make it about equal to grain as source of energy. Tapioca tubers should not supply more than one third dry matter in the rations of animals. Starch of tapioca is fermented rapidly in the rumen and thus it is a good source of fermentable energy for the rumen microbes to improve the non-protein nitrogen sources. Some concentrate mixtures containing tapioca products are presented here (Table 3). Tapioca starch waste is a byproduct obtained during the manufacture of starch from tapioca tubers. It is high in fibre.

Tapioca thippi: It is a byproduct obtained during the manufacture of sago. Deskinned tubers are soaked in water and crushed for extraction of milk. The milk is passed through sieves to remove the fibrous material. This dried fibrous material is known as tapioca thippi.

Tapioca milk residue: It is dried second grade starch that could not get together to form the crystals of sago.

Table 3. Examples of Grain-less concentrate mixtures with tapioca

Feedstuffs (%)		1	2	3	4	5
Wheat Bran		30.75	41.31	17.85	23.07	23.29
Rice Bran		30.75	0	17.85	23.07	23.29
Groundnut Cake		12.75	25.69	0	10.85	10.41
Gingelly Cake		12.75	0	16.30	0	0
Tapioca Flour		10	30	15	10	20
Gram Husk		0	0	30	30	20
Mineral Mixture		2	2	2	2	2
Salt		1	1	1	1	1
	DCP	18.29	15.7	10.15	8.60	8.60
Nutritive Value						
(%)	**TDN**	73.67	62.83	61.59	61.52	62.41

Molasses

Cane or blackstrap molasses: This is the byproduct of sugar industry; about 25-50 kg molasses is obtained from production of 100 kg refined sugar.

Beet sugar: This is obtained as a byproduct of the manufacture of beet sugar. The protein content is higher (6-10%).

Citrus molasses: When orange or grape fruits are processed for juice, there remains 45-60% of their weight in the form of peel, rag and seeds as wastes. The liquid obtained from pressing these wastes contains between 10-15% soluble solids of which 50-70% is sugar. This material can be concentrated into citrus molasses. It has about 30% moisture, 14% protein and has a bitter taste. This bitter taste does not affect its usefulness in cattle feeding.

Wood molasses: By giving high pressure at high temperature in the presence of dilute acid, wood is converted to molasses. One ton of wood will yield about 0.5 tons of sugar. In the manufacture of paper, fibre-boards, pure cellulose from wood, there results an extract which contains soluble carbohydrates and minerals of the wood material which may also be processed into molasses for livestock feeding. This molasses has a bitter taste but highly acceptable to cattle, particularly used for beef cattle.

Molasses addition more than 1to 3% in poultry usually produces loose excreta because of high potassium content. It is a rich source of pantothenic acid, riboflavin, niacin and choline.

Protein rich concentrates

Plant proteins: oilseed meals **a.** groundnut cake/meal, **b.** linseed meal, **c.** mustard cake, **d.** cottonseed cake (whole pressed cottonseed cakes i.e., undecorticated; dehulled i.e.,decorticated), **e.** coconut cake **f.** sesame meal, **g.** sunflower cake h. corn gluten meal **i.** soybean meal. All these byproducts, left after extraction of oil from oil seeds, are used for feeding of all kinds of livestock. The three methods of oil extraction are ghani, expeller and solvent extracted and accordingly nomenclature cake and meal have come.

Groundnut or peanut cake/meal: It is usually made from the kernels. If this is made from whole pods (occasionally may be made) the byproduct is known as undecorticated groundnut cake/ meal. Groundnut cake is an excellent source of arginine, but low in lysine, methionine, cystine and tryptophan. It is rich in pantothenic acid, niacin and choline. Groundnut cake, on account of its higher availability, has been the conventional vegetable protein supplement extensively used in preparing mixed feeds for the various classes of poultry. However, groundnut cake protein is not balanced in amino acid pattern desirable for fast growth of broilers with deficiencies of methionine, tryptophan and lysine. Often it contains aflatoxins and is adulterated with groundnut hulls.

Sunflower meal: It is a better source of arginine and methionine than soybean meal, but poor in lysine, cystine and glycine. It is an excellent source of pantothenic acid and niacin. It is high in fibre. The use of this in poultry rations has been associated with appearance of characteristic egg shell stains which develop after laying.

Linseed meal: Extracted linseed meal is the finely ground residue remaining after oil extraction of flax seed/linseed. The meal is satisfactory for all classes of livestock except for poultry where if fed in more than 5%, it has a depressing effect on the growth. It contains cyanogenic glycoside. The toxicity can largely be eliminated by boiling the linseed for 10 minutes or by soaking the meal in water for 24 hours or by adding pyridoxine (B6). It should not be fed more than 2-3% to poultry, if not processed. The meal has a very good reputation as a feed for ruminants due to high content of mucilage (3-20%). The compound is capable of absorbing large amounts of water which results in higher retention time in the rumen and give a better opportunity for microbial digestion. The lubricating character of the mucilage also protects the gut wall against mechanical damage and together with the bulkiness, regulates excretion, preventing constipation without causing loose motion.

Sesame meal: There are three varieties of til cakes: white, black and red. Nutritive value is highest in white variety and lowest in the red variety cakes. Til cake is richest among all oil cakes in calcium content, being 2.3%. But it has high levels of oxalates and phytates and hence availability is questionable.

Cottonseed meal: Cottonseed meal contains gossypol. Nonruminants and immature ruminants (functionally undeveloped rumen) are particularly susceptible to gossypol toxicity. However, there are cases of gossypol toxicity in mature dairy cows and deaths of cows have been reported. Gossypol causes discolouration of egg yolks and cyclopropenic fatty acids impart pink colour to egg whites. The use of ferrous sulphate at the rate of four parts to one part of free gossypol, up to a maximum of 400ppm, will overcome the problem of yolk discolouration.

Rapeseed meal: It contains about 36-39% protein, which compares favourably with SBM protein in amino acid balance. Rapeseed meal protein is somewhat lower in lysine and higher in methionine than the protein of SBM. Rapeseed meal has been limited in its use as a high-protein feed over the years.

(1) Meals produced from the earlier grown varieties of rapeseed were high in glucosinolates, the hydrolytic products of which (e.g., isothiocynates, oxyzolidinethiones, and nitrites) are more or less toxic to most livestock, causing lowered performance and possibly goiter when used as a major source of protein in the ration.

(2) Rapeseed meal is high in CF (11-13%) and low in digestible energy.

Canola meal: Canola is rapeseed developed in Canada for food and feed applications. Canola meal is derived from extraction (usually solvent extraction) of double zero (low glucosinolates and low erucic acid) varieties of *Brassica napus and Brassica campestris*. By definition canola meal must contain less than 30 micromoles per gram total glucosinolates (mixture of 3-butenyl glucosinolate, 4-pentenyl glucosinolate, 2-hydroxy-3-butenyl glucosinolate, and 2-hydroxy-4-pentenyl glucosinolate) and less than 1% erucic acid in the oil. Plant breeding and also the heat and steam involved in oil extraction have reduced the levels of glucosinolates. Canola meal from Canada and Australia contains 10 -16 micromoles of total glucosinolates per gram.

Canola meal must contain a minimum of 35% CP, a maximum of 12% crude fibre, and a maximum of 30 µmol of glucosinolates per gram (AAFCO, 1992). Canola meal has 65% protein and this protein contains an excellent balance of essential amino acids. But it has high levels of fibre and antinutritional factors, particularly phytates. MCN Bioproducts, Inc (Canada) developed a process for the aqueous fractionation and processing of oil-extracted canola. CanPro-IP65 is a specialty canola meal with over 90% digestibility of CP, more than fish meal itself.

Canola meal (the oil-free residue of low glucosinolate, low erucic acid rapeseed) is a good source of protein for animals and is a particularly rich source of the sulphur amino acids, methionine and cystine. Prepress-solvent extracted canola meal is characterized as having lower and less consistent/more variable amino acid digestibility than soybean meal (NRC, 1994). Canola meal is also characterized as having a lower metabolizable energy level than of other protein sources such as soybean meal (NRC, 1994). The lower apparent metabolizable energy (AME) is at least partially due to the higher fibre content of the meal and also due to the reduced apparent ileal digestibility of nutrients especially amino acids through Maillard reactions that occur in the extraction process.

Prepress-solvent extraction of canola involves 10 stages, including cleaning, drying, conditioning, flaking, expelling, cooking, solvent extraction with hexane, desolventization/toasting, drying and cooling. The average processing conditions are as follows: clean the seed by aspiration, dry it with warm air (for 45 -60 min, final temperature about 52° C), the seed is then conditioned for 30 min at 75-78° C, it is flaked, cooked at 90° C for 20-30 min, solvent extracted in hexane at 50 - 60° C for 90 min, desolventized/toasted (total residence time 60 min, exit temperature 100-110° C), dried/cooled (15 min residence, exit temperature 34° C). Prepress-solvent extraction is currently the most effective method of extracting oil from canola meal. But Newkirk et al. (2003) reported that the commercial desolventization/toasting can reduce the content and coefficient of apparent ileal digestibility (CAID) of many amino acids in canola meal and increase the level of variability in nutritional value between canola meal samples.

Crambe meal: Crambe meal is the seed meal of *Crambe abyssinica* obtained after the removal of oil from the seed and hull. The oil may be removed by prepress solvent extraction or by solvent extraction alone. The resulting seed meal is heat-toasted and shall contain not less than 24% CP, not more than 11% moisture, not more than 4% oil, and not more than 26% crude fibre. It is to be used only in the feed of feedlot cattle, and at a level not to exceed 4.2% of the diet. Further specifications on crambe meal are: glucosinolate calculated as epiprogoitrin, not more than 4%; goitrin, not more than 0.1%; nitrile, calculated as 1-cyano-2-hydroxy-3-butene, not more than 1.4%. At least 50% of the nitrogen shall be soluble in 0.5 M sodium chloride. Mirosinase enzyme activity shall be absent.

Merits of soybean meal over groundnut cake or fish meal

Fish meal, which is commonly used as an animal protein supplement, is often contaminated with high level of sand, silica and salt. Steam sterilized fish meal which is subjected to heat treatment for longer duration may contain a toxic substance called 'gizzerosine'. This substance causes severe gizzard erosion and ulcers in chickens.

Soybean meal: Production of soybean meal is increasing consistently in India. The amino acid pattern of SBM is most desirable to meet the dietary requirement of broilers and layers, among all vegetable protein supplements. Methionine, which is relatively deficient, may be supplemented easily. It contains least crude fibre and silica among all vegetable protein sources. Digestibility of soybean meal protein is around 97%. If fish meal is to be replaced completely with SBM in chicken feeds, methionine, vitamin B12, selenium, Ca and P requirements are to be taken care of.

Soybeans and soybean meal in ruminant rations

Soybean meal is the most commonly used protein supplement in beef and dairy cattle diets. It is very palatable and has a good amino acid balance and high availability. Its bypass amino acid index is just next to ruminal microbial protein beating all other undegradable protein sources. Relative to other commonly used feed proteins, soybeans are rich in lysine but methionine, valine and isoleucine are the first, second and third limiting amino acids, respectively. In fact, SBM, out of the common plant proteins used in animal feeds, has one of the highest percentages of essential amino acids (47.6%) as a percent of CP. When soybeans are fed with maize (whose first limiting amino acid is lysine), the combination provides a well balanced protein.

Soybeans as a protein supplement are also an economical and convenient way to provide dietary fat. Full fat soybean has 18% fat, 5% fibre and 38% protein. However, soybeans and SBM have relative low protein efficiency because of extensive ruminal degradation. It is estimated that only 25% to 34% of protein in soybeans and SBM escapes rumen fermentation. Their use is becoming limited in diets of rapidly growing and high-producing ruminant animals. Therefore, improvement in ruminal escape characteristics of soybeans and SBM is of major importance to both beef and dairy producers and the soybean industry.

Methods used to increase the bypass protein content of SBM

Various methods have been used to treat soybeans and SBM in order to increase their ruminal bypass protein content. Of these methods, roasting, extrusion, expeller and lignosulfonate treatments are most commonly used in the U S feed industry. All these methods involve the Maillard reaction. Controlling this reaction by optimizing the heating process is the key to successful protection of soybeans and SBM. The properly treated soybeans or SBM produced through each of these processes significantly reduced its ruminal protein degradation without affecting its intestinal protein digestion and absorption. Substantial benefits in terms of increased milk production and improved growth can be obtained by feeding properly treated soybeans or SBM as a protein supplement to dairy and beef cattle over untreated soybeans or SBM.

Roasting: There has been growth in the use of heat processed soybeans as a protein and energy supplement for beef and dairy cattle in the US. Roasting and extrusion are the two commonly used methods to process full-fat soybeans, of which roasting of SB is the predominant process. Roasting of SB involves a revolving finned cylinder which lifts the beans through jets of flame. Roasting is popular because of a high through put (3 to 12 tons per h) and roasting equipment is mobile resulting in on-farm processing of beans. One drawback of this process is that many times roasting is done subjectively based on the degree colour of the beans exiting the roaster. This results in a large variation in the amount of heat that SB are exposed to when processed by commercial suppliers. Heating of SBM at 149° C for 2, 4 and 6 h increased the amount of ADIN (as a percentage of total N) from 1.9% in SBM to 4.6%, 8.9 and 19.7%, respectively.

Extrusion: Extrusion is another commonly used method to treat full-fat SB for ruminant diets. In this method, SB are fed into an extruder barrel, where a central revolving shaft forces the beans through the extruder. The SB are treated by the heat generated through friction and /or steam which is frequently injected during the process. No oil is removed from the SB during extrusion. SBM can also be processed through extrusion. Extrusion usually results in a product that is more uniform in quality than does roasting but through put (1- 10 tons/h) is relatively slow, mobility of the processing equipment is poor, and the cost of the treated product is high.

Expeller method: In this method, soybeans are initially cleaned, cracked and dried. The SB are then transported to tempering devices and heated uniformly. From the tempering bins, the SB are fed into expeller presses. A central revolving shaft creates pressure within the press, causing the extraction of oil from the ground SB. The extracted beans leave the presses in the form of flakes, which are subsequently ground. Expeller processing is a method that involves heating to a maximum 163° C which results in the Maillard reacton between sugar aldehyde groups and free amino acids. If the extent of the reaction can be controlled by regulating the amount of heat applied, ruminal protein degradation can be decreased without adversely affecting intestinal protein digestion. Expeller SBM contains 42 to 46% of CP and 4.5 to 6% of fat on as-fed basis.

Lignosulfonate treatment: Soybean meal is treated with 7% (wt/wt) calcium lignosulfonate and then heated at 95° C for 1 h before it is dried. A higher temperature of 100° C for 30 min is used in a commercial process of lignosulfonate-treated SBM. Lignosulfonate is a term used to describe any product derived from the spent sulfite liquor that is generated during the sulfite digestion of wood and containing a percentage of lignosulfonic acid or its salt as well as hemicellulose and sugars. Calcium lignosulfonate is produced from hardwoods via the acid-sulfite wood pulping process and contains a variety of wood sugars, main sugar being xylose. Initially, lignin present in the spent liquor was thought to protect the protein in the feed, when it was mixed with 0.25-3.0% spent sulfite liquor, from ruminal microbial degradation. However, later it was concluded that calcium lignosulfonate itself does not play any active role, rather heat and the presence of wood sugars, mainly xylose, are necessary for protein protection. In this process, the amount of sugar added, temperature, pH, moisture and time of reaction are critical to obtain the optimal effect.

Animal proteins: a. fish meal, **b.** meat meal, **c.** blood meal, **d.** meat and bone meal **e.** feather meal, **f.** hatchery byproduct meal

Single cell protein (SCP): SCP is obtained from single cell organisms, such as yeast, bacteria and algae that have been grown on specially prepared growth media. Production of this type of protein can be attained through the fermentation of petroleum derivatives or organic wastes or through the culturing of photosynthetic organisms (algae) in special illuminated ponds. Bacteria (*Methanomonas methanica*), algae (*Chlorella vulgaris, Spirulina maxima and Scenedesmus obliquus*) and yeast (*Saccharomyces cerevisiae, Torulopsis utilis, Candida lipolytica*) are useful microorganisms.

Petroprotein is a term used for crude or refined source of protein produced from fermentation of petroleum hydrocarbons available from distillation of crude oil in oil refineries by using *Candida lipolytica.* SCP is a fine, odourless and pale yellow powder. It has about 53% CP, 2.4% EE, 0.9% CF, 35% NFE, 1.5% P and 0.5% Ca on DMB. It is completely devoid of mineral oil residues and can be stored for at least one year at room temperature. It is palatable and can be used up to 20% level in concentrate mixture of adult bullocks for maintenance.

How to bridge the gap between the demand and supply of feed resources?

The area under fodder crops has been estimated to be 3.3% and 4.41% of total cultivable area as reported by two independent estimates. The area under green forage production is likely to be further reduced and most of the land would be used for cereal, pulses, oilseed crop cultivation. This would thus result in increased crop residues for animal consumption. At some places, area under crops has been diverted to aquaculture as well.

Several steps had been taken to bridge the gap between the demand and supply of animal feed resources in the country. They are

1. ICAR initiated an **AICRP on the Utilization of Agricultural Byproducts and Industrial Waste Materials for Evolving Economic Rations for Livestock** in 1967at 4 centres, GAU, Anand; KAU, Trissur; GBPUAT, Pantnagar and OUAT, Bhubaneswar.

2. In the V Plan 4 more centres were started at PAU, Ludhiana; BAU, Ranchi; JNKVV, Jabalpur and BAIF, Uruli-Kanchan (Pune) with a coordination centre at JNKVV, Jabalpur.

3. In the VI Plan two more centres were added at APAU, Hyderabad and AAU, Guwahati.

4. In the VII Plan, the scope of the Project was expanded and the title was modified to "Determination of the Availability of Animal Feed Resources and Their Utilization with Special Emphasis on Crop Residues, Byproducts of Industries, Forest, Aquatic and Slaughter house in Origin and Animal Organic Waste for Evolving Economic Rations for Livestock and Poultry".

5. During this VII Plan three more centres were added at HAU, Hisar; Konkan Krishi Vidyapeeth (KKV) at Bombay Veterinary College, Bombay and TNAU at Madras Veterinary College, Madras. Two centres one at Jabalpur and the other at Bhubaneswar were closed and the Co-ordinating Unit was shifted to the NDRI, Karnal. Thus the project functioned at 11 centres during the VII Plan and the coordinating centre was shifted to Hisar later.

6. An Indo-US Project, "Conversion of Biodegradable Animal Wastes for Animal Feed" was sanctioned (during VII Plan) as a support to the Project and functioned at 5 centres, viz. NDRI, Karnal; PAU, Ludhiana; HAU, Hisar; KKV, Bombay and KAU, Trissur.

7. In the IX Plan the project was renamed as **"Network Programme on Agricultural Byproducts as Animal Feeds – Complete Feeds"** and functioned at only four centres, APAU, Hyderabad; BAIF, Uruli-Kanchan (Pune); GAU, Anand and HAU, Hisar.

8. In the X Plan, the 3 network projects viz-Micronutrients in Animal Nutrition and Production, Agricultural byproducts as Animal Feed and Crop based Animal Production Systems had been converged into the ICAR - AICRP entitled **"Improvement of feed resources and nutrient utilization in raising animal production"**. NIANP is the coordinating unit for this project with 22 participating centres including SAU's, sister ICAR institutes and NGO's covering almost all parts of the country. The objectives and activities of this project are to address different farming systems and livestock production systems in the country through nutritional intervention in raising animal productivity and profitability.

Non-conventional feed resources (NCFR): Some examples

Roughages: Top feed resources include forages available from trees and shrubs. These are conventional feeds for goats. During scarcity tree leaves serve as roughages for livestock. Tree leaves and fallen tree leaves such as banyan, pipal, mango, teak, bamboo, neem, gliricidia, banana, cassava, mulberry, khejri, etc. are useful.

Other examples are groundnut shells, paddy husk/hull, coffee seed husk, cotton straw, cotton seed hull bran, safflower straw, sunflower straw and heads, maize cobs, bajra cobs, sorghum cobs, legume pod husk-husks of bengalgram, blackgram, greengram, redgram, etc. cocoa pod husk, water hyacinth, sugarcane trash, sugarcane tops, bagasse, molasses and pressmud (is a byproduct of sugar industry during precipitation. It can be utilized as a mineral supplement for large ruminants). The use of these husks and hulls, bagasse, tree leaves in combination with nonprotein nitrogen (NPN) sources of protein (urea) and molasses can meet the nutritional needs of animals during scarcity periods.

Concentrates: Ambadicake, castor bean meal, mangoseed kernal, neemseed cake, prosopis pods, rubberseed cake, sunhemp seed, tamarindseed, tamarindseed kernal, tamarindseed hulls, dehulled tamarindseed, tapioca waste/cassava waste, water melon seed cake, salseed meal, safflowerseed cake/kardy cake, nigar seed cake, spent tea waste, spent coffee seed cake, mahua cake, kosum cake, karanj cake, etc.

Energy sources: Sal seed meal, tapioca flour, tamarind seed powder, mango seed kernel, babul seeds and pods, prosopis pods, rain tree pods,

Starch Industry waste: Maize germ, maize bran, maize gluten and maize oil meal

Dehulled ground tamarind seed: Tamarind seeds have been processed to obtain white kernel and red testa (hulls). The white kernels have been powdered and used to replace maize to the extent of 10% in the concentrate feeds of growing cattle and sheep.

Tamarind seed hulls: The red testa (hull) covering tamarind seed is also comparable in energy and protein content to maize. The hulls can be incorporated in the concentrate feeds of growing calves to the extent of 10% replacing cereal grains without any adverse effect on growth or nutrient utilization. Higher levels may not be advisable due to its high tannin content. Incorporation at 10% level is also useful for better utilization of groundnut cake protein since tannin of tamarind seed protect the proteins of groundnut cake from rumen degradation.

Deoiled salseed meal: It can safely be incorporated in the concentrate feeds of growing cattle and sheep at 10% level and at 5% level in the rations of swine replacing maize without adversely affecting their growth rate and nutrient utilization.

Prosopis juliflora pods: Prosopis juliflora trees give fruits twice in a year and each tree yields about 20 kg mature yellow pods per year. Mature yellow pods contain about 16% protein. The ground pods were supplemented in the concentrate mixtures of sheep and cattle from 10 to 40% level in place of wheat bran and the results suggested that pods can be economically utilized to the extent of 20% without affecting their performance. It is suggested that the pods should not be fed as sole ration. It is necessary to grind the pods in hammer mill so as to ensure proper grinding of the seed otherwise the seed will be voided in the faeces.

Bamboo (*Dendracalamus strictus*) seed: The raw bamboo seeds contain 6.7% hulls when dehulled in a domestic flour mill. The seed contains 10.0% CP, 11.0% CF and 75.4% NFE. The proximate composition of the seed is comparable to coarse cereal grains.

Dried rumen digesta: Huge quantities of reticulo-rumen contents are available every day from the slaughter houses. These half-digested materials contain about 10%-15% protein. It is a good source of essential amino acids and B-complex vitamins. This material is comparable in composition to some of the commonly grown fodders like napier, sorghum or maize and superior to straws. Sun-dried rumen digesta can be incorporated in the rations of weaned piglets up to 10 - 15% level replacing wheat bran.

Spent coffee seed cake: It is a byproduct from the instant coffee industry and contains about 18% CP. It can be incorporated in the concentrate mixtures up to 10 to 20% level for growing cattle in place of wheat bran without affecting growth rate or nutrient utilization.

Protein supplements

Vegetable protein supplements: guar meal, niger cake, karanja cake, neem seed cake, rubber seed cake , kapok seed cake, sunnhemp seed, daincha seed, cassia tora seed, safflower seed cake, mahua seed cake, tobacco seed cake, water dammar seed cake, bijada cake

Ambadi (Hibiscus cannabinus) cake: Ambadi seed contains 20% oil, while the residual cake contains 28.5% CP and 21.4% CF. Ambadi cake contains 2.93% lysine as compared to 2.99% in the groundnut cake. Ambadi cake can safely replace groundnut cake protein in the concentrate feeds of dairy cows without affecting quality and quantity of milk production. Similarly it can replace the entire groundnut cake of broiler and layer rations, though the efficiency of feed utilization is poor in broilers.

Animal protein supplements: hatchery byproduct meal, poultry byproduct meal, liver residue meal, frog meal, prawn/ shrimp waste, crab meal, hydrolysed feather meal, squilla meal

Marine and aquatic waste: Fish waste, Frog meal (leftovers of the frog leg industry), and seaweed meal (agar-agar is being extracted from sargussam sea weed and its byproduct can be used for livestock feeding. It contains 33% ash and 10% protein).

Slaughter house byproducts: Blood meal, meat meal, meat and bone meal, tankage (a fat free product obtained by cooking of meat in water), rumen contents.

Blood meal: The total quantity of blood in an animal amounts to 1/11 to 1/14 of the body weight. However, all is never recovered from the body. Blood meal of 5 to 7 kg per 100 kg live weight is possible as fresh and 5 kg fresh blood gives 1 kg dried blood.

Poultry industry byproducts: Feather meal, offal meal/poultry waste meal, hatchery waste.

Animal wastes: These are fallen and slaughtered animal wastes, animal organic wastes (excreta) and animal byproduct wastes. **Abattoir wastes** are blood meal, tankage, meat scrap, feather meal, horn and hoof meal. **Animal organic wastes** include poultry litter/ dried poultry waste, caged poultry droppings/ dried poultry manure, cow manure, pig excreta,

Rendering

Rendering is the recovery of fat from animal material by heating. During rendering, fat recovered from fresh and healthy parts is used for edible purposes while the one recovered from decomposed material is used for industrial purposes, such as greases.

Slaughter house offals are converted into stock feeds, fertilizers and fats, although greater emphasis is needed to produce stock feed as it commands a higher price. The rendering process must comply with three general principles.

1. Sterilizing and making the product safe for feeding
2. Reducing the moisture to a minimum, thus creating conditions unfavourable for bacterial growth and therefore preventing decomposition
3. Recovering the fat from sterilized and dried meal, which would otherwise cause rancidity

Rendering is of wet rendering and dry rendering. The name wet rendering is applied where the raw material is processed with added water or condensate derived from steam. In dry rendering, all the unwanted moisture is eliminated without the loss of any nutrient. The steam is applied to the jacket only and not to the material to be processed, as in wet rendering.

High moisture agroindustrial byproducts

High moisture feedstuffs can deteriorate rapidly during warm weather, which will reduce palatability and quality. Fruit and vegetable factory byproducts, dairy whey, pulp and papermill residues, brewery waste (brewer's grains), distillers grain, condensed molasses solubles, yeast sludge, single cell protein, animal waste, such as excreta and rumen contents from slaughter house

Generally high moisture (70-80%) food processing wastes should be used shortly after processing as moisture content makes processing and storing difficult and expensive. They are low in protein and fibre. Animal wastes usually have high protein content. Residues from the pulp and paper industries are partially delignified and are thus potentially good sources of feed. Aquatic plants vary in nutritional value. Algae are high in protein and low in fibre. Water hyacinth is high in fibre.

Food-processing residues

Fruit and vegetable factory byproducts: apple pomace, mango peels and kernels, pineapple wastes, banana wastes, citrus processing waste (citrus peels, dried citrus pulp, citrus meal and fines, citrus molasses), dried cocoa pod husk, oil palm byproducts, tomato processing wastes (tomato pomace, etc), potato processing wastes, vegetable wastes.

Certain food waste has low levels of calcium or high levels of P that may cause an imbalance in the Ca to P ratio. This imbalance and dietary phosphorus level in excess of calcium can cause urinary calculi. Some food waste contains high levels of salt. Fruit- and vegetable-processing waste may contain pesticide residues such as halogenated pesticides (lindane, hepatochlor, dieldrin, aldrin, etc.), organophosphate pesticides (malathione, etc). Potato screenings and peels may contain excessive levels of sodium that will limit the effectiveness of monensin (a commonly used feed additive that improves feed to gain ratios in beef cattle, sheep and goat diets), and reduce DMI when fed at high levels.

Non-conventional roughages

Sunflower straw and heads: Sunflower straw contains about 2.8% CP, 31.0% CF and 52.2% NFE. Sunflower heads after removal of seeds contain about 7.2% CP, 16.6% CF, 62.6% NFE and 1.4% calcium. Low-cost ready-made balanced feeds have been formulated and processed utilizing sunflower heads (33 to 48% level) and subabul (30%) for sheep. It was also demonstrated that sunflower heads or straw (at 50% level) can work out as the sole source of roughage in the formulation of complete feeds for sheep and crossbred cattle. Supplementation of subabul meal replacing 45% of groundnut cake protein in the sunflower straw rations further reduced the feed cost without affecting the performance of the animal and feeding quality of the ration.

Groundnut shell: Soak groundnut shell in water overnight and mix it with groundnut cake in 9 to1 proportion. This is to be ground and pressed or fed directly to livestock.

Fallen tree leaves: Low-cost complete feeds were formulated utilizing mango leaves (30-50%, fallen teak leaves (50%) in place of conventional roughage (mixed grass) and these feeds were successfully tested among sheep. Feeding of these rations did not affect feed intake, palatability, nutrient digestibility and utilization. Supplementation with 0.5% CaO improved the utilization of nutrients. The cost of processing i.e., grinding, mixing and pelleting of fallen leaves is lowest as compared to the conventional roughages. Therefore, during scarcity situations low-cost ready-made balanced feeds can be processed commercially utilizing fallen tree leaves, as nonconventional roughage source (Anonymous, 1989).

Oil palm byproducts	CP	CF
Palm press fibre (PPF)	4	36
Palm kernel cake (PKC)	19	16
Palm oil sludge (POS)	10	18
Palm oil mill effluent	–	–

Utilization of sugarcane byproducts in animal feeding

The major byproducts from sugar industry are sugar cane tops (25-30% of sugar cane harvested), molasses (3% of sugar cane), bagasse (10-15% of cane crushed) and press mud. Of these, press mud or filter mud (3.4% of sugar cane) is used as a fertilizer. It contains, on a dry basis, about 1% phosphorus and 1% nitrogen.

Sugarcane tops: Abundant quantities of sugarcane tops as green forage are available every year during the harvesting season i.e., October to March. Sugarcane tops contain 5.5% protein, 36% fibre, 48.5% soluble carbohydrates, 8% total ash and 0.4% calcium. The tops contain 2.7% DCP and 45.7% TDN. Silages were prepared by enriching sugarcane tops with 1% urea wet and dried poultry droppings to supply approximately 15 and 30% of the total dry matter. From the results of the study in crossbred ram lambs, it was concluded that enriching sugarcane tops with dried poultry droppings at 30% on dry basis along with molasses at 1% and salt at 0.5% and then ensiling for 62 days appeared superior. This silage had 18.7% CP, 12.6% DCP and 55.1% TDN (Kutty and Prasad, 1980).

Liquid feed: Liquid molasses containing 2 to 3% uniformly mixed urea fortified with minerals and vitamins is named as 'liquid feed'. Such feed comprises urea, fresh water, mineral mixture, salt and molasses at 2.5, 2.5. 2.0, 1.0 and 92.0 per cent, respectively. Vitamins A and D are added at a level of 25g per 100 kg liquid feed.

Enrichment of straws/bagasse with urea-molasses liquid feed

Urea of 2 kg and 10 kg molasses are mixed together and dissolved in 100 litres of water. This mixture is sprayed on 100 kg of straw/bagasse provides nitrogen and a readily available source of energy to the rumen microorganisms and help to maximise the rumen fermentative digestion of the straw/bagasse.

Urea-molasses blocks

The animals lick such block and meet part of their daily nutrient requirements. The level of urea in these blocks is generally 10%. Different binding materials have been tried such as quicklime, cement, dolomite, bentonite, magnesium oxide and starch. Main problem with such blocks is the maintenance of consistency. If it is soft, the animal consumes more material which may result in toxicity. If it is hard, the animal may not get the required nutrients.

Survey on feeding practices

The feeding systems commonly practised in Rajendranagar Mandal (Hyderabad district, A P) were grazing for about 8 hours a day followed by feeding of 'Kutti' for milch and work animals. The dry animals were maintained only on grazing. The 'Kutti' consisted of chaffed sorghum straw, rice/wheat bran and oil cakes (groundnut cake/ cotton seed cake etc). The concentrates and chaffed sorghum straw are usually mixed at 1:2 or 1:3 proportions, respectively. These feedstuffs are mixed manually after adding 10-15% water. This type of complete feed, called locally as kutti was prepared, stored overnight before feeding. About 3-4 kg of kutti was being fed to the animals at the time of milking. Common salt is added to kutti but mineral mixture is not included (Anonymous, 1989).

Feed resources to meet the increased demand for animal products

The major feed resources are grass and grazing, crop residues, AIBPs (byproducts of oilseed processing, grain milling and other agroindustrial activities), NCFRs, forage and fodder from food crops, field crops, plantation crops and coconut groves, foliage from trees/shrubs and cultivated fodders. Feeding on cereal straws and natural grazing alone results in reduced live weight and perpetual low productivity in most animals. One solution to these problems is strategic supplementation (Reddy, 2001) with feeds that provide additional energy, proteins and minerals to meet maintenance and production requirements. Leguminous fodder is handy for the farmers. The much studied plants are *Leucaena leucocephala* and *Gliricidia sepium*.

Increasing human population and changes in dietary habits associated with urbanization and higher incomes are causing increased demands for food of animal origin. Delgado et al. (1999) estimated that between 1993 and 2020, the demand for livestock products will double and meat and milk production in developing countries will grow at annual rates of 2.7 and 3.2%, respectively. The inadequate feed supply, quantitatively as well as qualitatively, to feed the livestock is the major constraint in meeting future demands for meat and milk. Improving the feed supply, both in yield and quality, is an effective means to build assets and increase livestock productivity.

Importance of crop residues among the feed resources

Small farmers who rear one to five animals possess few resources to feed their animals. They generally feed their animals with crop residues, roadside grass and occasionally grasses collected from field bunds. Crop residues are the most important feed for ruminants in small-holder crop-livestock production systems in tropical and sub-tropical developing countries. In the early days of cereal crop improvement, the feed value of crop residues has been largely ignored and this has resulted in development of dwarf, high-yielding (grain) varieties. However, recognizing the need for crop residues as feed for livestock, the emphasis has been shifted to dual-purpose cultivars. The International Crop Research Institute for the Semi-Arid Tropics (ICRISAT), Patancheru (India) and the International Livestock Research Institute (ILRI), Ethiopia have implemented collaborative research on the genetic improvements of fodder value of food-feed-crops, with emphasis on sorghum and pearl millet because of the following reasons: Traditionally sorghum has been of critical importance in the crop-livestock systems of the semi-arid regions of India. Pearl millet is the most drought tolerant of all domesticated cereals

Crop residue-based rations
Processing complete feeds and compressed feed blocks

In an effort to utilise the AIBP and NCFR in a more intensive way these are processed and complete rations have been developed for ruminants. All the feed ingredients inclusive of roughages are processed (chaffing, grinding and pelleting) and mixed into a uniform blend that discourages selection (Raj Reddy, 1987). Blending the coarsely ground (8mm) crop residues, AIBPs, NCFRs in the form of complete feeds / total mixed rations (TMR) helps in developing low-cost feed, avoids refusal of unpalatable portion or selective feeding, improves utilization of supplemental urea or uric acid of poultry droppings resulting in efficient feed resource use These complete rations provide adequate and balanced nutrients in an optimum ratio of roughage to concentrates. Complete feeds have a particular relevance and considerable future potential when viewed in the context of a shift towards more intensive systems of production of milk and mutton. The latter is distinctly likely, given the diminishing availability of land and the need to have more intensive feeding systems and efficient feed resource use.

Crop residues such as sorghum stover, maize stover, sunflower straw, cotton straw, groundnut straw, agroindustrial byproducts such as bagasse, groundnut hulls/ shells or forest grasses such as *Sehima nervosam* hay, *Heteropogon contortus* hay were used to formulate several complete rations (Table 4). The crude protein percent varied from 12.82 to 13.7. These rations were fed to goats and sheep and voluntary dry matter intake per kg metabolic body size was 41.4 to 85.5 g. Goats utilized fibrous residues more efficiently than sheep. Of all the roughages tested, maize stover appeared to be a potential roughage source both for goats and sheep (Krishna and Prasad, 1990). Some more examples of complete rations are given in Table 8.

Table 4. Complete rations for small ruminants

Feedstuff	Parts
Crop residue*	25
Groundnut haulms	25
Wheat bran	20
Maize	11-18
Groundnut cake	9-16
Mineral mixture	2
Salt	1

Sehima nervosam hay/ Heteropogon contortus hay/ Sorghum stover/ Maize stover/ Bagasse/ Sunflower straw/ Cotton straw/ Groundnut straw/ Groundnut hulls or shells

In an effort to make use of cotton seed hulls in place of conventional forest dry grass, two complete rarions were formulated (Table 5). These diets were compared among the weaned Deccani lambs in a 150-day growth experiment. The diet containing cottonseed hulls recorded higher daily gain and feed efficiency as compared to the forest dry grass (Reddy and Reddy, 1990).

Table 5. Ingredient composition, chemical composition and nutritive value of complete diets

Feedstuff/ Constituent	%	%
Forest dry grass	40	----
Cotton seed hulls	---	40
Groundnut cake	15	15
Maize	10	10
Deoiled rice bran	13.5	13.5
Poultry droppings	10	10
Molasses	10	10
Mineral mixture	1.0	1.0
Salt	0.5	0.5
Crude protein	12.5	12.7
Ether extract	2.1	1.8
Crude fibre	18.0	20.4
Nitrogen free extract	53.9	54.8
Total ash	13.6	10.3
Acid insoluble ash	6.0	3.5
Calcium	0.98	0.82
Phosphorus	0.41	0.54
Feed intake, g	775	796
Feed intake, % BW	4.3	4.3
Average daily gain, g	55	70
Dry matter intake/kg gain	11.7	9.1

Krishna Mohan et al. (1985) conducted experiment with weaned native and crossbred lambs from 91-180 days of age and noted that groundnut straw/haulms (CP 9.1%) can be included up to 60% in complete ration. In another trial, groundnut straw (CP 10.4%) was used at 20, 40, 60 and 80% of complete rations (Table 6) for Nellore ram lambs in a 84-day growth trial. The growth data and nutrient digestibility revealed that optimum level of inclusion was 40% (Durga Prasad et al., 1986). Two horse gram based complete rations were formulated using horse gram hay at 40% level and concentrate mixture with conventional or unconventional ingredients (Table 7). They were fed to ram lambs in a growth trial and ADG of 130-150 g was obtained (Anjaneya Prasad et al., 1983).

Table 6. Some examples of complete rations and performance of lambs

Feedstuff/ Constituent	%	%	%	%	%
Groundnut straw	60.0	40.0	50.0	----	----
Redgram straw	----	---	---	----	50.0
Banyan tree leaves	----	---	---	50.0	----
Maize	18.0	24.0	27.0	27.0	27.0
Groundnut cake	8.0	6.0	5.0	14.0	8.0
Deoiled rice bran	10.4	28.8	16.0	7.0	13.0
Molasses	2.4	---	----	----	----
Mineral mixture	0.8	0.6	1.5	1.5	1.5
Salt	0.4	0.6	0.5	0.5	0.5
Crude protein	12.4	13.1	18.25	17.04	18.23
DCP	7.6	7.8	10.78	8.33	10.08
TDN	60.0	60.0	59.3	45.0	57.6
Average daily gain, g	73	72	75	72	97
Feed efficiency (feed/gain)	10.28	9.94	10.57	13.6	9.53
Dry matter intake, g	870	656	715	865	843

Groundnut straw CP 11.5%; redgram straw CP 9.32%; banyan tree leaves CP 5.23%.

Table 7. Horse gram hay based complete rations for lambs

Feedstuff/ Constituent	%*	%*
Horse gram hay	40.0	40.0
Maize	30.0	----
Groundnut cake	10.2	----
Wheat bran	18.0	----
Tamarind seed waste	----	30.0
Sunflower cake	----	4.8
Niger cake	----	6.0
Safflower cake	----	3.0
Cotton seed hull bran	----	8.4
Molasses	----	6.0
Mineral mixture	1.2	1.2
Salt	0.6	0.6
Crude protein	16.19	15.88
DCP	11.39	9.28
TDN	71.55	59.20
Average daily gain, g	136	159
Feed efficiency (feed/gain)	5.73	6.51
Feed consumed, g	755	1024

*Anjaneya Prasad et al., 1983

Compressed feed blocks / Densified feed blocks

Densification of such complete feeds (compressed feed blocks) reduces the volume of feed which makes its handling, storage and transportation easy. For the production of 'feed blocks', the mixture of roughage and concentrate is compressed in a machine. Dr.Amar Singh and his team of scientists from IARI, New Delhi developed a prototype of 'block making machine', which has been patented as well. Complete feed blocks for medium and high yielding dairy animals are commercially available now.

Example of Compressed feed block (Reddy, D.V., 1989)

Ingredient Composition	%	Nutrient composition
Urea ammoniated wheat straw	73	CP: 8.4%
Wheat bran	10	DCP: 5.1%
Molasses	15	TDN: 58.82%
Minerals + Salt	2	ME: 2.07Mcal/kg DM
Vitamin AD_3	10 g per 100 kg	

Expander-Extruder processing of complete feeds

The nutritive value of the complete feeds could be further improved by expander extruder technology. This is a system which combines the features of expanding (application of moisture, pressure and temperature to gelatinize the starch portion) and extruding (pressing the feed through constrictions under pressure). The feed material is conditioned to 16-17% moisture by adding sufficient quantity of water and then fed to the machine. The Expander-Extruder is a single continuous barrel with about 5.25 inches internal diameter and of approximately 2.56 meter working length.

The feed material enters into the barrel and is pushed in forward direction. The feed material is subjected to steam and pressure leading to rise in temperature to about 100°C, as the material is extruded through the 16 mm die holes present at the other end of the barrel. The pellets coming out of die holes are cooled and collected into sacks. This process increases the bulk density, ensures detoxification of antinutritional factors and destruction of microbes.

Expander extruder processing is simple to operate with less maintenance cost and high production efficiency. Further, it ensures complete gelatinization of the feed material comprising roughage and concentrate when compared to conventional pellet mill. Dr.G.V.N.Reddy and his team of scientists standardized the technology at CVSc, Hyderabad as part of the TOE on Feed Technology and Quality Assurance (NATP) ending 2003.

Table 8. Straw based (%) complete diets and their nutritive value

Ingredients	Name of the crop residue				
	Dry forest grass	Sorghum straw	Wheat straw	Cotton straw	Sunflower straw
Dry forest	47.5	-	-	-	-
Sorghum straw	-	46.0	-	-	-
Wheat straw	-	-	50.0	-	-
Cotton straw	-	-	-	45.0	-
Sunflower straw	-	-	-	-	35.0
Tapioca chips	-	20.0	-	-	-
Groundnut cake	10.0	10.0	10.0	10.0	-
Maize grain	10.0	-	-	-	-
Cage layer droppings (dried)	-	10.0	15.0	-	-
Cottonseed cake	-	-	-	-	25.0
Molasses	10.0	12.0	13.0	15.0	8.5
Deoiled rice bran	-	-	10.0	-	10.0
Wheat bran	20.0	-	-	10.0	10.0
Rice polishings	-	-	-	17.0	10.0
Urea	-	0.5	0.5	1.5	-
Mineral mixture	1.8	1.0	1.0	1.0	1.0
Common salt	0.7	0.5	0.5	0.5	0.5
Nutritive value					
DCP (%)	7.7	7.0	7.3	9.5	5.3
TDN (%)	63.1	56.4	51.8	48.6	56.2

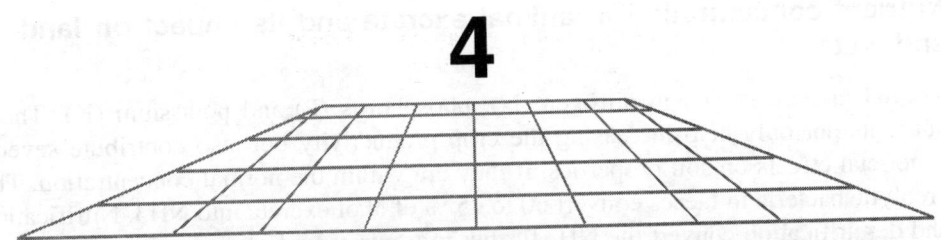

Low Pollution Feeds for Environment-
Friendly Animal Production

INTRODUCTION

Intensive farming and intensive animal production alone are able to meet the rising consumer demand for more animal products. Therefore the demand for animal feed will continue to grow all over the world.

Efficient production of livestock and poultry and the maintenance of normal health in animals require that essential nutrients be provided in appropriate amounts and in forms that are biologically utilizable. The objective of nutritional management of animals in the present intensive animal production systems is to maximize the output of products like milk, meat, eggs, etc., with little or no attention being paid to the output of less desirable products such as faecal and urinary excretion of nitrogen, phosphorus, etc., or the loss of carbon dioxide, methane (CH_4), ammonia (NH_3) and other volatiles. The nutrients present in animal excreta and the expired gases contribute considerably to their concentration in soil, water and air. Large amounts of phosphorus and nitrogen, to a greater extent, in swine and poultry wastes are considered as environmental pollutants. With the increased public awareness in environment, nutritional management can also be used as a tool to help control environmental pollution.

Eutrophication

Runoff from farms and towns carries a heavy load of silt, nutrients, and other pollutants. The nutrients trigger blooms of algae, which taint drinking water. Death and decay of the algae depletes oxygen, kills fish and bottom-dwelling animals, and thereby creates "dead zones" in the body of water. Ecologists call this syndrome of excessive nutrients, noxious algae, foul water, and dead zones as eutrophication.

Earlier no one knew for sure what caused eutrophication, even though the symptoms were well described in scientific literature. The confusion was resolved by series of experiments (Schindler, 1977) and the results showed unequivocally that P, and not N or C, caused eutrophication. It is now generally accepted that P inputs must be decreased to mitigate eutrophication of lakes and reservoirs.

Nutrient concentration in animal excreta and its impact on land and water

Animal manure is rich in nitrogen (N), phosphorus (P) and potassium (K). These nutrients not only help increasing the crop productivity but also contribute several beneficial effects on soil properties, if they are within the normal concentration. The ureolytic bacteria in faeces convert 60 to 75 % of N of excreta into NH3. Nitrification and denitrification convert the NH_3 further into nitrate and gaseous nitrogen [nitrous oxide (N_2O), nitrogen oxide (NO) and nitrogen dioxide (NO_2)]. Nitrates when present in excess are considered as pollutants and similarly nitrous oxide damage the ozone layer. Reactive N emissions are involved in greenhouse warming, smog, growth of weedy terrestrial plants, and human health impacts from air and groundwater pollution. It is reported that nitrate concentration beyond 50 mg/litre drinking water is deemed to be dangerous to human health. Higher N concentration in the water causes overgrowth of algae in channels, estuary, etc., displacing wading birds and killing many of the invertebrates that underpin the food chain.

Nitrogen and total salts content usually limit the land application rate of poultry manure. Soil nitrates in excess of 1000 mg/kg of soil have occurred with high application rates. Potassium and phosphorus are rated second and third as nutrients most likely to accumulate in soils. Phosphates are a key nutrient for algae and higher phosphorus in water and soil leads to overgrowth of algae in water, which can significantly harm aquatic life.

Excess potassium can increase the incidence of gross tetany in cattle grazing pastures fertilized with high level of poultry manure. That means, the higher potassium causes a magnesium deficiency by lowering magnesium absorption.

Trace minerals such as zinc in the manure possibly induce heavy metal pollution of soil. It was reported that long term applications of broiler litter and swine manure increased zinc concentration in soil and forages. Such high concentration of zinc suppresses the growth and yield of food crops. Compared to dietary zinc content in swine feeds, zinc retention is extremely small and the apparent absorption of zinc is almost negligible. When dietary zinc content was 100 mg/kg and apparent dry matter digestibility was 80%, faecal zinc concentration was estimated to be 500 mg/kg dry matter. Therefore zinc concentration in feeds should be minimized (Matsui and Yano, 1998).

Impact of Swedish ban on "infeed-antibiotics" (which had been in vogue since 1986) resulted in zinc pollution because zinc oxide had been used to treat enteritis in piglets at levels as high as 2500 ppm and increased the excretion of phosphates and nitrates from livestock and poultry because of the unchecked metabolic activity of bacteria in the gut.

How to reduce the N losses in Animal Excreta?

These are possible through better nutritional management.

1. **Reducing the N losses from rumen**

   In ruminants N losses from the rumen are reduced by using a reduced dietary N level, a reduced rumen degradable N (RDN) or a more efficient capture of RDN by rumen microbes, by using a complete diet, by increasing the frequency of feeding, etc.

2. **Reducing the N losses from small intestine**

   Some N losses from the small intestine occur because of incomplete digestion of feed nitrogen due to the presence of antinutritional factors like lectins, protease inhibitors in certain legume seeds or due to the excretion of endogenous protein caused by neutral detergent fibre and other non-starch polysaccharides (NSPs). These losses can be reduced by employing the needed processing techniques to such feeds and by application of relevant enzymes. The NSPs, protein, phytic acid and various minerals are present as complex compounds in the cell walls of plants. Nutrients bound to NSP or phytate are released by NSP degrading enzymes or phytases so that the digestibility of the protein and of various minerals (Ca, Mg, Zn, etc.) can be improved as a concomitant effect.

   In monogastric animals, enzymes such as proteases, amylases, lipases are produced and there is a need to supplement them in young animals and in adults (when fed on certain feeds) to further their digestive capacity. Enzymes such as β-glucanases, pentosanases (xylanases), α-galactosidases, phytases are not produced by monogastric animals and these are to be added to digest the NSP, oligosaccharides and phytates. Beta glucans and pentosans (which are mainly present as arabinoxylans in rye and wheat) belong to the non-starch polysaccharides. Alpha galactosides (e.g. raffinose, stachyose, verbascose) are the oligosaccharides present mainly in certain legumes.

3. **Reducing the N losses in intermediary metabolism**

   The nitrogen losses in intermediary metabolism can be reduced by following the concept of 'ideal' protein for monogastric animals. Phase feeding is also followed since protein requirements vary with age and physiological state. Phase feeding, for instance in pigs, refers to the practice of offering a series of feeds during the growing and finishing life stages of pigs. Piglets have greatest requirement for amino acids in proportion to dietary energy as the fuel for gaining lean tissue. The requirement for amino acid, more importantly lysine, decreases as the animal advances in its age. Phase feeding reduces feed costs as well as nitrogen excretion. Diet acidification promotes a more effective digestion of protein, since the conversion of pepsinogen to pepsin is inhibited by increase of pH above 4.

   A more efficient intermediary metabolism will reduce N excretion in urine whereas a reduction in losses from gastrointestinal (GI) tract will reduce excretion both in faeces and in urine.

4. **Use of nutrient repartitioners**

   Nutrients supplied to farm animals are usually partitioned between fat and protein which is largely controlled by the animal's endocrine balance.

Endocrine balance is influenced by its physiological status, plane of nutrition and environmental temperature. Nutrient repartitioners (hormones and β-agonists) improve N deposition in growing pigs by reducing the urinary N excretion.

5. **Use of antibiotic growth promoters**

Use of antibiotic growth promoters in pig rations can help to reduce at least one percentage point in protein levels (Yen and Veum, 1982) and this would lead to a reduction in N and P excretion in their excreta.

Reduction of emission of Ammonia

Non-starch polysaccharides (NSP) are reported to reduce the emission of ammonia in pigs through a change in nitrogen excretion, away from urine and towards the faeces. The NSP are physiologically active in promoting beneficial gut development and have laxative action and anticholesterolemic effect. The NSP are fermented by intestinal bacteria in the large intestine to produce volatile fatty acids and microbial protein. The NSPs are called as 'prebiotics' and microorganisms are known as 'probiotics'. Microbial protein goes into the manure and is less likely to release ammonia than the N in the urine. e.g. Sugarbeet pulp, soybean hulls, alfalfa meal.

Development of low pollution feeds

It is apparent that a certain amount of N and P that come from animal excreta / manure originates from feed source. The N and P of the manure contributed their content to soil and water and reached alarming levels leading to call them as environmental pollutants. Hence there is a need to develop low pollution feed by using either a highly utilizable feed resource or by using feed additives to enhance the utilization of that feed resource.

Bioavailability of a nutrient from a feed source can be influenced by animal species (e.g. phytate phosphorus is unavailable in monogastrics) and by nutrient demand of the animal in relation to dietary intake. Any physiological function or state that may increase nutrient demand can increase absolute nutrient utilization, especially when dietary intake of the nutrient is less than the animal's minimal requirement.

Synthetic amino acids: They help to enhance the digestibility of amino acid (nitrogen) and nitrogen excretion could be reduced significantly. Small amounts of synthetic amino acids (0.1-0.3%) could spare dietary protein by 2-3% (Han et al., 1998). Nitrogen excretion can drop by 30% where synthetic amino acids are used to compensate for a lower dietary level of crude protein. To assure the profitable use of synthetic amino acids as feed additives, it is essential to know both the absolute requirements for the respective amino acids and also the relative proportions in which they should be given to the animals. The efficiency of one amino acid depends on the level of another in the diet.

While formulating low pollution feeds, it is essential to keep in mind the relationships among amino acids (e.g. methionine + cystine and lysine), amino acid imbalances (e.g. arginine and lysine) and amino acid antagonism (e.g. leucine-isoleucine and valine).

Enzymes: At least a 25% reduction in P content of manure is obtained by including phytase in monogastrics because of an increase in P digestibility. The use of NSP degrading enzymes (β-glucanases and xylanases especially endo-β-glucanases and endo-xylanases) reduced the viscosity of gut contents and improves the nutrient utilization, which reduces nutrient excretion (N, P, etc.) by an average 5% and further results in higher faecal dry matter level. Similarly supplementation of amylase, protease and lipase reduces the excretion of nutrients. Hence enzymes make a significant contribution to a better environment- and resource- friendly animal production (sustainable animal production).

Organic forms of minerals: Proper mineral nutrition controls animal wastes. In case of bioavailability of mineral elements, chemical form and degree of solubility can have a profound effect on utilization of supplemental sources. Organic forms of minerals (Zn, Cu, Se, Mn,) and substances stimulating their absorption (for example, dietary citric acid in case of zinc) may also be applied as feed additives.

Leanness enhancer: Bovine somatotropin (BST), porcine somatotropin (PST), beta agonist, or chromium supplement may also be added to enhance the nitrogen deposition in body tissues.

5

Global Climate Change - Its Effect on Livestock and Mitigation Measures

Climate change

Climate change can be defined as the misbalance of customary weather factors such as temperature, wind and rainfall characteristic of a specific region on Earth. Climate change is likely to be one of the main challenges that humankind will face in the current century (Rowlinson et al., 2008). International Conference "Livestock and Global Climate Change" was held in 2008 Hammamet, Tunisia, and the proceedings were published by editors P. Rowlinson, M. Steele and A. Nefzaoui.

The major scientific studies have shown that increasing average temperature of the Earth is now a reality and the increased concentrations of greenhouse gases (GHG) in the atmosphere, mainly the emissions of carbon dioxide resulting from combustion of fossil fuel contribute to the enhancement of global greenhouse effect, the disturbance of the radiative forcing, and consequently the intensification of climate change phenomena.

Climate experts expect that climate change would have serious impacts on ecologic equilibriums, human health, and sustainable development in general, especially in developing countries which do not possess necessary means of adaptation to these global phenomena. Considering the expected impacts of Earth temperature increase on ecosystems, natural resources, and economic activities in the medium and long run, the international community has given the matter great importance through an international agreement on climate change at the Earth Summit in Rio de Janeiro, 1992.

Greenhouse effect (Gaseous atmospheric pollution)

The "greenhouse effect" is a natural phenomenon of keeping the earth in a temperature range that allows life to sustain. The sun's enormous energy warms the Earth's surface and its atmosphere. As this energy radiates back toward space as heat, a portion is absorbed by a delicate balance of heat-trapping gases in the atmosphere, among them are carbon dioxide and methane which creates an insulating layer. But when these heat-trapping gases increase in amount resulting in a rise in the Earth's temperature, it causes "global warming". The theory behind this effect is that the earth is gradually warming due to problems encountered in the destruction of parts of our environment. The effect was named for the extra heat inside a house made from glass or greenhouse.

The greenhouse effect on the Earth is generated mostly by water vapour and opaque to infrared radiation and contributes about 65%, CO_2 33% and other GHG such as ozone, methane and nitrous oxide 2%. Earth is warming (0.75° C in the last 100 years; 1900-2000) due to emission of GHG as a result of human activity mainly CO_2 emitted by burning the fossil fuels. Higher concentration of carbon dioxide, methane in the atmosphere causes the heat from the sun to become more intense and the temperature of the earth to be raised. The Global Carbon Project (GCP) released the figures of rise in atmospheric CO_2 level. The average annual mean growth rate of atmospheric CO_2 during 1980-2000: 1.5 ppm per year; 2000–2007: 2.0 ppm; of this, year 2006 accounts for 1.8 ppm while 2007 accounts for 2.2 ppm.

Green house gases and atmospheric brown clouds

These manmade aerosols (air pollutants) are referred to as atmospheric brown clouds (ABCs; V.Ramanathan and Y.Feng, 2008). GHGs, metaphorically, act like the blanket that keeps us (the planet) warm on a cold night by trapping the body heat (the heat radiation from the planet). This heat (heat radiation) would have otherwise escaped to the surrounding room (outer space). The build-up of GHGs caused by human activities has thickened this blanket by ≈2%. Many aerosol species in ABCs, e.g., sulphates and nitrates, **reflect visible solar radiation**, which gives rise to the hazy skies, while black carbon aerosols, a major constituent of soot, absorb visible solar radiation, which gives rise to the **brownish colour of the haze**. The reflecting aerosols in ABCs act like tiny mirrors on the GHGs blanket and make the planet brighter, which will have a climate cooling effect. On the other hand, the black carbon in ABCs will make the blanket brownish by absorbing more UV and visible sun light, which in turn warms the blanket and the surface. The current understanding is that the **global cooling effect of the mirrors** is much larger than the warming effect of the brownish soot with the result that ABCs have masked a significant fraction of the **warming effect of the GHGs** blanket. However, ABCs are a shorter-term problem, first because their lifetimes are few weeks or less, and next because of being implementation of 'clean air acts' to their negative impact on health and ecosystem. Thus, ABCs are bound to decrease significantly in that time period, while many GHGs continue to increase and hence, the need for reducing CO_2 emissions becomes even more urgent.

Global Warming and Climate Change

In general, global warming is attributed to anthropogenic releases of carbon dioxide, methane and oxides of nitrogen and their accumulation in the atmosphere. The accumulation of the greenhouse gases in the atmosphere has been gradually increasing due to the burning of fossil fuels to meet the energy needs of an increasing population and greater wealth. Global warming is mother of all challenges. It exacerbates the challenges of poverty and environmental degradation and together they pose a threat of far reaching consequences to societies around the world. Agriculture, the mainstay for developing economies, is far more susceptible to climate-induced disasters.

The three main GHGs are carbon dioxide (CO_2), methane (CH_4), and nitrous oxide (N_2O) (Steinfeld *et al.* 2006). The capacity of GHG to trap heat in the atmosphere is described in terms of their global warming potential (GWP), which compares their warming potency to that of CO_2 (with a GWP set at 1). The atmospheric abundance of methane is about 200 times smaller than that of carbon dioxide. But methane has relatively high GWP, which is 23 times higher than that of CO_2. The GWP of N_2O is 296.

If we place emphasis on the sustainable use of energy, the temperature could rise by about 1.8° C by the turn of this century (2100). If not, the temperature could rise by 6° C with even greater probability of causing abrupt or irreversible impacts. In 2007, the UN's Intergovernmental Panel on Climate Change (IPCC) had warned that an increase of between 1.8° and 5.4° C could trigger massive environmental changes, including melting of the Greenland ice sheet, the Himalayan-Tibetan glaciers and summer sea ice in the Arctic.

Anthropogenic influences

Although some natural occurrences contribute to GHG emissions, the overwhelming consensus among the world's most reputable climate scientists contends that human activities are culpable for a majority of this increase in temperature. An IPCC report issued in April 2007 concluded "with high confidence that anthropogenic warming over the last three decades has had a discernible influence on many physical and biological systems". While transportation and the burning of fossil fuels have typically been regarded as the chief contributors to GHG emissions and climate change, a November 2006 report, Livestock's Long Shadow: Environmental Issues and Options, by the Food and Agriculture Organization (FAO) of the United Nations highlighted the farm animal production sector's substantial role.

H. Steinfeld and coworkers (FAO, 2006) presented a valuable assessment of the environmental consequences of livestock production, climate change and use of the natural resources in the face of the increasing demand for foods of animal origin. The report gave descriptions as well as quantitative data of the full impact of the livestock sector on environmental problems in both developing and developed countries. Identifying it as "a major threat to the environment", the FAO found that the animal agriculture sector emits 18 percent, or nearly one-fifth, of human-induced GHG emissions, more than cars, SUVs, and other vehicles (Steinfeld *et al.* 2006). However, it has been felt that these statements are not accurate. Yet their wide distribution through news media has led to much of the public confusion over livestock's role in climate change.

Livestock and livelihood

The livelihood contribution of livestock has been well acknowledged. But there are increasing concerns on the likely negative impacts of livestock on the environment. In a country like India, where more than 60% of the geographical area is arid and semi-arid, livestock's contribution towards risk reduction and adaptation to climate variability is significantly higher than their negative impacts. Almost 80% of milk in India is produced in integrated mixed crop-livestock farming systems. A well managed integrated crop livestock system has the potential to create a win-win situation for both farmers and the environment.

Milch animals play significant role in the lives and livelihoods of urban and periurban dwellers, as well as rural households. Urban livestock production is promoted as an integral factor to the development of sustainable and environmentally-friendly cities. Livestock are increasingly recognized for their value in recycling waste, as well as in providing products needed by the urban markets, and thus offering a source of living for those struggling to make both ends meet.

Animal products, even in tiny quantities, support physical and intellectual development of young people and pregnant mothers (Waterlow, 1998). Instinctively people recognized the nutritional role of animal products which provided essential amino acids and micronutrients, deficient in cereal based diets. Thus animal production is not simply a matter of producing food, it is also relieving the ill health of resource poor people resulting from essential nutrient deficiencies in mainly cereal based diets. In the following discussion, it is argued that herbivorous animal, particularly ruminants, but also small herbivores, fed on agro-industrial or under-utilized feeds will need to dominate the meat and milk production requirements of future generations with measures to minimize their "long shadow" (Steinfeld et al., 2006).

Effects of climate change

Global warming's many impacts are already detectable. As glaciers retreat, the sea level rises, the tundra thaws, hurricanes and other extreme weather events occur more frequently, and penguins, polar bears, and other species struggle to survive (Topping 2007), experts anticipate even greater increases in the intensity and prevalence of these changes as the 21st century brings rises in GHG emissions. Increasing sea levels will undoubtedly remove considerable areas of fertile delta farm lands. Warming also carries with it the risk of decreased crop production as rice yield decrease by 10% for every °C rise in night time temperature.

It is important to remember that changes in climate are not limited merely to an increase in temperature, but in fact involve several impacts such as an increase in intensity and frequency of floods, droughts, heat waves and extreme precipitation events. Therefore, these pose serious implications for the availability of water in several parts of the world and could have negative impacts on the yields of several crops.

Effects of climate change on livestock production

Climate change, especially increases in temperature, has a direct impact by increasing heat stress in animals. This results in both a loss of production (largely through reduction of feed intake) and reduced reproductive efficiency. Changes in the pattern of rainfall and ranges of temperature affect feed availability, and weed, pest and disease incidence.

"Impact of climate change and environmental changes on emerging and re-emerging animal disease and animal production" was the theme of 77th General Session of the International Committee of the OIE (Office International des Epizootes, World Organisation for Animal Health) held at Paris, France during 24-29 May, 2009. It was envisaged that climate change and environmental changes are a subset of the larger set of ecosystem changes that are promoting the emergence and re-emergence of animal diseases. Globally there is a need to fully examine the potential impact of the extension to the ranges of mosquitoes, tsetse fly and ticks that are anticipated as a result of temperature increases. Both animal and human health will be increasingly vulnerable to insect-borne disease risks. A temperature rise of 2°C over the pre-industrial period cannot be avoided. Hence to contain the rise to 2°C, greenhouse gas emissions will have to be reduced by about 40% by 2020.

Impact of livestock on climate change

Whenever the causes of climate change are discussed, fossil fuels top the list. Oil, natural gas and especially coal are indeed major sources of human-caused emissions of carbon dioxide and other greenhouse gases (GHG). For GHG reporting, total anthropogenic GHG emissions are considered under five major sectors: energy, industry, waste, land use and land use change and forestry and agriculture. According to FAO (Steinfeld et al., 2006) about 12% of total emission of greenhouse gas is related to livestock production. This contribution is even higher (18%) when the deforestation related to the expansion of livestock production area is also considered (to meet the growing demand of animal products). Livestock contribute about 9% of total carbon dioxide (CO_2) emissions, but 37% of methane (CH_4), and 65% of nitrous oxide (N_2O).

Animal production may have adverse effects on many environmental aspects including air and water pollution, degradation of soil quality, reduction of biodiversity and global climate change. The emission of greenhouse gas in livestock production systems originates mainly from the animals (enteric fermentations), the manure, and the fields used for the production of feed and forages. To be specific, livestock sector emits 37% of anthropogenic methane and most of that comes from enteric fermentation by ruminants. Methane emissions come from agriculture, power station, coal mining. Methanogens are archaea (bacteria like prokaryotes) that are capable of producing methane under oxygen-limiting conditions. Most methanogens are capable of using carbon dioxide as their source of carbon, and hydrogen as the reducing agent to produce methane. A number of methaongens are commonly found in guts of animals (ruminants), wetlands and in the marine environment.

Livestock emits 65% of anthropogenic nitrous oxide, the great majority from manure. Livestock are also responsible for almost two-thirds (64%) of anthropogenic ammonia emissions, which contributes significantly to acid rain and acidification of ecosystems.

On the eve of a major international climate summit at Copenhagen, Denmark during December 11-18, 2009, a European campaign called "Less Meat = Less Heat" was launched. This was countered by a University of California authority on farming and greenhouse gases. "Smarter animal farming, not less farming, will equal less heat. Producing less meat and less milk will only mean more hunger in poor countries, where growing populations need more nutritious food" hence what is needed is efficient animal production.

Mitigation measures

A key risk factor for climate change is the growth of human population and increased population of livestock and poultry. Efforts are made to slow the climate change through renewable energy and energy efficiency. However, only relatively modest amounts of renewable energy and energy efficiency have been developed (along with more nuclear- and fossil-energy infrastructure).

Mitigating the impacts of climate change on livestock production

Heat stress is a major problem affecting the overall productivity. Where economics allow, mechanical interventions such as use of artificial shade, and evaporative cooling systems in animal enclosures may be provided to ameliorate environmental impacts.

Considerable opportunity exists to breed animal genotypes adapted to the changing conditions resulting from climate change. The CSIRO livestock improvement programme based in Rockhampton, for example, has introduced tropically adapted cattle breeds (crossbred cows of African, European and Indian origins) into northern Australia and greatly improved reproductive efficiency and meat production (Frisch and O'Neil 1998). Major livestock enterprises in Australia have used this genetic diversity to develop composite breeds of cattle adapted to the production systems and imparting greater disease resistance, heat tolerance, better capacity to graze and high reproduction rates.

Animals can also be selected on the basis of increased overall feed-use efficiency (Alford et al., 2006) to lower the GHG emissions.

Mitigating the impacts of livestock production on climate change

GHG emissions have increased since the Kyoto protocol was signed in 1992 and climate change has accelerated. GHG emissions from animal agriculture have been long recognized to be a function of the efficiency of production (productivity) and of total numbers. Thus improved productivity is required to reduce emissions. Leng (1993) promoted 'environmentally friendly' livestock production system which means that production increases should be met by improved productivity, and not by an increase in animal numbers nor expansion of land area under production.

Species differences do exist with reference to the production of GHG emissions (Table 1) and accordingly cows and buffalo for milk are desirable

Substituting one meat product with another that has a somewhat lower carbon footprint is a promising strategy.

Some feel that an effective strategy must involve replacing livestock products with better alternatives.

There are a variety of emission reduction options, which include reduction of methane emissions from ruminant production, in particular, dairy cattle and buffaloes, reduction of methane and nitrous oxide emissions from animal waste. This means that mitigation can be achieved in different ways related to animal feeding and management, manure collection, storage and spreading (through energy recovery (biogas) and improved animal waste management) and management of crops for feed production, and also by more drastic changes of the whole production system.

Reduction of GHG emissions of ruminants through nutritional strategies

Ruminants produce GHG in a number of ways: directly through enteric fermentation (methane), nitrogen excretion (nitrous oxide) and stored manure (methane and nitrous oxide); indirectly through use of fossil fuels and electric power in animal production systems, and through use of feedstuffs for their feeding that have incurred emission of GHG in their production.

Rumen nitrogen metabolism produces hydrogen and is channeled out via methane synthesis by rumen methanogens. Strategies to reduce enteric methane production can therefore seek to reduce the production of hydrogen, inhibit methanogenesis and redirect hydrogen into alternative products, or provide alternative sinks for hydrogen. Hence interventions to reduce GHG include nutritional means, chemicals (e.g. halogenated analogues) and biotechnological products (e.g. immunization, bacteriophages and bacteriocins, enzyme additives, yeast additives).

Nutritional abatement strategies are to be aimed at reduction of methane emission per kg milk or meat. Aim for improved animal performance through better nutrition (energy for maintenance is reduced as a proportion of total energy requirement, and methane associated with maintenance is reduced), which led to reaching target slaughter weight at a younger age and the total lifetime methane emissions are reduced. There is a need to work out the effect of mitigation strategies at a whole system level on the full production system, i.e. a life-cycle analysis.

Diet quality

Higher proportion of concentrate in the diet leads to a reduction in methane emission as a proportion of energy intake due mainly to an increased proportion of propionate in ruminal VFA. This was reported by K.L.Blaxter and L.Clapperton in 1965. Structural carbohydrates (cellulose and hemicellulose) ferment at slower rates than non-structural carbohydrates (starch and sugars) and yield more methane per unit of substrate fermented due to a greater acetate:propionate (Czarkawski, 1969). It has also been suggested that non-structural carbohydrates should be further subdivided as soluble sugars have a higher methanogenic potential than starch. This suggests that cereal feedstuffs will result in lower emissions than byproduct feedstuffs with higher fibre levels.

Adding lipid to the diet

Czerkawski et al reported in 1966 that methane emissions decreased with increasing fat and oil supplementation. Oils containing lauric and myristic acids are particularly toxic to methanogens. Lipids cause the depressive effect on methane emissions by toxicity to methanogens, reduction of protozoa numbers and therefore protozoa associated methanogens. But lipids, at higher level, also cause depression in fibre digestibility eventually could impact on total tract digestibility leading to reduction in DMI. Hence total dietary level is to be kept below 6-7% level in the diet.

Forage species

Animals fed legume forages have been observed to emit less methane compared emissions from grass-fed animals.

Plant secondary compounds and plant extracts

Saponins have been shown to possess strong defaunating properties both *in vitro* and *in vivo*, which could reduce methane emissions. K.A.Beauchemin, T.A.McAllister et al reviewed literature in 2008 and concluded that there is evidence for a reduction in methane from at least some sources of saponins. They also reported that there is evidence that some condensed tannins (CT) can reduce methane emissions. Some legunes contain CT, but unfortunately these may reduce forage digestibility. Extracts from plants such as rhubarb and garlic could decrease methane emissions. D.N.Kamra and coworkers have been doing work on plant secondary compounds and extracts as mitigation strategies.

Organic acids

R.J. Wallace, C.J. Newbold and coworkers use fumaric and other organic acids as alternative sink for hydrogen and reduce the amount of hydrogen used in methane formation. Organic acids are generally fermented to propionate in the rumen, and in the process reducing equivalents are consumed. A dose-dependent response to fumarate in sheep was reported. Wallace et al (2006) described a proportional reduction of 0.4-0.75 when encapsulated fumaric acid (0.1 of diet) was fed to sheep.

Ionophores

Monensin is antimicrobial which is widely used in animal production to improve performance because of a shift in rumen VFA proportions towards propionate and a reduction in ruminal protozoa numbers.

Technical efficiency in production systems should be optimized so as to minimize emissions per kg of milk or meat produced. Here comes a key role for animal nutrition in achieving this optimization. In view of lower proportion of GHG emissions (Table 1) small ruminants, pigs and poultry may be preferred for meat and egg production while dairy animals for milk production

Table 1. Species contribution to GHG emissions (millions t of methane per year)*

Species	Enteric	Manure
Dairy	15.69	3.08
Beef	50.16	4.41
Buffalo	9.23	0.34
Sheep and goats	9.44	0.34
Pigs	1.11	8.38
Poultry	-	0.97

* Source: Steinfeld et al. (2006)

Disasters

Disasters are undesirable and often sudden events causing human, material, economic and/or environmental losses, which exceed the coping capability of the affected community or society. They are caused either by natural forces/processes (known as 'natural disasters') or by human actions, negligence, or errors (known as "anthropogenic disasters").

Natural disasters: Natural disasters are generally classified into three major groups (CRED, 2009): (i) 'geophysical disasters' (e.g., earthquake, volcanic eruption, rockfall, landslide, avalanche, and subsidence); (ii) 'hydro-meteorological disasters' (e.g., flood, drought, storm, extreme temperature, wildfire, and wet mass movement); and (iii) 'biological disasters' (e.g., epidemic, insect infestation, and animal stampede).

Anthropogenic disasters: Anthropogenic disasters are broadly classified into two major groups (http://en.wikipedia.org/wiki/Disaster): (i) 'technological disasters' (e.g., disasters due to engineering failures, transport disasters, and environmental disasters); and (ii) 'sociological disasters' (e.g., criminal acts, riots, war, stampedes, etc.).

Drought hazards

Droughts are manifestations of significant shortages in all domains of the water cycle. They have adverse impacts on the environment, water availability and water quality, water supply system, hydropower generation, navigation, groundwater balances, vegetation cover, agricultural production, etc. of the affected region. Drought is a regular part of natural cycles and single-most weather related natural disaster affecting livelihoods, developmental activities, natural resources (water, soil, and biodiversity) and economy of a country (http://en.wikipedia.org/wiki/Drought). Although droughts may persist for several years, even a short, intense drought can cause significant damage and severely affect local economy. This global phenomenon has a widespread impact on agriculture. Indeed drought is one of the most serious problems arising from climate variability for human societies and ecosystems (Yurekli and Kurune, 2006).

The occurrence of droughts is not limited to a particular region. It has been observed that their impact has been completely different in developed and developing nations because of several socio-economic and political factors influencing both behavioural and management patterns. Even within the developing countries, the effects of droughts can vary significantly, but the fact remains that the economically weaker countries or groups in a country are most severely affected by the droughts.

G. Ravindra Chary et al. (2010) presented, in their book "Drought Hazards and Mitigation Measures", a raft of measures that can mitigate, if not reverse, the impact of global warming on the resources we have.

6

Nutrient Partitioning

PRODUCTIVE EFFICIENCY

The goal of farming is the improvement of economic and productive efficiency of farm animals, for example dairy cows in case of dairy farming. Hence livestock are fed for production, and generally not for maintenance. Calculations (NRC, 1989) revealed that nutrient requirements per litre of milk production decreased from 151 g protein and 2.37 Mcal ME to 102 g protein and 1.24 Mcal ME as the milk yield enhanced from 5 litres per day to 15 litres per day (Reddy and Krishna, 2009). This is possible because of increased productive efficiency that occurs in genetically superior cows and it is principally due to a dilution of maintenance requirement.

Food from animals should be safe, environmentally friendly and produced in a (animal) welfare friendly system. This means that emphasis is less on maximizing production but increasingly on optimizing production. Emphasis is on optimum utilization of nutrients.

Bauman et al. (1985) reviewed the sources of variation and prospects for improvement of productive efficiency in the dairy cow. Productive efficiency, simply, is the yield of milk obtained in ratio to the nutritional costs associated with maintenance, milk synthesis and loss of body condition during lactation because the cow has to return to the level of body condition that existed before the onset of lactation.

Optimum productive efficiency

An understanding of the several biological processes is vital for improving efficiency by systematic manipulation of metabolism. The biological processes are divided into digestion and nutrient absorption, maintenance requirement, utilization of metabolizable energy for production and nutrient partitioning. Improvements in efficiency could occur as a result of changes in digestion and absorption of nutrients, maintenance requirement, and utilization of ME for production or nutrient partitioning.

Little variation is observed among cows in their digestion and nutrient absorption, maintenance requirement and utilization of ME for production and hence, such factors do not respond to selection for increased milk yield. However, individual cows differ substantially in feed intake and in the partitioning of absorbed nutrients among body tissues (Swan, 1976; Bauman and Currie, 1980; Hart, 1983).

Partitioning of nutrients

The term 'nutrient partitioning' refers to the processes by which available nutrients are channelled, in varying proportions, to different metabolic functions. The partitioning of nutrients to various body tissues involves two types of regulation, homeostasis and homeorhesis. Homeostasis control involves maintenance of physiological equilibrium, i.e. constant conditions in the internal environment. There are many well established examples of homeostasis, such as regulation to maintain constancy of body temperature (Kennedy, 1967). An example in metabolism deals with intake of food and partitioning of nutrients during absorptive and postabsorptive periods (Tepperman and Tepperman, 1970).

Homeorhesis is the second type of control in partitioning nutrients. Bauman and Currie (1980) defined homeorhesis as the orchestrated or coordinated changes in metabolism of body tissues necessary to support a physiological state. The most pronounced example of homeorhesis would be in a dairy cow where initiation of lactation dramatically alters metabolism of many maternal organs in order that the mammary gland be supplied with nutrients necessary for synthesis of milk. Friggens and Newbold (2007) referred to this aspect of nutrient partitioning as teleophoretic rather than homeorhetic since it is in the service of genetic drives, or goals (Fig 1 B).

The classic work of J. Hammond (1947) was in reality dealt with homeorhesis when he emphasized different tissue priorities in partitioning of circulating nutrients in farm animals. G.C.Kennedy in 1967 introduced the term homeorhesis incidentally in his review on the thermoregulation of intake. His illustration depicted homeorhesis as the "tendency to home on to a direction or pathway of change" (i.e., partitioning of nutrients to muscle during physiological state of growth), whereas homeostasis was defined as maintenance of equilibrium within a physiological state (i.e., thermoregulation of intake).

Nutrient partitioning during pregnancy

Pregnancy imposes a substantial cost to the animal, because total requirements for nutrients at the end of pregnancy are about 75% greater than in a nonpregnant animal of the same weight. Striking maternal adaptations are required to meet these metabolic requirements and are achieved by regulatory influences arising in the conceptus. Thus, in keeping the concept of directed partitioning of nutrients of Bauman and Currie, needs of the conceptus are accorded high priority by the homeorhetic controls it transmits to the dam. Pregnancy includes not only development of the feotus but also growth of foetal membranes, gravid uterus, and mammary gland.

Nutrient partitioning during lactogenesis

Nature has accorded a high priority to lactation, since the ability of mammals to synthesize milk is essential for survival of the newborn. The functional mammary

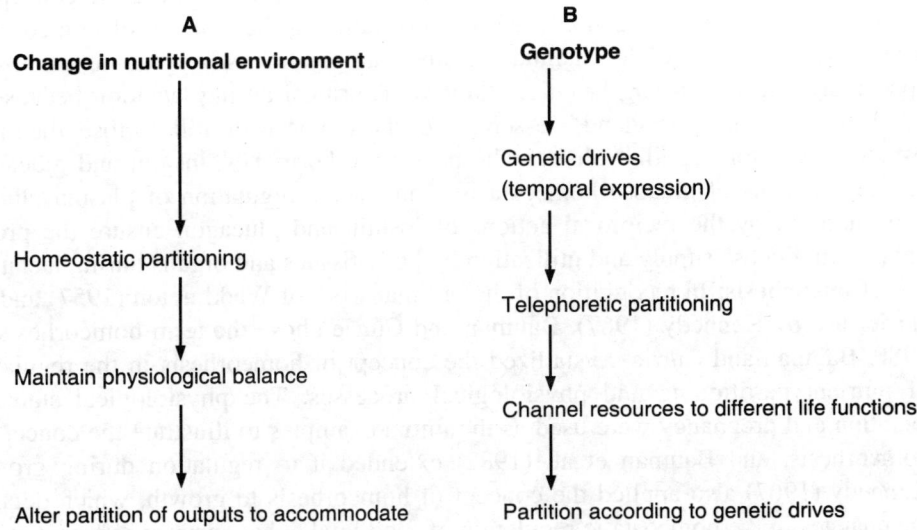

Figure 1. A schematic representation of the two types of nutrient partitioning, homeostasis and telephoretic (N.C.Friggens and J.R.Newbold, 2007: Animal,1: 87-97)

gland is one of the most highly differentiated and metabolically active tissues in the body (Davis and Bauman, 1974). The period of lactation in which the animal's ability to coordinate partitioning of nutrients assumes the most critical role is during the onset and development of copious milk secretion. At the initiation of lactation, marked alterations in the general partitioning of nutrients and metabolism of the whole animal must occur to accommodate demands of the mammary gland.

It is well documented that partitioning of nutrients changes with stage of lactation, and lipolysis and lipogenesis are up or down regulated at different stages of the reproductive cycle. The net result of such changes is that nutrients are channelled to differing extents to different organs and life functions such as growth, milk yield, body lipid reserves, reproduction, immune function etc. Nutrient partitioning that takes place with changes in stage of lactation / reproductive cycle is not as a function of changing nutritional environment but rather as a function of (physiological) time. The onset of lactation provides the classic example of this homeorhetic, or teleophoretic mechanism with the uncoupling of growth hormone (GH) and insulin-like growth factor (IGF) and the resulting channelling of nutrients to the mammary gland (Bauman 2000). This emphasizes that there is an aspect of nutrient partitioning that is genetically driven and the animal has genetic drives.

Concepts of regulation

Homeostasis: While the concept of homeostasis is universally accepted today, it resulted in substantial debate over several decades following its introduction (Waddington, 1942, 1953; Lerner, 1954; Lewontin, 1956). Now the concept of homeostasis is well known to biologists, and there are many systems where the positive and negative feedback controls to preserve steady state are well established.

Glucose was an example used by Bernard (1878) in developing the concept of milieu *interieur* and by Cannon (1932) in crystallizing the concept of homeostasis. The homeostatic controls to maintain steady-state conditions for glucose are also of special significance during lactation. Glucose is critical during lactation because its uptake by the mammary gland is essential for the synthesis of milk lactose, the major osmotic regulator of milk volume. The pancreatic hormones, insulin and glucagon, are key controls of glucose homeostasis. Thus, acute regulation of plasma glucose concentration by the reciprocal actions of insulin and glucagon ensure the proper balance in glucose supply and utilization by body tissues and organs during lactation.

Homeorhesis: In recognition of the original work of Waddington (1957) and the earlier use by Kennedy (1967), Bauman and Currie chose the term homeorhesis. In 1980, Bauman and Currie crystallized the concept of homeorhesis in the regulation of nutrient partitioning and physiological processes. The physiological states of lactation and pregnancy were used as the initial examples to illustrate the concept of homeorhesis, and Bauman et al. (1982) extended it to regulation during growth. Kennedy (1967) also applied the concept of homeorhesis to growth, which detailed the changes in the homeostatic regulation of food intake that occur at different stages of development.

The concept of homeorhesis relates to the ability of the animal to adjust biological processes in a manner to support a dominant physiological state for animal well-being and survival of the species. The general concept represented by homeorhesis has been extended to an impressive range of biological situations encompassing many different physiological, nutritional and even pathological states, examples include lactation, pregnancy, growth, puberty, ageing, hibernation, egglaying, chronic undernutrition, chronic illness.

Adaptations to lactation

A key physiological state in the survival of mammals is lactation. In all species, the extent of nutrient use for milk synthesis requires integrated regulation of the metabolism of the mammary glands and other body tissues. Many physiological adaptations (Table 1) occur during lactation. The net effect is that the increase in mammary gland metabolic rate and nutrient use which occurs during lactation coincides with alterations in the metabolism of other body tissues so that an adequate quantity and pattern of nutrient to support milk synthesis is ensured.

During lactation, food intake is increased in many species. Corresponding adaptations do occur in the size and absorptive capacity of the gastrointestinal tract, thereby allowing for an increased absorption of nutrients (Bauman and Elliot, 1983; Vernon, 1989). Increases in feed intake and digestive tract size occur in dairy cows, with the magnitude of the increase in voluntary intake being related to milk yield (Bauman and Elliot, 1983). However, the increase in feed intake occurs over a longer interval in high-producing dairy cows so that they may not achieve a positive energy balance until 8 - 12 weeks post-partum (Bauman and Currie, 1980).

Despite adjustments in feed intake, many species rely on body reserves during early lactation. In cow, goat and pig, the use of body reserves is more extensive during the lactation cycle. For example, lactational yields in dairy cows are related to the magnitude of body reserve utilization (Bauman et al., 1985). High-producing dairy cows can mobilize body fat during the first month of lactation, which can be equivalent to over one-third of the milk produced (Bauman and Currie, 1980).

Table1. Partial list of physiological adaptations which occur in lactating dairy cows*

Process ort issue	Response
Mammary gland	Increased number of secretory cell
	Increased nutrient use
	Increased supply of blood
Food intake	Increased quantity
Digestive tract	Increased size
	Increased absorptive capacity
	Increased rates of nutrient absorption
Liver	Increased size
	Increased rates of gluconeogenesis
	Increased glycogen mobilization
	Increased protein synthesis
Adipose tissue	Decreased de novo fat synthesis
	Decreased uptake of preformed fatty acids
	Decreased re-esterification of fatty acids
	Increased lipolysis
Skeletal muscle	Decreased glucose utilization
	Decreased protein synthesis
	Increased protein degradation
Bone	Increased mobilization of Ca and P
Heart	Increased cardiac output with a larger percentage going to the mammary glands
Plasma hormones	Decreased insulin
	Increased somatotropin
	Increased prolactin
	Increased glucocorticoids
	Decreased thyroid hormones
	Decreased IGF-I

* Source: D.E.Bauman Chapter 18 Regulation of nutrient partitioning during lactation: Homeostasis and homeorhesis Revisited. IN: CAB International 2000.Ruminant Physiology: Digestion, Metabolism, Growth and Reproduction (ed.P.B.Cronje)

Mechanisms for nutrient partitioning

The metabolic adaptations occurring with the onset of lactation are undoubtedly related to the plethora of hormonal changes occurring throughout this period. Some of the hormones undergoing major changes are listed in Table 1. Alterations to homeostatic controls occur in several of the tissues and processes (Table 2) during lactation. Feed intake provides a general example, and a number of homeostatic controls for regulating feed intake have been identified (Forbes, 1996; Langhans, 1999). These homeostatic controls are obviously functioning in non-lactating and lactating animals, but in species such as the rat and cow the set points are altered during lactation. Thus, homeostatic controls of feed intake still occur but the altered set-points allow for a greater voluntary intake so that nutrient supply more adequately meets the nutrient requirement.

Table 2. A partial list of adaptations in metabolic regulation which occur during lactogenesis and early lactation in ruminants (Bauman, 2000)

Tissue/processes	Homeostatic control	Response to altered set-points
Feed intake	Multiple controls	Increased appetite and satiety set point
Adipose tissue	Insulin	Decreased lipogenesis
		Decreased uptake of preformed fatty acids
	Catecholamines	Increased stimulation of lipolysis
	Adenosine	Increased inhibition of lipolysis
Skeletal muscle	Insulin	Decreased glucose uptake
	Insulin (?)	Decreased protein synthesis
		Decreased amino acid uptake
		Increased protein degradation
Liver	Insulin	Increased gluconeogenesis
Pancreas	Insulinotropic agents	Decreased insulin release
Whole animal	Insulin	Decreased glucose oxidation
		Decreased glucose utilization by non-mammary tissues

Insulin is an especially powerful mediator of many different physiological effects, most of which serve to acutely maintain metabolic equilibrium in the face of short-term variations in nutrient supply and demand. Thus, this acute regulatory signal is a pivotal target for chronic metabolic adaptations. Many tissues have specific responses to insulin (Table 2) which are attenuated with the onset of lactation. This includes liver (gluconeogenesis), adipose tissue (fat synthesis), skeletal muscle (glucose uptake) and whole body (glucose oxidation) (Vernon and Sasaki, 1991). An attenuated response is not observed for all acute regulatory functions of insulin. For example, the antilipolytic effect of insulin is greater in lactating sheep compared with non-lactating sheep (Vernon et al., 1990), and the inhibition of whole-body rates of protein degradation is enhanced during early lactation (Tesseraud et al., 1993). Thus, the changes in response to insulin are specific for certain tissues and certain biochemical processes within those tissues, rather than representing any generalized phenomenon. Overall, the physiological adaptations in the response of various processes to insulin have the net effect of enhancing hepatic production of glucose, and sparing glucose use by non-mammary tissues, consistent with the increased glucose requirement of the mammary gland.

Somatotropin (ST) is the homeorhetic control for which mechanisms have been most extensively investigated. In dairy cows, it was demonstrated that exogenous bovine somatotropin resulted in an increase in milk yield of the treated animal and a series of coordinated adaptations in body tissues to support the greater use of nutrients for milk synthesis.

Overall, the changes which occur with the onset of lactation or the initiation of bST treatment allow for a chronic alteration of nutrient utilization. When a meal is consumed and circulatory insulin increases, less nutrients are directed to body fat reserves and other non-mammary tissues because of their altered response to insulin, and more nutrients are taken up by the mammary gland consistent with the increased milk synthesis. Likewise if nutrient supply is inadequate the coordinated responses require a greater mobilization of energy reserves to meet the requirements associated with the increased milk synthesis, and this is accommodated by a greater response to signals which stimulate lipolysis. Thus, adaptations in the response to homeostatic signals affect metabolic processes in an orchestrated manner to match the mammary gland need for nutrients for milk synthesis.

Coordination of biological processes

Coordination represents a key feature of biological regulation. Bauman (1999) demonstrated that bST treatment of dairy cows resulted in a series of coordinated responses and now it is used commercially in many countries. The use of bST improved lactational yield and persistency consistently over the 4-year period of commercial use, and animal well-being was maintained as indicated by performance, milk quality, stayability and herd-life (Baumjan et al., 1999).

Tepperman and Tepperman (1970) were among the first to elaborate specific examples of coordination relative to metabolic processes. They referred to this as the **'Sherrington metaphor'** based on Sir Charles Sherrington's (Sherrington, 1947) famous 'principle of reciprocal inhibition of antagonistic muscles'. Examples of the Sherrington metaphor provided by Tepperman and Tepperman (1970) included the coordination between metabolic pathways within a cell (e.g. lipogenesis and gluconeogenesis in the rat hepatocyte) and between organs in different nutritional states (e.g. nutrient flow during fasting and re-feeding).

D.E. Bauman (2000) used the 'Sherrington metaphor' to explain the coordination of biological processes that occur during lactation. Coordination occurs among biochemical pathways within a cell as indicated by the reduction in the pathways of fatty acid synthesis and the increased importance of the pathways of lipolysis which occurs in adipose tissue with the onset of lactation (Table1). The substantial mammary demand for glucose which occurs with the onset of lactation is provided for by a series of orchestrated adaptations which include increased hepatic synthesis of glucose, reduced glucose uptake by several non-mammary tissues and an overall reduction in whole-body oxidation of glucose (Table1). If these adaptations fail, then a chain of metabolic events occurs leading to a metabolic disease, ketosis, and a compromise in animal well-being.

Concerns over animal welfare

Some research workers (Rauw et al., 1998; Broom, 1999) assume that genetic selection and improved management practices lead to evolving of more efficient, high-producing animals which are at variance with the physiological controls for animal well-being/ animal welfare. Some have expressed concerns that practices to improve the productive efficiency of dairy cows may be pushing them too far, thereby compromising animal health and shortening the lifespan. But Hammond (1952) and Bauman et al. (1985) did not share that concern.

Bauman (2000) stresses that genetic selection and management improvements are successful because they have altered the biological controls in a coordinated manner. The fact is that biological regulation involves a series of orchestrated responses and it is the improvements in the biological control systems which are responsible for the increases in milk yield and the gains in productive efficiency, rather than the biological controls being at discord with increased performance.

Role of coordinated responses in metabolic regulation

As our knowledge of biology increases we appreciate even more the remarkable system for the regulation of metabolic processes which occurs in different physiological states. The coordination of metabolic regulation needs to be considered in evaluating research results. An example is research relating to the low-fat milk syndrome in dairy cows (Davis and Brown, 1970).

What causes milk fat depression (MFD)?

The low-milk fat syndrome is characterized by a marked reduction in both yield and percentage of milk fat, and diets which cause milk fat depression typically result in a more positive energy balance, an increase in circulating insulin, and an increase in body fat accretion. Variations in circulating insulin have no acute effects on mammary lipid metabolism of dairy cows, but they can affect adipose tissue rates of lipogenesis and lipolysis.

Glucogenic-insulin theory: One theory for the cause of MFD is the glucogenic-insulin theory which postulates that when diets cause an increase in circulating insulin, the mammary gland is deprived of milk fat precursors due to vigorous competition by adipose tissue. D.E.Bauman and coworkers (Griinari et al., 1997) evaluated this theory using a 4-day hyperinsulinaemic-euglycaemic clamp. This technique involves intravenous infusion of insulin to achieve a constant elevated concentration and simultaneous infusion of sufficient glucose to maintain normal blood concentrations. Despite the substantial challenge to the mammary gland supply of lipogenic precursors imposed by the fourfold increase in circulating insulin, body metabolism was coordinated so that the rate of milk fat synthesis was relatively constant during the insulin clamp (Mackle et al., 1999). Thus the experiment demonstrated the coordinated regulation of nutrient partitioning, but it provided no support for the glucogenic-insulin theory.

Direct inhibition of mammary fatty acid synthesis: Another theory proposes that MFD is caused by a direct inhibition of mammary fatty acid synthesis by products from incomplete or unusual biohydrogenation of polyunsaturated fatty acids in the rumen. Trans fatty acids have received special attention as the cause, and more recently Bauman and group have expanded the causes to include trans fatty acids and related metabolites (Griinari et el., 1998). Consistent with the trans fatty acid theory, MFD is observed when partially hydrogenated vegetable oils are abomasally infused and there is a close relationship between the decrease in milk fat percentage and the increase in milk fat content of trans-C 18:1 (trans vaccenic acid) over a wide range of diets (Erdman, 1996; Griinari et el., 1998). The typical ruminal biohydrogenation of linoleic acid to stearic acid produces cis-9, trans-11 CLA and trans-11 C18:1 as intermediates. However, diets which caused MFD showed a shift in ruminal biohydrogenation: reduction in milk fat percentage had a corresponding increase in the milk fat content of trans-10 C18:1 and trans-10, cis-12 CLA (Griinari et el., 1998, 1999). The reader may refer chapter on 'milk fat depression' pp 135–142 for more details.

Role of the conjugated linoleic acid (CLA)

Baumgard et al. (2000) infused abomasally CLA isomers to directly examine the role of the CLA on milk fat synthesis. The cis-9, trans-11 CLA isomer had no impact on milk fat whereas a 4-day abomasal infusion of less than10 g of trans-10, cis-12 CLA per day resulted in over a 40% reduction in milk fat content and yield. Thus, the results are consistent with diet-induced MFD involving a direct inhibition of milk fat synthesis by intermediates formed in rumen biohydrogenation of polyunsaturated fatty acids.

In this scenario the increase in body fat accretion which is particularly evident with MFD induced by *high grain-low fibre diets* would represent a shift in nutrient partitioning which occurs as a consequence rather than a cause of the reduced mammary fat synthesis. Dietary addition of CLA has also been shown to inhibit body fat accretion in several species, but the required dose appears to be 10-20-fold greater than the dietary level which achieves MFD (Baumgard et al., 2000).

Several research groups led by Dale Bauman at Cornell University, Rich Erdman and Bev Teter at the University of Maryland, and Joe Herbein at Virginia Tech University discovered the powerful suppressive effects of various microbially derived fatty acids having trans-10 double bonds on fat synthesis in mammary gland and adipose tissue. The cis-9, trans-11 isomer CLA is known for its anticarcinogenic effect. Since it is produced by the rumen microorganisms, focused research had been conducted on CLA or its precursor, trans monounsaturated fatty acids to enhance their content in milk and beef. The findings confirmed the hypothesis of Carl Davis and Dick Brown in the late 1960s that trans fatty acids produced in the rumen of cows fed *high-grain diets* might be responsible for milk fat depression.

Conclusion

Lactation provides an impressive example of homeostasis and homerhesis in action, and examples were used to provide an overview of the integrated mechanisms. Overall, the homeostatic and homeorhetic mechanisms provide a coordinated regulation of the metabolism of different organs and tissues to ensure the proper nutrient supply to the mammary gland.

SECTION II
Ruminant Animal Nutrition

SECTION 3
Economic Impact Analysis

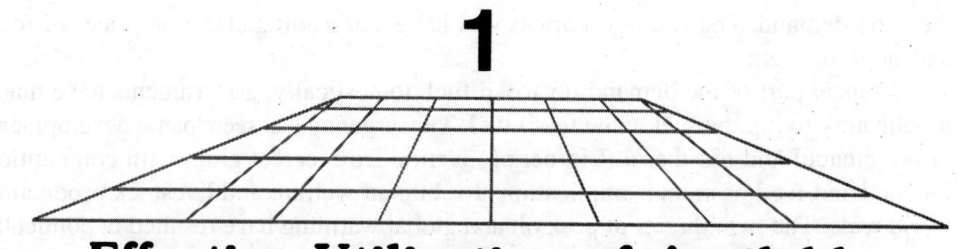

1

Effective Utilization of Available Feed Resources

INTRODUCTION

R.A.Leng in his lecture "Decline in available world resources-implications for livestock production systems" in FAO/IAEA International Symposium June 2009 held at Vienna, Austria, discussed the three simultaneous and interrelated/interactive crises that the world is facing: climate change, peak oil (end of inexpensive energy) and global resource depletion. Burning of fossil fuels is the major source of greenhouse gas emissions.

Climate change

The most significant effects of climate change on agriculture arise through changes in weather patterns and instances of droughts and inundating rains. Increasing temperatures in tropical countries can have a slowing effect on photosynthesis and hence plant growth. Recent models suggest that global warming is likely to reduce world agricultural output by between 16 and 3%. However, the effects will not be spread evenly and productivity in the tropical, developing countries likely to be reduced disproportionately by 21 - 9%.

Peak oil

The primary resource depletion is fossil fuel energy. Earlier oil production and oil demand were finely balanced. But oil production has **out paced** new discoveries since 1981. The world has been using more fossil energy than is being discovered and it appears that the reserves of energy that can be cheaply mined are now at peak production (half these resources have been combusted). The upward trend in oil price has been building for several years and Dr Colin Campbell in 2005 predicted a vicious cycle of -price shock- recession- demand fall- price collapse - recovery - price shock. The 'easy to extract' fossil fuels have been depleted and increasing world demand for fuel will inevitably force world fuel prices to rise, but with a saw-tooth pattern over time, as periodic recessions lower demand and price, allowing both to rise again thereafter. As oil reserves are depleted, prices will rise continuously with the extra demand. The rise in oil prices will have a cascading effect on prices of food and nonfood items.

To meet part of the demand for fossil fuel domestically, governments have made it obligatory to mix biofuel in the fossil fuel. This urgency has seen 'panic development' of bio-ethanol and bio-diesel. Biofuel production from cereal grain with competition for food and feed has major implications for human welfare and livestock production world wide. The twin threats of peak oil and global warming have resulted in politically driven development of large scale production of biofuel from sugar cane in Brazil, and maize in USA. One litre ethanol is produced from 2.6 kg maize grain/5.45 kg fresh cassava roots/14 kg fresh sugarcane stalk. The major sources of biodiesel are the oils produced from oilseed crops (soybean, rapeseed, sunflower and sesame) and from trees such as *Jatropha curcas* and Castor bean (*Ricinus communis*).

Livestock farming

Livestock farming began with early hunters and gatherers as they settled into crop production and harnessed livestock (primarily cattle and buffalo) for transportation and tilling the land. Ruminants are also used as source of milk and meat production. Similarly birds and pigs were initially scavenging animals, feeding on left-over or spilt food, byproducts and natural fauna. Like this animals mostly remained an integrated component of farming. But with the advent of inexpensive energy (fossil fuel energy) and therefore feed (energy and protein), the livestock (and poultry) production diverged from their integrated roles in food production to industrialized production systems.

The shift in the relationship between fossil fuel energy and food and meat or milk production began around 1970 with major changes in the cost of oil. L.R. Brown (2009) stated that a bushel of wheat costs about the same as that of a barrel of oil during 1950-1970 but the equivalent cost increased 4 fold in recent times.

Food and feed resources—Preferred animals

The twin threats of peak oil and global warming has resulted in policy decisions for biofuel production. Production of biofuel from cereal grains and food sources with competition for food and feed has major implications for human welfare and livestock production world wide. The food and feed requirements and the resources to meet the projected human and livestock population appear to be unattainable unless certain prudent measures are taken. The production of bio-fuels and its effect on land use and grain availability is blamed for at least 30% of the price hike that has occurred in world food prices.

As fossil fuel energy becomes scarce it appears that food production costs will escalate and increasingly divert a higher proportion of income in the developed countries/ industrialized countries to maintenance of energy of people including their food and transport costs. Species with high efficiency of conversion of grain /feed to meat such as poultry, herbivorous fish, pig for meat and dairy cattle for milk may be initially favoured. People may reduce their over consumption of expensive animal products but retain funds for transport. In the less rich societies, the cost of food may develop into major famine risk and all countries will need to develop their own food security measures.

Use of sugarcane, cereal grains and oilseeds for biofuel production has global consequences for animal nutrition and will certainly be that less quality feed (byproducts from biofuel industry) will be available for livestock. Ruminants and rabbits reared on crop residues with strategic supplementation of deficient nutrients are the logical animals for future meat and milk production in developing countries. Farming of herbivorous fish (carp), poultry and pigs are likely to be continued with newer technologies of high efficiency.

Feed resources and their effective utilization

From the aforementioned discussion, it can be deduced that the major feed resources are grass and grazing, crop residues, agro-industrial byproducts (AIBP; byproducts of oilseed processing, grain milling, food processing and other agro-industrial activities), non-conventional feed resources (NCFR), forage and fodder from food crops, field crops, plantation crops and coconut groves, foliage from trees / shrubs and cultivated fodders. However, cereal grains and millets do need in the feeding of poultry and swine.

Crop residues must become a major resource for livestock production in the future

Straw has a number of uses: it is fed to ruminants as it is, straw is fed with treatment and supplementation, it may be burned to facilitate multiple cropping practices or ploughed back into the land. Much speculation has centred on the prospects for producing second generation cellulosic ethanol fuel from straw. Straw is the feed of future and feeding straw to ruminants increase animal protein in the future. Straw feeding returns the lignin part of the straw organic matter to soil through application of animal dung/faeces since lignin is 100% excreted by the animal. Thus straw feeding retains the soil carbon.

Small farmers who rear one to five animals possess few resources to feed their animals. They generally feed their animals with crop residues, roadside grass and occasionally grasses collected from field bunds. Crop residues are the most important feed for ruminants in smallholder crop-livestock production systems. However, feeding on cereal straws and natural grazing alone results in reduced live weight and perpetual low productivity in most animals. One solution to these problems is strategic supplementation (Reddy, 2001) with feeds that provide additional energy, proteins and minerals to meet maintenance and production requirements. Leguminous fodder is handy for the farmers. The much studied plants are *Leucaena leucocephala* and *Gliricidia sepium*. The tree leaves are classed as emergency fodder for livestock in general, but they form an integral part of goat feeding. Nutritive value of tree leaves and their supplementary effect, supplementary effect of green fodders (legumes as well as nonlegumes), hays (legumes as well as nonlegumes), and legume straws on cereal straws, native pastures has been studied extensively.

To bridge the gap between availability and requirement of nutrients, efficient utilization of the available feedstuffs is of paramount importance. Blending the coarsely ground (8 mm) crop residues, AIBPs, NCFRs in the form of complete feeds helps in developing low-cost feed, avoids refusal of unpalatable portion or selective feeding, improves utilization of fertilizer urea or uric acid in poultry droppings resulting in efficient feed resource use. Densification of such complete feeds (Compressed feed blocks) reduces the volume of the feed which makes its handling, storage and transportation easy.

Increased productivity through strategic supplementation
Concept of strategic supplementation

Fibre-rich, low-protein forages and crop residues are the most abundant and appropriate feeds for ruminants in India and other developing countries in the tropics. Slow rate of evacuation of indigestible material from the rumen (Van Soest, 1982) and the degree of fill in the reticulo-rumen (Campling and Balch, 1961) have been suggested as some of the dominant factors limiting voluntary intake of roughages. Dr R A Leng challenged the description of crop residues as being of low quality. He preferred to relate to them as imbalanced forages (Leng 1990).

The ruminant animal is treated as a two compartment system in which there is
1. A microbial fermentative digestion system that functions efficiently when there is a balanced supply of microbial nutrients within an appropriate ecosystem.
2. The animal relies on the products of the microbial fermentative digestion system and those digestible feed components that escape the rumen fermentation.

Creating an efficient rumen ecosystem for fermentative digestion of fibre and balancing the products of fermentative digestion with rumen un-degradable nutrients (largely protein) have been emphasized in order to optimize ruminant productivity on straw based rations (Preston and Leng, 1987). Differences in the rate and potential degradability of straw have been associated with different rumen environments created by manipulation of feeding through supplementation with both rumen nutrients (mainly ammonia, sulphur and phosphorus) and bypass (escape) nutrients (Purushotham Reddy et al., 1996; Prakash et al., 1996; Reddy, 1996).

Strategic supplements that accommodate the requirements of the rumen microorganisms and balance the absorbed nutrients to the animal's requirement are to be chosen. Supplements such as caged poultry droppings (CPD), sugarcane molasses, deoiled rice bran, drought-tolerant green forages, legume straws, tree foliages that are locally available have been used as nutrient resource for rumen microbes as well as the host ruminant. Smallholder livestock raising on such feed resources in integrated farming systems' approach has the potential to become the environmentally sustainable alternative to industrial livestock production. Strategic supplementation increases the efficiency of ruminant productivity on straw-based diets (Leng 1991) and thus paves the way for developing 'environment-friendly' livestock production system.

Science Behind Supplementation

The term "supplementation" is sometimes used inappropriately. Supplement is an addition to the diet which supplies deficient nutrients. An ideal supplement should maintain or increase intake of the basal diet rather than substitute for it. As a result of 'substitution' the objective of utilizing the straw to its maximum cannot be achieved, the reason being that straw (which is difficult to consume, digest and passage) is supplemented by a feedstuff which is palatable, easy to consume and highly digestible. So naturally animal prefers the supplement to the fibrous basal diet. Hence the supplement meant is to be offered in restricted amount.

Dietary supplementation is the most obvious way of manipulating the supply of absorbed amino acids, glucose and glucose precursors. Most supplements are expensive and their use in ruminant nutrition competes with monogastric animal and human nutrition. It is mandatory that research should produce response relationships to distinguish economic from biological optima. As a rule of thumb, the role of the supplement ceases to be "catalytic" when it exceeds about 30% of the diet dry matter. The amounts of supplement to be provided will be dictated by the marginal value of animal product added per unit of additional supplement. This in turn will be determined by the shape of the response curve between output and input.

Straw diets typically give rise to a high rumen production rate of acetate relative to that of propionate. This is usually accompanied by a reduced supply of amino acids and negligible amounts of glucose and lipids which results in a high proportion of acetate relative to glucose precursors in the absorbed nutrients. Preston and Leng (1987) proposed that an insufficient supply of glucose relative to acetate may reduce the efficiency with which acetate is utilized. A viable explanation for this may be that glucose precursors such as propionate provide a source of NADPH (via gluconeogenesis and the pentose phosphate cycle) necessary for the conversion of acetate to fatty acid, in the absence of which acetate would be diverted to futile cycles and lost as heat. Other explanations include the availability of oxaloacetate, activity of acetyl CoA carboxylase and effects of insulin. Hence there is a need for some measure of balance between the availability of acetate and precursors of glucose (protein, starch).

The studies of Leng and his team (Cronje *et al.*, 1991) showed that the metabolism of excess acetate is responsive to the dietary supply of glucose precursors, and provide support for the concept that additional glucose precursors are necessary for the efficient utilization of acetate when roughage diets low in protein are fed.

Surprisingly high levels of production can be achieved when the two 'rules of thumb' concerning supplementation i.e. 1. to achieve optimal rumen microbial growth and 2. supply of protein (primarily) and energy postruminally, are applied to diets based on straws. Strategic supplements that accommodate the requirements of the rumen organisms and balance the absorbed nutrients to the animal's requirements are to be chosen.

Straw treatment-Ammoniation

To unlock the energy of cellulosic material, whose gross energy equals to that of starch in cereal grains, delignification and simultaneous reduction of cellulose crystallinity is imperative. Of all chemicals including oxidizing agent hydrogen peroxide (Reddy et al 1989), ammonia treatment through urea hydrolysis is a promising method because of simple technology and low cost involved. Ammonia treatment of wheat straw significantly enhanced the soluble phenolics by 52% and decreased the total cell wall phenolics by about 12% (Reddy and Singh 1992). The CP content was enhanced to 10.37% from 2.59 while ME content was enhanced to 1.99 Mcal/kg DM from 1.62. Voluntary intake of feed may be increased not only by physico-chemical treatment (chopping and ammoniation) but also through enhanced rumen fermentative digestibility by supplementation of critical nutrients (Reddy 1989), which stimulates intake of feed.

Complete diet was formulated with ammoniated wheat straw (72.8%), molasses (15%), wheat bran (10%), fish meal (1%), and mineral mixture and salt (1.2%) fortified with vitamins A and D_2 (Reddy 1989) because complete diet system reduces diurnal variation and improves efficiency of microbial protein synthesis in the rumen. Knowledge of quantitative nutrition has clearly shown that substantial increases in productivity of ruminants on forage-based diets can be obtained through the balanced nutrient approach that considers the efficiency of the rumen ecosystem and the availability of dietary nutrients postruminally (Leng 1993). Hence strategic supplementation of poultry droppings at 5.2% level in complete diet enhanced rumen degradation kinetics (Reddy et al 1990) and nutrient digestibility and feed intake (Reddy and Singh 1991) while 3 kg green berseem per day to buffalo bulls fed on ammoniated wheat straw diets provided optimum conditions for improved rumen degradation of straw (Reddy et al 1991) and daily feed intake (Reddy et al 1992).

Effect of catalytic supplementation of critical nutrients on the nutritive value of Rice straw in buffaloes

Ammoniation of straws through urea hydrolysis, though simple, could not become popular among the farmers. The most practical approach would be to use rice straw and supplement it with several strategic supplements to ensure efficient rumen function and balance the fermentation end products with bypass nutrients postruminally (Reddy 1995).

Supplementation of rice straw with 30g mineral mixture and 30g salt daily (Purushotham Reddy et al 1996) to buffaloes enhanced the nutritive value of rice straw to 0.81% DCP and 49.9% TDN (Table 1). Further supplementation of 500g caged poultry droppings (sun-dried and ground) and 250g molasses significantly (P<0.01) increased the rice straw intake. However, the diet had maximum CP of 5.0% only which is less than the 6.9 to 8.8% CP considered necessary to optimize intake of forages (Blaxter and Wilson 1963). Supplementation of 1 kg deoiled rice bran (Reddy 1996) maximized (P<0.05) the utilization of rice straw.

The ratio of N / digestible organic matter (N / DOM) for this diet was 0.021, while the optimum should be 0.032 g N per g DOM (ARC 1980). Further addition of protein meals non-significantly increased rice straw and significantly (P<0.10) increased the total DM intake (Prakash et al 1996). Among the protein meals, animals fed fish meal diet had lower urinary N excretion and higher (P<0.01) N retention. The increase in dry matter intake in fish meal-rice straw fed buffalo bulls may be

Table 1. Effect of strategic supplementation on feed intake and nutritive value of rice straw diets in buffalo bull calves (Rice straw was offered ad libitum)**

Supplement		Dry matter intake (g per day)		Nutritive value of the diet		
		Rice straw	Total diet/kg $W^{0.75}$	CP %	DCP %	ME Mcal /kg DM
60 g minerals and salt[1]		2434	56.78	3.92	0.81	1.804
60 g plus 500g CPD, 250 g SM[1]		2798	71.40	5.00	2.72	2.038
810 g CPD, SM,minerals plus 1kg DORB[2]		3104	95.54	7.44	4.11	2.042
1810 g plus 100g protein meals[3]						
Groundnut cake		3244	88.9	8.65	4.52	1.754
Soybean meal		3335	89.6	8.77	4.56	1.706
Fish meal		3374	91.0	8.77	4.59	1.730
1910 g plus 1 kg legume straw[4]						
Blackgram	734 g*	3889	103.80	8.52	3.77	1.921
Greengram	892 g	3694	103.12	8.10	3.43	1.802
Redgram	746 g	3461	97.55	8.49	3.61	1.755
1910 g plus 3 kg green fodder / tree foliage[5]						
Cenchrus ciliaris	1092 g*	3484	93.47	7.46	3.62	1.934
Stylosanthes hamata	938 g	3181	88.99	9.94	5.18	1.996
Subabul	900 g	3393	87.69	9.81	5.15	1.884

1 Purushotham Reddy et al 1996; **2** Reddy 1996; **3** Prakash et al 1996; **4** Reddy 1997; **5** Reddy 1998; **CPD:** caged poultry droppings; **SM:** sugarcane molasses; **DORB:** deoiled rice bran; **CP:** crude protein; **DCP:** digestible crude protein; **ME:** metabolizable energy

* Actual amount of dry matter consumed;   * D V Reddy and N Krishna, LRRD, 21, 3, 2009.

attributed to the rumen undegraded protein content of fish meal, which has been reported previously (Egan 1977; Lee et al 1985). This kind of strategic supplementation in an integrated poultry - buffalo farming system supports moderate levels of productive functions on rice straw without recourse to the use of grain based concentrates.

The legume straw-supplemented diets apparently provided rumen degradable N to satisfy the N requirements of the rumen microbes. Though statistically insignificant, rice straw intakes were depressed by the legume straw supplements (Reddy 1997), while blackgram straw increased (P<0.10) the protein digestibility and N retention. Green forage supplementation did not influence the total intake of the animals, although they decreased (P<0.01) the rice straw intake compared to that of control diet (Reddy 1998). Legume pasture or tree foliage were better supplements.

The downside of ruminant production from poor quality roughages

In developing countries the majority of ruminants are supported on forages of poor nutritional value. In general, growth rates, milk production and reproductive rates in these systems are extremely low compared with the genetic potential of these animals.

Slow growth, low milk yield and poor reproductive performance result in poor feed conversion and a large methane output relative to product output (Leng, 1991).

Potential of nitrate as fermentable N source for ruminants fed poor quality forage

Recent studies suggest that the fermentable nitrogen requirements of ruminants on diets based on low protein cellulosic materials can be met from nitrate salts (Trinh et al., 2009) and this potentially reduces methane production to minimum levels (Leng, 2008). Trinh et al. (2009) demonstrated that with adaptation, young goats given a diet of straw, tree foliage and molasses grew faster with nitrate as the fermentable N source as compared with urea. This is a major step forward in ruminant nutrition which should create a paradigm shift in animal protein production. If methane production is lowered significantly when nitrate is fed in low protein diets consumed by ruminants, it will remove a major barrier to replacing much of the monogastric production lost because of the unavailability of feed grain in the future.

The supply of animal protein can be enhanced using the rabbits by feeding forages (Lukefahr, 2007), since rabbits have ability to utilize cellulosic biomass efficiently, coupled to a high fertility with ability to breed every 6 weeks producing multiple offspring.

Supplementary feeding of goats

Goat plays a unique role in supporting the livelihood of some of the poorest people in India. It has huge potential for the economic transformation of rural poor from poverty to prosperity (Peacock, 2005). The goats in India are reared under extensive system on range feeding. Their poor performance is largely due to their sustenance on low nutrition roughages available on range.

Stall-feeding of goats with Napier Bajra hybrid green fodder (Co-3) could meet the digestible protein requirement, but not the energy requirement (Elanchezhian and Reddy, 2009). It indicated that there was a need for supplementary feed to meet the deficit in energy requirement. Supplementation of 100 g of wheat bran per goat per day to Napier Bajra hybrid green fodder (Co- 3) not only provided the nutrients needed for maintenance of the goats (15 kg), but also for a little growth (Elanchezhian et al., 2011).

Small-hold farmers do not always purchase concentrate for their animals because of economical reason and hence extensive system is the most prevailing practice of rearing goats. This has a telling effect on their productivity since feeding and nutrition is the principal determinant of their performance among the non-genetic factors. Increasing the total dry matter intake can be done by correcting nutrient deficiencies, which is dependent upon enhanced rumen fermentative digestibility due to supplementation of critical nutrients (Reddy, 1989) and thus stimulate intake.

Studies on voluntary feed intake, nutritive value and growth rate of male kids on Napier Bajra hybrid green fodder diet (*ad libitum*) with supplementation of different kind of tree leaves e.g., subabul (*Leucaena leucocephala*), sesbania (*Sesbania grandiflora*), acacia (*Acacia auriculiformis*), jack (*Artocarpus heterophyllus*), yellow gold mohur (*Peltophorum ferrugineum*) and cashew (Anacardium occidentale) at the rate of 300 g per day per goat have revealed that tree foliage from sesbania, jack, subabul and acacia had high potential supplementary effect in meeting the nutrient requirements of the kids to support a moderate growth (Reddy et al., 2009; Table 2).

Deterrents of tree leaf utilization in ruminant nutrition

Trees of several species could provide palatable and nutritious fodder during drought and scarcity periods by lopping their branches (Reddy 2006). There are many advantages of the forages from multi-purpose tree crops (Devendra 1992). The leaf fodder of some trees is almost as nutritious as that of the leguminous fodder crops. However, presence of antinutritional factors (ANF), especially tannins limits their use as animal feed.

Based on their structures and properties, tannins are distributed into two major classes-hydrolysable tannins (HT) and condensed tannins. Condensed tannins (CT) are hydrolytically cleaved to anthocyanidins and related compounds and are more correctly called proanthocyanidins or proflavanoids. Tannins are hydrosoluble polymers that form complexes with proteins, starch, cellulose and several minerals (Makkar 2003). These complexes are broken under conditions of high acidity (pH < 3.5) or high alkalinity (pH > 7.5) (Jones and Mangan 1977).

The anti-nutritional effects of condensed tannins include complexing with microbial extra cellular enzymes leading to impaired rumen function and depressed feed intake. The negative effects of tannins may be overcome by dosing of animals with polyethylene glycol.

Table 2. Voluntary feed intake and nutritive value of tree leaves and Napier Bajra hybrid green fodder (Co-3) diets in goats (Reddy *et al.*, 2009)

Feed/ Parameter	Green fodder alone	Supplemental Tree leaves + NB green fodder ad libitum					
		Subabul	Sesbania	Acacia	Jack	Yellow gold Mohur	Cashew
Dry matter intake (g) per day							
Supple-ment	---	97	86	126	117	115	116
NB green fodder	344	283	359	332	360	309	236
Total DMI	344	380	444	459	477	424	352
DMI (g) % BW	2534	2940	3414	3502	3592	2950	2507
DMI (g)/kg W 0.75	48.6	55.7	64.8	66.6	68.6	57.3	48.5
Nutritive value of Diets							
DCP %	6.65	8.55	10.60	7.46	7.07	4.58	5.84
TDN %	49.55	54.80	63.88	66.67	53.59	54.22	52.53

Condensed tannins may confer protection from degradation of leaf protein in the rumen and thus increase the bypass protein content. Hence condensed tannins may be used as organic protectant of protein from rumen degradation. Condensed tannins also increase transulphuration of methionine to cysteine and reduce the gastrointestinal parasitism. Anthelmintic effects are also reported. In view of several beneficial effects of tree leaves, this is a fertile ground of research to improve them as sustainable forage resources.

Potential of tree leaves in ruminant feeding

Some common trees of Puducherry area are selected to study the fibre components, non-fibre components and various phenolic fractions of their leaves for assessing their potential in feeding ruminant animals (Reddy and Elanchezhian, 2009; Elanchezhian et al., 2011). These trees are *Acacia auriculiformis* (Australian wattle), cashew (*Anacardium occidentale*), *Gliricidia sepium*, guava (*Psidium guajava*), jack (*Artocarpus heterophyllus*), *Sesbania grandiflora*, subabul (*Leucaena leucocephala*) and yellow gold mohur or copper-pod tree (*Peltophorum ferrugineum*). The leaf fodder of some trees is almost as nutritious as that of the leguminous fodder crops and can serve as supplementary feeds to poor quality crop residues.

NDICP and ADICP

The calculated difference between NDICP and ADICP is christened as B3 while the ADICP is called as C in the CNCPS (Cornell net carbohydrate and protein system) fractionation of protein in feedstuffs (Sniffen et al 1992). In the parlance of CNCPS, B3 is slowly (rumen) degraded true protein and C is undegraded true protein. Among the tree leaves studied, *Sesbania grandiflora* had highest amount of slowly rumen-degraded protein followed by gliricidia, subabul, and acacia. The intestinal digestibility coefficients for B3 (0.80) and C (0.00) are not always as indicated. This is particularly true for the assumption that fraction C always has a digestibility of 0.00. Several studies indicate that variable amounts of ADICP are digested in the small intestine (NRC 2001; McNiven et al 2002). Refer Appendix for further details on these components of CNCPS.

Carbohydrates of tree leaves

Rumen microbes and animals utilize the different fractions of protein, non-fibre carbohydrate and structural (fibre) carbohydrate fractions differently and their estimation in the feedstuffs elucidates more information about their availability (Sniffen et al 1992). Inadequacies in the nitrogen free extract of the Weende analysis have been addressed by development of methods to quantify the nonstructural carbohydrates (NSC), which are mainly starches and sugars.

The calculation of non-fibre carbohydrates (NFC or neutral detergent soluble carbohydrates, NDSC) and ratio between NFC: NDF (see appendix for data) throws light on the suitability of these tree leaves as sole diets when available in plenty as well as supplementary feeds in ruminant feeding. The NFC values for two pools of microbes exist in the CNCPS and microbial growth is a function of carbohydrate (NDF and NFC) availability at the given quantity of appropriate nitrogen sources (Russell et al 1992). Nitrogen must be supplied as NPN or free AA and peptides. Fermenters of NDF can only utilize ammonia while fermenters of NFC also need slowly degraded protein to meet their peptide requirement, which is provided by B3 fraction.

The optimal concentration of non-fibre carbohydrates (NFC) is important in ruminant diets to avoid acidosis and other metabolic problems. Diets with excess NFC can cause ruminal upsets and health problems (Nocek 1997). From the NRC

(2001) recommended maximum NFC and minimum NDF concentrations for lactating cow diets, the calculated ratio between NFC and NDF varies from 1.76 to 1.01.

Polyphenolic compounds

The leaves of cashewnut were found to be most tanniniferous as they contained highest total phenolics, total tannin phenolics and condensed tannins (see appendix for details). Total phenolics of acacia, cashewnut, gliricidia, guava, jack, sesbania, subabul and yellow gold mohur, respectively, were 13.4, 20.3, 5.6, 17.0, 15.6, 9.4, 11.3 and 12.5%. Sesbania, subabul and gliricidia were kept in best category in view of their higher protein (34.9, 22.0 and 24.4), lower lignin and phenolics, while acacia, jack and yellow gold mohur (CP levels: 15.5, 12.9 and 12.4) in the next best category. Cashew leaves (CP = 9.4) were kept in the last category in view of relatively lower protein and higher lignin and phenolics, which were responsible for the low nutritive value of them in goats. However, considering the beneficial effect of condensed tannins in protecting protein from rumen degradation, cashew or other leaves may be incorporated at appropriate level in the ruminant diet.

Studies of Kamra et al (2009) also revealed the potential of plants containing secondary metabolites as rumen modulators for controlling methane emission in ruminants. The data generated for the commonly fed tree foliages related to their CP, protein content of NDF and ADF and the calculated B3 fraction, fibre and the non-fibre carbohydrates along with the phenolic fractions help to evaluate the tree leaves as ruminant feedstuff for sustainable and ecofriendly animal production. Tree leaves could be considered promising and interesting sources for incorporation into ruminant diets.

2

Feeding of dairy cows and buffaloes

INTRODUCTION

The following information is needed for feed formulation
1.   Nutrient requirements
2.   Information on feed ingredients

The reader may refer the companion textbooks on animal nutrition by the author for the information on feeding standards, nutrient requirements and feed ingredients (See section 'General Animal Nutrition').

Formulating feeds for ruminants using tropical feed resources requires an understanding of the relative roles and nutrient needs of the two-compartment system (Preston and Leng, 1987) represented by the symbiotic relationship between rumen microorganisms and the host animal.

*   A microbial fermentative digestion system that functions efficiently when there is a balanced supply of microbial nutrients within an appropriate ecosystem
*   The animal relies on the products of the microbial system and those digestible feed components that escape the rumen fermentation

Relevance of Feeding Standards

In order to formulate feeds and develop feeding systems, it is necessary to relate information on the nutritional characteristics of feed resources to the requirements for nutrients, depending on the purpose and rate of productivity of the animals in question.

Fibre-rich, low-protein forages and crop residues are the most abundant and appropriate feeds for ruminants in the tropics. The relevance of feeding standards for developing countries, particularly those in the tropics, has been questioned from the socio-economic (Jackson, 1980) and technical (Preston, 1983) viewpoints. It has been apparent for many years that feeding standards based on assigned nutritive values (e.g., net energy) are misleading when unconventional feed resources are used, since the levels of production achieved may be considerably less than the level predicted. This often led to the rejection of many available feed resources because they apparently are too low in digestible energy to supply the energy needed for production.

1. The efficiency of the rumen ecosystem cannot be characterized by any form of feed analysis. The recently developed CNCPS is based on the rumen occurrences.
2. Feed intake on some diets bears no relationship to digestibility and is much more influenced by supplementation.
3. Supplementary feeds provide critical nutrients for rumen microbes and thus enhance the potential of imbalanced tropical feeds.

For these technical reasons, it has been proposed to develop feeding systems that aim to optimize the utilization of locally available feed resources and to build on traditional practices, which is more appropriate for developing countries. The objective is to "match livestock production systems with the resources available" (Preston and Leng, 1987). However, one should not lose sight that feeding standards should be considered as guides and flexible rules in computation of rations to individual animals and groups of animals in a farm.

Nutrient requirements of dairy animals
Dry matter

Dairy animals have an enormous potential to produce animal carbohydrates, protein and fat in terms of milk, but they also have very high nutrient requirements to achieve this potential. Dairy animals must be able to consume up to 4% of their live weight as dry matter each and every day.

Energy requirements

A pregnant animal needs extra energy for the maintenance and development of the calf inside her. From conception through the first five months of pregnancy, the additional energy required is about 1 MJ / d (0.1 kg TDN) for each month of pregnancy. Energy requirements for pregnancy become significant only in the last four months.

Energy is the most important nutrient to produce milk. The energy needed depends on the composition of the milk (i.e. fat and protein content).

When environmental temperatures exceed body temperature (tropical environment) the resultant heat stress causes a rise in basal metabolic rate and the catabolism of protein. In practice, this means that the requirement for protein (amino acids) per unit of energy substrate will generally be greater for ruminants in tropical environments than for those in temperate environments. When animals are heat stressed to the point that they are panting, their energy requirements for maintenance can be increased by up to 10%. Cold stress may influence the energy requirements as per its intensity.

Body condition scoring

A very thin cow might score 3 or lower while a fat cow might score 6 or greater.

Generally, the amount of weight gain required to increase the cow's condition by one condition score is about 8% of its live weight.

When an adult animal puts on body weight, it is mostly as fat. Some of this fat is apparent on the backbone, ribs, hip bones and pin bones and around the head of the tail. This extra subcutaneous fat gives rise to a system of body condition scoring by visual appraisal. Alternatively the animal can be weighed. It is more accurate. It takes longer to notice visual changes in body condition (four weeks at least) than it does to monitor changes in live weight (one to two weeks).

Gaining 1 kg in the dry period takes more energy than gaining it in late lactation. Hence, it is more efficient to feed extra energy during late lactation to achieve the desired condition score prior to drying off the dairy animal.

Protein requirements

The amount of protein a dairy animal needs depends on her size, growth, milk production and stage of pregnancy. Of all these, milk production has major influence on protein needs. Protein is measured as crude protein, which is the sum of rumen degradable protein (RDP) plus undegraded dietary protein (UDP).

Dairy animal needs to meet the N requirements of rumen microorganisms i.e. its inhabitants in the rumen and its amino acid requirements. Hence, when calculating the protein requirements, CP, RDP or UDP figures can be used. But remember that the requirements of RDP and UDP are only 'guesstimates'.

There is a limit to the rumen's capacity to use RDP to produce microbial protein, which is available for digestion and absorption at the intestine level. Microbial protein synthesized in the rumen can sustain milk production up to a certain level. Above that, some protein in the diet must be UDP. However, with poorer quality forages of the tropics, UDP generally stimulate milk yields through enhancing the feed intake.

Fibre

Ruminant animals need a certain amount of fibre in their diet to ensure that the rumen functions properly and to maintain the fat level in the milk. The minimum percentage of fibre needed in the diet of a dairy animal for healthy rumen function is 30% NDF, 19% ADF and 17% crude fibre. Low-fibre, high-starch diets cause the rumen to become acid. Crude fibre is commonly analysed because it is required in the calculation of TDN. It is now considered an unacceptable measure because it does not take into account the digestible fibre which is nutritionally useful to the animal, both a source of energy in the diet and as a substrate for some of the rumen bacteria.

Vitamins and Minerals

Vitamins A and E are important while animals obtain vitamin D upon exposure to sun. Macrominerals such as calcium, phosphorus, magnesium, sodium, potassium, chlorine and sulphur and microminerals such as cobalt, copper, iron, iodine, manganese, zinc, selenium and molybdenum are to be furnished to the dairy animals.

Types of energy

Energy can come from various components of the feed namely carbohydrates, fats and oils, and even protein can provide energy. Forages contain 2 to 3% fat. Ruminant animal diet should not have more than 5% fat, beyond which fat coats the fibre particles interfering its digestion by the rumen microorganisms. Fats are energy dense nutrients and are provided in the diets of high milk yielders, as rumen inert fats.

Fibre carbohydrates

Carbohydrates of feeds and fodders are comprehensively discussed elsewhere (see pp 185). Crude fibre, acid detergent fibre and neutral detergent fibre are the most common measures of fibre used for routine feed analysis, although none of them are chemically uniform. Neutral detergent fibre measures most of the structural components in plant cells (cellulose, hemicellulose and lignin) generally considered to comprise fibre. Acid detergent fibre does not include hemicellulose, and crude fibre does not quantitatively recover hemicellulose and lignin. Neutral detergent fibre, therefore, is the best expression of fibre available currently, though recommendations are also given for ADF because of its widespread use.

On average NDF is less digestible than nonfibre carbohydrates (NFC; starch, sugar and pectin) resulting in negative correlation between the concentration of NDF and energy concentration of the diets. The chemical composition of NDF (proportions of cellulose, hemicellulose and lignin) affects the digestibility of the NDF fraction. Therefore, feedstuffs or rations with similar NDF concentrations will not necessarily have similar NEL concentrations, and certain feedstuffs or rations with high NDF may have more NEL than other feedstuffs or rations with lower concentrations of NDF.

The maximum amount of NDF concentration of the ration will be determined by the NEL requirement of the cow. The minimum amount of dietary NDF needed is based largely on ruminal and cow health because the majority of dietary NDF is from forage with a physical structure that promotes chewing and saliva production, which helps in maintenance of optimal ruminal pH and thus ruminal health. Long-term effects of poor ruminal health may include instances of laminitis and displaced abomasum.

Bacteria that digest structural carbohydrates produce a large proportion of acetic acid, important in the production of milk fat. These bacteria are sensitive to fats and acidity in the rumen. Reduction or elimination of these bacteria reduces the digestibility of the fibre, and thus reduce the intake of feed.

NDF versus NFC: The major nutritional differences between NDF and NFC are their site, rate, and extent of digestion. Usually more than 90% of the digestion of NDF occurs in the rumen. Depending on the feed, between 60 and 80% of digestible NFC is digested in the rumen and 20 to 40% is digested in the small intestine. The rate of digestion in the rumen is usually rapid for NFC and slow to moderate for NDF. Total tract digestibility of NFC is usually greater than 90% and 30 to 60% for NDF. These differences between NDF and NFC must be considered when formulating diets.

Cows do not have a requirement for NFC, but because NFC is highly digestible it is a primary energy source for cows. Because NFC is digested rapidly (may increase rumen acidity), increasing NFC usually increases dry matter (DM) intake. The same properties (rate and extent of digestion) that make NFC desirable can be detrimental to the health and long term productivity of cows.

NDF versus ruminal pH

The concentration of NDF is inversely related to ruminal pH because NDF generally ferments slower (less acid production in the rumen) and is less digestible than NFC.

Forage is usually a primary source of NDF and the physical characteristics of most forages stimulate chewing which increases saliva flow helping to buffer the rumen. The NDF in feed that promotes chewing is called effective NDF. No uniform method of measuring effective NDF has been adopted. Therefore, concentrations of effective NDF cannot be measured. To overcome this problem the NRC (2001) adopted a simple approach of dividing NDF into NDF provided by forages and NDF provided by other feedstuffs. In general NDF from forage is about twice as effective at maintaining rumen pH as NDF from nonforage sources.

NDF from forages: Forages that are long or coarsely chopped provide NDF in a form that is distinctly different from NDF in nonforage sources.

NDF from nonforage sources: Nonforage sources include soyhulls, beet pulp, maize gluten feed, grains. Many nonforage fibre sources have a relatively large pool of potentially degradable NDF, small particle size, and relatively high specific gravity. Nonforage fibre sources have similar or faster passage rates than many forages, and many have rates of NDF digestion that are similar to or slower than those of forages. A large proportion of the potentially available NDF from nonforages may escape ruminal fermentation resulting in less acid production in the rumen (Firkins, 1997). Most sources of nonforage NDF are significantly less effective at maintaining milk fat percentage than are forages. NRC (2001) gave an average effective value of NDF from nonforage sources (e.g., soyhulls, beet pulp, maize gluten feed, grains) as 50% of that for NDF from forages based on the published reports.

NDF recommendations

The minimum recommended concentration of total dietary NDF for cows was set at 25 % of dietary DM with the condition that 19 % of dietary DM must be NDF from forage, along with maximum dietary NFC of 44% and minimum dietary ADF of 17%. These recommendations are for specific situations: when the diet is fed as a total mixed ration, the forage (being lucerne or maize silage predominantly) has adequate particle size, and ground maize is the predominant starch source. Diets that contain less fibre (forage NDF, total NDF or total ADF) than these minimum values and more NFC than 44 % should not be fed (NRC, 2001). To avoid acidosis and other metabolic problems, the maximum concentration of NSC should be approximately 30 to 40 % of the ration dry matter (Nocek, 1997). The acceptable concentrations for NFC are probably 2 to 3 percentage units higher than for NSC.

NDF recommendations vary as per the particle size of forage, ruminal availability of starch: Particle size of forage as well as concentration of NDF in the ration has an impact on ruminal pH.

Particle size: Allen (1997) reported that when finely chopped forage was substituted for coarsely chopped forage, salivary buffer flow decreased by nearly 5 %, but an increase in forage NDF in the diet from 20 to 24 % increased salivary buffer flow less than 1%. The mean particle size of alfalfa hay necessary to maintain rumen pH, chewing activity and milk fat percentage appears to be about 3 mm.

Ruminal availability of starch: Rations containing steam-flaked maize, steam-flaked sorghum, high moisture-maize, barley grain or other sources of starch that have high ruminal availability should contain more than 25% NDF and less than 44% NFC.

Milk fat percentage, ruminal pH and ruminal VFA profile are often altered when starch availability in the rumen is increased (e.g., steam-flaked vs. dry processed grains, high moisture vs. dry grains, or barley vs. maize) even when the concentration of dietary NDF is not altered. These alterations in ruminal fermentation and milk fat percentage suggest that the NDF requirement increases when sources of readily rumen available starch increases.

Cows fed rations based on barley grain should contain about 34% NDF (Beauchemin, 1991), since barley grain has high ruminal available starch.

The minimum recommended NDF concentration is increased as the amount of forage NDF in the diet decreases.

The NDF concentration in the diet must be higher when the forage is finely chopped.

Inclusion of supplemental buffers may decrease the amount of NDF required in the diet.

Furthermore, the minimum recommended concentrations of NDF should not be considered the optimal concentration.

Lower producing cows require less energy, and diets should contain NDF concentrations greater than the minimum.

Minimum amount of roughage DM in total mixed ration or complete diet

Feeding large amounts of concentrates to high yielding cows, e.g. over 70% of the ration in urban dairies can lead to acidosis and impaired rumen fermentation, depressed intake and depressed butterfat content of the milk. In those cases, it is necessary to provide **a minimum quantity of fibre, e.g. approximately 30% NDF in the total DM** provided to the animal.

If a ration consists of a concentrate mixture of about 14% NDF, the minimum amount of roughage DM that is to be provided is

25% if the roughage contains 70% NDF, e.g. rice straw

30% if the roughage contains 60% NDF, e.g. maize and sorghum stover

39% if the roughage contains 50% NDF, e.g. lucerne, berseem and cowpea

Effective fibre, effective NDF and physically effective NDF

The origin of the effective fibre concept was to meet the minimum fibre requirement that would maintain milk fat percentages (Mertens, 1997). The effective fibre concept is an attempt to formulate rations not only for NDF but also for the ability of a diet to stimulate chewing. Chewing response is an important characteristic of feeds (Balch, 1971).

For animals in early lactation, ruminal pH is a more meaningful response variable for determining fibre requirements than are other factors. Mertens (1997) proposed that two terms should be used to distinguish between the effectiveness of fibre in maintaining milk fat percentage or in stimulating chewing activity.

Effective NDF (eNDF) was defined as the sum total ability of the NDF in a feed to replace the NDF in forage or roughage in a ration so that the percentage of milk fat is maintained.

Physically effective NDF (peNDF) is related to the physical characteristics of NDF (primarily particle size) that affect chewing activity and the biphasic nature of ruminal contents. Physically effective NDF (peNDF) concept is a step towards the quantification of the chemical and physical attributes of fibre into a single measurement.

Study conducted by German workers Zebeli et al. (2006) indicated that accounting for dietary physically effective fibre is a more efficient procedure to assess effective fibre adequacy of dairy cow rations than simply taking into account dietary NDF or forage NDF. High-concentrate diets for high-yielding dairy cows must contain sufficient physically effective fibre (i.e., fibre that stimulates rumination, saliva production, and rumen buffering) to prevent ruminal dysfermentation and subacute ruminal acidosis (SARA). The concept of physically effective fibre was created to amalgamate the chemical characteristics and particle size of forages, and to quantify its value to rumen function (Mertens, 2000). However, the NRC (2001) provides no recommendations for inclusion of peNDF because of the lack of a standard, validated technique to quantify the physically effective properties of fibre in a diet.

Types of protein

Dietary protein is commonly termed 'crude protein' (CP). Crude protein is not measured directly but is calculated from the amount of N in a feed (N X 6.25). Nitrogen is from two sources: true protein and non-protein nitrogen (NPN). The microbes in the rumen are able to convert this NPN into microbial protein (true protein) if sufficient energy is available to them. Because of this, both sources of nitrogen can be used as protein sources by the ruminant.

Crude protein is the sum of rumen degradable protein (RDP) plus undegraded dietary protein (UDP). RDP is any protein in the diet that is fermented and used by the microbes in the rumen. RDP includes NPN and degradable part of the dietary proteins. UDP is any protein in the diet that is not digested/fermented in the rumen and passed on the abomasum and small intestine for digestion. That is why UDP is also called 'bypass protein'.

Microbial protein

Rumen microbes are the major source of protein in the ruminant's diet. Rumen bacteria break down RDP to amino acids, then ammonia. The bacteria also convert NPN to ammonia. Bacteria are engulfed by protozoa. The rumen microbes are continually 'flushed' from the rumen, through the omasum to the abomasum, where they are killed and digested by the animal. The amino acids produced from the digested microbial protein are absorbed through the small intestine. The amount of microbial protein synthesized in the rumen depends on the synchronous availability of energy and ammonia in the rumen.

If energy is limited, rumen bacteria become less efficient at using ammonia. Ammonia is absorbed across the rumen wall into the bloodstream. In the liver, ammonia is then converted to urea. Most of this urea is excreted in the urine although some is recycled back into rumen as NPN in the saliva and also into large intestine.

How do feed requirements change during lactation?

Energy, rather than protein, is the most common limiting nutrient for the milking cow in most tropical feeding systems. Energy requirements and intake capacity of dairy animals change at different stages of lactation. Following calving the milk production of a cow / buffalo starts rising and reaches to a peak by about seven weeks into lactation then gradually fall by the end of lactation. Although her maintenance requirements will not vary, she will need more dietary energy and protein as milk production increases, then less when production declines. However, to regain body condition in late lactation, she will require additional energy.

Once the animal becomes pregnant she will need some extra energy and protein, which become significant after the sixth month. The calf doubles its size in the ninth month, so at that stage a considerable amount of feed is needed to sustain its growth.

Cows / buffaloes use their own body tissues for about 12 weeks after calving, to provide energy in addition to that consumed. The energy released is used to produce milk, allowing them to achieve higher peak production than would be possible from their diet alone. To make this possible, cows / buffaloes must have sufficient body condition available to lose, and therefore they must gain body weight in their late lactation stage (in the previous lactation) or during the dry period. Thus animals in early lactation tend to lose weight to divert additional nutrients towards milk production while those in late lactation tend to repartition nutrients to replace previously lost body reserves.

Energy needs of the dairy cow during early lactation

Some species (rodents and humans for example) lose very little body weight or condition during the periparturient period because they rely primarily on increased feed intake to meet the increased energy demands of lactation (Bauman, 2000). Other species (seals, bears, and baleen whales) rely almost entirely on mobilized tissue to meet the energy demands of lactation (Oftedal, 1993). Dairy cows belong to a group of species that rely upon both increased feed intake and mobilized body tissue to meet their energy needs during early lactation. High merit cows partition a greater proportion of their available energy to milk than body tissue (Bauman et al., 1985). As cows transition through the postpartum period, they receive signals that result in gradual increases in intake until intake meets their metabolic needs for continued milk synthesis and replenishment of tissue mobilized in early lactation.

Adjustments in feed intake occur more slowly than the periparturient increases in milk yield. The cow, therefore, enters a period of negative energy balance. However, duration of negative energy varies considerably among cows. Some cows achieve positive energy balance very early (before week 4), most by week 7 to 10, and others later in lactation. This is an interactive process and, especially during early lactation, homeorhetic mechanisms within the cow function to increase energy intake to meet the increased demands of milk synthesis in a coordinated manner. The cow can accept and adapt to an episode of negative energy balance, but if energy intake is limited, production will be limited. This is an insidious problem for the farmer in that the cow appears healthy, appears to be performing well with no outward or obvious indication that production is limited by an insufficient energy supply.

Retrospective analysis indicates that every unit increase in peak yield equates to an additional 127-unit increase in total milk yield for the lactation (Baumgard et al., 2006). Although feed intake needs to be maximized so that peak milk yield is maximized, if the process is disrupted by disease or metabolic disorders, the magnitude of negative energy balance can becomes excessive or the interval prolonged and incidence of reproductive problems increased.

Lactation curve

Lactation curve has a characteristic shape.

First phase 10-12 weeks: During the first phase of the first 10-12 weeks of lactation milk production increases rapidly while milk fat percentage inversely follows the lactation curve. Dry matter intake rises after calving but lags behind the needs of the rapidly increasing milk production. The cow is able to consume less energy than she is expending. This is a most difficult phase for feeding and the cow / buffalo loses body weight over this period. Higher weight loss may lead to metabolic disease and impaired fertility.

At calving, appetite is only about 50% to 70% of the maximum at peak intake. This is because during the dry period, the growing calf takes up space, reducing rumen volume and the density and size of rumen papillae is reduced. After calving, it takes time for the rumen to 'stretch' and the papillae to regrow. It is not until weeks 10 to 12 that appetite reaches its full potential. By providing a high quality diet during early lactation, the physical restrictions of appetite would be reduced.

Second phase 12 -24 weeks: During phase two DMI is at its maximum. The cow / buffalo should no longer be in negative balance.

Third phase week 24 till end of lactation: Phase three is the period when yield begins to fall. During this period the cow / buffalo should be able to restore weight lost in early lactation as well as supporting the increasing demands of the developing fetus. It is generally more profitable to improve the condition of the cow / buffalo in late lactation rather than in the dry period, since lactating cows use energy more efficiently for weight gain (75% efficient) compared to dry cows (59% efficient).

Fourth phase - dry period: Phase four is the dry period of 60 days. The dry period is between the end of one lactation and the beginning of the next. The purpose of a dry period is to allow the cow's udder an opportunity to regenerate secretory tissue and to allow the digestive system to recover from the stress of high levels of feed intake. Rations are predominantly based on good quality forage and should be supplemented with vitamins and minerals.

Steaming Up: During the latter weeks of the dry period (14 days prior to calving) the rumen of the cow / buffalo should be prepared for the diet it is going to be fed in early lactation. Rumen microflora and fauna take 10-14 days to adjust to a new substrate i.e., post-calving diet. Feeding large amounts of concentrates before calving is necessary so that the cow / buffalo can store sufficient resources to be drawn on in early lactation. This proactive feeding is known as 'steaming up'. Feeding concentrates is helpful to stimulate the restoration of the rumen papillae which in turn increases post-calving absorption from the rumen.

Lead feeding / challenge feeding

Calving to peak milk production: Once the pregnant animal calves the milk letdown is initiated and the milk production in dairy animals increase for 80-90 days. As the animal increases production during the first 3 months, it is beneficial to calculate her production needs and continue to add little extra nutrients to take care of the increasing production. Feeding a bit more then, is what is called lead feeding. This is also called challenge feeding. High milk producing animals are fed increasing quantity of feed challenging them to produce at their maximum potential. Best grades of hay, high grain level, undegradable intake protein (UIP) to meet as much as one-third of the total protein requirements, sodium bicarbonate as a rumen buffer to avoid acidosis are offered.

Dietary cation-anion balance (DCAB)

Dietary cation-anion balance is the difference between the concentrations of inorganic cations (sodium, potassium, magnesium and calcium) and anions (chlorides) in the feed. Normally, rations fed to herbivores have a positive DCAB value, as evidenced by the alkaline urine commonly encountered in such animals. The calcium loss in alkaline urine is low. Metabolic alkalosis predisposes cows and buffaloes to milk fever and subclinical hypocalcaemia. Metabolic alkalosis is largely the result of a diet that supplies more cations than anions to the blood.

A negative DCAB gives rise to loss of calcium in the urine. This calcium loss enhances calcium turnover in bone i.e., enhances bone resorption and increases calcium absorption.

Acidifying the diet (through salts such as ammonium chloride, magnesium sulphate, calcium chloride) of the dairy animal during the last part of pregnancy will therefore prime it for the sudden increase in calcium demands at parturition, and for maintaining plasma calcium in the normal concentration range at parturition, when faced with calcium losses through colostrum.

Milk fever

Milk fever can be prevented by increasing calcium absorption and enhancing bone resorption before parturition. Both processes are stimulated when a diet that leads to a negative calcium balance is fed during the last part of pregnancy. Acidifying the diet leads to negative DCAB that result in a negative calcium balance which is a desirable feature of diets used before calving in dairy animals prone to develop hypocalcemia.

Diets contributing less than 15 g calcium per day, and fed for 10 days prior to parturition, can reduce the incidence of milk fever. The modus operandi of this management technique is that such calcium-deficient diets stimulate increased production of the parathyroid hormone (PTH) prior to parturition.

Action of PTH

Parathyroid hormone stimulates mobilization of bone mineral (Ca and P). PTH increases 1, 25 dihydroxy cholecalciferol synthesis, which stimulates both intestinal Ca and intestinal P transport. Calcium is reabsorbed in the kidney under the influence of PTH and 1, 25 dihydroxy cholecalciferol. PTH causes a phosphate diuresis. Therefore, under the condition of a hypocalcaemic signal, plasma calcium only rises while keeping the plasma phosphorus level constant. But remember, low magnesium (hypomagnesia) can reduce PTH secretion, which, in turn, can decrease calcium availability.

Major advances in applied dairy cattle nutrition

Estridge (2006) reviewed the major advances in applied dairy cattle nutrition (mostly from USA and those published in Journal of Dairy Science) occurred during 1980-2005. Milk yield per cow has increased about 2% per year. DMI has increased to supply the increased demand for nutrients through diets of higher nutrient density. It is common in USA, for herds to average 12,500 kg milk per lactation with feed intake of 25 to 27 kg DM per day. Some of the advances made in dairy cattle feeding practices are mentioned in the following:

Protein: Among the nutrients, protein has been studied to a greater extent. Balancing rations has been changed from CP of the diet to balancing for RDP and RUP fractions. Rumen protected protein sources have become common in dairy animal diets. The RDP fraction is even further defined to most rapidly degraded (soluble protein: usually at 25 to 30% of CP). From the 1989 NRC to the 2001 NRC, equations for protein requirements are altered and emphasis is shifted to balancing diets for metabolizable protein (MP).

Concentrations dietary protein to feed cows of prepartum versus during different stages of lactation has received considerable attention. Close-up dry cows (last 2 to 3 week of gestation) should generally be fed diets with 14 to 15% CP, with response to balancing for RUP being minimal.

Milk and blood urea nitrogen (MUN, BUN) have been related to efficiency of nitrogen use. More information is now available on the amino acid needs of dairy cattle, especially methionine and lysine. Protein sources are selected to provide a complement of amino acids in diets and rumen-protected amino acids are supplemented.

Fat: The practice of fat supplementation has increased to meet the energy requirement of high milk-yielding animals. Feeding fat is common during summer months when DM intake is likely be depressed because of its energy density and no contribution to heat increment. However, excessive concentration of unsaturated fat interferes with fibre digestion in the rumen and eventual DM depression. This led to supplementation of rumen inert fats sources like calcium salts of fatty acids. The natural sources of fat such as oilseeds are added to diets to take the advantages of their inherent fatty acids to enhance the healthful fatty acid content of their products.

Vitamins: Supplementation of niacin at 6 to 12 g/day prevented ketosis in dairy animals. Biotin supplementation at about 20 mg/day can improve hoof health, and may increase milk yield. Supplementation of rumen-protected choline may increase milk yield and improve the transport of lipids, thereby reducing the incidence of ketosis.

Bovine Somatotropin: Bovine somatotropin (bST) daily injections (which were introduced in 1994) are replaced with sustained-released products (once in 14 days). Several studies have clearly demonstrated a positive response in milk yield, no change in milk composition, and a 3- to 4-week lag in the increase in DMI with the use of bST. Diets are formulated as usual for high-producing animals. The response to bST will not continue unless diets are formulated to provide adequate concentrations of nutrients (especially adequate energy).

3

Transition Period – Metabolic Changes – Optimizing Transition Animal Diets

Physical and metabolic stress during transition period

Transition period is the period 2-4 weeks prior to calving through 2-4 weeks after calving. The transition period is also called as periparturient period. Depression of feed intake pre-calving and slow intake increase post-calving is observed during this period. During transition from pregnancy (dry period) to lactation, the dairy animal is under enormous stress both physically and metabolically. Moe and Tyrrel (1972) reported that the energy requirements of the dairy cow increase by 23% to support foetal and gravid uterus growth in the last month of pregnancy. Further, mammary uptake of glucose increases by 400%, acetate uptake by 180% and blood flow increases by 200% from one week prior to parturition to 1 day before calving (Bell, 1995). But DM intake starts to decline approximately 3 weeks before parturition and reduces dramatically in the last 7 days. The level of decline has been as high as 30% (Bertics et al., 1992).

Metabolic disorders and infectious diseases

The dairy animal has to adjust from eating a high fibre low energy diet during the dry period to a high energy low fibre diet in early lactation. There is also the need to compensate for a dramatic increase in mineral turnover. Failure to achieve a smooth transition from the dry period to early lactation stage may result in poor milk productivity, metabolic disease and impaired fertility. Most metabolic disorders and infectious diseases occur during this time. Milk fever, ketosis, retained fetal membranes, metritis, and displaced abomasum primarily occur during the periparturient period.

Negative energy balance and Nonesterified fatty acids

J.K. Drackley and coworkers (Drackley, 1999) did pioneering work on biology of dairy cows during the transition period. The **metabolic hallmark of the transition** from pregnancy to lactation in high-yielding dairy cows is a massive mobilization of nonesterified fatty acids (NEFA) from adipose tissue during and after parturition. The rapid mobilization of lipid and protein stores is to support the sudden onset of high milk production. But the situation in most dairy cattle prior to calving is declined energy intake due to appetite depression and consequent decreased dry matter intake. Hence such animals experience negative energy status during the final week before calving. Then, a phenomenon known **as negative energy balance (NEB)** occurs in transition dairy animals.

The need for increased energy requirements are compensated by lipolysis: break down of adipose tissue. The released fatty acids reach the blood and are reversibly bound to albumin. These are referred to as NEFA to distinguish them from triacylglycerol fatty acids in chylomicrons and lipoproteins. NEFA can be used directly for energy by many tissues especially the peripheral tissues such as muscle. It has been reported that at least 80% of dairy animals are in NEB during early lactation. Negative energy balance during early lactation is the major nutritional link to low fertility in lactating dairy cows. Negative energy balance delays recovery of postpartum reproductive function and exerts carryover effects that reduce fertility. The degree of NEB in early postpartum period has been correlated with both the level of milk production and the number of days to first ovulation.

Analyzing data published by Nielsen *et al* (2003) of 400 cow lactations, Friggens and Newbold (2007) reported that the cows were in substantial negative energy balance at 14 days after calving and feed intake on that day was only 80% of the maximum intake attained. It was concluded that the observed body lipid mobilization in early lactation was largely genetically driven. High milk yields in dairy cows are related to the ability to mobilize body energy reserves (See Reddy and Krishna, 2009). Animals of high genetic merit produce more milk, have greater voluntary intakes and use more of their body reserves in early lactation than those of low merit. Marked mobilization of body reserves during early lactation, and replacement of these reserves in late lactation, is an important component of the increased productive efficiency that genetically superior cows achieve by dilution of maintenance. Excessive lipid mobilization from adipose tissue is linked with greater incidences of periparturient health problems.

Indicators of negative energy balance (NEB)

- Elevated level of serum NEFA in postpartum dairy cows
- Increased plasma concentration of beta-hydroxybutyrate
- Decreased plasma glucose concentration
- Decreased amount of insulin and insulin-like growth factor-1 (IGF-1)
- Decreased concentration of plasma leptin and
- Fatty liver due to accumulation of triacylglycerol in the liver

Serum NEFA levels in transition cows

Plasma NEFA concentration increases a few days before parturition and peaks around parturition and rises to higher levels than prepartum until about two weeks postpartum. Drackley suggested that NEFA levels may be used as a tool to monitor energy balance in transition dairy cows. Drackley reported less than 0.2mM as normal NEFA levels for cows in positive energy balance. These values increased slowly, as the cow approached calving, to 0.5 - 1.0 mM on the day of calving due to hormonal changes and the stress of calving. After calving, NEFA levels decrease and values greater than 0.7mM indicate severe negative energy balance and by six weeks after calving, values are again below 0.3 mM. Field study results revealed that cows with high plasma NEFA levels had postpartum disorders.

Beta-oxidation of NEFA: Mitochondrial β-oxidation and Peroxisomal β-oxidation

Oxidation of NEFA provides ATP needed for gluconeogenesis. The major site of fatty acid oxidation in animal cells is the mitochondrion. Mitochondrial β-oxidation is an oxidative pathway for NEFA, central to the provision of energy. An alternate pathway for hepatic oxidation of NEFA occurs in peroxisomes, which are subcellular organelles present in most organs of the body. Peroxisomal β-oxidation may play a role as an "overflow" pathway to oxidize fatty acids during extensive NEFA mobilization. The main function of peroxisomal oxidation is the shortening of the NEFA chains, for example those larger than 22-24 carbon atoms preparing them for β-oxidation by the mitochondrial system. Peroxisomes do not contain a respiratory chain linked to ATP formation and hence it is not regulated by energy demands of the cell. The initial oxidative step in peroxisomes is catalyzed by an oxidase, which results in the production of hydrogen peroxide rather than reduced NAD. These characteristics make peroxisomal oxidation well suited to partially oxidize fatty acids that are poor substrates for mitochondrial enzymes.

Complete oxidation of NEFA generates acetyl CoA that can be used to generate energy via the Krebs cycle or tricarboxylic acid cycle. This spares glucose for oxaloacetate formation in the major peripheral tissues, which facilitates the entry of acetyl CoA into the Krebs cycle through citrate formation. However, if the Krebs cycle gets overloaded, the acetyl CoA is shunted off to produce ketones (acetoacetic acid, ?-hydroxy butyrate and acetone) to avoid accumulation of acetyl CoA. That is, incomplete oxidation yields ketones, primarily acetoacetate and ?-hydroxy butyrate as an additional strategy to compensate for insufficient intake of glucose precursors.

NEFA's role in lactogenesis

Nonesterified fatty acids are utilized for about 40% of milk fat during the first days of lactation. In ruminants the fatty acids in milk arise from two sources: uptake from the circulation and de novo synthesis within the mammary gland epithelial cells. The free fatty acids taken up from circulation by the mammary gland are derived from circulating lipoproteins and NEFA that originate from the absorption of lipids from the digestive tract and from the mobilization of body fat reserves, respectively.

Utilization of NEFA during exercise

It has been suggested that walking activity or daily exercise improved the well-being of dairy cows in the transition period by reducing the concentration of plasma NEFA in blood circulation (Adewuyi, 2004). Excessive NEFA may be lost through mitochondrial β-oxidation during increased activity or muscular exercise.

Optimizing transition animal diets

During the transition period, dairy cows undergo large metabolic adaptations in glucose, fatty acid and mineral metabolism to support lactation and avoid metabolic dysfunction. The practical goal of nutritional management during this timeframe is to support these metabolic adaptations. Strategies to optimize metabolic health during transition period include feeding of transition animals with appropriate diets. Diet formulation recommendations for transition animals vary widely due to conflicting experimental results. Literature review supports division of 'dry animals' into two groups-early dry period (all dry cows except those within two or three weeks of calving), and late dry period (dry cows within two or three weeks of calving). Minimize overfeeding of nutrients during the early dry period while increasing nutrient supply to facilitate metabolic adaptation to lactation during the late dry period.

Dry matter intake is of the order of 1.8 to 2.2% of body weight for the former while the latter consume less, which is 1.5 to 1.8%. Reasons for a reduction in DM intake include physical factors such as restricted feeding space, chemical feedback from high levels of blood NEFA, etc. Due to this decrease in DM intake, buffaloes/ cows within two to three weeks of calving should be placed on a more nutrient dense feeds to meet the requirements of advanced pregnancy.

Increasing the amount of energy supplied through dietary carbohydrates during prepartum period and early lactation results in generally positive effects on metabolism and performance of transition animals. Remember steaming up and challenge feeding of transition animals, a continuity in their journey for a successful lactation. Starch sources with lower ruminal digestibility/ fermentability should be highly digestible in the small intestine to provide the greatest yield of glucose precursors. Hence, choose less rumen fermentable starch / more bypass starch sources, such as ground maize grain in the feed. Amino acids mobilized from tissue are important contributors to glucose production following calving. Glycerol part of mobilized fat is a glucose precursor and is expected to stimulate oxidation of acetyl CoA less than propionate. Although glucose production must increase in early lactation, and propionate production needs to be enhanced from rumen fermentation, it is essentially imperative to maintain healthy ruminal pH by including digestible fibre sources and providing adequate effective fibre to increase ruminal retention of small fibrous particles, increasing their digestibility.

Physically effective fibre (peNDF)

The physically effective fibre is a good indicator of the rumination potential of the feed. Zabeli *et al.* (2006) indicated from the results of their studies in early lactating cows fed total mixed rations that accounting for dietary physically effective fibre were a more efficient procedure to assess fibre adequacy of dairy cow rations than simply taking into account dietary NDF or forage NDF. The physically effective fibre (peNDF) of a feed is the product of its physical effectiveness factor (pef) and

NDF concentration. Physically effective fibre (peNDF) could be measured either as a proportion of DM retained by the 19- and 8- mm Penn State Particle Separator screens multiplied by dietary NDF content or as the proportion of DM retained by a 1.18-mm screen multiplied by dietary NDF using a dry sieving technique.

Feeding of protein for optimum reproductive performance

It is known that serum urea nitrogen concentration is found to be negatively associated with conception rate in dairy cows (Ferguson et al., 1993). **Diets high in CP** (17 to 19%) are typically fed during early lactation to both **stimulate and support high milk production**. However, feeding high protein diets have been associated with reduced reproductive performance (Butler, 1998). As a result of feeding high protein, increased plasma urea concentrations may interfere with the normal inductive actions of progesterone on the microenvironment of the uterus and, thereby cause suboptimal conditions for support of embryo development (Butler, 2001).

Rhodes *et al.* (2006) evaluated the quality of embryos flushed from superovulated lactating cows having moderate (15.5 mg/dl) or high (24.4 mg/dl) plasma urea nitrogen (PUN) concentrations; subsequent embryo survival was determined after transfer to recipient heifers with either low or high PUN. Their results indicated that high PUN concentrations in lactating dairy cows decreased embryo viability through effects exerted on the oocyte or embryo before recovery from the uterus 7 days after insemination.

Considerations for diet formulation

- Feeding a high fibre low energy diet prior to calving and gradually change to a high energy low fibre diet in early lactation enable the transition animal to control energy intake appropriately.
- Forage fibre is much more important than non-forage fibre to meet the peNDF requirement.
- Diets with high concentration of grain, non-forage fibre, and finely chopped forages fed through the transition period should be avoided because of low ruminal pH and the consequential health problems.
- Grass and straw diets with high potassium concentrations might require anionic salts in prepartum diets to reduce milk fever following calving.
- Starch sources with moderate ruminal fermentability and high digestibility in the small intestine, such as ground maize, will provide glucose precursors and less propionate.
- Milk yield increases rapidly following calving, and over the next several weeks, plasma glucose increases, insulin increases, and fat mobilization decreases, decreasing plasma NEFA. Since less NEFA is available for oxidation, the acetyl CoA concentration in the liver decreases thereby decreasing ketone output by the liver.
- Rumen protected protein and protected fat provide a practical feeding strategy to regulate nutrient and energy partitioning thereby increase the milk yield and improve reproductive performance.

Feed additives for transition buffaloes and cows

Feed additives such as propionate production promoters, propionate enhancers (fumarate, malate), ketosis controlling agents, methyl donors, rumen inert fats / rumen bypass fat, rumen bypass protein, biotin, niacin, vitamin B_{12}, pantothenic acid, riboflavin are included in their diets. Propionate is converted to glucose in the liver of ruminants by a series of enzymatic reactions which require biotin, vitamin B_{12}, niacin, pantothenic acid and riboflavin. Rumen-protected niacin decreases fat mobilization. Trace mineral chromium increases sensitivity, and supplemental chromium has been demonstrated to decrease plasma NEFA concentrations in lactating cows.

4

Feeding to Minimize Maintenance Requirements and Increase Milk Production

In 2001, the NRC published the Seventh Revised Edition of the Nutrient Requirements of Dairy Cattle. The NRC book is an excellent resource for people involved with dairy cattle nutrition. The conceptual framework of energy metabolism is the basis for the estimate of maintenance energy described by the NRC (2001) for dairy cattle. Values are based on measures in mature dry cows at 0.73 Mcal /kg BW $^{0.75}$ and allow for an adjustment for activity of 10% so that the values used are 0.80 Mcal /kg BW $^{0.75}$.

Dr. William P. Weiss (2002) gave an overview of the 2001 NRC dairy cattle requirements. Substantial modifications had been made in the methods used to calculate nutrient requirements. The approaches taken account for more sources of variation than previous versions and, in many cases, they are clearly more biologically sound.

Energy feeding systems

It is obviously desirable that the units used in feeding standards should be the same as those used in the evaluation of feeds.

The NE value of a feed depends on whether it is used for maintenance, fattening, growth or milk production. Metabolizable energy is used with different degrees of efficiency for maintenance and body gain in non-lactating animals but is used with similar degrees of efficiency for maintenance and milk production in lactating animals. For this reason NRC tables (1988) gave three NE values for feeds: NE_m, NE gain and NE lactation. NEm is the value of feeds for the maintenance of non-lactating animals (dry animals). NE_g is the NE value of feeds for the deposition of body tissue in growing males and females and mature bulls. $NE_m + NE_g$ = total energy needs for growing cattle. In lactating animals, the NE value of feeds as well as requirements for all physiological functions is described in terms of single value as NEl, since energy is used with similar degrees of efficiency for maintenance and milk production.

NEL Requirements

The daily NEL requirement for a lactating cow is a function of body weight (BW), milk yield, milk composition (fat, protein, and lactose), stage of gestation, and whether the cow is grazing. Body weight is used to calculate the maintenance requirement (increasing BW increases maintenance requirement). The maintenance requirement includes the NEL needed to maintain the cow plus the NEL expended for normal activity. Daily yields of milk fat, milk protein, and lactose are used to calculate lactation requirements. For most cows the lactation requirement will be the largest component of total NEL requirements. For lactating cows, stage of gestation has only a small effect on NEL requirements (usually less than 10% of total requirements). No gestation requirement is calculated until a cow has been pregnant for 190 days. The total NEL requirement is maintenance + lactation + gestation + grazing (if any).

Feed NEL values

Although NE based systems can account for most sources of energy loss during digestion and metabolism of consumed feed, NE systems have limitations. Most of these occur because procedures required to measure NE of feeds are expensive in both time and resources. As a result, NE values for most feeds have been estimated rather than measured directly.

In previous versions of NRC, feed NEL values were calculated directly from reference TDN values. The previous NRC (1989) system overestimated the NEL content of feeds by an average of 7%. Because of these problems, the NRC (2001) developed an entirely different method to estimate NEL concentrations of feeds.

The National Research Council (2001) converted to a chemical based system to estimate feed NEL values and incorporated a more dynamic approach to adjust for the effect of feed intake on energy availability. The DE and TDN (at maintenance) concentrations of feeds are calculated (Conrad et al., 1984; Weiss et al., 1992) using concentrations of neutral detergent fibre (NDF), crude protein (CP), ash, lignin, crude fat (or fatty acids), acid detergent insoluble CP (ADICP), and neutral detergent insoluble CP (NDICP). For most feeds, actual values should be used for NDF, CP, ash, and lignin, and table values can be used for fat, ADICP, and NDICP. If a feed has an appreciable concentration of fat (e.g., cottonseeds), a fat analysis is recommended. Concentrations of ADICP and NDICP should be measured in heat-damaged forages and in byproducts that have high concentrations of NDF and CP (e.g., brewers' grains). The TDN values obtained are only used to calculate the discount factor. TDN is not used to directly calculate other expressions of energy.

Digestible energy (DE) and TDN concentration of feeds when fed at maintenance intake is calculated from feed composition data. Digestibility decreases as feed intake increases. Therefore DE calculated for maintenance intake is not appropriate when feeds are fed at higher intakes and in mixed diets. A discount factor (since the higher dry matter intake of lactating dairy cows depress the digestibility of feed) is calculated based on dry matter intake and TDN of the total diet to estimate DE at productive levels of intake. The discount increases as intake and diet digestibility increases. The DE (at maintenance) is multiplied by (1 - Discount) to obtain DE at productive levels of intake. Feed ME concentrations are calculated from discounted DE concentrations and NEL values are calculated from the ME concentration. On average, NEL concentrations are about 5% lower than those in the 1989 version.

Because feed processing can affect digestibility, but not necessarily feed composition, a method was needed to account for processing effects. A processing adjustment factor was used to account for processing effects on the starch digestibility.

Review of the NEL System

The underlying basis of the NEL system is the first law of thermodynamics and all things, including cows, must obey that law (William P Weiss, 2008). In terms relevant to animal nutrition, the first law of thermodynamics can be stated as: **Energy input must equal energy output plus or minus any change in body energy.** If we can accurately estimate the NEL of a diet and NEL requirements, then energy balance can be calculated and we can project changes in body energy reserves (i.e., body condition). The health and long term productivity of a cow depends on proper management of body condition. On an average, about one-third of the energy consumed is lost via faeces, about one-fourth is lost via heat and only about one-third of the energy consumed is converted to NEL.

Net energy for lactation is the energy consumed by a cow that actually does something It is the energy secreted in milk, retained in the body (fat, growth, fetus), and used to perform maintenance functions. It is calculated as ME minus the heat generated by the inefficiency of transforming energy from one form to another (i.e., the heat increment). Heat increment cannot be measured directly. It is calculated from total heat production measured using a whole animal calorimeter. Because these instruments are extremely expensive and only a few are available in the entire world, measured NEL data are extremely limited. Type of carbohydrate and concentrations of dietary fat and protein affect the efficiency of converting ME to NEL. As fibre and protein increase, the efficiency of converting ME to NE usually decreases and as fat and starch increase, efficiency increases. Measurement of NEL is the least accurate measure of energy because it includes all errors associated with measuring GE, DE, and ME plus the errors associated with measuring heat increment.

Protein Requirements

Protein requirements are presented on a metabolizable protein (MP) basis (Weiss, 2002). Metabolizable protein is defined as the total component of amino acids (on a crude protein equivalent basis) that have been absorbed by the intestine and are used for productive purposes. The total MP requirement for maintenance calculated using the 2001 NRC will be similar but generally lower (2 to 3%) than maintenance requirements in the previous version (NRC, 1989). This is because of higher efficiency assumed in 2001 NRC. The MP requirement for pregnancy is a function of BW and day of gestation (no requirement is estimated until gestation day is greater than 190). Overall, total MP requirements calculated using 2001 NRC is about 3 percent lower than values calculated using the 1989 system.

Protein Supply

Method of calculating MP: The 2001 NRC uses a completely different method of calculating MP supply than used previously. The amount of crude protein broken down in the rumen (rumen degraded protein, RDP) is calculated from *in situ* data and software-estimated rates of passage. To estimate RDP, feed crude protein is partitioned into three fractions using *in situ* techniques. The A fraction is readily soluble in water and is measured as the amount of crude protein washed from the bag before ruminal incubation. The A fraction is considered all RDP. The C fraction is the crude protein that will not be degraded in the rumen after at least 48 hour of incubation. The C fraction is all RUP. The B fraction is the remaining crude protein and it will be degraded in the rumen at a given rate. The proportion of B that is RDP depends on the rates of degradation and passage. Feeds with a rapid rate of degradation will have more RDP derived from the B fraction than feeds with slow rates of degradation.

The amount of microbial protein synthesized is then calculated from RDP supply and energy intake. The amount of rumen undegraded protein (RUP) is simply CP minus RDP. The amount of MP provided by RUP is calculated using an efficiency of 0.67 and variable digestibility constants. Digestibility constants are a function of feedstuff and range from 0.5 to 1.0. Estimated RUP digestibility for the more common feedstuffs ranges from about 0.65 to 0.9.

When RDP is limiting, microbial protein (g/day) = 0.85 × RDP intake (g/d). When RDP is not limiting microbial protein is calculated from intake of discounted TDN. Because discounted TDN is used, the marginal increase in microbial protein usually decreases as dry matter intake increases. The practical consequence of this is that as milk production increases resulting in increased feed intake, the marginal increase in RDP requirement is reduced and the marginal increase in RUP requirement is increased. High producing cows at high intakes will require a higher proportion of the crude protein as RUP than cows at lower intakes. However, supply of RUP will also increase at higher intakes because of increased rate of passage and reduced degradation in the rumen.

On average, the 2001 NRC protein system will result in higher RUP supply and higher RUP requirements than the 1989 system. In general total crude protein requirements were reduced slightly (Weiss, 2002).

Minerals

With reference to minerals, the NRC (2001) contains no safety factors. The calculated requirements assume normal, healthy cows fed diets with few mineral antagonists. On average, dietary Ca requirements are increased, dietary P requirements are reduced slightly and requirements for the other macrominerals are similar between the 2001 and 1989 versions. Requirements for Fe and Mn are substantially lower in the 2001 version, requirements for Co, Cu and Se are similar, and requirement for Zn is higher.

Vitamins

The 2001 NRC presents requirements for vitamins A, D, and E and they are expressed as the amount of supplemental vitamin needed. Vitamins provided by basal feedstuffs are generally not considered. This approach has been followed because the concentrations of vitamins in feedstuffs are extremely variable and are rarely measured in field situations. Requirements for vitamins A and E are increased substantially from the 1989 version but the requirement for vitamin D is not changed (Weiss, 2002).

Historical B-vitamin research identified that alteration of dietary forage to concentrate ratios, dietary CP source, and grain processing in ruminating animals altered ruminal B-vitamin concentrations. Past B-vitamin research led to the general dogma that dietary supply and ruminal synthesis are sufficient to meet dairy cow requirements (NRC, 2001). Although ruminal B-vitamin synthesis appears to be sufficient to prevent clinical deficiencies in most situations, supplementing dietary thiamin, biotin, niacin, and folic acid increased lactation performance. However, lactation performance was not always improved by supplemental folic acid, niacin, or biotin. Possible reasons for lack of consistent responses to B-vitamin supplementation are numerous, but a potentially important factor is variable amounts of ruminally synthesized B-vitamins. The NRC (2001) estimates of ruminal B-vitamin synthesis in lactating cows were extrapolated from steer data of Miller et al. (1986) and Zinn et al. (1987) as lactating dairy cow data were not available.

Increasing dietary forage and nonfibre carbohydrate (NFC) contents influenced B-vitamin intakes, duodenal flow, and ruminal apparent synthesis (AS) (Schwab et al., 2006). Thiamin, riboflavin, and folic acid AS appear to be increased when overall dietary intake and digestibility and microbial N production increase; B6 and niacin AS are enhanced with increased dietary NFC content. Negative AS values for biotin suggest minimal ruminal synthesis and/or appreciable ruminal degradation. Vitamin B12 AS was highest for 35% forage-30% NFC diets and was increased with increasing dietary sugars.

The effect of dietary forage and nonfibre carbohydrate (NFC) on ruminal apparent synthesis could be due to changes in populations or functions of ruminal microbial species, their interrelationships, and subsequent effects on microbial B-vitamin metabolism.

Feeding to minimize nutrient requirements for maintenance

Feed costs represent a large portion of the costs of producing milk. Hence factors that impact the efficiency of conversion of feed to milk are of considerable importance. These include several biological processes, environmental influences, genetic factors. The main components of energy requirements are the costs associated with maintenance, body composition changes, and production (growth, reproduction and lactation). Maintenance energy needs are a priority in the animal. Maintenance is the physiological state in which there is no net change in body energy or alternatively when energy balance is zero. Increased maintenance costs have a direct impact on the efficiency of conversion of feed to milk or tissue deposition. A decrease in maintenance requirements or a dilution of maintenance in cows that are capable of producing greater amounts of milk is, therefore, an important goal in the dairy enterprise.

Components of Maintenance

The components of maintenance include the energy required for basal metabolism; energy of thermal regulation; the energy costs associated with digestion, absorption and assimilation of meals at maintenance intake; and the energy associated with waste production. Basal metabolism is essentially equal to fasting heat production (**FHP**) or the heat production of an animal in a postabsorptive state in a thermoneutral environment in an inactive (lying or standing with no activity) state (Baldwin, 1995).

Factors that affect FHP are due to differences in sex, breed, physiological state, level of production, and previous plane of nutrition. The importance of plane of nutrition is highlighted in experiments where sheep were shifted from a high nutritional status to low nutritional status. The observed maintenance requirements were 32% greater than when shifting animals to the opposite diet sequence. It can be explained by a high correlation between FHP and weight of the major digestive organs (primarily liver and gastrointestinal tract).

Factors Affecting Maintenance Requirements

The adjustment to maintenance requirements for lactating cows includes the effect of activity, terrain, and level of feed consumption (NRC, 2001). These adjustments recognize the increased overhead maintenance requirements associated with additional physical activity and the energetic costs associated with increased nutrient digestion and absorption. For heifers, the impact of growth, thermal loss due to cooling, body composition, coat condition, and heat stress are all recognized as adjustments to maintenance requirements.

Type of diet: high fibre diets

Animals on diets with high fibre contents spend more time on chewing and rumination than those on diets with less fibre. This would have increased the energy costs of maintenance. Higher maintenance requirements on forage-based diets could result from higher energy requirements (higher heat production) of the gastrointestinal tract to digest the feed. Oxygen consumption in the intestines has been shown to increase on diets rich in forage (Reynolds et al., 1991).

Nitrogen content of the diet

Excess nitrogen content in the diet increases the NEm requirements. High concentrations of CP may be found in grass, and surpluses of nitrogen have to be excreted. The synthesis and excretion of urea in sheep requires 21.8 kJ/g excreted N (Martin and Blaxter, 1965).

Condition of the cows

The condition of the cows may also play a role in increased maintenance requirements. Lean cows may have higher maintenance requirements than fat cows, because of the higher rate of turnover of protein compared to body fat (Kirkland and Gordon, 1999).

Lean body mass is associated with greater metabolic activity and is positively correlated with basal energy expenditure (Speakman et al., 2004).

Breed effect

There is considerable evidence to suggest differences in maintenance requirements among beef breeds (NRC, 1996). A portion of the breed effect on maintenance requirements in beef cattle is due to inherent differences in lean tissue as a fraction of total body weight (BW) among breed types. Early experiments suggested a similar scenario for dairy breeds (Van Es, 1961), but a more recent comparison of Holstein and Jersey cattle indicates that although milk production was greater for Holstein cows, the energy requirements per unit of metabolic weight were the same for both breeds (Tyrrell et al., 1991). Similarities in lean mass percentage among dairy cattle breeds may be one of the underlying biological effects that obviate a breed adjustment for maintenance requirement. The NRC (2001) accepts a lack of variability due to breed in assigning maintenance energy requirements.

Immune challenge

One of the challenges in animal nutrition is in understanding how energy is partitioned among physiological processes. There is a paucity of research that directly examines the impact of immune challenges on maintenance energy expenditure. However, it is well recognized that sub-acute disease affects productivity. Therefore, it is reasonable to assume that a portion of the costs of an immune challenge are reflected in increased maintenance costs.

Visceral organ size

Visceral organ size plays a critical role in determining energy expenditure. Liver represents approximately 1.6% of empty BW but it receives 30% of cardiac output and is responsible for 25% of FHP (Baldwin, 1995). Therefore, a small change in liver size or metabolic activity may have a tremendous impact on maintenance requirements. For example, liver weight is greater in lactating cows compared to nonlactating cows. Most of this 25% increase in liver size is needed to accommodate the increased needs for gluconeogenesis and ureagenesis that accompany lactation. Smith and Baldwin (1974) suggested that maintenance requirements for lactating cows are about 10% higher than for non-lactating cows because of bigger internal organs (heart, lungs, stomach and intestines), and a higher feed consumption in lactating animals.

Relationship between BMR and visceral organ size: The close relationship between basal metabolic rate and visceral organ size is highlighted in laboratory mice that have been subjected to divergent selection for a high and low basal metabolic rate (Ksiazek et al., 2004). Food consumption was greater for high BMR mice, and organ weights were also greater when expressed either as absolute weight or as portion of lean body mass. Greater liver weights were associated with greater BMR. The fact that BW did not differ between these lines of mice but BMR was clearly different indicates the importance of visceral tissue to the whole body maintenance requirement.

Selection of animals for low maintenance requirement

The coefficient of variation for maintenance for cows under controlled conditions is 8 to 10% (Van Es, 1961). Therefore, this variation could represent an opportunity to select animals with an inherently low maintenance requirement, and thus existence of a high potential efficiency for channeling nutrients to milk or tissue gain.

Effects of early life events on maintenance requirements

Considerable data indicate that events during certain critical periods of gestation can have a lasting impact on the metabolism of the offspring (Barker and Clark, 1997; McMillen et al., 2001). The **fetal programming hypothesis** of metabolic diseases has evolved from epidemiological data that linked low birth weight, maternal nutrition, and increased prevalence of adult disease (Barker and Clark, 1997).

It is becoming increasingly obvious that **epigenetic inheritance**, or non-DNA based forms of heritability, may also be part of the fetal programming puzzle (Bogdarina et al., 2004). It appears that a portion of these changes may involve alterations in BMR. Although these effects have not been specifically documented for dairy cattle, the available evidence suggests that the potential exists in this regard.

A study in mature human subjects identified a correlation with body composition and energy expenditure that is linked to fetal growth and birth weight (Kensara et al., 2006). Specifically, low birth weight individuals displayed less fat free body mass as adults and had lower resting energy expenditure. Similar programming effects may exist for dairy cattle and may impact requirements for maintenance, production, or both (Donkin, 2008.

5

Optimizing Nitrogen Efficiency in Ruminant Animals; Enhancing Milk Nitrogen Efficiency

INTRODUCTION

A major advantage of ruminants is their ability to convert vast quantities of otherwise human inedible, low digestibility plant material (forages, crop residues) into high quality human edible food products. The down side, however, is that ruminant converts only 5 to 35% of dietary nitrogen (N) into products such as milk, meat and wool (compared to 45-50% in case of pigs and poultry). As a consequence of this low efficiency, ruminants excrete significant amounts of N as manure into the environment. The excess nitrogen excreted can result in both water and air pollution.

However, there is much greater potential to improve N efficiency of ruminants, and reduce manure wastes through a better understanding of the urea recycling process. One of the main areas where significant losses of N occur, and where there is large potential for improvement, is ammonia absorption (46-47% of the N available in the gut lumen) and excretion of N (30-70% of urea production) into urine as urea. Ammonia utilization can be improved and thus urea excretion can be minimized. Numerous feeding strategies have been evaluated with the focus on improving nitrogen efficiency. All these improvements in efficiency should lead to reduce feed costs associated with expensive protein supplements.

Improving N efficiency through enhanced efficiency of N recycling

Urea is recycled to the gastrointestinal tract (GIT) through plasma, endogenous secretions and saliva and in ruminants this process is a major mechanism to ensure high rates of microbial protein synthesis and to maintain the supply of a high quality protein (microbial protein) for meat, milk and wool synthesis. Thus, urea recycling or N recycling is of tremendous importance to ruminants. Now let us know the fates of urea entering GIT, mechanism of urea transfer to the GIT and the factors affecting urea-N recycling and utilization in ruminants.

I. Amounts of ammonia absorbed from the gastrointestinal tract

In both ruminants and non-ruminant animals, ammonia is generated in the GIT lumen (rumen, small intestines, lower gut) from microbial activity. However, in ruminants, ammonia-N represents from 37 to 66% of the total N sources (amino acid-N and ammonia-N) absorbed, whereas in pigs ammonia-N represents a smaller proportion (about 26%; Lenis *et al.*, 1996).

In ruminants, absorbed ammonia-N is converted to urea by the liver, with the urea either excreted into urine or recycled to the rumen for use in microbial protein synthesis. The extent that absorbed ammonia is partitioned between these two fates is variable and largely unpredictable in ruminants. Given the magnitude and potential that recycling of urea to the rumen has on overall N economy, efforts have been made to summarize current knowledge of the mechanisms controlling and dietary factors influencing the urea recycling process as a first step towards defining the contribution of this process to N economy and the protein nutrition of dairy cows, and for ruminants in general (Brian J. Bequette and Nishanth E. Sunny, 2005).

Nitrogen recycling

The term "urea recycling" is not strictly correct because it is not the urea molecule that is recycled, but rather it is N that recycles. Gastrointestinal N recycling occurs in mammals (via urea) and to some extent in poultry (via uric acid transport to the colon and caeca by retrograde peristalsis). In ruminants, however, the proportion of urea transferred to the GIT is higher (10-80%) and of much greater importance to overall N economy than in other species.

Urea recycling (also known as "the protein regeneration cycle") has long been recognized as a major mechanism to improve protein quality of animals, especially in ruminants fed low protein or low quality roughage-based diets. Urea is synthesised mainly by the liver as the end product of ammonia and amino acid metabolism in all mammals. In all mammals, the amount of urea produced by the liver is much greater than the amount of urea excreted into the urine. Urea that is not excreted into the urine has two potential fates: 1. It can be partitioned to the rumen where urea is rapidly hydrolyzed to ammonia and used by microbes for protein synthesis which subsequently can be digested and absorbed in the small intestines and 2. Urea may be partitioned via the blood to the lower GIT (caecum, large intestines) where the N is lost to the faeces as microbial protein-N.

Fates of urea entering the gastrointestinal tract

In rumino-reticulum: Urea is water soluble and distributed throughout all body fluids. Thus, urea has the potential to enter all compartments of the GIT through normal GIT secretions (i.e. saliva, gastric juice, bile and pancreatic juice) and by diffusion from blood (Kennedy and Milligan, 1980; Egan *et al.*, 1986). Estimates in sheep are that 27-60% of GIT entry is directed to the rumen (via saliva or blood transfers) (Kennedy and Milligan, 1978; Koenig et al., 2000). Ruminants rely heavily upon the presence of a large and active microbial population in the rumen to enhance the transfer (via rumen wall and saliva) of urea to the rumen for capture by microbes for protein absorption. However, depending upon diet characteristics that may shift fermentative activity throughout the GIT, urea transfer to the rumen is also variable. Most of the urea entering the GIT is hydrolyzed to NH_3 by the action of urease in the bacteria that localise at the luminal surfaces of the rumen, small intestines, caecum and large intestines. The released ammonia is either reabsorbed into blood as ammonia or it is utilized as a N source for microbial protein synthesis, some of which may be excreted into the faeces (about 10%).

In caecum or large intestine: By contrast, if bacterial synthesis from the hydrolysed urea occurs in either the caecum or large intestines, sites where amino acids are not known to be absorbed, then recycled urea will be lost to the faeces. The NH3 not captured by the bacteria and absorbed from the GIT is removed by the liver and again converted to urea. Similarly, the amino acids of bacterial origin, derived from recycled urea-N, may also be absorbed and catabolized by the liver to yield urea (Sarraseca et al., 1998; Milano et al., 2000), and the cycle continues. The fractional contributions of recycled urea-N towards each of these fates depends upon various conditions in the rumen (pH, ammonia/ammonium concentration, fermentable energy) which themselves are determined by dietary factors such as protein content, nitrogen solubility, the concentrate:forage content of the diet, available or fermentable energy, and others.

Efficiency of N or urea recycling

Urea transfer to the rumen: Kennedy and Milligan (1980) suggested that rumen clearance of urea (theoretically the same as rumen urea entry), which is the product of rumen epithelial permeability to urea and the functional area of rumen epithelia, is greater in sheep than in beef cattle. This may be due to a greater permeability of sheep rumen epithelia to urea (1.7 times that of cattle) or due to differences in the papillary bed (e.g. more surface area in sheep). These observations suggest that sheep may be more efficient in utilizing recycled urea for anabolic purposes compared to cattle. It is reported that buffaloes are more efficient in recycling urea into the rumen, which means that buffalo rumen epithelium must have a greater permeability to urea. It is to be explored.

Wallace et al. (1979) proposed a hypothesis based on the urease activity in the rumen. Here, bacterial urease incorporates into the cornified ruminal epithelium, allowing urea to be rapidly broken down to ammonia. This creates a large concentration gradient of ammonia, thereby "pulling" urea molecules into the more acidic rumen environment. Studies as early as 1965 also suggested that urea transport across ruminal epithelium followed saturation kinetics, implying that there may exist an active transport system for urea. Indeed, recently, carrier mediated facilitative urea transport mechanisms have been identified in rumen epithelia and ovine colon, which aides in the bidirectional transport of urea by these tissues (Marini and Van Amburgh, 2003).

Urea transfer to the small intestines: Up to 70% of recycled urea has been reported to enter post stomach tissues (small intestine and large intestine) (Reynolds and Huntington, 1988; Huntington, 1989).

Most of the urea-N entering the small intestines is converted to ammonia and returned to the liver, rather than being used for microbial protein synthesis. Observations have been made in pigs and humans, where ^{15}N forms of either urea or ammonia were infused into the intestine or colon, that luminal-generated or derived [15]NH_3 appears in **lysine** and **threonine** of animal proteins. Because these two **amino acids cannot undergo transamination** in the animal body, they would have been synthesised by microbes in the hind-gut and absorbed into the body. In humans, who are most often fed to maintenance, the net supplies of lysine and threonine from intestinal or hind-gut bacterial synthesis can contribute about 10% to amino acid requirements. Lapierre and Lobley (2001) have argued that the net supply of amino acids from hind-gut bacterial synthesis in ruminants probably occurs, but is unlikely to make a substantial contribution to whole body amino acids requirements, especially under growing or lactating conditions when net growth requirements for amino acids are 3-4 times that of maintenance.

Urea transfer to the caecum and large intestines: Studies by Dixon and Milligan (1984) in sheep and Bergner *et al.* (1986) in bulls suggest a minimal role for the lower digestive tract (cecum, colon) in the degradation of urea and reutilization of the N by hind gut microbes for net amino acid absorption. They found that most of the urea-N transferred to the hind-gut appeared in the faeces, most likely bound in the microbial biomass. However, provision of fermentable energy to the caecum increases the proportion of urea entry to the GIT that is lost to faeces (10-25%), and this probably explains **why the feeding of large amounts of resistant starch results in higher faecal N excretions.**

Mechanisms of urea transfer to the GIT
Diffusion or Transport of urea from blood

It is known that high plasma urea concentrations lead to greater diffusion and urea recycling to the GIT. A recent comprehensive analysis across studies by Lapierre and Lobley (2001) showed that this relationship occurs only at plasma urea concentrations of < 6 mM for sheep and < 4 mM for cattle, and that above these concentrations urea entry is inhibited, presumably by **boundary layer effects** by rumen ammonia (Egan et al., 1986). Lapierre and Lobley (2001) also pointed out that the correlation between plasma urea concentration and GIT entry of urea was very low when plasma urea exceeded 6 mM.

To distinguish the effects of boundary layer (i.e. rumen events) from the animal's capacity to transport urea across the GIT tissues, Sunny *et al.* (2004) manipulated blood urea by infusion and followed the fates of urea with [^{15}N] urea in sheep. In the absence of dietary intake and crude protein effects that may disturb rumen fermentation, Sunny et al. (2004) observed a highly significant linear correlation between plasma urea concentration (2.5 to 14 mM) and urea entry to the GIT. These data suggested that (1) urea diffusion or transporter activity probably do not limit urea transfer to the GIT and (2) ruminants, or at least the sheep in this study, have a very large capacity to recycle urea to the rumen.

Salivary transfer of urea to the GIT

Factors that affect salivary flow rate: Saliva is also a significant route (15-100%) of urea-N transfer to the rumen, the extent of which will depend upon type of diet (e.g. concentrate vs. forage) (Huntington, 1989). As recycling of urea through saliva can be measured as the product of saliva flow rate and urea concentration, factors affecting salivary flow rate, for example rumination activity, feed intake, etc., will affect urea transfer via saliva (Egan et al., 1986). For example, a diet high in fibre or a dry forage stimulates rumination activity which in turn increases salivary flow to the rumen. Marini and Van Amburgh (2003) observed an increase in salivary transfer of urea with high levels of N intake. The amount transferred were approximately 3-4% of the total urea GIT entry. Generally, salivary transfer dominates when the animal is fed a forage diet (about 70%) compared to a concentrate diet (about 23%; Lapierre and Lobley, 2001).

Factors that affect urea-N recycling and utilization in ruminants

Ammonia produced in the GIT from the hydrolysis of urea entering the GIT can be reutilized for synthesis of amino acids which can be reabsorbed and used for productive purposes. The percent of recycled urea used for bacterial protein synthesis within the rumen ranges from 46% to 63%, depending on the level of intake, type of diet, and fermentable energy intake (Sarraseca et al., 1998; Lobley et al., 2000; Archibeque et al., 2000). However, it is possible for the ammonia from rumen hydrolysis of urea-N to be reabsorbed and re-enter the liver ornithine-urea cycle several times without being excreted in the urine. Thus, multiple entries of the same urea-N into the ornithine cycle will increase the probability of capture and bacterial use of urea-N within the rumen for protein synthesis. The extent that urea-N recycles from rumen to liver to rumen is highly dependent upon prevailing conditions in the rumen, and type of fermentation characteristics promoted by diet ingredients.

1. **Dietary protein intake**
    In general, at low protein intakes and when low quality roughage diets are fed, ruminants tend to have lower blood concentrations of urea, lower urinary urea excretion and increased transfer of urea to the GIT (Huntington, 1989; Marini and Van Amburgh, 2003). Archibeque et al. (2001) evaluated the effects of two forage species, each having two levels of N, on urea kinetics and N metabolism. They concluded that the efficiency of N use is greater at low N intakes even though the absolute movements of N through the body (i.e. urea flux) increased with N intake. By contrast, in sheep fed low quality hay, urea recycled to the GIT accounted for 80-90% of hepatic urea synthesis and a higher proportion of absorbed N was retained (Bunting et al., 1987).

2. **Energy intake and fermentability of the diet**
    Increasing the fermentable carbohydrate fraction of the diet increases urea recycling to the rumen (Kennedy, 1980; Kennedy and Milligan, 1980; Huntington, 1989) but decreases urea transfer to post gastric tissues (Reynolds and Huntington, 1988). Thus, supplemental grain, starch, dried pulp and sucrose provided as energy sources significantly increases urea degradation

in the GIT, particularly in the rumen. This response may be due to a combination of factors including a reduction in rumen ammonia concentration, and an increase in the quantity and rate of fermentation of dietary organic matter in the rumen (Kennedy and Milligan, 1980).

Intraruminal infusion of sucrose was found to increase propionate production in addition to lowering the rumen ammonia and plasma urea concentration, all of which promoted increased urea recycling to the GIT. In turn, propionate was available for glucose synthesis, thus sparing amino acids for tissue growth (Obara and Dellow, 1993; Seal and Parker, 1996). Propionate itself may also play a role in regulating urea recycling. In sheep given an infusion of propionate into the abomasum (post-rumen), urea entry to the GIT increased and the sheep retained more N (+5 g/d) (Kim *et al.*, 1999).

However, it is to be ascertained, whether the effect of propionate relates to an energy response, a stimulation of insulin secretion or some specific affect of propionate on rumen tissues.

3. Feed processing

Theurer et al. (2002) observed an increase in urea-N recycling to the GIT with a resultant decrease in urinary urea-N output in growing beef steers fed **steam-flaked sorghum** compared to **dry rolled sorghum**. This response may be due to the fact that steam-flaking increases starch and crude protein digestibility. Processing of feed may result in better synchrony of starch and N fermentation in the rumen, which consequently made, rapid capture and lowering of rumen ammonia to allow greater diffusion of blood urea to through the GIT wall (Huntington, 1997).

4. Rumen ammonia concentration

Rumen ammonia concentration may have a direct effect (decrease permeability of ruminal epithelia) on urea entry to GIT or it may affect concentrations of other fermentation products that impede urea entry to the GIT. Rumen ammonia concentrations may depress urease activity (Egan *et al.*, 1986), but to date no direct evidence exists to support this contention. They hypothesized that a **'boundary layer effect'** of ammonia and carbon dioxide at the rumen liquid may occur at the epithelial interface that inhibits urea entry to the rumen. This suggestion was based on observations that with high urease activity at the rumen epithelial interface, high levels of ammonia are generated at the rumen epithelial surface. The movement of ammonia into the rumen biomass or into the blood will therefore depend upon the pH at these two locations and the ammonia gradient generated between the extra cellular fluid of the rumen wall and the rumen liquid.

5. The rumen pH

The ratio of ammonia (unionised, NH_3) to ammonium (ionized, NH^{4+}) ions and carbon dioxide to bicarbonate ions also may be **potential determinants of entry of urea** to the rumen. Feeding greater soluble carbohydrates lowers rumen pH to about 5.5-6.0, thus shifting the proportion of ionized to unionized ammonia more towards the ionized form. As it is only the unionized (NH_3)

form that diffuses across the rumen epithelial wall into the blood, ammonia absorption will be impeded and ammonia will build-up locally at the rumen wall surface. Thus, recycled urea will be rapidly hydrolyzed due to the high urease activity of bacteria adhering to the rumen wall, creating a further 'boundary layer effect' from the local build-up of ammonia (Egan *et al.*, 1986). Egan *et al.* (1986) reasoned that the boundary layer effect is one of the major impediments to the entry of urea from the blood to the rumen, in consequence, incr asing the fraction of urea entry excreted in the urine.

II. Enhancing nitrogen efficiency in lactating dairy cows

Numerous studies show that dairy cows utilize feed CP (N × 6.25) much more efficiently than other ruminant livestock but still excrete about 2 to3 times more N in manure than in milk. Inefficient N utilization necessitates feeding large amounts of supplemental protein, increasing milk production costs, and contributing to environmental N pollution (Glen Broderick, 2005).

Requirement for metabolizable protein and monitoring the cow needs

Crude protein is the term that has been used to formulate and evaluate dairy rations for many years. Dairy cattle do not have a CP requirement but do need absorbable amino acids to meet requirements for maintenance, growth, pregnancy and milk production.

The function of dietary CP is to supply the cow with metabolizable protein (MP) as absorbed amino acids (AA), but any extra dietary CP that does not contribute to absorbed AA that are used in production will be largely lost in the urine. Urinary N is the most polluting form of excretory N because much of it is lost as atmospheric ammonia or into surface and ground water. Hence a number of refinements have been added over the years to increase the usefulness of the CP system. These include considering soluble protein, rumen degraded protein and rumen undegraded protein (RUP). The NRC (2001) Dairy publication proposes that metabolizable protein (MP) be used for ration formulation rather than CP. Metabolizable protein is basically the sum of microbial protein and RUP. Requirements for metabolizable protein (MP) are the sum of protein necessary to support maintenance, lactation, growth and gestation. In dairy cows, the requirement for MP for production is milk true protein yield divided by 67%.

Use of milk urea nitrogen (MUN) as a practical tool for monitoring herd performance

When supplies of RDP and rumen undegradable protein (RUP) are balanced for milk production, plasma urea will fall within a specific range for a group of cows (Roseler *et al.*, 1993). In addition, milk urea is as useful as blood urea to monitor protein status (Baker *et al.*, 1992; Roseler *et al.*, 1993). Urea moves into milk via passive diffusion from blood and rapidly equilibrates with blood values (Baker *et al.*, 1992). Based on work by Baker and Roseler, it was proposed that the mean optimal urea values for a group of cows would fall between 10 to 14 mg/dl and 95% of the individual cows in the group would range +/- six units from the mean milk urea nitrogen (MUN) value (DePeters and Ferguson, 1992). The minimum value of 10 mg/dl agrees with Hof *et al.* (1997) observation for the minimum MUN value below which rumen available N may impair performance. Higher values of MUN would be associated with reduced efficiency of protein utilization and would be wasteful. Therefore, MUN serves as a useful tool to assess protein feeding efficiency (Hof *et al.*, 1997; Jonker *et al.*, 1998). In nonlactating cattle, blood samples would need to be used to assess urea-N concentrations, but the same principles would apply.

Precision feeding

Dairy cattle diets can be adjusted to improve nitrogen efficiency. Precision feeding reduces N and P inputs to the levels required to maintain optimum production, resulting in 20-40% reductions in the nutrient content of manure. It has been demonstrated that through proper feeding management practices and careful nutritional formulation, N inputs can be reduced without compromising animal performance.

A close matching of diet to nutritional requirements of the animal, feeding only enough RUP to meet cows' metabolizable protein requirements, reducing particle size to increase ruminal digestion of grain starch and increase microbial protein formation optimizes microbial protein synthesis, maximizes feed N conversion into milk and minimizes urinary N excretion. Ammonia emissions from dairy cow stalls can be reduced by using bedding materials and using the floor configurations that physically separate faeces (which contains urease) and urine.

Factors that affect efficiency of feed N transformation into milk

Ruminants obtain the metabolizable protein (MP) required for maintenance and production from microbial protein synthesized in the rumen plus dietary protein that escapes the rumen undegraded. The amino acid (AA) pattern of this protein is better than the feedstuffs commonly fed to domestic ruminants (Schwab, 1996). Optimizing microbial protein formation in the rumen plus feeding only enough rumen-undegraded protein (RUP) to meet the cow's MP requirements are the best strategies for maximizing N transformation into milk(J.M. Powell and G.A. Broderick, 2009).

1. Optimizing synthesis of microbial protein in the rumen

Ammonia level: Ruminal bacteria utilize peptides, AA and ammonia for protein synthesis. *In vitro* research showed that microbial protein formation was not improved by ammonia-N concentrations greater than 5 mg/dL (Satter and Slyter, 1974). However, *in situ* studies suggested that ammonia-N levels as high as 20 mg/dL (Mehrez *et al.*, 1977) may be required to maximize carbohydrate digestion in the rumen. Ammonia derives largely from deamination of AA released from rumen-degraded protein (RDP) and ammonia production parallels formation of peptides and free AA.

Protein degradation products other than ammonia: The NRC (2001) feeding model assumes that RDP from nonprotein N (NPN) sources, such as urea, are equivalent to RDP from true protein. However, protein degradation products other than ammonia stimulate microbial protein synthesis. Recently, it was demonstrated that replacing RDP from true protein (soybean meal; SBM) with that from urea depressed yields of milk, fat and protein. These responses were due to reduced ruminal outflow of nonammonia N (NAN) and total AA that resulted from reduced microbial protein formation (Broderick and Reynal, 2009).

There are substantial differences in ruminal fermentability among dietary sources of fibre (Coblentz and Hoffman, 2009), starch (Herrera-Saldana et al., 1990) and other carbohydrates. For example, effects of reducing maize particle size on extent of ruminal starch digestion are much greater than effects on total tract digestibility (Owens et al., 1986).

Particle size and ruminal starch digestion: It was found that grinding high moisture maize through a 1-cm screen optimized ammonia uptake *in vitro* and feeding this high moisture maize grain (with 1.7 mm mean particle size) reduced *in vivo* ammonia concentration in the rumen and increased milk yield (2.4 kg/d) and protein yield (120 g/d) compared to control high moisture maize (with 4.3 mm mean particle size) (Ekinci and Broderick, 1997).

Reducing mean particle size of dry shelled corn from 3.5 to 0.6 mm increased ruminal starch digestibility from 54 to 70% (Remond et al., 2004). Charbonneau et al. (2006) observed that replacing cracked corn with ground corn or ground corn plus cornstarch increased milk yield (10%) and protein yield (14%) in lactating dairy cows.

2. Optimizing amount and composition of rumen degraded protein – practising phase feeding

Dietary CP that is not utilized by the cow gets excreted largely as urinary N, regardless of whether the CP is digested in the rumen or the intestine.

Diets with 3 energy densities (36, 32, and 28% NDF in dietary DM) at each of 3 levels of CP (15.1 to 16.7, and 18.4% of DM, added as solvent SBM) were fed to cows (Broderick, 2003). Cows responded to CP the same at all 3 energy levels: milk and protein yield increased from 15.1 to 16.7% CP, but there were no production differences between 16.7 and 18.4% CP. However, marked increases in urinary N excretion (virtually all as urea) were observed with added CP.

In a later trial, dietary CP was increased, in steps of about 1.5 percentage units, from 13.5 to 19.4% CP (Olmos Colmenero and Broderick, 2006). Milk urea N reflected the linear increase in urinary N excretion, and linear decrease in milk N/N-intake, that occurred with elevated CP. Production was highest on 16.5% CP and quadratic responses indicated that milk and protein yields were maximal at, respectively, 16.7 and 17.1% CP. Greater than those levels of CP reduced yields, a surprising result in view of the common practice of feeding lactating cows diets with 18% or more CP (Shaver and Kaiser, 2004). Depressed production at higher CP may have occurred because high moisture maize grain was replaced with SBM, which diluted dietary energy, and because of the metabolic cost of excreting excess N as urea (NRC, 1989). Most of these trials were short-term reversal studies in which diets are switched after a few weeks.

Wu and Satter (2000) conducted a study for the entire lactation period following the phase feeding of protein. They found that the dietary CP regime supporting optimum yield of fat-corrected milk (FCM) over the whole lactation involved feeding 17.4% CP for the first 16-weeks after calving, followed by 16.0% CP for the remaining 28 weeks. Increasing CP to as much as 19.3% during the first-phase, or to 17.9% CP during the second phase, did not improve yield of FCM, but only increased N excretion.

3. Feeding enough RUP

Compared to an isonitrogenous diet supplemented with urea, it was found much greater production when feeding 1 of 3 true proteins that differed in RUP and AA content (Brito and Broderick, 2007). Although flow of RUP and total protein from the rumen was greatest on cottonseed meal, intermediate on canola meal and lowest on SBM (Brito et al., 2007), protein and fat yield both were highest on canola meal, intermediate on SBM, and lowest on cottonseed meal. Enhanced production on different sources likely was related to the AA pattern of the RUP being complementary to microbial protein (Broderick, 1994).

Importance of rumen-protected methionine: Methionine and lysine are the essential AA most often limiting for lactating dairy cows (Schwab, 1996). Responses to rumen-protected methionine (RPM) have been more consistent than to rumen-protected lysine (Armentano et al., 1997). Similar protein yield, and even greater yield of milk and FCM were obtained, when RPM was fed in diets containing 17.3 and 16.1% CP versus an 18.6% CP diet without RPM (Broderick et al., 2008). Moreover, production on 15.8% CP plus RPM was about equal to that on 17.1% CP without RPM in a recent study (Broderick et al., 2009). The results of other trials confirm that RPM supplements will correct the methionine limitation without adding dietary CP.

How to reduce nitrogen excretion in dairy cows?

Nitrogen excretion is a function of protein feeding. Reducing dietary protein decreases nitrogen excretion, and it may-but does not have to-reduce milk yield. Reducing dietary protein, while concomitantly balancing for amino acids, can result in an equivalent or greater milk yield.

Feeding low CP rations to dairy cows without affecting their milk yield

Dairy producers should consider lowering crude protein (CP) levels in rations for two primary reasons. One is to improve profitability by increasing the efficiency of converting feed nitrogen (N) intake to milk N output while maintaining milk production. A second reason is that feeding lower CP rations decreases the excretion of N to the environment. On many of farms, there is an opportunity to lower ration CP by 0.5 to 1.5 units with minimal risk of lowering milk production (Chase et al., 2009).

A number of trials testing various levels of CP in diets were conducted and found that, generally, there were no increases in yields of milk, fat-corrected milk, or protein with more than 16.5% dietary CP. In one trial, reducing CP to 15.6%, but adding rumen undegraded protein (RUP) as heated soybean meal (SBM), did not support production equal to 16.6% CP. However, fish meal, especially low soluble fish meal, and canola meal were found to be more effective sources of RUP than SBM or cottonseed meal.

Milk N efficiency (MNE)

In simple terms, nitrogen consumed in the feed is either used as a nutrient source to support productive functions (maintenance, growth, pregnancy, milk) or it is excreted via urine and faeces. The dairy cow has a limited ability to store N compared with energy. Milk N efficiency (MNE) is one index that can be used to assess the efficiency of N use in the dairy cow. This index is simply the ratio of the quantity of N excreted via the milk as a percent of the quantity of feed N consumed. The MNE values observed in commercial dairy herds usually ranges between 20 and 35%. This implies that 65 to 80% of the consumed N is excreted in the manure. As ration CP increases, the MNE value tends to decrease.

The following salient findings can be drawn from a research trial in which rations ranging from 13.5 to 19.4% CP were fed (Olmos Colmenero and Broderick, 2006).

- The quantity of N excreted in the milk changed very little for all levels of ration CP used in this trial.
- Total manure N excreted per day increased as ration N intake went up.
- The portion of the total manure N found in the faecal portion varied little with increasing ration CP levels.
- As total N excretion went up with higher levels of ration CP, urinary N was the main route of excreting excess N.
- Milk N efficiency decreased as ration CP increased.

Formulating diets for achieving efficient and economical milk production

Formulating diets for specific target levels is a fundamental and practical approach for achieving efficient and economical milk production (Dave Byers, 2007). Formulate for specific nutrients, which can be measured in a laboratory.

1. Fibre carbohydrates: The most important nutrient to formulate for in dairy rations is the fibre. It is necessary for the health of the rumen, the health of the animal, and the efficiency of fermentation. Formulate for 32 - 34% NDF. This is higher than many recommendations and slightly higher than the NRC (2001). Furthermore, aim for effective NDF.

2. Nonfibre carbohydrates (NFC): After meeting the fibre requirement, the objective is to liberally feed glucose precursors, primarily starches and sugars, to drive milk production. This produces the following cascade of events: starches & sugars >>> propionate (rumen) >>> glucose (liver) >>> lactose (mammary gland).

Milk production varies directly with the production of lactose, because it is the osmotic regulator of milk yield. Optimizing the levels of starch and sugars is necessary for the best possible milk performance (Broderick and Radloff, 2004).

3. Protein: Formulate for balancing for three protein fractions. First, balance for RDP, It is as follows: RDP = NFC (lb) / 3.30. Target for a balance of -0.30 to -0.50 lb/d. The reason for a negative balance is that it permits feeding/diets lower in crude protein. Second, formulate for the amino acid, lysine. The target level is a balance of +4.0 to +8.0 g/d. Lastly, formulate for the amino acid, methionine. The target level is a balance of -2.0 to -4.0 g/d. The typical strategy is to formulate diets with feeds that are relatively rich in rumen undegraded, lysine, and if necessary or beneficial, supplement with rumen protected, methionine.

4. Fat: Since fats are not sources of fermentable energy for rumen microbes, use minimal levels of fat. There is, however, a level of fat needed to support reproductive efficiency (3.0 - 5.0% is adequate). Where possible, follow fat levels in the lower part of this range (3.0 - 4.0%). The literature does tend to show two disadvantages of liberally fat feeding (>5.0%). One, DMI is generally depressed, especially with Ca salts of FA. This seems to be the result of unsaturated fat increasing satiety and reducing gut motility. Two, protein test is generally depressed 1 - 2 points.

5. Ash: Try to restrict the level of ash below 7% in rations. This gives ration space in order to feed extra fermentable carbohydrates.

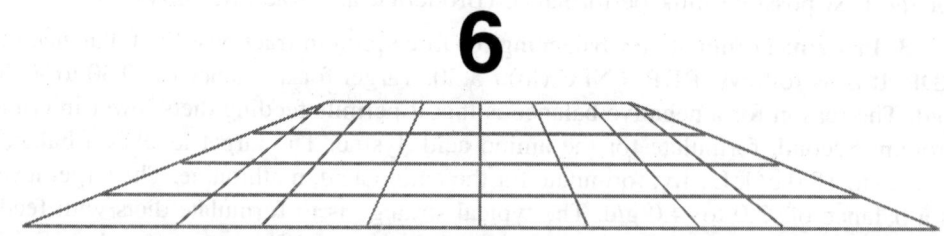

6

Diet and Milk Production; Maximizing Milk Components and Metabolizable Protein Utilization

INTRODUCTION

The ability of cows / buffaloes to produce milk depends largely on water and feed eaten and intake of nutrients (dry matter, energy, protein and fibre). The feed must first be digested for the products of digestion to be absorbed into the blood from the digestive tract. The ability of animals to produce milk depends on how they use or partition (see chapter on 'Partitioning of Nutrients' pp 63) these products of digestion for maintenance, pregnancy, milk production or growth / body condition. Feed intake and their capacity to use or partitioning of the absorbed products of digestion to metabolic activities influence the volume and composition of milk produced.

The products of digestion are VFA, microbial protein, undegradable dietary protein (UDP / RUP), fats. Others include ammonia, carbon dioxide, methane and undigested fibre, of which ammonia and undigested fibre are utilized mostly in large intestine. These products of digestion reach blood through rumen and intestines for their ultimate utilization for maintenance and to form tissue for growth or milk in the udder. **Fats** are formed from acetate, butyrate and fats in the diet, **glucose** from propionate, and **amino acids** from microbial protein and UDP / RUP those reach blood circulation of the animal, and they becoming available for their role in metabolic processes.

Milk production process

Milk is formed in the mammary gland by the udder tissue. About 500 L of blood pass through the udder to produce 1 L of milk. Cells in the udder tissue use these substrates to form and secrete milk which is made up of water, minerals, lactose, milk fat and milk protein. The level of fat and protein in milk varies with many factors such as the breed of cow / buffalo, stage of lactation, body condition and the diet. The total lactation yield of an animal depends on quantity of milk at peak lactation and the rate of decline from the peak. In temperate dairy systems, total milk yield for a 300-day lactation can be estimated by multiplying peak milk yield by 200.

Lactose production in the udder

The udder makes lactose from glucose arriving in the blood. The lactose secreted into the udder attracts water with it, at roughly constant proportions. The lactose content of milk is about 4.8% and hardly varies. Therefore, the quantity of glucose arriving at the udder determines how much lactose is produced, hence what volume of milk produced. The relationship between quantity of glucose reaching the udder and volume of milk produced can be described as follows:

More Blood Glucose → More Lactose → More Milk → Constant Lactose Content
(Kg)   (L)

Fat production in the udder

The secretory cells in the udder make milk fat from the fat carried in the blood. These blood fats come from acetate and butyrate (mainly from fibre in the diet), from the fat that is mobilized body tissue, or from fats in the diet. Fat percentage in milk varies greatly. It depends on the type of energy in the diet, the stage of lactation, body condition of the cow/buffalo and energy intake.

The type of energy in the diet: Fat percentage is higher in diets high in fibre, when the blood carries more acetate while it is lower in diets high in starch, because the blood contains more glucose (from the propionate), which is used for lactose production. On a high starch diet, not only is less milk fat produced, but the extra lactose produced increases the milk volume, diluting the fat even more.

The stage of lactation: Fat percentage is likely to be lower in early lactation when milk volume is at its highest.

Body condition of the animal: In animals of good body condition, body condition loss in early lactation may help maintain milk fat concentration as yield increases.

Energy intake: When energy intakes are high, rumen fermentation rates are also high, the rumen is more acidic, and the starch-digesting microbes which produce propionate will work better than the fibre-digesting microbes which produce acetate. With more propionate, there will be more lactose produced and, therefore, a greater volume of milk. With less acetate, there will be less milk fat.

Protein production in the udder

The udder makes milk protein (casein) from the amino acids and glucose carried in the blood. Amino acids are the building blocks, and the glucose provides the energy needed to form the protein.

Supply of amino acids to the udder is plentiful, but there is no enough glucose energy available to build them into protein: In this situation, some of the amino acids are converted to glucose, and used to provide energy. This is not an efficient use of feed because it wastes the protein-producing potential of the amino acids.

Glucose is plentiful but amino acids are in short supply: In this situation, the building of milk protein will be limited. The surplus glucose may produce some lactose, but most will be stored. Cows will then put on body weight rather than produce more milk. This is also not an efficient use of feed.

Milk protein and lactose production (and hence milk volume) are related because glucose in the blood is needed to produce both lactose and milk protein.

A well-balanced diet high in energy furnish appropriate amounts of amino acids and amount of glucose in the blood, ready for protein and lactose production for milk production.

Diets with higher level of concentrate feeds

With intensification of small holder dairying in many peri-urban areas (due to government schemes under poverty alleviation for landless people and other sections of the society), shortage in availability of roughage (see chapter on 'Feeding Practices') has led to increasing amounts of concentrate feeding. This kind of feeding inappropriate amounts of brans and oilseed cakes and roughages has dramatic effects on milk composition.

Sanh (2001) conducted a series of feeding trials using crossbred Friesian cows fed diets based on varying proportions of Napier grass, brewer's grain, and local byproducts such as rice bran, cassava meal, maize bran, and groundnut cake. Forage: concentrate ratios varied from 70:30 to 30:70. When the forage ratio decreased from the highest to lowest, the cows responded with higher daily milk yields as the concentrate amount increased. In, addition, contents of milk protein increased and of milk fat decreased with increasing percentage of concentrates, of which milk fat was more affected than milk protein.

Milk production – body condition – hormones

Body condition of cow/buffalo at calving has a large effect on milk production and fertility. The animal either stores body fat or mobilizes it, depending on the level and type of feed and the stage of lactation. Two hormones namely **insulin** and **growth hormone** that circulate in the blood of the animal cause body fat to be used or stored. Insulin regulates the storage of body fat from the fats and glucose in the blood. Insulin is produced by the pancreas and is in higher concentrations in the blood when cows are being fed well and glucose is plentiful in the blood. **Growth hormone** regulates the release of body fat to produce milk fat. Growth hormone is produced by the pituitary gland and is in the blood in higher concentrations in early lactation or when cows are not fed well.

Effect of nutrition on milk composition

Nutrition remains an integral part of expressing the genetic potential. To the extent that milk pricing is linked to milk components, farmers / milk producers will continue to exploit nutrition of the cow as a means to modify milk composition for maximum economic return. The greatest opportunities on the horizon for manipulating milk composition will be directed at using milk for delivery of nutraceuticals (see chapter on 'Designer Milk and Milk products pp 150) to enhance human health and to combat clinical diseases, such as obesity, lactose intolerance, or osteoporosis.

Because of the greater sensitivity of milk fat to dietary manipulation than either protein or lactose, nutritional control of milk fat content and fatty acid composition received a great deal of attention. The discovery of conjugated linoleic acid (CLA) as a potent anticarcinogen also led to extensive work on enhancing its concentration in milk through nutritional manipulation and discovering the physiological effects of specific CLA isomers. New protected fats have been developed in recent years to resist biohydrogenation and enhance the concentration of unsaturated fatty acids in milk.

New insights have been tested on modes of action whereby **fat supplements caused a decline in protein concentration**. Forage to concentrate ratio, the amount and source of dietary protein, and the amount and source of dietary fat are found to influence on milk protein content.

Changes in milk lactose concentration occur only in extreme and unusual feeding situations, but the basic biology of lactose synthesis and regulation are still being explored using modern molecular techniques.

Protein Recommendations

Although variation exists, the RDP requirement for most cows will be met if diets contain about 10% RDP (DM basis). Because the cost of under feeding RDP (reduced intake causing reduced milk production) is greater than the cost of slightly overfeeding RDP (slightly increased feed costs, small increase in excretion of nitrogen via urine, and slightly increased risk of reduced reproductive performance) a small excess of RDP (5 to 10%) should be fed (approximately 10.5 to 11% of DM). Once the RDP requirement is met, RUP supply must be evaluated. The supply of RUP can be increased by increasing the total CP content of a diet or by selecting feeds with high RUP concentrations. When choosing an RUP source, the digestibility of the RUP must be considered (Table 1). Lysine or methionine is generally the first limiting amino acid for milk protein production. Diets with large amounts of maize products (maize silage, maize grain, distillers grains) will be lysine limited, and diets with high amounts of lucerne protein usually are limited in methionine.

In many cases, providing slightly more CP than required to meet RUP requirements is the most economical alternative. However, this option increases excretion of nitrogen via manure, and environmental regulations may make this option less economically feasible. Cows in early lactation and high producing cows usually require substantial amounts of RUP. The RUP supplement used should be highly digestible and provide the proper balance of amino acids.

Excess dietary RDP may reduce milk yield

Milking cows require diets containing 12 to 18% CP, depending on their stage of lactation and milk yield. Roughages are generally the cheapest feeds available. But in peri-urban areas byproduct feeds are readily available and purchased roughages are expensive. Hence byproduct feeds are offered liberally. This may lead to excess

Table 1. Average digestible RUP of some feeds

Feedstuff	RUP % of DM	RUP Digestible %	Digestibility RUP, % of DM	Amino acid Class*
Blood meal, batch dried	73	65	47.5	Lysine
Blood meal, ring-dried	73	80	58.4	Lysine
Brewers grains, dtied	16	80	12.8	Neither
Corn gluten meal	47	92	43.2	Methionine
Distillers grain	15	80	12.0	Neither
Fish meal	44	88	38.7	Lys / Met
Soybean meal, heat treated	31	93	28.8	Lysine
Soybean meal, 48% CP	22	93	20.5	Lysine
Cottonseed meal, 50% CP	21	92	19.3	Neither

*Amino acid class designates whether a given feed contains above average concentrations of lysine or methionine. When diets are limited by lysine, feeds classified as lysine should be used, and when diets are limited by methionine, feeds classified as methionine should be used. Source: W.P.Weiss (2002) Protein and carbohydrate utilization by lactating dairy cows. P44 In: North Caroline Dairy Nutrition Management Conference Proceedings

protein, with much of this protein as rumen degradable. Some times, excess dietary protein result from feeding of immature grasses or legumes with concentrates rich in RDP.

High levels of RDP lead to excess rumen ammonia, which must be detoxified in the liver in order to be excreted as urea in the urine. The metabolic costs associated with this process require energy, which would otherwise be used to produce milk. This 'urea cost' may result in 1 to 2 litres less milk per day. Feeding energy supplements high in readily fermentable carbohydrates will allow rumen bacteria to capture this RDP and synthesise microbial protein, for ultimate use by the animal to produce milk.

Balancing dairy cow rations for metabolizable protein and amino acids

Based on results of research with non-ruminant animals, Heger and Frydrych (1989) concluded that when the essential amino acids (EAA) are absorbed in the profile as required by the animal, the requirements for total EAA is reduced and their efficiency of use for protein synthesis is maximized. Research with lactating dairy cows has been shown many times that increasing predicted concentrations of lysine and methionine in metabolizable protein (MP) to recommended levels increases efficiency of use of MP for milk protein synthesis. This should not be a surprising observation in feeding situations where lysine and methionine are the first two limiting amino acids. Therefore, it is reasonable to conclude that maximizing milk components and MP utilization in lactating dairy cows requires providing a profile of amino acids in MP that matches the profile required for the combined functions of maintenance, reproduction, and milk production, and that the MP is provided in amounts that meets but doesn't exceed requirements for optimal health, reproduction and milk production (C.G. Schwab and G.N. Foster, 2009).

Research to date indicates that of the twenty amino acids that occur in proteins, only the amount and profile of EAA in MP are of concern. Providing a mixture of nonessential AA (NEAA) to post-weaned dairy calves (Schwab et al., 1982), or lactating dairy cows (Whyte et al., 2006), where one or more EAA were shown to be limiting, were without benefit. It was also observed that infusing the 10 EAA into the abomasum of lactating cows fed protein deficient diets resulted in increases in yields of milk protein that were similar to the yields that were obtained when casein was infused. Collectively, these observations indicate that when amino acids supplies approach requirements for total absorbable amino acids, requirements for total NEAA are met before the requirements for the most limiting EAA.

Concentrations of lysine and methionine in MP: Because lysine and methionine had been shown to be the first two limiting EAA for lactating dairy cows fed diets common to North America, NRC (2001) published dose-response plots that related changes in measured percentages and yields of milk protein to model-predicted changes in lysine and methionine concentrations in MP. By using a rectilinear model to describe the dose-response relationships, breakpoint estimates for the required concentrations of lysine and methionine in MP for maximal content of milk protein were determined to be 7.2 and 2.4%, respectively; corresponding values for maximal protein yield were 7.1 and 2.4%. These were the first estimates ever presented by a Dairy NRC Committee to evaluate a diet for adequacy of AA concentrations in MP, and have proven exceptionally useful for routine users of the NRC (2001) model in their quest to increase milk component yields with similar or lower predicted flows of MP. Because they can be rather easily achieved, target levels for lysine and methionine in MP have typically been 6.6 and 2.2%, respectively. Both values approximate 96% of the concentrations needed, according to NRC (2001), for maximal content and yield of milk protein.

It is recognized that histidine has been identified as the first limiting AA when grass silage and barley and oat diets are fed, with or without feather meal as a sole or primary source of supplemental RUP. Based on NRC (2001) predicted concentrations of lysine, methionine, and histidine in MP for the diets fed in these experiments, Schwab and Foster (2009) speculated that histidine may become the third limiting AA rather quickly in some diets, particularly where barley and wheat products replace significant amounts of maize in the diet.

Steps to maximize milk components and MP utilization: C.G. Schwab and G.N. Foster (2009) considered the following 5 steps as being important to maximizing milk components and MP utilization. A brief discussion of each step is also given.

Step 1: Feed a blend of high quality forages, processed grains, and byproduct feeds to provide a blend of fermentable carbohydrates and physically effective fibre that maximizes feed intake, milk production, and yield of microbial protein

Microbial protein, based on research to date, has an excellent AA composition for lactating dairy cows. The average reported concentrations of lysine and methionine in bacterial true protein approximate 7.9% and 2.6%, respectively. Realizing maximal benefits of feeding a balanced supply of fermentable carbohydrates on feed intake, milk production, and yields of microbial protein requires use of high quality feeds, adequate intakes of physically effective fibre, well-balanced and consistent diets, unlimited supplies of fresh water, and superior farm management.

Step 2: Feed adequate but not excessive levels of RDP to meet rumen bacterial requirements for AA and ammonia

Realizing the benefits of feeding a balances supply of fermentable carbohydrates on maximizing yields of microbial protein also requires balancing diets for RDP. Rumen degraded feed protein is the second largest requirement for rumen microorganisms. It supplies the microorganisms with peptides, AA, and ammonia that are needed for microbial protein synthesis. The amount of RDP required in the diet is determined by the amount of fermentable carbohydrates in the diet. The NRC (2001) model typically predicts RDP requirements of 10 to 11% of diet DM. Monitor feed intake, faecal consistency, milk/feed ratios, and milk urea nitrogen (MUN) to make the final decision. A common target value for MUN is 10-12 mg/dl (see 'Clinical Nutrition' section). A deficiency of RDP will suppress the ability of the microorganisms to reproduce, but they can continue to ferment carbohydrates. This results in higher feed intake, but milk/feed ratios will be low because of lower than expected synthesis of microbial protein.

Avoid over-feeding RDP to the point that rumen ammonia concentrations markedly exceed bacterial requirements. It results in wastage of RDP and decreases flows of microbial protein to the small intestine. It impairs the uterine environment and affects fertilization.

Step 3: Feed high-lysine protein supplements to achieve a level of lysine in MP that comes as close as possible to meeting the optimal concentration.

If protein supplementation is required, select high quality, high-lysine protein supplements (e.g., soybean and canola meals, blood meal, and fishmeal). Feeding low- lysine feeds such as distiller's grains or maize gluten meal as sources of additional protein is not consistent with balancing for AA. Another option is supplementation of rumen-protected lysine sources available in the market, to at least partially compensate for the low content of lysine in the RUP fractions from forages, grains and distiller's grains.

Step 4: Feed a "rumen-protected" methionine supplement in the amounts needed to achieve the optimal ratio of lysine and methionine in MP.

Feeding a rumen-protected methionine supplement, in conjunction with one or more of the high-lysine protein supplements, is almost always necessary to achieve the correct Lys/Met ratio in MP. Lys to Met ratios in MP of 3.3 or higher are often observed and values as high as 3.5 and 3.6 are not uncommon. "Out of balance" Lys to Met ratios lowers the efficiency of use of MP for protein synthesis and the more "out of balance" the ratios, the less efficient the use.

Step 5: Don't overfeed RUP

Three factors determine the cows' requirement for RUP. These are: 1) supply of microbial protein, 2) RUP digestibility, and 3) AA composition of RUP. Field experience indicates that cows are more responsive to changes in diet RUP content when RUP has a good amino acid balance.

Benefits of balancing diets for lysine and methionine in metabolizable protein

The adoption of the concept of balancing diets for AA continues to increase. Benefits include 1) reduced need for supplemental RUP for a given level of milk and milk production, or increased milk yield and milk protein production with the same intake of RUP, 2) reduced N excretion per unit of milk or milk protein produced, 3) more predictable changes in milk and milk protein production to changes in RUP supply, 4) improved herd health and reproduction, and 5) increased herd profitability. Increases in milk protein (0.1-0.25 percentage units) and fat (0.1-0.15) concentrations have been obtained. Increases in milk yield are more common in early lactation cows than late lactation cows, and can be rather significant if balancing for lysine and methionine is started before calving. With high feed costs and low milk prices, an important benefit of AA balancing has been the opportunity to increase milk and milk component yields with less RUP supplementation and similar or lower feed costs.

If metabolizable protein (MP) levels are optimized, the level of lysine (6.6 percent of MP) and methionine (2.2 percent of MP) will meet amino acids needed for high producing cows. Methionine has several key roles including to improve milk yield and components, source of methyl donor (similar to choline) to improve fat mobilization from the liver, and reduce the level of ketone bodies. When feeding legumes (such as lucerne, clover, and soybean meal) metabolizable methionine can be limiting when balancing amino acids. Maize products (such as maize silage, maize grain, and maize byproducts) may require both metabolizable lysine and methionine.

Heat treatment of feedstuffs and monitoring of lysine damage

Of all amino acids in feed protein, lysine is generally the most susceptible to damage during heat processing. Blood meal is often specifically fed to increase concentration of lysine in metabolizable protein.

Heat processing of feeds is commonly used in the production of byproduct ingredients. It is also utilized to decrease ruminal degradation of feed protein and increase the proportion of RUP (rumen undegraded protein). Heat application for this process needs to be carefully controlled because excess heat can destroy lysine and depress intestinal lysine digestibility. Monitoring the effect of heat treatment on intestinal digestibility of lysine in RUP (RUP-Lys) is especially important for lactating cows as lysine is often co-limiting with methionine (Met) or second limiting for milk and milk protein production when diets high in maize products are fed. When feeds are heated to decrease the proportion of RDP and increase the proportion of RUP, the greatest benefit will be observed if the RUP is readily digested and RUP-AA (RUP amino acids) are readily absorbed by the animal. Processing methods that increase RUP supply without damaging RUP-Lys should be used.

Heat damage of protein and amino acid in feedstuffs primarily results from three major reactions: Maillard reaction, AA racemization reactions, and protein cross-linking reactions (Meade et. al., 2005).

Of the reactions that occur during heat processing of foods and feeds, the Maillard reaction generally has the greatest impact on nutritional quality. The reaction most commonly occurs in feeds between carbonyl groups of reducing sugars and the free amino group present on the side-chain of lysine. Therefore, one of the major nutritional consequences of the Maillard reaction is the destruction or loss of lysine, an essential AA (EAA) that is often limiting for livestock production. The early Maillard reaction is characterized by the destruction of lysine, but as the reaction progresses, cross-links within and between protein molecules form, reducing digestibility of the entire protein molecule or fragments of the molecule.

Identifying an accurate **in vitro** method that can be used to rapidly and economically analyze more samples for RUP-AA digestibility, particularly RUP-Lys digestibility, may allow ruminant nutrition models to more accurately predict MP-Lys supply from individual feed ingredients.

Monitoring lysine damage that results from heat processing conditions can also be useful in monitoring quality of protein feeds supplied from various sources.

Low starch diets for lactating dairy cows

Maize grain can be replaced with byproduct feeds in lactating cow diets and the resulting low-starch (18 to 21%) diets have no adverse effects on ruminal fermentation and lactation performance. In particular, diets containing NFFS (Nonforage fibre sources include wheat middlings, dried brewers' grains, soy hulls, beet pulp and citrus pulp) that provide digestible NDF can support excellent production and feed efficiency with lower than commonly recommended amounts of starch.

Diets with sufficient fermentable NDF often maximize milk production and growth in sheep by increasing intake without sacrificing rumen health. Including soy hulls in diets increases feed intake and production in ruminants. This is likely due to the high fraction of fermentable neutral detergent fibre (FNDF) found in soy hulls, which may optimize VFA production for rumen health.

Rapidly and slowly degradable starches

It is generally recommended that dairy rations for high yielding animals contain 21-27% starch. At the same level of total dietary starch, however, one ration containing a large amount of fast fermenting starches such as barley, high-moisture maize, or bakery product may result in acidosis, whereas a ration containing a more slowly degradable starch like maize meal may not. A high extent of starch availability is desired but a combination of rapidly and slowly available starches will help with acidosis control.

Microbial protein yield

For efficient growth of the rumen microbes to occur, the availability of carbohydrate and protein to the microbes must be synchronized on an hourly basis. Work with continuous cultures of rumen microbes showed that microbial yield decreased curvilinearly from 34.2 to 10.3 g bacterial nitrogen per kg DM digested as the nonstructural carbohydrate / rumen degradable crude protein ratio widened from 1.9 to 8.9. Aldrich et al. (1993) showed that microbial protein yield was highest (262 g/ d) when a rapidly digestible protein source as fed with a rapidly digestible starch source and lowest when a slowly digestible protein source was fed with a rapidly digestible starch source (214 g/d).

Starch digestibility

Particle size: Grinding increases the amount of surface area that the rumen microbes can attach to. Thus, grinding increases starch digestibility. Maize grain may be ground either coarsely or finely. It has been recommended that 67% of maize meal should pass through a sieve of ~1.18 mm. This equates to an average particle size of 1100 microns (Hutjens, 2008). High-moisture maize should be rolled prior to feeding if it is 28–32% moisture but it should be ground to a smaller particle size if it has less than 25% moisture.

Starch type: Maize starch type also effects digestibility. Taylor and Allen (2005) increased rumen starch digestibility of maize grain in lactating dairy cows from 35 to 57% when maize grain with a floury endosperm was fed rather than vitreous maize grain.

Kind of processing: Heat and pressure make starches more rapidly fermentable (Huntingdon, 1997). Steam flaking, extrusion, and pelleting all cause starch to gelatinize. However, the degree of "cook" is highly dependent on the amount of moisture, pressure, and heat actually obtained during each of these processes.

High sulphur content of diets can be dangerous to ruminants

Rumen microorganisms and the host ruminant animal require many macro and micro minerals for normal growth and development. Among these minerals, sulfur is a necessary component of the amino acids cystine and methionine that are building blocks of proteins. In ruminants, many inorganic forms of sulfur (e.g. potassium sulfate and calcium sulfate) can be used because sulfate is reduced in the rumen to sulfide by a group of bacteria referred to as the sulfur reducing bacteria and subsequently incorporated into microbial protein. However, excess production of sulfides in the rumen may be detrimental because high levels can cause polioencephalomalacia (PEM). Polioencephalomalacia is a disease condition characterized by necrosis of the cerebrocortical region of the brain. A thiamine deficiency has been the most common cause of PEM in ruminants. Excess sulfur or sulfate in feed (Table 2) or water has been the second most reported condition associated with PEM. Consumption of excess lead (Christian and Tryphonas, 1971) and water deprivation (Sullivan, 1985) can result in the disease in some instances.

Table 2. Sulphur content of feedstuffs

Feedstuff	Sulphur, %
Lucerne hay, early bloom	0.28
Barley malt sprouts, dehydrates	0.85
Brewers grains, wet	0.32
Maize distillers grain, dry	0.46
Maize gluten meal, 60%	0.72

Table 2. Sulphur content of feedstuffs (Contd.)

Feedstuff	Sulphur, %
Molasses, cane	0.47
Rapeseed meal	1.25
Whey, dehydrated	1.12
Turnip root	0.43
Ammonium sulphate	24.10
Calcium sulphate	18.62
Copper sulphate	12.84
Potassium sulphate	17.35
Sodium sulphate	09.95

Source: Limin Kung, Jr (2008) Burping can be dangerous if you are a ruminant: Issues with high sulphur diet. P.30 in: Four-State Dairy Nutrition and Management Conference Proceedings.

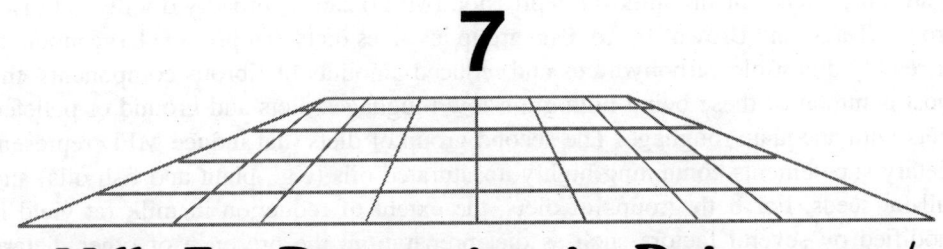

7

Milk Fat Depression in Dair cows/ buffaloes

INTRODUCTION

Fat and fatty acid digestion and metabolism in dairy animals are of considerable interest due to several reasons: (1) The increasing use of dietary fat supplements to increase the energy density of diets to meet requirements of the high producing dairy cow/buffalo (2) it is now recognized that fatty acids, both of dietary and rumen origin, can have specific and potent effects on ruminant metabolism and human health and (3) it is now recognized that specific fatty acids produced in the rumen are potent regulators of milk fat synthesis in the mammary gland.

Supplementation of fat: Rumen inert fatty acids

Fat supplements are used as a means to increase the energy density of the diet and many of these are referred to as inert. In this case, inertness simply means that the fat or fatty acid supplement has minimal affects on rumen fermentation. Although deemed inert at the level used, they can still be hydrolyzed if they are in the form of a triglyceride, or hydrogenated if they are in the form of unsaturated fatty acids. Often, calcium soaps of palm fatty acids or canola are referred to as 'protected'. However, these are not protected from ruminal biohydrogenation, but they are rather ruminally inert with regard to their effects on the microbial population (Palmquist, 2006). Factors such as low rumen pH and increased unsaturation of the fatty acid can lead to dissociation of the Ca fatty acid complex, allowing biohydrogenation to occur (Demeyer and Doreau, 1999). Thus, the feeding of a Ca-salt of unsaturated fatty acids will "protect" against adverse effects on microbial fermentation, but in most cases, it will not increase either the bypass of these fatty acids to the duodenum (Lundy et al., 2004) or their content in milk fat (Castañeda-Gutiérrez et al., 2005) compared with the feeding of the parent oil.

Milk Fat Depression (MFD)

Milk fat is the most variable of milk components and is highly responsive to nutrition. Over the last 50 years there has been substantial research addressing the low-milk fat syndrome. Diets causing milk fat depression (MFD) can be broadly divided into two groups (Davis and Brown, 1970). One group involves diets that provide large amounts of readily digestible carbohydrates and reduced amounts of fibrous components, the most common of these being high grain-low roughages diets and ground or pelleted diets with adequate roughage. The second group of diets that induce MFD represent dietary supplements containing highly unsaturated oils (e.g., plant and fish oils) and full-fat seeds. For both groups of diets, the extent of reduction in milk fat yield is modified by several factors such as diet preparation, the presence of other dietary components, feeding frequency and level, stage of lactation and body condition of cow.

Much of the classical work on milk fat depression was linked to the National Institute for Research in Dairying (NIRD) at Reading, UK (R.J.Dewhurst, 2005). Drummond et al. (1924) first demonstrated MFD by feeding 200 g of cod-liver oil per day. The fact that this was related to rumen effects has been demonstrated by feeding 'rumen-protected' fat supplements (Bines et al., 1978), which could increase milk fat content. Powell (1939) showed that restricting hay intake and increasing the level of concentrate feeding led to milk fat depression and Loosli et al. (1945) suggested that this may be related to effects on rumen fermentation.

Sutton and Morant (1989) explained 92% of variation in milk fat content using predictions based on feed acid detergent fibre (ADF) and dry matter intake, using results from a series of experiments conducted at NIRD. The effect of long-fibre on milk fat content is now so well characterized that it forms the basis of the physically effective NDF (peNDF) scheme developed by D.R.Mertens (1997).

Milk fat depression (MFD) refers to a marked reduction in milk fat yield with no change in milk yield or yield of other milk components. The MFD has been observed over a range of feeding situations, including diets supplemented with fish oils or plant oils, and diets high in concentrates and low in fibre (HCLF) (Bauman and Griinari, 2001). The fat content of milk can also be affected by the **physical characteristics of the roughage** (e.g. grinding or pelleting) or **use of ionophores such as monensin**.

Milk fat depression is commonly observed in ruminants fed highly fermentable diets or diets that contain high concentrations of PUFA. Altered fermentation of these diets results in rumen outflow of unique biohydrogenation intermediates, some of which reduce lipid synthesis in the mammary gland.

How is MFD diagnosed?

The MFD is properly diagnosed by an observed reduction in milk fat yield, as milk fat percentage can be influenced by a change in milk volume with no actual change in milk fat produced. Several general characteristics have been identified that provide insight into the biology of MFD (Bauman and Griinari, 2003).

- First, the changes that occur with diet-induced MFD are specific for milk fat; fat yield can be reduced by 50% or more with little or no change in milk yield or the yield of lactose or protein.
- Second, the yield of most of the different fatty acids in milk fat is reduced, but the decline is greatest for de novo synthesized fatty acids. As a result, milk fat composition shifts toward lower proportions of short chain and medium chain fatty acids (<16 carbons) and a greater concentration of longer chain fatty acids (>16 carbons).
- Third, changes in ruminal microbial processes are an essential component for the development of MFD. These changes in the rumen environment are often associated with a decrease in rumen pH and a shift in the acetate:propionate ratio.
- Fourth, for MFD to occur, the diet must contain unsaturated fatty acids and the pathways of their biohydrogenation in the rumen must be altered.

Thus, the induction of MFD is centered on both an altered rumen environment and an alteration in the rumen pathways of PUFA biohydrogenation.

Mechanisms of milk fat depression

A large number of theories have been proposed to explain MFD over the years. The two broad origins of MFD, high levels of readily fermentable carbohydrate with low fibre and marine oil supplementation, were well recognized by the time of the review of Davis and Brown (1970). Griinari et al. (1998) linked these effects and showed that dietary PUFA are required for low fibre diets to lead to MFD. The fundamental problem in describing the cause of MFD is one which is central to many issues in nutritional science. Diets (or absorbed nutrients) are complex mixtures in which increases in one area are necessarily balanced by reductions in another (Parks 1982). As a result it is easy to be misled by the results of univariate analysis that do not take into account variation in other attributes. Since changes in acetate, propionate, vitamin B12, insulin, trans fatty acids and other unspecified factors are all correlated, it is extremely difficult to assign causality.

Building up the evidences

Davis and Brown (1970) were among the first to recognize that increases in the milk fat content of *trans* fatty acids (TFA) was associated with MFD caused by feeding HCLF diets. Later, it became evident that MFD was often related to an increase in the TFA content of milk fat across a wide range of diets (Griinari et al., 1998). However, the basis for MFD had to be more complex than a simple relationship to the ruminal production of TFA. With the help of improved analytical techniques it was understood that diet-induced MFD occurred more due to the pattern of trans 18:1 isomers rather than total TFA that was correlated to MFD. Specifically, Griinari et al.(1998) demonstrated that MFD was associated with a marked increase in the milk fat content of trans-10 18:1. Thus, under certain dietary situations, a portion of the linoleic acid undergoes biohydrogenation via a pathway that produces trans-10 18:1 (Figure 1). Trans-10, cis-12 CLA is also an intermediate in this pathway, and it was found that the milk fat content of this unique CLA isomer also increased in many dietary situations associated with MFD (Bauman and Griinari, 2001). Studies with pure CLA isomers revealed that trans-10, cis-12 CLA was a potent inhibitor of milk fat synthesis (Baumgard et al., 2000). Effects of trans-10, cis-12 CLA are specific for milk fat and its mechanism and that for diet-induced MFD involves coordinated reductions in key mammary enzymes involved in the regulation of milk fat synthesis (Griinari and Bauman, 2006). As shown in Figure 1, dietary components can impact the risk of milk fat depression in three predominant ways (Lock and Bauman, 2007). 1. through increasing substrate supply of 18-carbon unsaturated fatty acids, 2. by altering the rumen environment and biohydrogenation (BH) path ways, and 3. via changes in the rate of BH process.

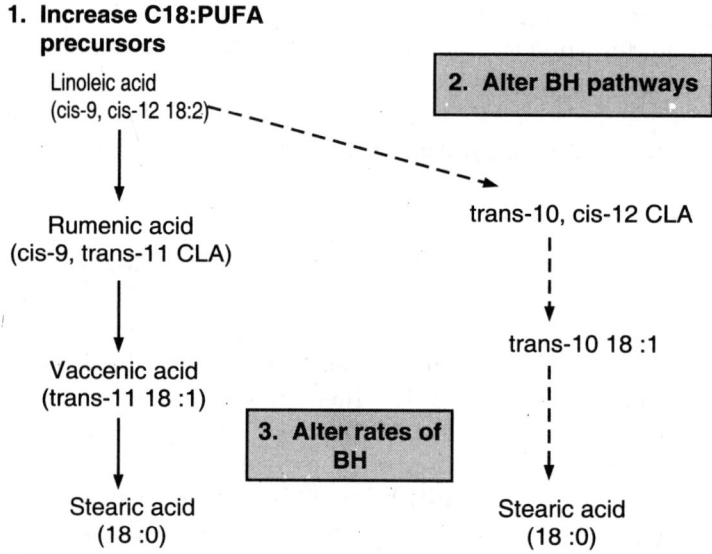

Figure 1. Generalized scheme of ruminal biohydrogenation of linoleic acid under normal conditions (solid lines) and diet-induced MFD (dotted lines) (Adapted from Bauman and Griinari, 2003)

Biohydrogenation theory

In view of these advances, Bauman and Griinari (2001) proposed the "biohydrogenation theory" to explain MFD and hypothesized that "under certain dietary conditions the pathways of rumen biohydrogenation are altered to produce unique fatty acid intermediates which are potent inhibitors of milk fat synthesis." Clearly, *trans*-10, *cis*-12 CLA represents one example, and results from several recent studies have led investigators to suggest the existence of additional fatty acid intermediates that inhibit milk fat synthesis. Of particular interest, milk concentrations of *trans*-10 18:1 are highly correlated with the extent of diet-induced MFD. Recent studies showed that *trans*-9, *cis*-11 CLA and *cis*-10, *trans*-12 CLA reduced milk fat synthesis in lactating dairy cows. Therefore, three CLA isomers have been identified as regulators of milk fat synthesis, and the production of these is increased in different types of diet-induced MFD.

Bauman and Griinari (2003) present a structured analysis of the various MFD hypotheses, looking particularly at studies in which single factors have been manipulated (by controlled infusions) and studies in which volatile fatty acid (VFA) production has been quantified. They pointed out those differences in rumen VFA proportions with low fibre diets reflect increased propionate production rather than a decrease in production of acetate and butyrate, so the hypothesis that these latter two are limiting for *de novo* fatty acid synthesis is weak.

How can dietary components impact the risk of milk fat depression?

The three predominant ways in which dietary components can impact the risk of milk fat depression are (1) through increasing substrate supply of 18-carbon unsaturated fatty acids, (2) by altering the rumen environment and BH pathways, and (3) via changes in the rate of BH at various steps in the BH process. These three areas are discussed in the following sections.

Supply of unsaturated fatty acids

Given that the specific fatty acids that cause MFD are intermediates produced during ruminal BH of PUFA, it is logical that the amount of initial substrate (linoleic acid and perhaps linolenic acid) may be related to the amount of the key BH intermediates that are produced. Linoleic and linolenic acids represent a large percentage of the fatty acids found in most of the forages and other plant-based feedstuffs fed to dairy cattle, with linoleic acid representing the predominant PUFA in maize and maize byproducts.

With the increased availability of maize byproducts (e.g. distillers' grains) an additional important consideration is their fat content because they can contain a considerable amount of lipid which is predominately linoleic acid. In particular, the fat content of maize distillers' grains is highly variable (e.g. about 5 to 15% of DM), and this degree of variation can significantly alter the dietary supply of unsaturated fatty acids to the dairy cow, thereby increasing the risk of MFD.

The feeding of supplement fat can be challenging since various lipids and fatty acids can trigger a number of changes in rumen metabolism. In general, as you increase the degree of unsaturation of supplemental fat and/or the availability of the fatty acids present (e.g. extruded vs. roasted oilseeds), the chances of MFD occurring will increase. Recently, Relling and Reynolds (2007) examined the impact of feeding rumen-inert fats differing in their degree of saturation on performance of lactating dairy cows. Cows were fed a Control mixed ration *ad libitum*, and treatments were the dietary addition (3.5% of ration dry matter) of 3 rumen-inert fat sources differing in fatty acid profile. As the unsaturation of the supplemental fat increased, this was associated with reduced milk fat content and yield.

Sometimes it may be appropriate to more broadly consider overall 'unsaturated load' in the rumen when troubleshooting MFD. Increasing the dietary supply of oleic acid (cis-9 18:1) from tallow or other sources (e.g. palm fatty acid distillate), will not directly increase the rumen outflow of 18:2 BH intermediates because these fat supplements supply very little PUFA. Hinrichsen et al. (2006) showed under some circumstances oleic acid can be fed at high levels without inducing MFD. In some circumstances, however, it would appear that the increase in unsaturated load from increasing oleic acid supply is sufficient to alter BH pathways to favour the production of trans-10, cis-12 CLA and related intermediates from the PUFA already in the diet. This hypothesis has been supported by a recent study using continuous cultures and 13carbon-labeled oleic acid. As expected, lowering culture pH to 5.5 reduced the concentration of trans-11 18:1 and increased trans-10 18:1 concentration. The 13carbon enrichment of trans-10 18:1, however, was lower at pH 5.5 compared with pH 6.5 indicating that more of the trans-10 at low pH originated from sources other than oleic acid (Abu-Ghazaleh et al., 2005). This must come from PUFA sources and will presumably be driven through BH pathways that also promote the formation of trans-10, cis-12 CLA or related intermediates, thereby increasing MFD risk (Lock et al., 2006).

Alteration of the ruminal environment

One major change in the rumen environment that leads to flux of fatty acids through alternate pathways of ruminal BH is low ruminal pH. *Factors that can result in marked changes in ruminal pH through any 24-h period include:* dietary carbohydrate profile and rates of degradation of the carbohydrate fractions as affected by source, processing, and moisture; physically effective NDF (peNDF) supply as affected by source and particle size; and production of salivary buffers as a function of peNDF supply and source (Shaver, 2005).

Although data are limited, changes in rumen pH are most likely associated with MFD because they cause a change in the bacterial population favouring those that have alternative BH pathways. A common misconception, however, is that acidosis is a prerequisite for MFD to occur. This is not the case and in most situations rumen health appears excellent and there are no overt signs of ruminal acidosis (Overton et al., 2006). For example, Harvatine and Allen (2006) reported increased duodenal flow of BH intermediates and MFD with no change in ruminal pH measured every 5 seconds over 4 days. Again, this highlights the fact that only small changes in the rumen environment can lead to increased risk of MFD.

Although the implications of low ruminal pH for production of the MFD-causing intermediates have been considered, it is probable that other factors can also cause changes in the rumen bacteria population resulting in an increased flow of fatty acids through alternate pathways of ruminal BH (Palmquist et al., 2005). Overton et al.(2006) hypothesized that factors such as ensiled feeds with abnormal fermentation profiles (particularly high acetic acid silages) or mouldy feeds may also cause the changes in biohydrogenation required to cause MFD.

What is the impact of changes in rate of passage out of the rumen on MFD? Cows with higher dry matter intake (DMI) have higher rates of passage which potentially will 'flush' more BH intermediates out of the rumen. Cows with higher DMI in general (e.g., higher producing cow/buffalo) are, therefore, more likely at risk of MFD.

Alteration of rates of biohydrogenation

Under some circumstances specific feed components can alter rumen fermentation in a manner that results in changes in biohydrogenation rates of fatty acids. Altering these rates can potentially increase the rumen outflow of trans-10, cis-12 CLA and related intermediates responsible for MFD, thereby increasing risk of MFD. This is a facet of troubleshooting MFD which is not typically considered when thinking about the traditional 'supply of PUFA' or 'altered fermentation' groupings, even though these changes are a result of changes in the rumen environment.

Monensin: Monensin is an example of a feed ingredient that can affect biohydrogenation rates through altering rumen fermentation and the bacterial species present. In some cases during established lactation, monensin supplementation can result in decreased milk fat percentage and yield (Duffield and Bagg, 2000). These effects are likely the result of interactions with other dietary or management factors that predispose cows to experience MFD.

Monensin increases maintenance requirements of gram-positive bacteria in the rumen which renders these bacteria less competitive in the ruminal environment (Duffield and Bagg, 2000). The net result is changes in the ruminal bacterial population that appear to decrease rates of biohydrogenation of PUFA in the rumen. Very few species of bacteria have been identified that can convert trans-18:1fatty acids to stearic acid (18:0) and most of these have been identified as being gram-positive. Thus the final step in biohydrogenation is already the 'rate-limiting' step; therefore decreasing the number of bacteria that can carry out this process can potentially lead to a 'buildup' of BH intermediates in the rumen thereby increasing their passage to the small intestine.

This was highlighted by Fellner et al. (1997) when they examined the effect of monensin on the formation of BH products when linoleic acid was infused continuously into rumen fermentors. With an unsupplemented diet the rate of 18:0 formation was 7.5 mg/L/hr whereas this decreased to only 2.7 mg/L/hr when monensin was supplemented (Fellner et al., 1997). It is important to remember, however, that an increased rumen outflow of BH intermediates will not be a problem if typical BH pathways are present. However, even if a small proportion of dietary PUFA are being biohydrogenated through pathways that produce trans-10, cis-12 CLA and related intermediates, Monensin can potentially increase the passage of these to the small intestine and increase the risk of MFD.

Dietary fatty acids: Dietary fatty acids can also modify ruminal fermentation and may shift BH towards the production of intermediates that cause MFD. For example, Harvatine and Allen (2006) reported that fat supplements affected fractional rates of ruminal fatty acid BH and passage in dairy cows; increasing the unsaturation of the fat supplement slowed down the BH of 18:1 to 18:0 while causing a significant reduction in milk fat yield. It is also well known from experimental diets that the addition of fish oil to the diet alters ruminal fermentation towards increased production of BH intermediates. Long chain n-3 PUFA present in fish oils appear to affect rumen bacteria catalyzing the terminal step in BH, thereby increasing the rumen outflow of these intermediates.

In vitro studies with mixed cultures of rumen bacteria have established that docosahexaenoic acid is a specific n-3 PUFA responsible for this effect (AbuGhazaleh and Jenkins, 2004), though it is likely that other fatty acids may have similar effects. This effect of fish oil on rumen lipid metabolism has been used as a method to facilitate the production of *cis*-9, *trans*-11 CLA enriched milk (e.g. Lynch et al., 2005). Interactions are once again play a key role; if normal BH pathways are maintained then the rumen outflow of *trans*-11 18:1 and *cis*-9, *trans*-11 CLA will increase. Small changes, however, in rumen fermentation as a result of fish oil feeding can alter these pathways thereby increasing the rumen outflow of intermediates that cause MFD.

This is highlighted by recent studies by Dale E.Bauman of Cornell University and coworkers that emphasize the impact of feeding pattern of fish oil on MFD risk. Infusion of fish oil into the rumen 4X / day has led to a 24% decrease in milk fat yield. However, a follow up study which utilized a similar basal diet but infused the fish oil 6X / day resulted in no MFD (McConnell, Lock and Bauman, unpublished). Due to these multifaceted interactions it has proven difficult to experimentally distinguish the effect of PUFA as increased substrate vs. its potential role as a modifier of rumen fermentation.

Application of molecular techniques to detect metabolic changes

Bauman et al. (2008) extensively studied and identified *trans*-10, *cis*-12 CLA as one of the bioactive fatty acids, which reduce milk fat yield up to 45% at a dose of 0.045 g/kg body weight. In their subsequent work, D.E.Bauman and group (Harvatine, Perfield and Bauman, 2009) demonstrated the application of molecular techniques to detect metabolic changes. They investigated expression of lipid-related genes in adipose tissue during acute *trans*-10, *cis*-12 CLA-induced MFD in the dairy cow. Trans-10, cis-12 CLA decreased milk fat synthesis through transcriptional down-regulation of genes involved in mammary lipid synthesis. Thus, a CLA dose resulting in near maximal inhibition of mammary lipid synthesis resulted in increased expression of lipid synthesis-related genes in adipose tissue. Results are consistent with energy spared from the reduction in milk fat synthesis being partitioned toward adipose tissue fat stores during short term MFD.

The results of the study showed that CLA treatment caused a reduction in both milk fat production and voluntary intake resulting in a net energy excess. This energy excess was accompanied by increased expression of lipid synthesis genes in adipose tissue and is consistent with an increase in energy partitioning to body fat stores during CLA treatment. Specifically it was observed that increased adipose tissue expression of genes involved in the pathways of lipid synthesis, including fatty acid synthase, lipoprotein lipase, stearoyl-CoA desaturase, and fatty acid binding protein4 (FABP4). Increased expression of these adipose tissue genes demonstrate coordinated upregulation of lipid synthesis pathways, including those for the uptake, synthesis, desaturation, and transport of FA during short-term CLA-induced MFD.

8

Effects of Heat Stress on Energy Balance and Metabolism; Strategies to Reduce the Negative Impacts of Heat Stress on Reproduction

INTRODUCTION

Heat stress negatively impacts milk yield, growth and reproduction. Advances in management such as use of cooling systems and nutritional strategies have alleviated some of the negative effects of thermal stress on animals, but production continues to decrease during the summer.

Effect of Heat Stress on Rumen Health

Heat stress has long been known to adversely affect rumen health (L.H. Baumgard et al., 2007). One way cows dissipate heat is via panting and this increased respiration rate results in enhanced CO_2 (carbon dioxide) being exhaled. In order to be an effective blood pH buffering system, the body needs to maintain a 20:1 HCO_3 - (bicarbonate) to CO_2 ratio. Due to the hyperventilation (increased respiration rate) induced decrease in blood CO_2, the kidney secretes HCO_3 - to maintain this ratio. This reduces the amount of HCO_3 - that can be used (via saliva) to buffer and maintain a healthy rumen pH.

In addition, panting cows drool and drooling reduces the quantity of saliva that would have normally been deposited in the rumen.

Furthermore, due to reduced feed intake, heat-stressed cows ruminate less and therefore generate less saliva.

The reductions in the amount of saliva produced and salivary HCO_3 - content and the decreased amount of saliva entering the rumen (the animals have reduced ability to neutralize the rumen) make the heat stressed cow much more susceptible to sub-clinical and acute rumen acidosis (see review by Kadzere et al., 2002).

Due to the reduced feed intake caused by heat stress and the heat associated with fermenting forages, nutritionists typically increase the energy density of the ration. This is often accomplished with extra concentrates and reductions in forages ("hotter" ration). However, this needs to be done with care as this type of diet can be associated with a lower rumen pH. Better option is supplementation of rumen inert fat.

Biological consequence of heat stress

The biological mechanism by which heat stress impacts production and reproduction is partly explained by reduced feed intake, but also includes altered endocrine status, reduction in rumination and nutrient absorption, and increased maintenance requirements (Collier and Beede, 1985; Collier et al., 2005) resulting in a net decrease in nutrient / energy available for production.

Reductions in energy intake during heat stress result in a majority of dairy cows entering into negative energy balance (NEBAL), regardless of the stage of lactation. Essentially, because of reduced feed and energy intake the heat-stressed cow enters a bioenergetic state, similar (but not to the same extent) to the NEBAL observed in early lactation. The

NEBAL associated with the early postpartum period is coupled with increased risk of metabolic disorders and health problems (Goff and Horst, 1997; Drackley, 1999), decreased milk yield and reduced reproductive performance.

However, it is not clear how much of the reduction in performance (yield, daily gain and reproduction) can be attributed or accounted for by the biological parameters affected by heat stress (i.e. reduced feed intake vs. increased maintenance costs).

Metabolic Adaptations to Reduced Nutrient Intake

A prerequisite of understanding the metabolic adaptations which occur with heat stress, is an appreciation of the physiological and metabolic adaptations to thermal-neutral negative energy balance (NEBAL) that occur during the transition period or underfeeding.

Cows in early lactation are classic examples of when nutrient intake is less than necessary to meet maintenance and milk production costs and animals typically enter negative energy balance. Negative energy balance is associated with a variety of metabolic changes that are implemented to support the dominant physiological condition of lactation (Bauman and Currie, 1980). Marked alterations in both carbohydrate and lipid metabolism ensure partitioning of dietary derived and tissue originating nutrients towards the mammary gland, and not surprisingly many of these changes are mediated by endogenous somatotropin which is naturally increased during periods of NEBAL (Bauman and Currie, 1980).

Key homeorhetic mechanism implemented by cows in NEBAL

One classic response is a **reduction in circulating insulin** coupled with **a reduction in systemic insulin sensitivity**. The reduction in insulin action allows for adipose lipolysis and mobilization of non-esterified fatty acids (NEFA; Bauman and Currie, 1980). Increased circulating NEFA are typical in "transitioning" cows and represent (along with NEFA derived ketones) a significant source of energy (and are precursors for milk fat synthesis) for cows in NEBAL. Postabsorptive carbohydrate metabolism is also altered by the reduced insulin action during NEBAL with the net effect of reduced glucose uptake by systemic tissues (i.e. muscle and adipose). The reduced nutrient uptake coupled with the net release of nutrients (i.e. amino acids and NEFA) by systemic tissues are key homeorhetic (an acclimated response vs. an acute/ homeostatic response) mechanisms implemented by cows in NEBAL to support lactation (Bauman and Currie, 1980). The thermal-neutral cow in NEBAL is metabolically flexible, in that she can depend upon alternative fuels (NEFA and ketones) to spare glucose, which can be utilized by the mammary gland to copiously produce milk.

Production Adaptations to Heat Stress

Heat stress reduces both feed intake and milk yield and the decline in nutrient intake has been identified as a major cause of reduced milk synthesis (Fuquay, 1981; West, 1994). However, the exact contribution of declining feed intake to the overall reduced milk yield remains unknown. Baumgard et al. (2007) evaluated this question by conducting experiments on lactating Holstein cows in midlactation. The experimental results indicate that the reduction in dry mater intake (DMI) can only account for about 40-50% of the decrease in production when cows are heat stressed and that about 50-60% can be explained by other heat stressed induced changes.

Despite the fact that producing additional milk results in extra metabolic heat production, bST has demonstrated to be effective in a variety of management and environmental conditions (Collier et al., 2005). The mechanism by which bST remains effective during heat stress is due to its homeorhetic properties as it causes increased milk production via coordinating metabolism in almost all body tissues (Collier et al., 2005). This coordination includes an increased capacity to sweat and thus an enhanced ability to dissipate heat (Manalu et al., 1991).

To evaluate the effectiveness of rbST (bST produced by recombinant DNA technology) during extreme heat stress, lactating Holstein cows in mid-lactation were administered POSILAC @ 500 mg dose. The administration of rbST increased milk yield by about 10% and 15% in heat-stressed and thermal neutral cows, respectively (Wheelock et al., 2006).

Similar to thermal neutral cows (Bauman, 1999), it was demonstrated that bST reduces systemic insulin sensitivity in heat-stressed cows. Comparable to thermal neutral cows, this reduction in insulin action partially explains the partitioning of nutrients to the mammary gland to support increased milk synthesis during heat stress.

Heat and maintenance costs

Considerable evidence suggests that increased maintenance costs are associated with heat stress (7 to 25%; NRC, 2001). Maintenance requirements are increased, as there is presumably a large energetic cost of dissipating stored heat.

Metabolic Adaptations to Heat Stress

Due to the reductions in feed intake and presumed increased maintenance costs, and despite the decrease in milk yield heat-stressed cows enter into a state of NEBAL (Moore et al., 2005). However, unlike NEBAL in thermal neutral conditions as noted in transition cow / buffalo, heat stressed induced NEBAL doesn't result in elevated plasma NEFA.

How do you explain the difference between NEBAL in thermal neutral conditions and heat stressed NEBAL?

Heat-stressed cows have a much greater insulin response. The differences can be explained by increased insulin effectiveness. Insulin is a potent antilipolytic signal (blocks fat break down) and the primary driver of cellular glucose entry. The apparent increased insulin action causes the heat-stressed cow to be metabolically inflexible, in that she does not have the option to oxidize fatty acids and ketones. As a consequence, the heat-stressed cow becomes increasingly dependant on glucose for her energetic needs and therefore less glucose is directed towards the mammary gland.

Theoretical reasons for altered metabolism

Well-fed ruminants primarily oxidize (burn) acetate (a rumen produced VFA) as their principal energy source. However, during NEBAL cows also largely depend on NEFA for energy. Therefore, it appears the post-absorptive metabolism of the heat-stressed cow markedly differs from that of thermal-neutral cow, even though they are in a similar negative energetic state. The apparent switch in metabolism and the increase in insulin sensitivity is probably a mechanism by which cows decrease metabolic heat production, as oxidizing glucose is more efficient. Typically *in vivo* glucose oxidation yields 38 ATP or 472.3 kcal of energy (compared to 637.1 kcal in a bomb calorimeter) and **in vivo** fatty acid oxidation (i.e. stearic acid) generates 146 ATP or 1814 kcal of energy (compared to 2697 kcal in a bomb calorimeter; Brody, 1999). Despite having a much greater energy content, due to differences in the efficiencies of capturing ATP, oxidizing fatty acids generates more metabolic heat (about 2 kcal/g or 13% on an energetic basis) compared to glucose. Therefore, during heat stress, preventing or blocking adipose mobilization / breakdown and increasing glucose "burning" is presumably a strategy to minimize metabolic heat production (Baumgardet al., 2009).

The mammary gland requires glucose to synthesize milk lactose and lactose is the primary osmoregulator and thus determinant of milk yield. However, in an attempt to generate less metabolic heat, the body (primarily skeletal muscle) appears to utilize glucose at an increased rate. As a consequence, the mammary gland may not receive adequate amounts of glucose and thus mammary lactose production and subsequent milk yield is reduced. This may be the primary mechanism which accounts for the additional reductions in milk yield that cannot be explained by decreased feed intake

Heat-stressed cows require special attention with regards to heat abatement and other dietary considerations (i.e. concentrate:forage ratio, HCO3 - etc.). They may also have an extra requirement for dietary or rumen-derived glucose precursors. Of the three main rumen-produced volatile fatty acids, propionate is the one primarily converted into glucose by the liver. Highly fermentable starches such as grains increase rumen propionate production, and although propionate is the primary glucose precursor, feeding additional grains can be risky as heat-stressed cows are already susceptible to rumen acidosis.

Heat stress in Transition cow / buffalo

High environmental temperatures result in significant thermal stress for the transition cow. Exposure to heat during the third trimester of gestation shifts blood flow to the extremities and away from the uterus, compromising placental and fetal growth. Calves often have lower than normal birth weights, putting them at higher risk for mortality (Shearer and Beede, 1990).

Hormone alterations due to heat stress affect mammary development and lactogenesis, reducing milk yield in the subsequent lactation (Shearer and Beede, 1990). Strategies to keep cows cool and comfortable during the transition period include providing shade for cows on pasture or utilizing sprinklers, misters, and/or fans in their stalls. Cows should also be provided with an easily accessible source of clean drinking water.

Clearly the heat-stressed animal implements a variety of post-absorptive changes in both carbohydrate and lipid metabolism (i.e. increased insulin action). The primary end result of this altered metabolic condition is that the heat-stressed lactating dairy cow has an extra need for glucose (due to its preferential oxidization by extra-mammary tissue). Therefore, any dietary component that increases propionate production (the primary precursor to hepatic glucose production), without reducing rumen pH, will probably increase milk yield.

Strategies to reduce the negative impacts of heat stress on reproduction

Two primary strategies are followed to minimize heat gain by reducing solar heat load and maximize heat loss by reducing air temperature around the animal or increasing evaporative heat loss directly from animals. Following are several strategies to potentially help reduce the negative impacts of heat stress on reproduction in lactating dairy cows (Bilby et al., 2008).

Cow Comfort and Cooling

Identification of hot spots: Locating where heat stress is occurring on the dairy farm by identifying hot spots is key to implementing the proper cooling or management strategy to eliminate these hot spots. Temperature devices can be used to monitor core body temperatures in cows by attaching a temperature monitor to a blank continuous intravaginal drug release (**CIDR®**, Pfizer Animal Health, New York, NY) device for practical on-farm use. The device is inserted into the cow's vagina, measuring core body temperature every minute for up to 6 d. This allows monitoring of the cow's body temperature and identification of where the cow is experiencing heat stress. This is mentioned to make the readers aware about availability of such devices.

Providing enough shade is vital for proper cow comfort. There should be at least 38 to 45 sq ft of shade/mature dairy cow to reduce solar radiation. Spray and fan systems should be used in the holding pen, over feeding areas, over the feeding areas. Improved cooling is still the most profitable and effective way to improve both milk production and reproduction during the summer months.

Nutritional Modifications

The nutritional impacts on reproduction are well documented. Reducing metabolic diseases will further enhance our ability to improve reproduction during the summer months. Some simple feeding and nutritional strategies can be implemented to reduce the negative effects of summer heat stress on reproduction.

The maintenance requirement of lactating dairy cows increases substantially as environmental temperature increases. When possible, increase the number of feedings in order to increase dry matter intake (DMI). In addition, feed the animals during cooler parts of the day and increase moisture content in the ration. Tree leaves may be added to the straws / stovers.

The heat stressed cow is prone to rumen acidosis and many of the lasting effects of warm weather can probably be traced back to a low rumen pH during the summer months. As a consequence, care should be taken when feeding **hot rations** during the summer. Obviously fibre quality is important all the time, but it is paramount during the summer as it has some buffering capacity and stimulates saliva production. Furthermore, **dietary HCO$_3$** - may be a valuable tool to maintain a healthy rumen pH.

Feeding dietary fat (**rumen inert/rumen bypass**) remains an effective strategy of providing extra energy during a time of negative energy balance. Compared to starch and fibre, fat has a much lower heat increment in the rumen. Thus fat provides energy without a negative thermal side effect.

Wheelock et al. (2006) demonstrated that maximizing rumen production of glucose precursors (i.e. propionate) may be an effective strategy to maintain production during heat stress. However, due to the rumen health issue, increasing grains should be conducted with care. A safe and effective method of maximizing rumen propionate production is with **monensin** (approved for lactating dairy cattle in 2004 in USA). In addition, monensin may assist in stabilizing rumen pH during stress situations.

Proplyene glycol is fed typically in early lactation, but may also be an effective method of increasing propionate production during HS. With the increasing demand for biofuels and subsequent supply of glycerol, it will be of interest to evaluate glycerol's efficacy and safety in ruminant diets during the summer months.

Having a negative **dietary cation-anion difference (DCAD)** during the dry period and a positive DCAD during lactation is a good strategy to maintain health and maximize production. It appears that keeping the DCAD at a healthy lactating level (approx. +20 to +30 meq/100 g DM) remains a good strategy during the warm summer months (Wildman et al., 2007).

Unlike humans, cattle utilize potassium (K^+) as their primary osmotic regulator of water secretion from their sweat glands (Bilby et al., 2008). As a consequence, K^+ requirements are increased (1.4 to 1.6 % of DM) during the summer and this should be adjusted for in the diet. In addition, dietary levels of sodium (Na^+) and magnesium (Mg^+) should be increased, as they compete with potassium (K^+) for intestinal absorption.

Possible solutions for improving summer fertility

Certain feed additives can partially alleviate heat stress through increased heat dissipation, thereby lowering internal body temperature.

Fungal cultures: In several studies, fungal cultures in the diet decreased body temperatures and respiration rates in hot, but not cool, weather (Huber et al., 1994).

Rumen protected niacin: A recent experiment in Arizona showed an increase in sweating rates and lower core body temperatures when encapsulated niacin was fed to lactating cows compared to thermal neutral controls (Zimbelman et al., 2007). A follow-up study was conducted on a commercial dairy farm during the summer months in Arizona with rumen protected niacin being fed to late lactation dairy cows. Results showed similar effects with lower core body temperatures during the hot part of the day with an additional increase in fat- and energy-corrected milk (Zimbelman et al., 2008).

9

Designer Milk and Milk Products; Effect of Nutrition on altering the Composition and Functional Properties of Milk

Dairy farmers have long been interested in milk fat due to its economic value. The composition and functional properties of milk are of considerable importance to the farmer, milk product manufacturer and consumer. Milk composition varies. Now there is interest in milk fat and hence designer milk products are promoted because of its healthfulness and functional properties. Some of the important are given below.

- Lauric, myristic and palmitic acids of milk fat are known to have hypercholesterolaemic effects. Hence products with reduced content of these can be designed.
- Conjugated linoleic acid (CLA), butyric acid and sphingolipids have anti-carcinogenic properties (Parodi, 1997). Hence products with increased amounts of these can be designed.
- Selenium is an essential trace element fundamental to mammalian health.
- Very long chain (VLC) n-3 polyunsaturated fatty acids (PUFA) are beneficial in the maintenance of human health and the prevention of chronic diseases.

Conjugated linoleic acid has been discussed elsewhere (pp 80) and the reader may consult it for better information.

Selenium is an essential trace element fundamental to mammalian health. Selenium deficiency is associated with loss of immunocompetence, particularly to viral infections, reduced fertility, and increased incidence of cancer and heart disease in humans (Raymon, 2000). Milk and milk products have the potential to provide significant amounts of bioavailable selenium, as selenomethionine and selenocystine, in human diets.

Omega-3 or n-3 Fatty acids and Health

Very long chain (VLC) n-3 polyunsaturated fatty acids (PUFA) are essential for growth and development and are beneficial in the maintenance of human health and the prevention of chronic diseases including cardiovascular disease, inflammatory diseases, and neurological disorders. The main dietary sources of eicosapentaenoic acid (EPA; 20:5n-3) and docosahexaenoic acid (DHA; 22:6n-3) are marine algae, fish, and fish oils.

There is a need to look for alternative food sources to increase consumption of VLC n-3 PUFA (Whelan and Rust, 2006).

"Learning acquired in youth arrests the evil of old age; and if you understand that old age has wisdom for its food, you will so conduct yourself in youth that your old age will not lack for nourishment."

—Leonardo DaVinci

Further, the role of n-3 fatty acids, eicosapentaenoic acid (EPA) and/or docosahexaenoic acid (DHA) in geriatric populations has been published. They nourish us well. Low in vivo concentrations of EPA and/or DHA predict an increased risk of death in frail, hospitalized octogenarians from Norway and an accelerated cognitive decline in free-living septuagenarians from France. Higher tissue concentrations of EPA and DHA are associated with slower mental decline (Samieri et al., 2008).

Role of stearoyl-CoA desaturase to turn fatty acids of milk fat into healthful

Milk fat of dairy cows is typically composed of 50 to 70% saturated fatty acids (SFA), 20 to 40% monounsaturated fatty acids (MUFA), and 1 to 5% polyunsaturated fatty acids (PUFA). These percentages are influenced mainly by nutrition, although variation has been reported between and within breeds. In addition to nutritional influences, the relative proportions of SFA and MUFA are influenced by stearoyl-CoA desaturase (SCD; also referred to as Δ9-desaturase; EC 1.14.19.1), which is the enzyme responsible for Δ9-desaturation of fatty acids (FA) in the mammary gland and other tissues. This enzyme adds a double bond in the Δ9 position and converts myristic acid (14:0) to myristoleic acid (*cis*-9 14:1), palmitic acid (16:0) to palmitoleic acid (*cis*-9 16:1), stearic acid (18:0) to oleic acid (*cis*-9 18:1), and vaccenic acid (VA; *trans*-11 18:1) to the conjugated linoleic acid (CLA) isomer rumenic acid (RA; *cis*-9, *trans*-11 18:2).

The main biological role of SCD in the mammary gland is to maintain fluidity of milk by conversion of 18:0 to cis-9 18:1 and, to a lesser extent, the other aforementioned SFA into their respective MUFA. Both 18:0 and 16:0 are solid at body temperature, hence the physiological need to convert a portion of each to *cis*-9 18:1 and cis-9 16:1 that are liquid. Several studies identified a large degree of between-cow variation in SCD activity, which was consistent across diets and suggests a genetic influence. The most reliable index of SCD activity (Garnsworthy et al., 2010) showed a heritability of 0.38, which is comparable to the heritability of milk yield (0.35). Desaturase activity could, therefore, be used in future breeding programmes to improve the FA profile of milk fat by increasing MUFA and CLA isomer rumenic acid concentrations and decreasing SFA concentrations.

Enhancing the natural level of n-3 fatty acids in the milk

Milk fat levels of n-3 fatty acids are typically very low, less than 0.5% of total fatty acids, and this is mainly α-linolenic acid (ALA). Conversion of ALA to VLC n-3 PUFA is necessary for other physiological functions, and essential for optimum health and the prevention of chronic diseases. The conversion of ALA to VLC n-3 PUFA requires Δ6-desaturase (Figure 1), an enzyme that is limiting in humans (Whelan and Rust, 2006). Stearidonic acid (SDA; 18:4n-3) is an n-3 fatty acid that humans are able to convert to EPA. Stearidonic acid, a product of Δ6-desaturation of ALA that overcomes the rate-limiting step in n-3 metabolism, is of interest as a possible precursor of VLC n-3 PUFA. All dietary manipulations favouring polyunsaturated FA incorporation in milk lipids increase the risk of lipoperoxidation, which can be efficiently prevented by use of dietary combined hydro- and lipophilic antioxidants in the diet. This needs to be kept in mind.

Genetic modification of soybeans: Genetic modification of oilseeds such as soybeans is an approach that can be used to increase the SDA in soybean oil (SBO; Ursin, 2003), and toxicology studies have confirmed the safety of SDA-enhanced

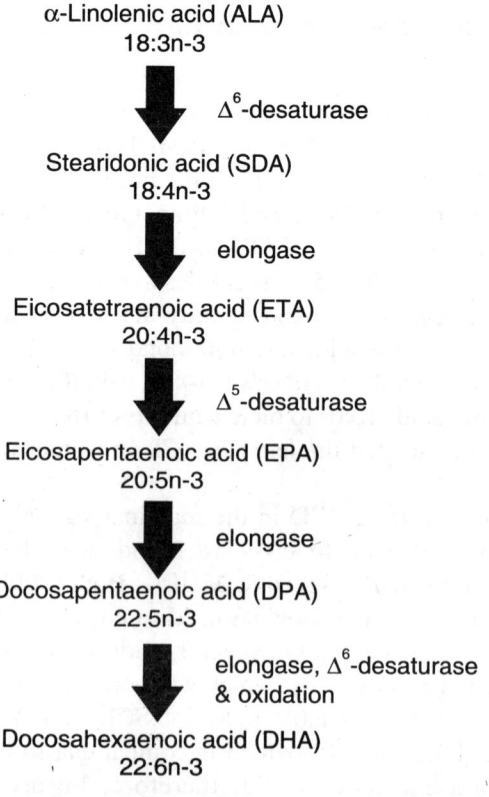

Figure 1. Biosynthesis of n-3 fatty acids

SBO (Hammond et al., 2008). D.E.Bauman and coworkers from Cornell University in collaboration with Monsanto company (G.Bernal-Santos et al., 2010) studied the effect of infusion of SDA-enhanced SBO into three Holstein cows. The study presented the first results on the uptake and transfer of stearidonic acid to milk fat in dairy cows. Further, their results also indicated that rumen-protected formulations of SDA-enriched SBO would be needed to achieve increases in the n-3 fatty acid content of milk fat. There is potential to utilize SDA-enhanced soybeans to produce n-3 FA-enriched milk and milk products which are of benefit to human health.

Effects of nutrition on milk protein

It is well established that milk protein concentration is positively correlated with ME intake, except with ME provided by digestible lipids (Sutton, 1989).

Effects of nutrition on milk fat

In ruminants, extensive ruminal biohydrogenation of unsaturated fatty acids results in numerous cis and trans isomers of 18:1 and of conjugated and non-conjugated 18:2, the incorporation of which into ruminant products depends on the composition of the diet (forage vs concentrate) and of dietary lipid supplements.

Supplementation with cereal grains

Supplementation of low quality roughage rations with cereal grains as a strategy to increase the metabolizable energy intake of lactating cows usually increases the ratio of amino acids and glucose relative to that of acetate and long chain fatty acid (LCFA) in the circulation, resulting in increased rates of synthesis of protein, lactose and, to a lesser degree, fat in the mammary gland (Sutton, 1989). At high cereal grain intakes, increased production of microbial protein and of propionate relative to acetate in the rumen are reported (Latham et al., 1974), while lipogenesis in mammary tissues may decrease leading to milk fat depression (Palmquist et al., 1993), as digestible lipid concentration of most cereal grains is low. Consequently, milk yield and milk protein concentration may increase, while milk fat concentration may fall.

Supplementation with lipids

The work of King et al (1990) showed that supplementing cows grazing pasture with both LCFA (0.5 kg/ cow/day) and cereal grain can reverse the reduction in milk fat concentration often caused by supplementing with cereal grain alone.

Palmquist (1988) reported that lactating cows can be offered 30-40 g supplemental LCFA/kg DM to increase the cow's total ME intake without significant reductions in DM intake or in the capacity of the rumen to digest fibre. Sunflower oil is high in linoleic acid, peanut oil is high in oleic acid and cottonseed oil contains malvalic acid and sterculic acid. Sterculic acid is an inhibitor of delta-9-desaturase in mammary and other tissues.

While reviewing the relationship between dietary fat supplementation and milk protein concentration, Wu and Huber (1994) observed increased milk fat concentration

154

and yield due to dietary fat supplementation, although milk protein concentration may be reduced when digestible lipids exceed 50-60 g /kg DM.

Methods to manipulate milk fat composition: Two methods

1. **Feeding protected lipid supplements:** The low amount of 18:3n-3 (?-linolenic acid) absorbed explains its limited incorporation in milk lipids. Its protection against hydrogenation has been an objective for several decades, but only encapsulation in a protein matrix is efficient. This method minimizes the action of microbial isomerases and hydrogenases on unsaturated lipid in the rumen.

2. **Feeding increased amounts of 18 C fatty acids in the diet:** This relies on increasing the amount of 18 C fatty acid substrate to delta-9-desaturase in the mammary gland and other tissues increase the concentrations of monounsaturated fatty acids (Rearon, 2001) in the milk fat (Fig 2 and 3) with changes to other fatty acids being highly dependent upon feeding conditions.

Targeted feeding strategies have achieved a good degree of control over the concentration and composition of milk fat and protein. These strategies include supplementing oil seeds, vegetable and fish oils, organic selenium sources (yeast enriched with selenium) and enable dairy farmers to produce milks with lower concentrations of fat or higher levels of unsaturated fats, including CLA, and / or high concentrations of selenoproteins.

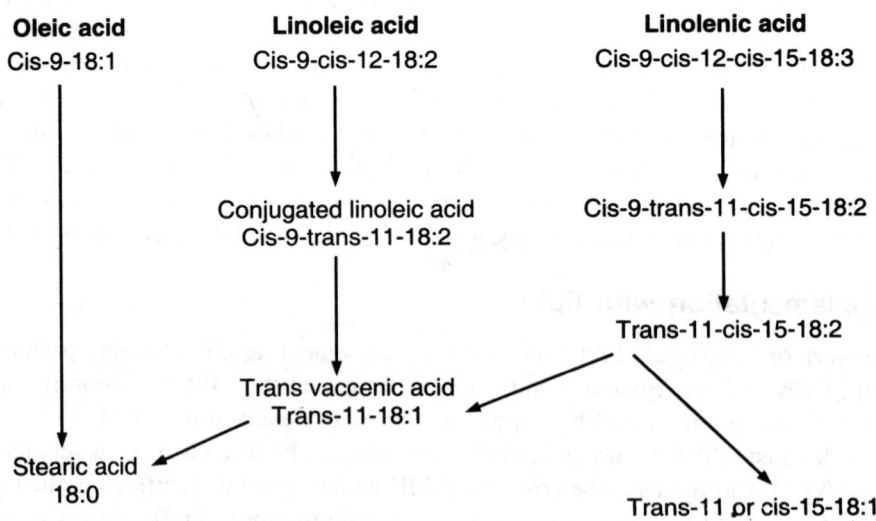

Figure 2. Putative pathways of ruminal biohydrogenation of oleic, linoleic and linolenic acids (Adapted from Bauman et al., 2001)

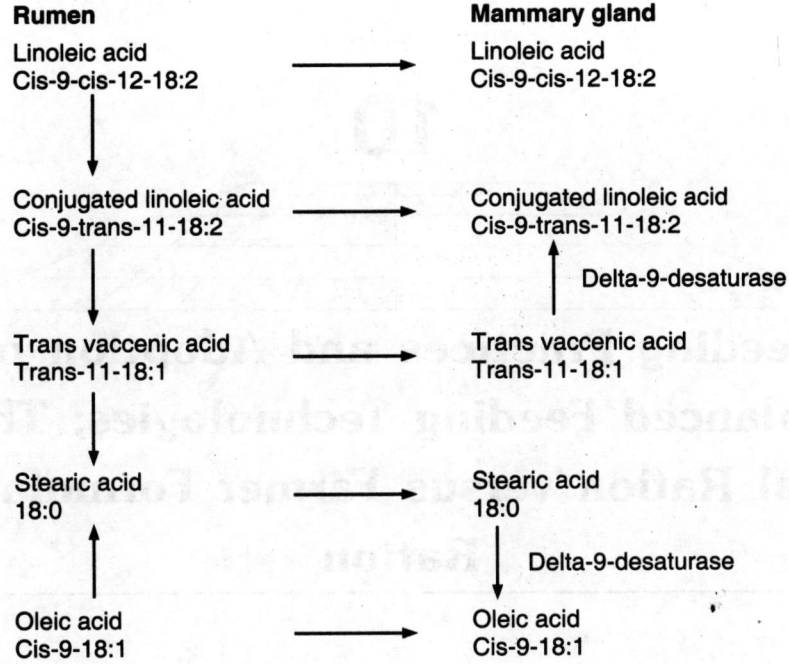

Figure 3. Pathways by which fatty acids derived from dietary oleic and linoleic acids can become available for milk fat production (Adapted from Bauman et al., 2001)

10

Feeding Practices and Adoption of Balanced Feeding Technologies; The Ideal Ration versus Farmer Formulated Ration

INTRODUCTION

Animal husbandry sector in India is mainly in the hands of small and marginal farmers and agriculture labourers, who maintain livestock as a means to meet part of their family food requirements and to earn supplementary income. Small farmers are the major contributors to livestock production. Smallholder crop-livestock mixed farming is the dominant livestock production system in India, which provides food security, income, employment, manure, draught power, fuel, savings and socio-cultural objectives, and is also used as insurance for urgent cash needs (B.R.Patil, 2006).

The study conducted by Dr. N.S.R.Sastry and his team from NIRD, Hyderabad for the development of livestock sector in the UT of Pondicherry (Sastry et al., 1993) revealed that the mean daily milk yield of cows varies from 4 to 6 kg and the lactation yield was estimated at 1400 kg in 270 days. The reproductive performance was also not ideal since 45 per cent cows were dry at any given time and the service period was as long as 185 days. Inadequate nutrition was identified as the cause of such poor performance.

UG Programme: Field visits

As part of UG education in Applied Nutrition courses, II B.V.Sc. & A.H students, [Rajiv Gandhi College of Veterinary and Animal Sciences (RAGACOVAS), Pondicherry] had been taken to a village each year and data was collected on feeding practices followed there by the farmers. Villages covered were Villianur, Uruvaiyar, Mettupalayam and Melthirukanchi. Dairy farms maintained by Aurobindo Ashram like Lakeview Farm was also shown to the students to have knowledge on the feeding practices followed in feeding animals at different physiological phases in organized dairy farms (Anonymous, 2005). The following observations were made.

Feeding practices in Pondicherry

In general, buffaloes, sheep and goats were let out for grazing while crossbred cows were stall fed. Buffaloes mostly are graded Murrah type and the remaining are nondescript type. Mostly crossbred (average exotic inheritance of 62.5% is maintained) cows are Jersy crosses while Holstein Friesian crosses are very few. The average milk yield in case of buffaloes was around 6 L/ day though some animals yield 10 L/day. In case of crossbred cows, the average was 5-6 L /day and very few animals yield 15 L/day.

Offering of commercial concentrate mixture was not a practice. However, some farmers offered concentrate mixture supplied by the Department of Animal Husbandry and Animal Welfare and The Pondicherry Co-operative Milk Producers' Union Ltd (Ponlait). The concentrates were usually offered regularly to milking animals. The commonly used concentrate feeds were deoiled rice bran, wheat bran, bengalgram husk, greengram husk, blackgram husk, gingelly cake, groundnut cake, sunflower seed cake, rice broken, *jowar* (sorghum) grain and bajra grain. Of all these the most popular ones in daily feeding were wheat bran, oil cakes such as gingelly and groundnut, rice bran and gram husk, in the order of preference. Salt was added in drinking water in selected few instances. Supplementation of mineral mixture was not followed as a regular practice though some farmers used it for milch animals.

Rice straw was the common roughage. Green sugarcane tops were fed whenever available. Some farmers offered **Agathi (*Sesbania grandiflora*)** green leaves to milch animals. Green grass from field bunds (bund grass) was offered selectively to few valued animals during periods of availability; otherwise feeding of green fodders was not a regular practice. Farmers did not perceive cultivation of green fodder as economical and hence most of the farmers had not taken up.

No grazing lands are available. Hence animals are allowed to graze on fallow lands/ community grazing lands, if any; otherwise animals graze on private lands or vacant house sites. In periurban and urban areas the animals may roam in the streets of the town and eat the little grass found on the vacant sites/ roadsides or feed from the garbage bins or feed on the wall posters.

It was observed that farmers feed more oilseed cakes than the requirement, which was later found in a systematic study (Ramkumar et al., 2003), while rice straw, the sole roughage, was fed in limited amount. This means incurring more cost in feeding the animal and less profit from dairy enterprise as feed alone accounts for about 60% of the cost of milk production.

Birthal and Jha (2005) also reported that lack of availability of green fodder had been the most critical nutritional constraint in realizing the production potential of crossbred cows, while mineral deficiency emerged as the most limiting factor for buffaloes and indigenous cows. Inadequate concentrate feeding had been the second most important nutritional constraint in improving the milk yields of buffaloes and indigenous cows.

Principal crops and their byproducts

Percentage of area under principal crops to the total area sown during the year 2000-2001 for the Pondicherry Union Territory is presented in Table 1 (Anonymous, 2000-2001). The byproducts of the crops and the byproducts from the food processing industries are available for animal feeding (Table 2).

Table 1. Percentage of Area under Principal crops to the Total area sown: 2000-2001 for the Pondicherry UT

Crop	%
Paddy	60.39
Ragi	0.29
Bajra	0.43
Sorghum	0.02
Total cereals and millets	61.13
Total pulses [blackgram, greengram, horsegram,	13.72
karamani (cowpea), panipayir (pillipesara)	13.72
Sugarcane	5.69
Other food crops	3.54
Total food crops	84.08
Groundnut	2.72
Sesamum	0.29
Coconut	5.16
Cotton	1.04
Casuarina	5.28
Other nonfood crops	1.43
Total nonfood crops	15.92

Livelihood security of landless livestock farmers in Pondicherry

To many a landless family in India livestock rearing is an important secondary occupation and the number of landless families is on the rise with increasing pressure on the land due to increased human population, industrialization and urbanization.

Dr. Kevin Waldie tried to rationalize the compound phrase 'landless livestock farmers'. People who have sold their land in recent memory/people whose families have been landless for generations/landless agricultural labourers who have access to common property resources/urban-dwellers who have adopted the intensive management and production system of 'zero-grazing' or 'cut and carry'. Hence 'landless' signifies a social problem and draws attention to issues of rural inequality, poverty and vulnerability as well as that land for grazing is largely absent in urban areas.

Survey of rural, peri-urban and urban areas: Ramkumar and Rao (2001) surveyed four selected villages of Pondicherry, two villages categorized under rural (T.N.Palayam and Uruvaiyar), one under peri-urban (Pitchaveeranpet) and one under urban (Reddiyarpalayam) to analyze the livestock situation in Pondicherry with reference to landless families. This forms part of the higher education link programme on "Livelihood security of landless livestock farmers in Pondicherry: Search for sustainable paradigm". The Indo-UK higher education link programme was between RAGACOVAS and University of Reading, U.K. funded by DFID.

Table 2. Feeds and Fodder available

Roughages

	Green roughages (green fodder)	Dry roughages (straw, hay, hull)
Leguminous		
Annuals	Cowpea, horsegram, groundnut haulms	Cowpea hay, horsegram hay/ straw, groundnut haulms/ straw, groundnut shells, husks and bhusa from gram crops
Perennials Pasture crops	*Stylosanthes hamata, S. scabra,* siratro, butterfly pea	Hay made from stylo, siratro, butterfly pea
Fodder trees	*Sesbania grandiflora,* subabul, glyricidia	Sesbania, subabul, glyricidia
Non leguminous Annual cereals	Maize (African tall variety), Jowar (M.P.Chari, COFS), Bajra	Rice straw, rice husk, cobs and stover of ragi, bajra and sorghum
Perennial cultivated	Sugarcane tops, napier bajra hybrid (Co-1,2,3), para, guinea	Sugarcane tops
Perennial range grasses	*Cenchrus ciliaris, C. setigerus, Heteropogon contortus*	Dry grasses

Concentrates

Cereal grains	Rice broken, jowar (sorghum), bajra, maize
Grain byproducts	Rice bran, wheat bran
Gram byproducts	Bengalgram husk, greengram husk, Blackgram husk, gram chuni
Protein supplements (PS) Vegetable PS	Gingelly cake, Groundnut Cake, Sunflower cake, coconut cake, cottonseed cake
Animal PS	Fish meal

A workshop was on conducted on the topic "Landless livestock farming: Problems and Prospects" on January 29th, 2001. The study had successfully documented the livestock production systems of the landless in the urban, peri-urban and rural areas of Pondicherry; milch animals play significant role in the lives and livelihoods of urban and peri-urban dwellers, as well as rural households; significant amount of milk is produced by them; brainstorming session brought out their problems which include low milk procurement prices, high cost of concentrates and acute shortage of green fodder.

Urban livestock production

The importance of urban livestock production has been recognized long back and a due mention has been found in the Government Policy in the First National Five Year Plan: "It is estimated that 60-70% of the fluid milk requirements of the urban areas is derived from milch animals maintained within the municipal limits. These animals are generally kept in unsanitary and congested conditions, which affect their health, milk performance and breeding capacity. They are also a source of nuisance to the surrounding residential areas. A majority of these animals, when become dry, are sent to the slaughter house. Maintaining animals in this manner is uneconomic and is a drain on the cattle wealth of the country."

Now after more than fifty years, this negative view is being challenged by a more positive discourse promoting the importance of urban agriculture as an integral factor to the development of sustainable and environmentally friendly cities. Cattle and other livestock, formerly perceived as pollutants, are increasingly recognized for their value in recycling waste, as well as in providing products needed by the urban markets, and thus offering a source of living for those struggling to make both ends meet.

Farmer-formulated rations

Based on the surveys from several farmers from several villages (Ramkumar and Rao, 2001) the following ranges of feedstuffs were found to be offered to an adult milch cow/ buffalo (BW 350 to 400 kg) per day.

Feedstuffs	Range, kg
Rice straw	4.74 to12.0
Green grass	1.30 to 12.93
Groundnut cake	0.0689 to 0.981
or	
GNC	0.07 to 0.54
& Gingelly cake	0.05 to 0.6
or	
Gingelly cake	Nil to 2.24
Rice bran	0.10 to 2.54
Wheat bran	2.70 to 3.90
Gram husk	0.06 to 1.23
Ponlait feed	Nil to 0.81
Tapioca thippi	Nil to 0.20 - 0.40
Sugarcane tops	Nil to 1.70 - 4.50

Farmers themselves play the role of experimenters in getting to know the effective feeding of their animals depending on their perceptions on feed ingredients. The cost calculations of their rations are presented in Table 3. These farmer-formulated rations need to be validated by research.

The ideal ration versus farmer formulated ration

A ration is formulated as per the nutrient requirements of the cow based on its body weight, milk yield and fat percentage and number and stage of lactation using the feed ingredients available to the farmers. This is called as a 'balanced ration', which takes care of the maintenance and production requirements of the cow. Of course, this is not a least-cost ration. Though it is 'an ideal ration', majority of the cattle

Table 3. Farmers' rations along with cost of the feedstuffs

Milk yield, l/day	T N Palayam 4.00		Uruvaiyar 5.69		Pitchaveeranpet 5.69		Reddiarpalayam 7.85	
	Cost Rs./kg	Feed Kg/day	Cost Rs./kg	Feed Kg/day	Cost Rs./kg	Feed Kg/day	Cost Rs./kg	Feed Kg/day
Roughages								
Rice straw	0.95	7.12	0.78	4.8	1.00	4.74	1.60	4.95
Green grass	-	7.46	-	12.0	-	12.93	0.40	1.30
Concentrates								
Groundnut cake	15.00	0.98	15.00	0.54	15.00	0.07	-	-
Wheat bran	6.50	2.81	6.50	2.70	6.50	3.46	6.50	3.90
Rice bran	2.50	2.54	2.50	0.49	2.50	0.69	3.00	0.10
Gram husk	6.50	1.23	6.00	0.06	6.50	0.33	6.50	1.18
Ponlait feed	4.54	0.88	4.54	0.81	-	-	-	-
Gingelly cake	-	-	14.00	0.05	14.00	0.60	14.00	2.24
Tapioca thippi	-	-	6.50	0.13	6.50	0.36	-	-
Sugarcane tops	-	-	0.50	4.54	1.00	1.72	-	-
Total concentrate feed, kg		8.44		9.32		7.23		7.42

owners are not adopting this for a variety of reasons. Hence, usually there always exists a gap between 'ideal ration' composed by the researchers and 'farmer formulated ration' used by the cattle owners. The ideal ration does not vary for similar cows under different farming system locations but the farmer formulated ration varies depending upon the farmers' perceptions and situation, social as well as economic.

A study was undertaken to understand the farmers' ration fed to milking cows (Ramkumar et al., 2003) in one of the peri-urban regions of Pondicherry, Thengaithittu. Information was collected with respect to the commonly used cattle feed ingredients in the region and the units of measurement used by the cattle owners. The terminologies of units of measurement used for the various cattle feed ingredients were identified; the feed ingredients were weighed in a weighing machine to get the accurate equivalence of the 'local feed unit' of the farmer in the SI system; the cost of the feed ingredients was obtained from the local grocery shop. Four case studies were conducted among the cattle owners to ascertain the ration they are providing to the milking cows. Balanced rations were formulated with the same feed ingredients used by the farmers. The cost of feeding in line with the two rations was compared. One example of the case study is presented in Table 4 for comparison.

The nutritional parameters, respectively, for farmer formulated ration and scientific recommendation are 11.01 and 10.0 kg dry matter, 859 and 700 g digestible crude protein (DCP), and 6.76 and 6.15 kg total digestible nutrients (TDN). Perusal of data in Table 4 and the nutritional parameters revealed that the farmer formulated ration was comparatively costlier and had more DCP and TDN compared to the one scientifically formulated.

Table 4. Comparison of farmer's ration with balanced ration for a crossbred cow (400kg) yielding 10kg milk per day

Feed ingredients	Farmer ration		Balanced ration	
	Quantity, g	Cost, Rs	Quantity, g	Cost, Rs
Wheat bran	3000	21.60	1000	7.20
Rice bran	2400	7.68	1000	3.20
Gram husk	2000	16.00	1000	8.00
Groundnut cake &				
Gingelly cake	900	13.95	1100	17.05
Bund grass	Approx. 3000	–	9000	–
Straw	3000	7.00	5.00	11.67
Salt	100	0.50	60	0.30
Mineral mixture	–	–	30	3.00
Total		66.73		50.42

Feed is the main culprit for poor production and productivity

Small holding livestock production, a predominant feature, is primarily based on crop residues and hence there is a need to provide good quality feed to the producing animals in order to improve their productivity, and profitability of the farmers. Survey studies conducted in several parts of the country (for example, Hisar district, Haryana; Lall et al., 1996) showed that the animals belonging to landless labourers, especially, did not meet the nutrient requirements including the minerals. Mineral content of feeds like local grass, wheat straw and wheat bran did not match the dietary requirement of zinc and manganese irrespective of dry matter intake through grazing ultimately resulting in increased incidence of anestrous. Another field study on blood P, Mg, Fe, Zn, Cu and Mn profile of anestrous and repeat breeder crossbred cows (Prasad and Rao, 1997) revealed that the animals were deficient in one or other minerals which are important for reproduction.

A rapid appraisal on "Repeat breeding in crossbred cattle in peri-urban regions of Pondicherry" by Dr Kandasamy and his team during Jan. 2004 made the following observations on feed and fodder: Only 3 kg paddy straw was fed against 7 kg requirement; some cut grass was fed to lactating animals along with grazing on roadside and uncultivated lands; concentrates like wheat bran, bengalgram husk, rice bran, groundnut cake, greengram husk were offered; few cattle owners offer readymade concentrate mixture; mineral mixture was not given to the cattle while common salt was given to the lactating cows. On the incidence of repeat breeding, the veterinarians felt that mineral supplementation alone could bring substantial improvement (74%) in the situation.

Department of Animal Husbandry and Animal Welfare, Pondicherry conducted 30 infertility camps during the year 2003. Analysis of the causes for repeat breeding showed that 55% (870/1500) of the infertility problems were due to nutritional causes, while 21.8% due to uterine pathology and 16.2% due to hormonal imbalance.

Adoption of balanced feeding technologies

Basunathe et al. (2010) carried out a survey among the dairy farmers in Nagpur district (Maharshtra, India) on the adoption behaviour and factors associated with the adoption of feeding concentrate mixture and mineral mixture technologies by farmers. The decision to apply an innovation and to continue to use that innovation has been termed 'adoption' (Van den Ban and Hawkins, 1988). Different stages in the adoption of technologies are awareness, interest, evaluation, trial and adoption. The balanced feeding technologies have to pass through these different stages before their final adoption by the end-users. The results of the study revealed that 73% and 12% of the respondents fully adopted concentrate feeding and mineral mixture feeding, respectively. The remaining respondents were classified under non-adoption, discontinuation or partial adoption categories.

Technologies associated with increased profitability, simplicity, low initial cost, observability of results and compatibility with the social system norms and customs would be adopted faster than other technologies (Rogers, 1983). The results of the study indicated that dairy farmers, logically, compared the relative advantages of the technologies before adopting them.

Dairy farmers-Scientist interaction

A regional workshop was organized by Animal Nutrition Society of India (ANSI)-South Zone in association with RAGACOVAS at Pondicherry on 8-9, October 2003 to provide an opportunity for the Scientists from different parts of our country to understand the dairy farming situation in Pondicherry vis-à-vis the specific problems being experienced by the farmers. This interactive workshop is a step in right direction in reducing the communication gap between the farmers and scientists to facilitate better understanding between them.

Conclusions

The following conclusions are drawn from the study on feeding practices. Farmers need to follow these guidelines to improve the productivity of their animals and gain more profits.

1. Chopping of green fodders to minimize wastage
2. Coarse grinding and soaking/cooking of grains and soaking of oilcakes, brans prior to feeding improve digestion and utilization.
3. Mineral mixture and salt supplementation help animals to express their potential for milk production and health.
4. Feeding least-cost balanced rations help realize more profit from dairy enterprise.
5. Feeding sugarcane tops may be followed to overcome shortage of green fodder/dry fodder.
6. Legume forage from fodder trees such as agathi (*Sesbania grandiflora*) and soundal (*Leucaena leucocephala*, subabul) form nutrient rich herbage, which can save costly concentrate feeds.
7. The drought-tolerant subabul plants can be grown on farm bunds, tank bunds, backyards of farmers' houses and in vacant lands.

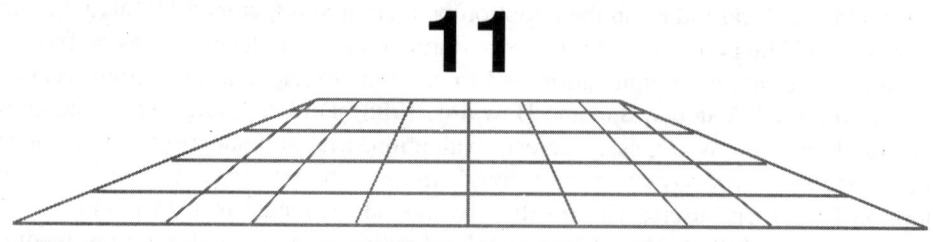

11

Utilization of Fibrous Feeds for Dairy Production
K Pradhan and N Krishna

INTRODUCTION

Animals are 'mediators' for high quality food production from the plant products, and dairy cattle are the most efficient converters of (human in-edible) feed protein and energy into milk. They can utilize large quantities of feed much of which cannot be used by human and other monogastric animals in its natural state. These feeds are highly fibrous in nature and sometimes constitute over 90% of feed resources in certain parts of the world. Wide variations are observed from different laboratories of the world regarding relative feed utilization by different dairy animals. This is particularly true for poor quality high fibrous diets. Feed is a major component of recurring cost input for growth and milk production. With technologically improved breeding, feeding and management, it should be possible to substantially increase the efficiency of conversion of nutrients into milk production from a variety of feeds that may significantly vary in their feeding value and quality. Generally, poor quality fibrous feeds and fodders are the major source of nutrients for ruminant animals in majority of developing countries.

Fibrous feed concept

Carbohydrates of feeds and fodder are broadly classified as either non-structural or structural compounds. Non-structural carbohydrates (NSC) are found inside the cells of plants and are usually more digestible than structural carbohydrates that are found in plant cell-walls. Feed fibre is the insoluble matter of plant cell organic compounds constituting both acid and alkaline resistant mixture and is not digested by animal enzymes. It is not a homogenous entity to be identified by a single value. Chemically, it is a complex of polysaccharides and other associated cellular components i.e., phenolic polymers which represent a part of feeds.

Plant tissues are composed of a heterogeneous population of cells, some metabolically active and others serve a structural function with extensively lignified cell-walls. The chemical constituents of the cell-wall are lignin, cellulose, hemicellulose, pectin, some protein, lignified nitrogenous substances, waxes, cutin and minerals which are further regrouped into insoluble substances (lignin, cellulose, hemicellulose and heat damaged protein) and soluble (pectin, waxes and protein) materials. Ruminants are capable of utilizing some of these components, which are otherwise indigestible by non-ruminants.

The evaluation of fibre in feed was first established by Henneberg and Stohmann in Germany in 1865 when they developed crude fibre (CF) analysis as part of proximate analysis, also known as the Weende method after the name of the experimental station. The detergent system (Van Soest and Wine 1967) of analysis was designed to replace the Weende system (proximate analysis) for determining the nutritional quality value of fibrous feeds by chemical methods. The most fundamental concept of the detergent system is based on the separation of feeds into fractions with uniform or non-uniform nutritional availability as defined by the Lucas test. Cell contents (neutral detergent solubles) and protein are feed fractions that usually have uniform nutritive availability. Cell-wall, cellulose and hemicellulose are feed fractions with non-uniform nutritive availability.

NDF, ADF and CF: Crude fibre, acid detergent fibre (ADF) and neutral detergent fibre (NDF) are the most common measures of fibre used for routine feed analysis, although none of them are chemically uniform. Neutral detergent fibre that measures most of the structural components in plant cells (cellulose, hemicellulose and lignin) is, generally, considered to comprise fibre. Acid detergent fibre does not include hemicellulose, and crude fibre does not quantitatively recover hemicellulose and lignin. Neutral detergent fibre, therefore, is the best expression of fibre available currently, though recommendations are also given for ADF because of its widespread use. Fibre fractions measured in terms of crude fibre, neutral detergent fibre and acid detergent fibre for important feedstuffs reveal wide variation in their chemical composition as presented in Table 1. NDF is further refined for its value as protector of rumen health (see later in this chapter PP 178 and in another chapter in this section pp 89.

High fibre feed resources potential

Major part of the feed consumed world over by cows, buffaloes, and other ruminant animals comes from roughages which include feeds from grassland, range land and cultivated green fodder as well as crop byproducts, namely straws and stovers. Concentrate feeds account for about one-fourth of the total feed available. The proportions of poor quality roughages available to these animals in developing countries are significantly higher. Crop residues and other byproducts provide the bulk. Also, the use of the byproduct feeds that are mostly fibrous in nature is increasing more rapidly than those of the cereal based feeds, mainly due to increase in food grain production and improved feed processing technology. In the recent past, animal feed consumption rate in developing countries expanded much faster than that in developed countries, because of the increasing demands for livestock products in the developing countries. Thus, improving livestock feed situation in developing countries may help ease the pressure on expanding the production of green fodder, grain, oil seed meal and other feed resources in future.

Table 1 Fibre components of some selected feedstuffs (% DM basis)

Feeds/fodder	NDF	ADF	CF
Green fodders			
Lucerne	37 – 51	31 – 40	16 – 35
Berseem	43 – 54	35 – 42	15 – 29
Maize	55 – 66	34 – 42	30 – 38
Sorghum	56 – 70	38 – 46	27 – 41
Pearl millet	57 – 70	39 – 43	24 – 33
Oat	47 – 70	30 – 38	18 – 37
Crop residues			
Wheat straw	76	53	53
Paddy straw	72	54	37
Oat straw	72	49	38
Gram straw	64	49	38
Pearl millet stover	78	54	38
Sorghum stover	78	51	36
Sugarcane bagasse	93	64	42
Byproducts			
Cottonseed hulls	89	71	38
Citrus pulp	28	22	13
Brewer grain	52	23	15
Maize cobs	88	39	36
Distiller grain	45	16	14
Grains/meals			
Maize (ground)	9	3	2
Barley (ground)	23	7	5
Soya bean meal	12	8	2
Groundnut cake	29	15	8
Cottonseed meal	64	40	18

Feed quality

High cell-wall constituents - low digestibility - voluntary consumption: It is evident that the shortage of feed ingredients has led to a greater use of over-grazed grassland, crop residues and agro-industrial byproducts by ruminant animals. Their feeding value for dairy cattle or buffalo is low and thus, requires improvement. These feeds contain a high proportion of cell-walls and are highly lignified. This results in the overall reduction in the digestibility of organic matter. The high cell-wall constituents and low digestibility would impose a limitation upon the voluntary consumption by the dairy animals. An application of appropriate technology in improving the quality of these feeds will go a long way in improving the food resource situation. A large number of unconventional and some of the conventional byproducts contain toxic principles like tannins, mimosine, saponins, nitrate, oxalates, etc., which may cause harmful effect to the animal system. They can be degraded to less toxic or non-toxic compounds, but the high cost of methodology does not find extensive field application. Therefore there is a wide scope of utilizing biotechnology in this area of research to develop simple and cost effective methods.

The fibrous agricultural and industrial byproducts, being poor in their nutritional worth, cannot support *per se* even the maintenance requirement of low producing dairy animals. Therefore, combining these feedstuffs with other essential supplements or developing a complete diet system is necessary for improving their utilization. While a large volume of research data has accumulated on the better utilization of crop residues and other agro-industrial byproducts for maintenance and production specially in cattle, buffalo, sheep and goat, the information on production parameters are based on a limited experiments of short duration. Most of the studies, however, are on rumen metabolism and fermentation behaviour in these animals fed straw based diets.

Straws and stovers: Crop residues as sources of animal feeds, mainly include byproducts from cereals, pulses, oilseeds, sugarcane and many plantation crops. Of all the crops, rice and wheat straws occupy the most prominent position in their availability, followed by stovers from sorghum, millets and maize crops. These residues are characterized by a low content of protein and less digestible cell wall carbohydrates (Table 2). These cellulosic plant materials are highly fibrous, poor in total digestible nutrients (TDN), digestible crude protein (DCP) and many essentials minerals. Their voluntary consumption is also very low. Dairy animals sustaining on them often suffer from under-nutrition.

Table 2. Nutritive value of major crop residues (% DM)

Straw/stover	DM	NDF	Protein		TDN	Energy (K cal/kg)		Ca	P
			Total	Dig.		DE	ME		
Paddy	91	71	4.2	1.0	48	2116	1735	0.24	0.90
Wheat	90	76	3.2	0.4	43	1896	1556	0.15	0.07
Maize	87	68	5.1	2.2	59	2801	2133	0.29	0.11
Sorghum	91	72	7.0	3.1	51	2294	1844	0.74	0.28
Pearl-millet	88	79	2.6	0.2	53	2352	1884	0.30	0.10
Barley	88	60	3.6	0.6	43	1896	1555	0.30	0.08
Gram	88	64	3.9	2.4	37	1632	1338	1.40	0.28

Higher lignin and silica contents also limit their consumption and digestibility. Lignin physically encrusts carbohydrates of plant materials thereby acting as a physical barrier against the action of microbial enzymes and digestive juices. The cellulose present in the crop residues is primarily crystalline in nature, and thus less reactive and accessible to the digestive juices. The rate of passage of these roughages through the digestive tract is also low, because of the presence of crystalline and lignified cellulose that stays for longer period in the reticulo-rumen for digestion. Plant silica, which is deposited within the matrix of the cell-wall adversely affects fibre digestibility. The insufficiency of available nitrogen, energy and minerals to satisfy the growth requirement of microbial population in the rumen has been one of the most serious limitations of these low quality roughages in influencing the poor digestibility and voluntary intake by ruminant animals.

Quality improvement

Various methods have been adopted during the recent years to improve the nutritive value of poor quality roughages in terms of digestibility and voluntary intake. These are physical processing methods like chopping, grinding and pelleting, chemical treatments with alkali and oxidizing agents, supplementation with deficient nutrients in various combinations and other physicochemical techniques. Their feeding value can also be improved by employing biological methods like ensiling and other microbial treatments (Table 3).

Physical, chemical and biological treatments: Physical processes such as chopping, grinding and pelleting, water soaking, radiation and steam treatments have been used to modify the structure of some of the refractory components of these roughages. These processes help increase the rate of passage and improve the microbial attack in the rumen. The chemical treatments using alkali and some oxidizing agents (H_2O_2) bring about changes in the cell-wall, which make their digestible components more accessible to digestible enzymes and, therefore, increase the intake and digestibility of these cellulosic materials. However, these methods have limited application due to economic reasons.

Supplementation of deficient nutrients: There is considerable evidence that the added dietary nitrogen (conventional or non-conventional), energy (molasses, starch and grains) and mineral elements have improved the voluntary intake and utilization of low quality roughages. Studies in crossbred calves fed wheat straw based ration supplemented with concentrate mixture and poultry litter as source of nitrogen show that nutritive value and dry matter intake are improved by enriching the straw with non-conventional source of nitrogen. The calves grew at a faster rate due to ration containing wheat straw and poultry litter compared to even the control (Table 4). Supplementing straws with molasses, urea and other proteinous feeds has invariably improved the feeding values of these poor quality roughages.

Ensilage process: Ensiling has been recommended to improve the nutritive value of poor quality roughages. During the process, the structure of fibrous materials is modified and as a result, a reduction of lignification due to breakage of acid-labile bonds of lignin occurs. The feeding value of wheat straw has been reported to increase after making silage in combination with green berseem or cowpea. Both intake and digestibility of feed dry matter are markedly increased. The milk production in cows on ensiled wheat straw diet has shown an upward trend suggesting a better utilization of straws. The production of biomass on crop residue is another biological approach in improving the feeding value of cellulosic materials. The protein content

Table 3: Effect of improving the nutritional value of poor quality roughages through various treatments

Treatment	Feed	Animal	DM Intake		Digestibility%				Reference
			%BW	g/kg W^{-75}	DM	CF	NDF	ADF	
Physical									
Chopping	Grass hay-chopped	Cow	--	--	72.8	--	79.1	--	Uden, 1998
Pelleting	Grass hay - pelleted	Cow	--	--	67.1	--	68.3	--	Anim. Feed Sci. & Tech. 19 : 145.
Grinding	Wheat straw -Ground	Buffalo	2.5	84.0	51.9	58.7	--	--	Chaturvedi et al. 1973. Indian J. Anim. Sci. 43:382
Chemical									
NaOH	Wheat straw-untreated	Buffalo	2.4	--	45.6	55.6	--	41.4	Jai Kishan et al. 1973. Indian J. Anim. Sci. 47 : 609
	Wheat straw-NaOH	Buffalo	2.2	--	52.5	66.6	--	48.1	
Urea-NH$_3$	Wheat straw-untreated	Heifer	1.8	60.0	48.4	51.9	47.9	47.2	Dahiya and Mudgal 1991 J. Anim. Sci. 61 : 218
	Wheat straw-urea-NH$_3$	Heifer	2.8	96.4	59.6	62.9	58.0	59.3	
Urea-NH$_3$	Paddy straw-untreated	Cattle	2.2	--	41.0	38.0	--	--	Reddy et al. 1989. Indian J. Anim. Nutr. 6:22
	Paddy straw-urea NH$_3$	Cattle	3.0	--	49.8	45.4	--	--	
Anhydrous-NH$_3$	Wheat straw-untreated	Steers	--	39.1	48.5	51.4	--	--	Horton, 1978. Canad. J. Anim. Sci. 58:471
	Wheat straw-anhy.NH$_3$	Steers	--	46.5	53.3	63.9	--	--	
Aqua-NH$_3$	Wheat straw-untreated	Heifers	1.8	60.0	48.4	51.9	47.9	47.2	Dahiya and Mudgal 1991 J.
	Wheat straw-Aqua-NH$_3$	Heifers	2.5	88.4	57.1	62.1	57.3	57.5	

Biological

								Reference
Silage								
Pearl millet-ensiled	Heifers	2.0	--	64.3	--	60.0	65.4	Jaster et al. 1985. Anim. Sci. 61: 218
Sorghum-ensiled	Heifers	2.5	--	60.1	--	61.1	57.0	Narang and Pradhan 1974. J. Dairy Sci. 68:2914
Fresh wheat straw & Cowpea	Cows	1.6	--	36.9	48.9	--	--	
Ensiled wheat straw & Cowpea	Cows	2.0	--	48.5	54.2	--	--	Indian J. Anim. Sci. 44:14
Fungal								
Urea treated-wheat straw	Goats	--	42.5	46.9	64.3	47.7	47.3	Gupta et al. 1988. Indian J. Anim. Nutr. 5:222
Fungal treated-wheat straw	Goats	--	50.7	48.3	55.9	37.9	39.4	

Table 4: Dry matter intake, digestibility and body weight gain in growing calves fed wheat straw (WS) based diets

Ration	DM intake (kg/d)	DM digestibility (%)	Weight gain (g/day)
WS + concentrate	3.79	53.9	386
WS + urea + molasses	2.80	59.7	46
WS + poultry litter	5.47	51.8	517
Silage (WS + lucerne)	5.17	59.6	280

Goel and Pradhan (1978)

and nutritional value of straws can be significantly increased by the growth of appropriate fungal strain after supplementing with a small amount of urea and molasses (Gupta *et al.*, 1988)

Urea-ammoniation technology: A successful technology for the nitrogen enrichment of straw has been adopted very widely. This technology improves the nutritive value without involving high cost or risk of any kind to the animal or environment. It improves the nitrogen content as well as available energy in treated straw. A number of studies conducted in India and elsewhere have demonstrated that 4 kg urea dissolved in 65 litres of water and sprinkled on 100 kg chopped straw and then, the wet material stored in the form of a stack for about 4 weeks, improves the DM digestibility of straw by about 40% and the voluntary feed intake by about 20%. The crude protein content increases from 4 to 8% in wheat straw and 5 to 12% in paddy straw. During the process, more than 70% of urea is degraded, part of which is utilized for the microbial protein synthesis. The increased temperature during fermentation helps ammonia penetrates into the cell-walls of the straw more efficiently. The processed straw with small quantity of protein, vitamins and mineral supplements can support the growth of dairy calves (Table 5) and also meet the nutrient requirements of low yielding cows (Reddy et al., 1991)

Table 5. Urea-ammonia treated paddy straw (TPS) for growing crossbred calves

Feeds	DM intake (kg/day)			DMI (kg/100 kg BW)	ADG (g/day)
	Straw	Concentrate/ berseem	Total		
TPS	3.95	0	3.95	1.71	246
TPS + Fish meal	3.46	0.16	3.62	1.66	237
TPS + Cotton seed cake	3.69	0.23	3.92	1.78	427
PS + Berseem	1.91	1.27	3.18	1.57	473
P S + Urea	2.83	0	2.83	1.26	111

Terminal Report (1967-85) of the AICRP on Utilization of Agro-Industrial Byproducts for Livestock, G. B. Pant University of Agriculture and Technology, Pantnagar

Feed fibre consumption and digestion characteristics: Differences between cattle and buffaloes

The consumption and digestibility of feeds are two most important aspects of nutrition, which determine the animal response. The fundamental characteristic of fibrous feeds is that the plant cell-wall contains digestible amount of cellulose and hemicellulose that contribute to the total digestive nutrients of the feed. As the forage matures, cell-wall digestibility declines because of increased lignification. The association of lignin with polysaccharide constituents of cell-wall limits microbial digestion, with lignin protecting about 1.4 times its own mass of cell-wall carbohydrates. The extent to which the feed is digested varies with the type of feed, particle size, NDF content, rate of cell-wall digestion and rate of passage. The hemicellulose, part of the NDF, not contained in ADF, is most sensitive to digestion. This may be the primary reason that NDF is associated with feed digestibility.

Consumption

The feed dry matter intake is affected by many factors including gut fill, chemostatic regulator, and digestibility of the ration. Neutral detergent fibre, which is inversely related to the feed intake, has been proposed by some researchers as good predictor of dry matter intake, because it contains all of the bulkier and less digestible portions of the feedstuff. Besides, NDF has been associated with many physical factors limiting feed intake, such as bulk density or volume, rumination time, total chewing time and the rate of particle size reduction required for feeds to escape from the rumen. Therefore, the use of neutral detergent fibre in formulating rations for dairy animals appears to have definite merits.

The eating pattern of dairy animals differs among various animal species due to fibrous feed sources. Buffaloes, irrespective of their physiological status are found to be slow eaters than cattle under poor quality high fibre feeding regime. It has been observed that a lesser quantity of dry matter (34%) was consumed by buffalo than cattle (46%) up to first four hours of feeding of *ad libitum* wheat straw and groundnut meal supplemented with mineral and vitamin mixture. In contrast, a relatively higher proportion of berseem hay, a good quality fodder, was eaten by buffaloes (78%) than cattle (58%) in early hours of feeding (Bhatia *et al.*, 1980). The experimental findings suggest that eating pattern of ruminants is a function of the nature of the fibrous diets and animal species.

The differences in dry matter intake and nutrient digestibilities have often been observed in cattle and buffaloes fed poor quality high fibrous diets. Based on a large number of feeding trials with crop residues, Pradhan et al. (1991) compiled the data on feed dry matter intake and digestibilities both in cattle and buffaloes and reported that buffaloes eat less feed dry matter per unit body weight or metabolic body size than the cattle (Table 6). However, in some isolated cases such differences do not exist. Extensive studies carried out by Krishna et al (1985) indicated that the differences in DM intake and nutrient digestibilities between cattle and buffaloes fed oat or berseem hays as a sole roughage source did not differ significantly. However, non-significant differences that exist were attributed to methodology adopted with respect to length of collection period, number of animals and species of animals used.

Fine grinding and pelleting of roughages generally result in a marked increase in dietary intake, but increasing the level of concentrate in the mixture reduces the effect. High concentrate or finely ground roughage diet may cause parakeratosis of the rumen papillae. Therefore, effort should be made with caution to derive gain from the information available in the literature.

Digestion

The digestibility of feed dry matter and nutrients is affected by the physical and chemical characteristics of feedstuffs consumed and animal types. The rumen ecosystem also plays an important role in nutrient degradation. The effect of roughage preparation on the rumen physiology has shown that crude fibre or cellulose digestion decreases when roughage is finely ground and pelleted, because of its high rate of passage through the gut. Higher concentration of volatile fatty acids is found in the rumen when roughage is finely ground and pelleted. There is also an increase in the concentration of propionic to acetic acid production.

Table 6: Dry matter intake and nutrient digestibility in cattle and buffaloes fed various roughage-protein diets*

Parameter	Cattle	Buffalo
Feed dry matter intake		
DMI (kg / d)	6.6 (3.5 – 9.4)	7.3 (3.3 – 9.1)
DMI (% BW)	1.8 (1.3 – 2.2)	1.6 (1.3 – 2.1)
DMI (g/W0.75 kg)	78.2 (58.2 – 101.0)	74.8 (56.8 – 85.7)
Digestibility (%)		
DM	53.3 (46.5 – 60.7)	55.4 (43.6 – 59.3)
CP	55.1 (29.3 – 76.4)	58.1 (30.3 – 77.8)
NDF	48.8 (37.7 – 60.7)	51.5 (41.7 – 59.7)
ADF	44.8 (39.5 – 51.5)	47.8 (39.7 – 57.0)
Cellulose	49.2 (38.0 – 64.0)	51.2 (36.7 – 64.0)
Hemicellulose	65.1 (45.1 – 79.0)	64.3 (44.3 – 77.7)

*Technical Bulletin, 1991. Relative rumen ecosystem and nutrient digestibility in cattle and buffaloes fed high fibrous diets. Haryana Agricultural University, Hisar

Buffaloes are reported to digest cellulosic poor quality feeds more efficiently than do cattle. The findings on the comparative functional rumen developments and rumen microbial activities have in general, led to the belief that buffaloes are efficient convertors of low-grade roughages.

Differences exist between cattle and buffaloes with regard to feed intake. But the nutrient digestibility of various low quality feeds remains largely unchanged due to animal species (Table 6). However, buffaloes appeared to be superior to cattle in digesting nutrients only with certain diets such as wheat straw-groundnut meal, wheat straw-berseem hay and chickpea straw-concentrate (Prasad and Pradhan, 1990). Irrespective of physiological stage, buffaloes digested relatively more feed nutrients from wheat straw-groundnut meal than cattle. The digestibility of feed nutrients from berseem hay also exceeded in growing buffaloes compared to those in growing cattle. However, adult buffaloes did not reveal this trend due to berseem hay diet, though significant differences in nutrient digestion were exhibited by mature buffaloes than mature cattle when maintained on wheat straw-berseem hay dietary regimen. Such differences may possibly be attributed to source and level of dietary fibre and protein in the maintenance ration of ruminant species.

Though inconsistent results on nutrient digestion between cattle and buffaloes are reported, it is generally believed that buffaloes are efficient convertors of low-grade roughages for different physiological body functions. The relatively lower feed intake associated with their lower fasting heat production may result in a higher production of net energy per unit feed consumed. Also, the feasibility of some diet characteristic(s) not discernible by conventional chemical analysis upon which the relative responses of ruminant species depend cannot be ruled out. This, however, is a complex phenomenon and requires further studies.

Metabolites

One of the primary functions of the rumen fermentation through its microbes is the breakdown of cellulose, hemicellulose and other polysaccharides into intermediary products. The bacteria and protozoa population, respectively, in the rumen is in the neighborhood of 1010 and 105 per gram of rumen contents, which may vary from one ruminant species to the other. Acetate, propionate and butyrate are the major volatile fatty acids produced from the polysaccharides of the fibrous feeds in the rumen and are utilized by ruminants for various physiological functions including growth and production.

Pentosans, which form about one-fifth of the total dry matter of grasses and hays, are digested in the rumen producing volatile fatty acids. A carefully formulated diet should provide conditions and environment that are required for maintaining proper pH, temperature, salivary secretion, rumination and rate of feed passage in the rumen, which help promote the development of proper microbial population and efficient microbial digestion. These conditions are influenced by the quantity and quality of dietary fibre.

The biochemical characteristics of ruminant animals due to various high fibrous diets have been extensively documented and their values in the rumen differ due to feeds and animal species (Table 7). Of varied rumen metabolites, higher ruminal ammonia concentration in buffalo than cattle has invariably been reported. Greater ability to synthesize urea by buffalo than cattle fed low quality roughages has been recorded (Norton et al., 1979). However, the trend for other nitrogenous fractions was not so different.

The metabolic profile in respect of fractionated volatile fatty acids (acetate, propionate and butyrate) in the rumen remains almost unchanged in cattle and buffaloes fed high fibrous poor quality roughages, although some reports suggest that buffalo has a variable, some times greater, concentration of volatile fatty acids than cattle due to source of diets. Though microbial profile, especially celluloytic bacteria (Wattanachantra et al., 1989) was better in the rumen of buffalo over that of cattle, the same did not reflect in the improved digestive function of the ruminant species, which indicated that factors (s) other than microbiota population size exert an influence on the feed digestibility. This confirms to the earlier view of Jung and Varel (1987) that fibre digestion can not be predicted from the decrease or increase of cellulolytic bacteria in the rumen.

No consistent differences exist in nutrient digestion between cattle and buffalo, though the population size of viable bacteria, cellulolytic bacteria and protozoal counts usually exceed in buffaloes over cattle (Pradhan et al., 1991). It may suggest that factors like basal metabolic rate, rumen volume, rumen fluid outflow rate and other physiological factors, not merely the rumen microbial status and profile, exert their influence on differential nutrient digestibility and degradation in the rumen of cattle and buffaloes.

Table 7: Nitrogen degradation and carbohydrate fermentation end products in cattle and buffaloes fed various low grade roughage protein diets*

Parameter	Cattle	Buffalo
Nitrogen metabolites (mg/100 ml)		
Total nitrogen	79.3	82.9
	(48.8 – 114.1)	(55.0 – 109.8)
Ammonia nitrogen	9.8	12.1
	(6.1 – 12.3)	(6.8 – 14.5)
Protein nitrogen	34.7	36.6
	(26.6 – 48.4)	(27.4 – 42.4)
Volatile fatty acids (meq/L)		
TVFA	109.4	116.9
	(75.7 – 199.9)	(87.5 – 193.9)
Acetate	85.8	91.3
	(58.0 – 157.0)	(67.3 – 143.2)
Propionate	13.9	14.9
	(9.6 – 26.2)	(9.5 – 26.3)
Butyrate	5.7	6.0
	(3.9 – 12.5)	(3.5 – 12.2)
pH	6.9	6.9
	(6.4 – 7.1)	(6.6 – 7.1)

*Technical Bulletin, 1991. Relative rumen ecosystem and nutrient digestibility in cattle and buffaloes fed high fibrous diets. Haryana Agricultural University, Hisar

Milk yield and composition

The production of milk and its composition always receive attention in order to make dairy enterprise profitable. Lactational response in terms of milk yield and composition is attributed to the genetic make-up of the animal and nutrient supply to meet the requirements for milk production and specifically for the precursors of milk constituents. Fifty five percent of the variation in milk components is due to heredity and 45 per cent due to nutrition. The response may also vary with the physiology and biochemistry of the secretary processes of mammary tissues depending on the short or long-term effect.

While milk lactose content varies within fairly narrow limits and is minimally sensitive to nutritional manipulation, milk fat and protein contents can be influenced by the nutritional factors. It is more pronounced on fat than on protein content of milk. The mechanism that influences the individual end products of digestion to milk fat and protein contents may relate to a simple relationship between the blood precursor supply and product synthesis or to a more complex system. The reader may refer chapter 'Diet and milk production' for more information. The concentration of acetate, butyrate and long chain fatty acids in the blood has a positive relationship with milk fat yield. It is rather apparent that acetate has a special role in mammary gland metabolism because of its position in the energy production cycle.

Importance of fibre: Energy and protein are the most limiting nutrients for high yielding dairy animals. However, other micro- and macro-nutrients are equally important for milk production. The fibre levels in the diet must be kept at a desired level in order to prevent health problems and low fat milk production. Milk production and composition generally relate to fibre level, physical form and concentrate to roughage ratio in the diet of dairy animals. It is an established fact that feeding high level of concentrate or pelleted forage to a cow results in depression of milk fat resulting from a low production of rumen acetate. It was first observed by Powell (1939) that the fat content of cow milk could be depressed as much as 60 per cent by feeding low roughage rations or by feeding roughages in a finely ground form.

There is apparently a positive correlation between the activities of the rumen and the composition of the milk produced. A high-energy ration low in fibre, produces less of acetate and more of propionate in the rumen. Thus, the ratio between the ruminal acetate to propionate concentration in respect of a ration is conclusively important for the milk fat synthesis. Milk fat depression in cows is usually associated with diets containing less than 17 per cent **crude fibre** or 19 per cent **acid detergent fibre.**

The presence of long fibre in the diets of cattle have a number of advantages, as such diets provide a more continuous flow of fermentable carbohydrates to rumen organisms and thus improve the overall utilization of the total diet. The quantity of long fibre in the diet of lactating cows should not be less than 0.5 per cent of body weight. Thus, a 500 kg cow should receive at least 2.5 kg of long fibre per day and more may be preferable.

Dietary fibre requirement

Feeds and fodders are available with widely variable quality attributes, sources of origin and are relatively less utilized by animals to their nutritional potentialities. This is further influenced by the relationship that exists between feed intake, nutrient availability and synthesis mechanism in animals. Factors intrinsic to the feed and animals may limit energy assimilation. Digestion inhibitors may also be present in some feeds. Thus, the net energy available from feeds for maintenance, growth, pregnancy and lactation is only a fraction of the gross energy ingested.

The output of milk and its constituents are sensitive to the nutrient supply and influenced by the mixture of the end products of digestion absorbed from the gut. The evidence available suggests that the yield of milk fat and protein will be maximized by rations giving high uptake of acetate, long chain fatty acids and amino acids. In practical terms, such diets will most commonly contain a large proportion of highly digestible forages or fibrous feedstuffs and some concentrates to provide energy and proteins. The protein supplements should maintain a proper balance between rumen degradable and undegradable proteins. A restricted amount of rumen soluble carbohydrate will promote ruminal acetate production and control levels of propionate and glucose.

Source and level of fibre

Experimental evidences are available to demonstrate that sources of neutral detergent fibre and starch affect the utilization of dietary nutrients. It has been observed by Weiss et al. (1989) that two diets (lucerne with barley or maize) containing a similar level of neutral detergent fibre (30% on dry matter basis) from two different sources have influenced the milk production. However, the intake in respect of dry matter, net energy and NDF remains similar between the diets. The digestibility of dry matter, NDF and crude protein are also not affected by the diets, but hemicellulose digestion was higher and cellulose and ADF digestion were lower in cows given lucerne-barley diets compared to lucerne-maize diets. Cows fed on the lucerne-maize diet had higher ruminal acetate to propionate molar ratio.

Woodford and Murphy (1988) reported that physical form of fodder has a direct relationship with chewing activities, dry matter intake and rumen functions of lactating dairy cows. In their research, they have observed that dairy cattle in early lactation require a minimum amount of effective fibre to optimize intake and milk production. This requirement was made when lucerne silage was 28 per cent of the diet dry matter. When this level was reduced to 12 per cent, the dry matter intake was significantly low. Also, rumen fluid dilution rate, volume and outflow, rumination time, chewing time and rumen acetate molar percentage decreased at low level of lucerne hay in the diet. Further, in long-term lactation studies (305 days), it has been confirmed that the level of fibre in the diet significantly influenced the milk yield of cows maintained on similar protein and energy level.

Crude fibre content of diet

The diets beyond 18 percent crude fibre level adversely affect the milk production. The lactating cows had the best performance in terms of milk production and composition due to a ration containing 18.7% crude fibre as compared to others having of 21.0 and 25.5% dietary fibre contents (Pasierbski and Warwarzynezak, 1987). The fibre requirement of dairy cows is also related to the stage of lactation. In the early period of lactation in mature cows, diet should contain 2 kg of structural fibre. This quantity should be increased to 2.75 kg during mid to late lactation. The average daily crude fibre intake for cows weighing 550kg has been suggested to be 0.5kg/100kg body weight. With high yielding cows the proportion of fibre in the diet may be less than the optimum 18 percent, but the amount of fibre, including the structural fibre, should be relatively constant at 3.0 to 3.5 kg.

NDF requirement

The optimum level of NDF and ADF in the diets for dairy cows varies with milk producing ability of the cow, stage of lactation and the nature of the feed. A minimum, of 28 per cent NDF and 21 per cent of ADF have been recommended for high producing cows during the first three weeks of lactation and thereafter, when milk production increases the dietary NDF (25%) and ADF (19%) contents get reduced (NRC, 1988) and then, increased during the later stage of lactation. Such data are not available for low milk yielding cows and buffaloes. In the revised edition (NRC, 2001), NRC recommended minimum dietary NDF for cows at 25 % of DM with the condition that 19 % of dietary DM must be in the form of NDF from forage (Table 8). Lower producing cows require less energy, and diets should contain NDF concentrations higher than the minimum.

Table 8: Recommended minimum concentrations (% of DM) of total and forage NDF and maximum concentrations (% of DM) of NFC in lactating cows fed total mixed ration

Minimum forage NDF	Minimum dietary NDF	Maximum dietary NFC	Minimum dietary ADF
19[a]	25[a]	44[a]	17[a]
18	27	42	18
17	29	40	19
16	31	38	20
15	33	36	21

[a]Diets that contain less fibre (forage NDF, total NDF or total ADF) than these minimum values and more NFC than 44 % should not be fed (NRC, 2001)

Physically effective fibre and ruminal pH

The concept of physically effective fibre (i.e., fibre that stimulates rumination, saliva production, and rumen buffering) was created to amalgamate the chemical characteristics and particle size of forages, and to quantify its value to rumen function (Mertens, 2000).

Despite the fact that milk fat percentage is an easily measured parameter, low fibre in the diet can detrimentally affect animal health without significant milk fat depression. Ruminal pH may be a better indication of ruminal health and optimal function, and a better basis for determining fibre requirements of dairy cows in early lactation than the maintenance of milk fat production. Zebeli et al. (2006) indicated that accounting for dietary physically effective fibre is a more efficient procedure to assess effective fibre adequacy of dairy cow rations than simply taking into account dietary NDF or forage NDF (FNDF).

Rations that bring about a significant positive response in milk protein yield may lower milk fat content. The effects of protein supplementation on milk fat content vary with the basal diet, but in many instances fat content is reduced, because milk yield is increased without a commensurate response in fat yield. While studying the effect of the type of ration on milk protein content, Grant and Patel (1980) observed that typical rations ranging in level of concentrate from 40 to 60 per cent had only slight variation in milk protein contents that could be attributed to the ration.

Limited information is available about the interaction of milk production, milk composition and dietary fibre when dairy animals are supplied a variety of high fibrous feeds including byproduct feeds at various stages of lactation and levels of milk production. Therefore, the fibre requirement values for milk production and composition, as reported in the literature should be utilized with caution. Also, any modification of the diets for dairy animals to alter the milk composition must be designed to maximize the economic efficiency of production.

Conclusion

In dairy enterprise the production of milk at a cheaper input cost is the primary aim of a dairy farmer. The feed resources that have direct relationship with milk yield and composition are the major limiting factors in dairy production system in most parts of the world for which the genetic potential of cows and buffaloes is inadequately exploited. Compared to dairy production in developed countries, the productivity of cows and buffaloes in developing regions is poor, as these animals are essentially maintained on poor quality natural grasses, crop residues and other byproduct feeds.

The grasslands including forage production situation in most part of the world is constantly declining. The availability of high-energy cereal grains and other food crops for livestock consumption has also shown similar trend, because of ever increasing human population growth. Therefore, the dairy animals, which used to consume in the past good quality high fibrous feeds, now depend largely on alternative feed resources of poorer quality i.e. crop residues and other byproducts for their maintenance and production purpose. Thus, it has become imperative to improve their nutritive value and utilize them for economic production of livestock.

The high fibrous feeds available in large quantities world over are ligno-cellulosic in nature, and are very poorly consumed and digested. The major barriers limiting their efficient utilization are highly structured cellulose and its association with lignin. Several methods have been developed to unlock the ligno-cellulosic bonding, but their field level applicability is limited due to high cost or environmental risk. However, a few technologies such as ammoniation or urea-ammonia treatment of straws have shown promise in improving their nutritive value to meet the energy and protein requirements for maintenance, growth and milk yield at low level of production in cows and buffaloes. Further, the present day science and technology must explore and help expand the feed resource position, preferably through their qualitative improvement. This demands a successful application of biotechnology in the production of nutrients for dairy animals.

REFERENCES TO THE LITERATURE (PARTIAL LIST)

Anonymous, 2000-2001. Season and crop report (July 2000-June 2001). Printed and Published by Directorate of Economics and Statistics, Government of Pondicherry, Pondicherry.

Anonymous, 2005. "A study on feeding practices at Pondicherry" conducted by Department of Animal Nutrition, RAGACOVAS, Pondicherry.

Basunathe, V.K., Sawarkar, S.W. and Sasidhar, P.V.K. 2010. Adoption of dairy production technologies and implications for dairy development in India. Outlook on Agriculture, 39, 2, pp134-140.

Bernal-Santos, B., O'Donnell, A.M., Vicini, J.L., Hartnell, G.F. and Bauman, D.E. 2010. Enhancing omega-3 fatty acids in milk fat of dairy cows by using stearidonic acid-enriched soybean oil from genetically modified soybeans. J. Dairy Sci. 93:32-37

Bhatia, S.K., K. Pradhan and R.Singh 1980. Rumen metabolic profile as influenced by dietary non-protein nitrogen and carbohydrates. Indian J. Anim. Sci. 50: 16.

Bilby, T.R., Baumgard, L.H., Rhoads, M.L. and Collier, R.J. (2008) Strategies to Improve Reproduction during Heat Stress. 2008 Mid-South Ruminant Nutrition Conference, Arlington, Texas

De Leeuw, P.N., Omore, A., Staal,S. and Thorpe, W., 1999. Dairy Production Systems in the Tropics. In: Smallholder Dairying in the Tropics (eds) Falvey, L.and Chantalakhana, C., ILRI, Nairobi, Kenya, pp19-37.

Garnsworthy, P.C., Feng , S., Lock , A.L. and Royal, M.D.2010. Heritability of milk fatty acid composition and stearoyl-CoA desaturase indices in dairy cows. J. Dairy Sci. 93:1743-1748.

Goel, S.C. and K.Pradhan. 1978. Use of wheat straw as major dietary component for growing crossbred calves. Indian J. Dairy Sci. 31: 350.

Grant D.R. and P.R. Patel. 1980. Changes of protein composition of milk by ratio of roughage to concentrate. J. Dairy Sci. 63: 756.

Gupta, B.N., T.K. Walli, S.N. Rai and Kishan Singh. 1988. Effect of feeding fungal treated wheat straw on dry matter consumption and nutrient utilization in crossbred goats. Indian J. Anim. Nutr. 5: 222.

Hammond, B. G., Lemen, J.K., Ahmed, G., Miller, K.D., Kirkpatrick, J. and Fleeman, T. 2008. Safety assessment of SDA soybean oil: Results of a 28-day gavage study and a 90-day/one generation reproduction feeding study in rats. Regul. Toxicol. Pharmacol. 52:311-323.

Huber, J. T., G. Higginbotham, R. A. Gomez-Alarcon, R. B. Taylor, K. H. Chen, S. C. Chan, and Z. Wu. 1994. Heat stress interactions with protein, supplemental fat, and fungal cultures. J. Dairy Sci. 77:2080-2090.

Jung, H.G. and V.H. Varel 1987. Adaptation of rumen microflora to different fibre types. J. Anim.Sci.65: 451.

King, K R, Stockdale, C R and Trigg, T E 1990. Influence of high energy supplements containing fatty acids on the productivity of pasture-fed dairy cows. Australian Journal of Experimental Agriculture 30, 11-16.

Krishna N, K Pradhan and S K Bhatia .1985.standardisation of digestibility trial using tropical forages using cattle and buffalo. Indian J. Anim.Sci.55(9):795-800.

Lall, D., Dixit, V.B., Chauhan, T.R. and Khanna, S., 1996. Indian Journal of Animal Nutrition, 13:95-100.

Mertens, D. R. 2000. Physically effective NDF and its use in dairy rations explored. Feedstuffs, April 10: 1-14.

National Research Council. 1988. Nutrient requirements of diary cattle. 6th revised edition. National Academy Press. Washington, D. C., USA.

Norton, B. W., J. B. Moran and J. V. Nolan. 1979 Nitrogen metabolism in Brahman cross, buffalo and Short Horn steers fed on low quality roughage. Australian J. Agri. Res. 30: 341.

Palmquist, D L 1988. The feeding value of fats. In 'Feed science' (Ed. E R Orskov) pp. 293-311. Elsevier Science Publishers: Amsterdam

Palmquist, D L, Beaulieu, A D and Barbano, D M 1993. Feed and animal factors influencing milk fat composition. Journal of Dairy Science, 76, 1753- 1771.

Pasoerbski, Z. and S. Warwrzynezak. 1987. The influence of level of fibre in feed ration on the milk yield of cows. World Review of Animal Production 23: 41.

Powell, E. B. 1939. Some relations of the roughage intake to the composition of milk. J. Dairy Sci. 22: 453.

Pradhan, K., S. K. Bhatia and D. C. Sangwan. 1991. Relative rumen ecosystem and nutrient digestibility in cattle and buffaloes fed high fibrous diets. Technical Bulletin. Haryana Agricultural University, Hissar, India.

Prasad, D. and K. Pradhan. 1990. Relative feed intake and nutrient digestibility n cattle, buffaloes and sheep due to various levels of concentrate in straw-based diets. Indian J. Anim. Sci. 60: 460.

Prasad, K.S.N. and Rao, S.V.N., 1997. Indian Journal of Animal Nutrition, 14:135-137.

Proceedings of the North-Carolena nutrition conference, Cornell nutrition conference, Tri-state dairy nutrition conference, Penn state dairy nutrition conference, Four-state dairy nutrition conference, Tennessee nutrition conference, Arkansas nutrition conference, Mid-Atlantic nutrition conference (formerly Maryland nutrition conference).

Raymon, M.P.2000.The importance of selenium to human health. Lancet 356, 233-241.

Ramkumar, S. and Rao, S.V.N., 2001. Cattle rearing as a livelihood activity of the landless in Pondicherry. In:"Landless livestock farming problems and prospects" (Eds) Ramkumar, S., Rao, S.V.N., Chris Garforth and Kevin Waldie. Proceedings of the workshop held at Rajiv Gandhi College of Veterinary and Animal Sciences, Pondicherry, on 29 January 2001, pp 53-73.

Ramkumar, S., Reddy, D.V. and Elanchezhian, N., 2003. Improving the farmer formulated rations: Problems and prospects pp25-33 In: "Dairy Farmers- Scientists Interaction on Animal Nutrition Issues" (Eds) Rao, S.V.N., Reddy, D.V. and Natchimuthu, K. Proceedings of the Workshop organized by Animal Nutrition Society of India (SZ) and Rajiv Gandhi College of Veterinary and Animal Sciences, Pondicherry, held on 8-9 October, 2003.

Rearon, A M 2001. Optimizing milk fat composition and processing properties. Australian Journal of Dairy Technology 56: 104-108.

Reddy, D. N., M. R. Reddy and M. Pasha Ali. 1991. Effect of feeding treated paddy straw to lactating crossbred cows on nutrient utilization and quality and quantity of milk production. Indian J. Dairy Sci. 44: 539.

Samieri C, Féart C, Letenneur L, et al. 2008, Low plasma eicosapentaenoic acid and depressive symptomatology are independent predictors of dementia risk. Am J Clin Nutr 88:714 -21.

Sastry, N.S.R., Reddy, D.P.R. and Hermon., 1993. Planning for Development of Animal Husbandry Sector, NIRD, Hyderabad and Book Link Corporation, Hyderabad.

Sutton, J D 1989. Altering milk composition by feeding. Journal of Dairy Science 72, 2801-2814.

Ursin, V. M. 2003. Modification of plant lipids for human health: Development of functional land-based omega-3 fatty acids. J. Nutr. 133:4271-4274.

Van Soest, P. J. and R. H. Wine. 1967. Use of detergent in the analysis of fibrous feeds. IV. Determination of plant cell-wall constituents. J. Asso. Off. Analy. Chem. 50: 50.

Walker, G.P., Dunshea, F.R. and Doyle, P.T. 2004. Effects of nutrition and management on the production and composition of milk fat and protein: a review. Australian Journal of Agricultural Research 55: 1009-1028.

Wattanchantra, C., M. Wanapat, S. Sarangbin and C. Chanthai 1989. A comprehensive study of rumen cellulolytic bacteria of swamp buffalo and cattle. Proc. Int Conference on the application of biotechnology to livestock in developing countries. University of Edinburg, UK.

Weiss, W. P., G. R. Fisher and G. M. Erickson 1989. Effect of sources of neutral detergent fibre and starch on nutrient utilization of dairy cows. J. Dairy Sci. 72: 2308.

Wheelock, J.B., S.R. Sanders, G. Shwartz, L.L. Hernandez, S.H.Baker, J.W. McFadden, L.J. Odens, R. Burgos, S.R. Hartman, R.M. Johnson, B.E. Jones, R.J. Collier, R.P. Rhoads, M.J. VanBaale, and L.H. Baumgard. 2006. Effects of heat stress and rbST on production parameters and glucose homeostasis. J. Dairy Sci. 89. (Suppl. 1):290-291. (Abstr.)

Whelan, J., and Rust, C. 2006. Innovative dietary sources of n-3 fatty acids. Annu. Rev. Nutr. 26:75-103.

Wildman, C.D., J.W. West, and J.K. Bernard. 2007. Effect of dietary cation-anion difference and dietary crude protein on performance of lactating dairy cows during hot weather. J. Dairy Sci. 90:1842-1850.

William S Harris 2008 n-3 Fatty acids and health: DaVinci's code, Am J Clin Nutr, 88: 595-6.

Woodford, S. T. and M. R. Murphy, 1988. Effect of forage physical form on chewing activity, drymatter intake and rumen function of diary cows in early lactation. J. Dairy Sci. 71: 674.

Zebeli, Q, 1 M. Tafaj, H. Steingass, B. Metzler, and W. Drochner 2006. Effects of physically effective fiber on digestive processes and milk fat content in early lactating dairy cows fed total mixed rations. J. Dairy Sci. 89:651-668

Zimbelman, R. B., J. Muumba, L. H. Hernandez, J. B. Wheelock, G. Shwartz, M. D. O'Brien, L. H. Baumgard, and R. J. Collier. 2007. Effect of encapsulated niacin on resistance to acute thermal stress in lactating Holstein cows. J. Dairy Sci. 86(Suppl. 1):231. (Abstr.)

Zimbelman, R. B., R. J. Collier, and T. R. Bilby. 2008. Effect of encapsulated niacin on resistance to acute thermal stress in lactating Holstein cows. J. Dairy Sci. 87(Suppl. 1):Abstr. in press.

SECTION III
Monogastric Animal Nutrition

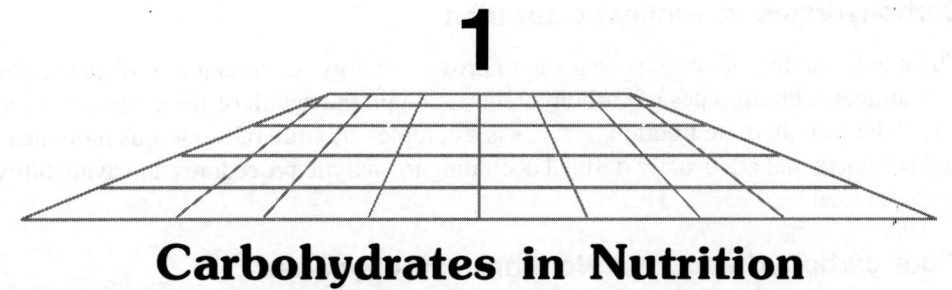

Carbohydrates in Nutrition

Carbohydrates of feeds and fodder

Plant tissue dry matter is about 75% carbohydrates. Carbohydrates are the main source of energy for livestock. The three types of carbohydrates are soluble, storage and structural.

Soluble carbohydrates

Soluble carbohydrates are the simple or individual sugars found in the cells of growing plants. They are found more in leaf than in stem. Soluble carbohydrates are digested and used almost instantly by the microbes in the rumen. The bacteria that ferment feeds high in soluble sugars (eg molasses, sugar cane, good quality grass) are similar to those that ferment starch. Sugary feeds need to be introduced to the ruminant's diet slowly.

Storage carbohydrates

Storage carbohydrates are found in grains, leaf and stem and in the bulbous roots of fodder crops. Starch is an example of storage carbohydrate. The bacteria that digest starchy feeds (e.g. cereal grains or tapioca / potatoes) are different from the cellulose-digesting bacteria. They are insensitive to acidity and produce mainly propionic acid. Starches are rapidly fermented, and the lactic and propionic acid they produce causes acidity to increase. The acidity caused by excess starch-digesting bacteria can suppress the bacteria which digest cellulose and so reduce the milk fat level.

Structural carbohydrates

Structural carbohydrates are fibrous components of plant cell walls. They provide the structural support that plants need to grow upright. Pectin, hemicellulose, and cellulose are all structural carbohydrates. Large amounts of them are found in mature grasses and crop residues / straws. Lignin and silica are often associated with structural carbohydrates in plants. They give structural support to plants but are indigestible and are not actually carbohydrates. Lignin and silica bind to the structural carbohydrates and make them less digestible.

Carbohydrates in ruminant nutrition

The main function of carbohydrates is to provide energy for rumen microbes and the host animal. Certain types of carbohydrates maintain the health of the gastrointestinal tract. The carbohydrate fraction of feeds is a complex mixture of numerous monomers and polymers that are usually defined according to analytic procedures and availability to the animal.

Fibre carbohydrates and Nonfibre carbohydrates

Carbohydrates are classified as either **fibre carbohydrates** (FC) or **nonfibre carbohydrates** (NFC). The FC is equal to the NDF and NFC is total DM minus sum of NDF (adjusted for NDICP), CP, fat and ash. Neutral detergent insoluble protein (NDICP) is deleted because it is the slowest to be degraded.

NDF can be equated with the cell wall constituents (CWC) of grasses and cereals. If preceded by a starch extraction, it can be equated with the CWC of many other feed ingredients. It underestimates the CWC of legumes. Legumes and other non-grass species contain relatively high concentrations of pectic polysaccharides (structural carbohydrate) that are extracted by neutral detergent and not included in their NDF fraction. Hence, NDF and cell wall constituents are not synonyms.

NDF is considerably higher than the conventional crude fibre (CF) values for some feeds since all of the lignin and hemicellulose are included in the NDF fraction. Fibre has come to be recognized as a required dietary ingredient for many herbivorous animal species and is necessary for normal rumen function in ruminants. Only coarse insoluble fibre is adequate for promoting rumen function. This corresponds to the NDF from forages and NDF is the preferred measure for ruminant feeds and dietary balancing programmes.

The nitrogen free extract (NFE) is calculated by summing up of the remaining five proximate principles and subtracting it from 100.

On dry matter basis NFE = 100 − [CF + CP + EE + ash]

Similar to NFE, the nonfibrous carbohydrates (Table 1) also can be calculated
NFC = 100 − [NDF + CP + fat + ash] OR
NFC = 100 − [(NDF-NDICP) + CP + fat + ash]

Carbohydrates are also broadly classified as either **structural or nonstructural**. Nonstructural carbohydrates (NSC) are found inside the cells of plants and are usually more digestible than structural carbohydrates that are found in plant cell walls.

Nonstructural carbohydrates (NSC)

The NSCs are those carbohydrates not included in the cell wall matrix and they are not recovered in NDF. Sugars, starches, fructans, galactans, beta glucans, organic acids, etc make up the NSC fraction and are major sources of energy for high producing dairy cattle. NSC and pectin are highly digestible and are generally increased

Table 1. The composition of Nonfibre carbohydrate (NFC) fraction of
certain feedstuffs (% of NFC)

Feedstuff	Sugar	Starch	Pectin
Maize grain	20.9	80.0	0
Barley	9.1	81.7	9.2
Soybean meal, 48% CP	28.2	28.2	43.6
Soyhulls	18.8	18.8	62.4
Grass hay	35.4	15.2	49.4
Beet pulp	33.7	1.8	64.5

in the diet at the expense of NDF to meet the energy demands of lactating dairy
cows. Nonfibrous carbohydrates (NFC) as calculated by difference and NSC as
measured by enzymatic methods are distinct fractions. Mertens (1988) reported that
the concentration of NFC and NSC are not equal for many feeds and the terms
should not be used interchangeably (Table 2).

Table 2. Nonstructural (NSC) and Nonfiber (NFC) analyses of
certain feedstuffs (% of DM)

Feedstuff	NDF	NFC[a]	NSC[b]
Maize grain	13.1	67.5	68.7
Barley	23.2	60.7	62.0
Whole cottonseed	48.3	10.0	6.4
Maize gluten meal	7.0	17.3	12.0
Soybean meal, 48% CP	9.6	34.4	17.2
Soyhulls	66.6	14.1	5.3
Mixed mainly grass hay	60.9	16.6	13.6
Alfalfa hay	43.1	22.0	12.5

[a]NFC, % = 100 - (NDF + CP + EE + ash); [b]NSC = nonstructural carbohydrates
determined using an enzymatic method (Smith, 1981). Modified enzymatic method
of Smith (1981) measures starch, sucrose, and fructans as NSC; in case of grasses,
NSC consists of fructans and sucrose; for beet pulp, citrus pulp and other byproduct
feeds, NSC is likely all sugars; for grains and byproducts, the NSC is nearly all
starch. In most feedstuffs starch comprises 50 to 100 percent of the NSC.

- NSC are higher than NFC only in grains. Much of the difference is caused
  by the contribution of pectin and organic acids.
- Pectin is included in NFC but not in NSC. Many carbohydrate chemists
  consider pectin in the *structural* group, but, for purposes of nutritional
  classification, it fits the NSP criteria. Pectins are important in grasses and
  cereals but are significant in dicotyledonous species, including forages and
  seed products.

The optimal concentration of NSC or NFC in diets for lactating cows is not well
defined. Alteration of dietary NFC influences ruminal fermentation patterns, total
tract digestion of fibre and milk fat percentage. To avoid acidosis and other metabolic
problems, the maximum concentration of NSC should be approximately 30 to 40
percent of the ration DM (Nocek, 1997). However, Minor et al. (1998) observed

increased percentage and yield of milk protein when NFC was increased from 41.7 to 46.5 % in the ration DM. Diets with excess NFC can cause ruminal upsets and health problems. The acceptable concentrations for NFC are probably 2 to 3 percentage units higher than for NSC.

Classification of nonstructural carbohydrates

1. The nonstructural carbohydrates (NSC) can be classified as water soluble and water insoluble. Water soluble NSCs include monosaccharides, disaccharides, oligosaccharides and some polysaccharides. Larger polysaccharides and resistant starches are insoluble in water.

   Cereal grains are very rich in carbohydrates and include sugars, starch and cell wall polysaccharides contributing the major energy yielding components of feedstuffs. The soluble NSC (soluble sugars-mono-, di-, oligosaccharides) are digested rapidly and almost completely fermented in the rumen (90 to 100%). The **insoluble, resistant starches** may escape. It can be argued that an NSC value including pectin is more appropriate because it is a rapidly digested carbohydrate. The general assumption that soluble substances are more easily and rapidly digested than insoluble ones is true only in a general sense. Some insoluble carbohydrates, e.g., unlignified amorphous cellulose in vegetable wastes, may be more rapidly fermented than some of the more soluble modified starches and hemicelluloses.

2. NSC can be subdivided into those carbohydrates (starch and sugar) capable of **yielding lactic acid** and those **not yielding lactic acid**, because lactic acid production has major impact on rumen efficiencies.

Nonstarch polysaccharides (NSP)

Cereal grains are very rich in carbohydrates and include sugars, starch and cell wall polysaccharides contributing the major energy yielding components of feedstuffs. Nonstarch polysaccharide (NSP) is a fraction of carbohydrate in feed and it does not include starch and free sugars. The NSP include cellulose, arabinoxylan, pectins, galactans and beta-glucans.

NSC – starch and sugars = Nonstarch polysaccharides (NSP)

Within the natural feedstuffs starch exists in hydrated polymeric form arranged in a crystalline lattice consisting of amylose (linear polymer of alpha 1-4, D-glucose units) and amylopectin having glucose units linked together by alpha-1, 4 and interspersing alpha-1, 6 linkages. The NSP are not fully utilized by the nonruminant species, especially birds (Table 4). The β-glucan is a glucose polymer containing a mixture of β1-3 and β1-4 linkages that make its physicochemical properties totally different from cellulose that is a straight-chain glucose polymer with only β1-4 linkages.

NSPs are beneficial to ruminants?

When large amounts of starch and sugar are added, the fermentation pathway can switch to lactic acid production, which can lead to acidosis. However, other soluble

NSP (Table 3), such as pectins, arabans, and β-glucans, are not fermented to lactate (Strobel and Russel, 1986). Hence, there is merit in distinguishing those feeds containing NSP because these can elicit good rumen efficiencies without the problems associated with too much starch (Van Soest, 1987). The β-glucans that occur in oats and barley contribute to gumminess and are objectionable in poultry diets but probably are beneficial in ruminant diets.

Table 3. The types and levels of NSP present in some cereal grains (% dry matter)*

Cereal grains	Arabinoxylan	β-Glucan	Cellulose	Pectins**	Total
Wheat					
Soluble	1.8	0.4		0.2	2.4
Insoluble	6.3	0.4	2.0`	0.3	9.0
Barley					
Soluble	0.8	3.6		0.1	4.5
Insoluble	7.1	0.7	3.9	0.5	12.2
Rye					
Soluble	3.4	0.9		0.3	4.6
Insoluble	5.5	1.1	1.5	0.5	8.6
Oats					
Soluble	0.8	2.8		0.2	3.8
Insoluble	14.7		10.1	0.3	25.1
Triticale					
Soluble	1.3	0.2		0.2	1.7
Insoluble	9.5	1.5	2.5	1.1	14.6
Sorghum					
Soluble	0.1	0.1		T	0.2
Insoluble	2.0	0.1	2.2	0.3	4.6
Maize					
Soluble	0.1			T	0.1
Insoluble	5.1	T	2.0	0.9	8.0
Rice					
Soluble	T			0.2	0.3
Insoluble	0.2	0.1	0.3	t	0.5
Millet					
Soluble	T	T		T	0.2
Insoluble	5.9		7.9	0.7	14.5

* Source: Choct, M. 2006. World's Poultry Science Journal 62, March 2006, 5-16.
** Pectins include mannose, galactose and uronic acid; t Trace

The Fibre Requirement

Ruminants generally and dairy cattle in particular require adequate coarse insoluble fiber for normal rumen function and maintenance of normal milk fat test. Normal rumen function in dairy cattle is associated with adequate rumination and cellulose digestion. These maintain rumen pH and cellulolytic microorganisms that characteristically produce the higher acetate to propionate ratios needed for normal lipid metabolism in the cow. Daily rumination time is directly proportional to coarse NDF intake and related to body size (Bae et al., 1979); Welch, 1982). Other estimations

Table 4. NSP content of common ingredients fed to poultry (% DM basis)*

Feed ingredient	Arabino-xylans	Cellulose	Pectin	?-glucans	Total NSP
Maize	5.2	3.1	1.0	----	9.3
Wheat	6.6	3.0	---	1.0	10.6
Sorghum	2.8	4.2	1.7	0.4	9.7
Barley	6.0	5.0	---	4.4	15.4
Deoiled rice bran	10.6	15.2	7.2	---	59.9
Soybean meal	3.8	5.7	6.1	---	23.5
Sunflower seed meal	11.0	22.7	4.9	---	36.7
Rapeseed meal	8.8	14.2	8.8	---	36.2

*A.Arun Kumar and A.K.Panda, Livestock International:April, 2006, 18-22.

of fibre, e.g., ADF or crude fibre are less well related, because only NDF quantitatively recovers insoluble matrix carbohydrates, including hemicellulose. The NDF is better related to intake and gastrointestinal fill than any other measure of fibre (Mertens, 1973; Van Soest, 1963), thus, the expectation that the fibre requirement is better expressed in terms of NDF rather than ADF or crude fibre. This point is illustrated by the experiments of Welch et al., (1969) at the University of Vermont, who examined the ability of various forages to promote rumination. The best relationship was with intake of NDF that was correlated at 0.99 with chewing time. Readers may refer ruminant animal nutrition section (pp 73–182) for greater details on fibre.

peNDF: Recently physically effective fibre (peNDF) is coined to amalgamate the chemical characteristics and particle size of forages, and to quantify its value to rumen function. The peNDF is a good indicator of the rumination potential of the feed.

Carbohydrates in non-ruminant nutrition

Some of the topics not covered in ruminants are mentioned here to take of their role in swine and poultry nutrition. In simple terms, non-starch polysaccharides (NSPs; Table 2 and 3) are hemicellulose, cellulose and pectin. The soluble NSP increases the viscosity of the digesta in the small intestine.

Water-soluble barley (1,3-1,4)-β-glucans are responsible for the high viscosity of β-glucan solutions. The water-soluble β-glucans (Table 3) cause problems in chicken feed, malting and brewing (Stone and Clark, 1992). Soluble β-glucans interfere with the diffusion of digestive enzymes and the transport of nutrients through the unstirred water layer adjacent to the mucosal surface. The water-insoluble fraction does not influence the viscosity.

Resistant starch (RS; named for its resistance to amylolysis) is starch or starch degradation products that are not digested by pancreatic amylase in the small intestine and reaches the colon. It was shown that the amylose component of barley meal could be partly converted into RS by extrusion technology under optimized conditions. Resistant starch can be fermented by human and animal gut microflora. Thus it is a major substrate for colonic fermentation and it is a good source of butyrate.

Starch has been classified into three types by Englyst, Kingman and Gummings (1992): RS1, starch entrapped within food matrix, RS2, granular starch structure and

RS3, retrograded starch formed by food processing. Granular starches synthesized by a number of food plants (native potato starch) provide examples of these resistant starches, being incompletely digested due to their size and molecular conformation (Vonk et al., 2000). Resistant starch increased the number of bifidobacteria, lactobacilli, streptococci and enterobacteria in the intestinal tract. The sum of R S and solubilized starch (nonresistant starch) is total starch. Resistant starch is generally considered to be one of the components that make up total dietary fibre.

Total Dietary Fiber (DF)

It is defined as the polysaccharides and lignin resistant to mammalian digestive enzymes and thus is relevant to most monogastric animals with hindgut fermentation. The fractions not recovered in NDF but resistant to mammalian *enzymes* are defined as **water-soluble NSP**. They include some legitimate cell wall components, such as β-glucans and pectins, as well as some storage polysaccharides, such as galactans in beans, other gums and mucilages.

Dietary fibre is essential components in human and animal nutrition. A high intake of DF is positively related to different physiological and metabolic effects. Barley grains are relatively rich in DF such as β-glucan, arabinoxylans and cellulose. It has been shown that blood cholesterol and lipoprotein concentrations can be reduced in humans and animals by β-glucan from barley or oats. Furthermore, β-glucan or β-glucan-enriched diets lowered the postprandial blood glucose and insulin responses in normal individuals.

Grain legumes: Oligosaccharides of raffinose series

Grain legumes (peas, faba beans, lupins (Blue lupin, Lupinus angustifolius) are an important component of both human and livestock diets. Oligosaccharides of the raffinose-series (namely raffinose, verbascose and stachyose: α-galactosides) are major components in many food legumes. Antinutritional activity of grain legumes is frequently associated with the presence of these oligosaccharides. Raffinose is a trisaccharide found in abundance in sugar beets and many other higher plants. It consists of galactose, glucose and fructose.

Raffinose-series oligosaccharides (α-galactosides) are not hydrolysed by digestive enzymes of monogastric animals in the upper gut due to the absence of α-galactosidase. In the hind gut, they are degraded by bacterial α-galactosidase and can cause flatulence and diarrhoea in animals (Delzenne and Roberfroid, 1994). Raffinose-series oligosaccharides are thus a factor limiting the use of grain legumes in monogastric diets. Raffinose, stachyose and verbascose (α-galactosides) are hydrolysed by α-galactosidase to galactose and sucrose.

Non-starch carbohydrates

= organic matter – (CP + EE + starch + sucrose + α-galactosides)

Sucrose and α-galactosides are analysed by HPLC (Quemener, 1988). Starch is analysed by using the amylo-glucosidase procedure according to Thivend et al. (1965).

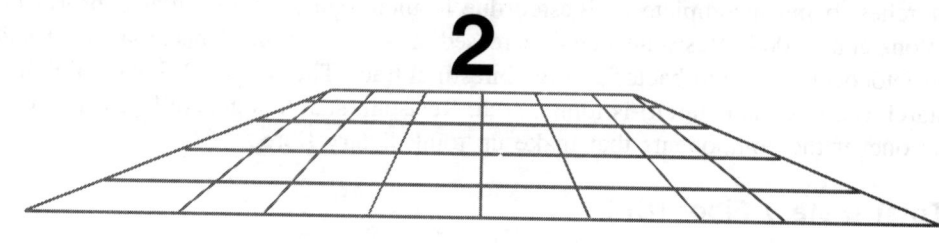

Feed enzymes

Enzymes are proteins with a highly complex three-dimensional molecular structure. Enzymes are highly effective biological catalysts which can be found in all biological systems acting under very specific pH and temperature on specific substrates. They are not spent during the reaction, but catalyse and return to their original state once the reaction is complete. For this reason the amount of enzyme required is small compared with the quantity of substrate. But enzymes are fragile proteins; extremes of temperature, pressure, friction, pH and microbial activity can degrade or destroy enzymes added to feed.

Classification of enzymes

Enzyme Commission (EC) classified the enzymes into six main classes namely 1. oxidoreductases/dehydrogenases/reductases/oxidases, 2. transferases, 3. hydrolases, 4. lyases, 5. isomerases and 6. ligases (synthetases) according to the type of reaction they catalyse. Among these, hydrolases are used as feed enzyme additives in animal nutrition.

Hydrolases

Hydrolases catalyse the cleavage of specific bonds including carbon-oxygen, carbon-nitrogen and carbon-carbon bonds, and oxygen-phosphorus bonds. Essentially these are

The following hydrolases can play an important role as feed additives.

E.C.3.1 Phosphatases (e.g. phytase)

E.C.3.2 Glycosidases (e.g. carbohydrases)

E.C.3.2.1 O-glycoside degrading hydrolases

E.C.3.2.2 N-glycoside degrading hydrolases

E.C.3.2.3 S-glycoside degrading hydrolases

Only O-glycoside degrading hydrolases are relevant for use in animal nutrition. Examples of some enzymes from the glycosidase group

E.C.3.2.1.1 α-amylase

E.C.3.2.1.3 glycoamylase

E.C.3.2.1.4 cellulase (1, 4-β-D-glucanase)

E.C.3.2.1.6 β-glucanase (1, 3-1,4- β-D-glucanase)

E.C.3.2.1.8 xylanase (1, 3-1,4- β-D-xylanase)

Enzymes produced by monogastric and ruminant animals include α-amylase, glucoamylase, maltase, isomaltase, maltotriase, β-glucosidase, while enzymes for substrates such as cellulose, 1, 3-1, 4- β-glucans, pentosans and phytates are not produced.

E.C.3.4 Proteases

Production of enzymes

Enzymes are produced by all living organisms such as microorganisms, plants and animals and thus are present in all cells as well as in extracellular spaces. Enzymes added to feedstuffs are broken down in the digestive tract in the same way as other proteins.

Commercially important enzymes are produced by microorganisms (fungi, yeasts and bacteria), from animal tissues (e.g. lipases and proteases from the pancreas) and plants (e.g. papain, a protease contained in the papaya fruit). Phytases are of two types: Aspergillus phytase (*Aspergillus niger*; 3-phytase) and non-aspergillus phytase (Peniophora phytase; *Peniophora lycii*; 6-phytase).

Commercial enzymes used in the livestock feed industry are products of microbial fermentation. Feed enzymes are produced by a batch fermentation process, beginning with a seed culture and growth media (Cowan, 1994). Compared to the fermentation extract, these enzyme products are relatively concentrated and purified, containing specific, controlled enzyme activities. They usually do not contain live cells. Enzyme products for animal diets are of fungal (mostly *Trichoderma longibrachiatum*, *Aspergillus niger*, *A. oryzae*) and bacterial (mostly *Bacillus* spp.) origin.

Submerged liquid fermentation

Most commercial feed enzymes are produced by using the submerged liquid fermentation (SLF) process in which microbes and substrate are suspended in a liquid nutrient solution containing essential cofactors for growth.

Solid state fermentation

In solid state fermentation (SSF) water binds to a solid substrate particle. Fungi or microorganisms seeded onto the substrate use the water to grow and break down the substrate for the nutrients. Air and water vapour circulate through the particles either by natural or forced aeration and because there is no free liquid, oxygen can more easily move to the microorganisms than in a SLF system.

Thermostability of enzymes

Enzymes are highly thermolabile. Thermostability of enzymes is influenced by various factors like types of enzymes, microbial source of enzymes, the exposure temperature and the length of exposure and the amino acid composition and their sequence. At the general pelleting temperature of 85°C, almost all enzymes in general get denatured with varying degree of 40-60%. Thermolability of all enzymes is directly proportional to the rise of temperature and length of exposure of temperature; higher the temperature and longer the exposure, higher is the loss of activity.

Now it is possible to genetically engineer the microorganisms to produce thermostable enzymes by inserting genes with high thermostability.

Different forms of feed enzymes: dry and liquid

Dry forms of enzymes: In dry form, the enzymes are manufactured in powder, granular and coated forms. Coated enzymes are stable. Such coated enzymes show no loss of activity in pelleted feed stored up to 3 months at 25°C. However, it is recommended to use pelleted feeds with enzymes as quickly as possible, since storing temperature is always higher.

Under conditions of normal steam conditioning, enzymes in dry form are alright. The stability of modern granular enzyme additives is much better because enzymes with inherent high stability are selected, new carrier materials are employed and novel manufacturing techniques such as protective encapsulation are used. As a result some granular feed enzymes have been shown to maintain efficacy after exposure to conditioning temperature above 90°C. Incorporating granular enzyme products is very similar to adding vitamins, trace minerals and other microingredients designed for inclusion directly in a batch mixing.

Liquid forms of enzymes: In case of feed manufactured using high temperature or superconditioning process, post-processing application of feed grade enzymes in liquid form are advocated (sprying onto the finished feed). But liquid enzymes are inherently less stable in storage than their dry, granular counterparts. Moreover, post-pelleting liquid micro proportioning and application can be a restrictive and expensive option, due largely to the complexity of the necessary equipment.

Feed enzyme additives

A key task for nutritionists is to achieve cost optimisation of feed formulations. High cost of feed ingredients spurred the pursuit of alternative ingredients. There is a global boom in the use of byproducts from non-food crop production as well as human food processing. However ways and means are to be found to use common feed ingredients more effectively. Here comes the enzyme additive to our aid. Feed enzymes act as biocatalysts to assist the digestion process and support the utilization of nutrients that otherwise may go unused.

Optimising digestion

Optimising digestive function is imperative to improve feed utilization in the animal system. This is more so in the present context in view of the following:

- Availability of low quantities of grains (e.g.maize) & protein supplements to feed the animals (poultry and swine, primarily) to meet the growing needs of humans for animal protein: This necessitates the search for alternate ingredients (e.g. barley, rye, oats; sunflower seed cake, lupin seed meal, etc) both to meet the demand of feed and to reduce cost of production.

- Restrictions for nitrogen and phosphorus excretion to avoid environmental pollution and thus follow eco-friendly animal husbandry practices.

Xylans, β-glucans and cellulose are a class of feed components from plants that cannot be fully degraded and utilized by monogastric animals. These are collectively known as non-starch polysaccharides (NSP). Levels of NSP in cereal grains are known to be dependent on genetics and growing or harvesting conditions of the grain (Jeroch and Danicke, 1995; Scott et al., 1998).

Viscous and nonviscous cereal grains

Cereal grains are broadly classified into two major categories, **viscous** (wheat, rye, triticale, barley, oats) and nonviscous (maize, sorghum, rice) cereals, according to their content of soluble NSP. The soluble NSP increases the viscosity of the digesta in the small intestine.

Wheat viscosity is related to the content of soluble non-starch polysaccharides (NSP) in wheat and is linearly related to the differences in *in vivo* digesta viscosity when wheat samples are fed to broiler chickens. Wheat starches are a mixture of amylase and amylopectin and the ratio of these two components can vary. The amino acid composition of wheat is poorly balanced relative to the requirements of the poultry, so the available energy content of wheat is the main factor that determines its economic value to the industry.

The total dietary fibre, including both soluble and insoluble constituents, is around 15% in barley, 25% in oats and 10% in wheat. The predominant non-starch polysaccharides in cereal grains are cellulose, arabinoxylans, and mixed-linked ?-glucans. In barley, and to a lesser extent oats, the endosperm cell wall contains a variable amount of viscous gel-forming β-glucan, an antinutritional factor causing sticky droppings (and thus greater litter moisture), reduced nutrient utilization and growth rate, especially in young poultry. The sticky droppings also lead to dirty eggs.

Beta-glucans are water soluble polysaccharides present in the endosperm of barley and other grains of graminae crops. These are formed of glucose units bound together by beta -1, 4 and beta-1, 3 linkages. The enzymes capable of disintegrating beta-glucans are known as beta-glucanases.

Feed enzyme supplementation: Why?

Enzymes are widely used in animal feed, especially for poultry and pigs, for more complete utilization of plant feed components. Addition of enzyme preparations containing (cellulolytic and hemicellulolytic enzymes) xylanases, β-glucanases, mannase, pectinase and cellulases to the feed reduce the antinutritional effect of NSP. It is believed that these enzymes degrade polysaccharide cage structure around proteins and reduce the viscosity of the intestinal contents of the animals. Feed enzymes are also able to upgrade sources of vegetable protein (such as soybeans, rapeseed, sunflower seed and legumes) in both pig and poultry diets. So enzyme supplementation improved the feeding value of these low energy feedstuffs for poultry.

Effect of enzyme supplementation is highest during younger age. e.g. β-glucanase had maximum positive effect on feed intake and growth rate of broilers on barley or oat-based diets during the first three weeks of life. Feed enzymes such as β-glucanases and xylanases have enabled nutritionists to incorporate up to 50 or 60% barley or wheat in poultry feeds. Feed costs can be reduced when barley or wheat are plenty and cheap and when maize is relatively scarce and expensive.

Enzyme supplementation could also be used to breakdown antinutritional substances found in raw materials, thus augmenting the digestive capacity of the animal, improving availability of feed nutrients, and increasing release of nutrients in the upper part of the gastrointestinal tract.

Phytase enzyme is not produced in monogastric animals such as poultry, swine etc. This results in utilization of only 12% of the phytin phosphorus in maize, wheat etc. This undigested phosphorus along with undigested nitrogen enters the environment via manure and can contribute to eutrophication of lakes and streams. Phytase enzyme supplementation increase phosphorus utilization and reduce its excretion in pigs and poultry.

A multi-enzyme preparation with cellulolytic and proteolytic activity can degrade the structural polysaccharides in the plant cell wall and the effects of such multi-enzyme product may be synergistic. Nitrogen excretion levels are also reduced. These N excretions are viewed increasingly as environmental contaminants. e.g. a multi-enzyme preparation consisting mainly of cellulases, β-glucanases and protease.

A combination of endo-1-4- β-galactanase and β-galactosidase could be used to improve the total ME for soybean meal in adult roosters by 7%. The enzyme combination increased the apparent ME by 3.9% in broilers on a diet of sorghum and soybean meal. However, used alone, the enzymes had limited effects.

Xylanase derived from Thermomyces is superior since this enzyme product withstood the high temperature (95°C) employed during pelleting and improved the apparent ME and fat digestibility of wheat-soya diets in broilers.

Mode of action of enzymes

Enzymes are naturally occurring proteins that act as biological catalysts. The mode of action of enzymes can be described by the "lock and key" principle. Imagine a substrate (the molecule on which an enzyme acts) as a kind of lock, and an enzyme as the only key which will open it. Put the two together and a rapid reaction takes place which breaks apart the substrate into two or more smaller parts. The enzyme key is then removed intact to play its role in another reaction.

Two main modes of action have been proposed for xylanase and β-glucanase in wheat- or barley-based diets. These include the viscosity theory and the so-called 'cage' effect (Bedford, 2002; Cowieson et al., 2006). However, currently research is focused on enzyme inhibitors and resistant starches.

Viscosity theory: The viscosity theory suggests that the incremental performance enhancement associated with the addition of the enzymes to poultry diets can be explained not only by the nutritive value of the released sugars but also by the increased digestibility of the other nutrients in the diet. As high-molecular weight soluble arabinoxylans and mixed-linked β-glucans have a high affinity for water, they have the ability to stimulate a geometric increase in the viscosity of the contents within the gastrointestinal tract (GI). High intestinal viscosity is negatively correlated with animal performance, nutrient digestibility and is also associated with detrimental changes in the microbial flora within the distal GI tract. Thus, facilitating a reduction in viscosity with exogenous enzymes confers a nutritional advantage to the animal. The negative effects of viscosity on animal performance are so pronounced that the viscosity of feed ingredients (such as wheat and barley) has been suggested as being a reliable indicator of the nutritional value of the ingredient and the efficacy of exogenous pentosanases. Furthermore, the effects of diet viscosity are more pronounced in young animals than in older birds, presumably associated with the maturity of the GI tract in older animals and the capacity to cope with soluble polysaccharides.

The 'cage' effect theory: This theory is associated with the effects of carbohydrases on cell walls, reducing their integrity and thus releasing nutrients that were previously encapsulated (Bedford, 2002).

Commerical enzyme products

Feed enzymes are produced from the large scale fermentation of naturally - occuring microorganisms (e.g. *Aspergillus niger*, a fungus). Commercial enzyme products are available in two basic forms.

1. A dry form of fat-coated, micro-granulated product, suitable for use in mash or pelleted feeds.
2. A liquid version, designed for spraying onto feeds which have been subjected to processing above 80°C.

Some examples: Avizyme series 1000, 1100, 1300, 2000 and Porzyme series from Finfeeds International Ltd.; Natugrain (endoxylanase & beta-glucanase), Natuphos (phytase), Vevozyme (α-amylase) from BASF corporation; Grindazym (pectinases) from Danisco Ingredients

Feed enzyme dose optimisation

Enzyme inclusion rates can be matched to cereal quality including its variability to maximise the cost-effectiveness of their use.

Soluble fibre concentration is variable due to genetics, crop location and storage period. For any variety, samples tend to be more viscous immediately after the harvest and this effect then decline throughout the storage period. Gut viscosity tends to be higher as intensity of processing increases (mash, pellet or an extrudate). Addition of fat also contributes to viscosity. As it is known, the more viscous the gut contents, the poorer are the utilization of nutrients.

Viscosity of the cereal can be determined with the help of an *in vitro* test (for example, aviCheck[TM]; Finfeeds International) and accordingly the dose of the enzyme is changed. This test is fast and the results correlate closely to *in vivo* results. The level of enzyme addition is accordingly fixed, to take care of the variation in cereal quality.

Wheat samples	Viscosity values	Optimum Avizyme 1300 dose
Highly viscous (20%)	22 CPs (Centipoise)	1.22 kg/MT
Average (40%)	11 "	1.00 "
Low (40%)	6 "	0.86 "

Exogenous enzyme supplementation: Examples

Exogenous enzyme supplementation (EES) has become a practice in intensive animal production to increase the efficiency of digestion (to 100%) and hence, it can be seen as an extension of the animal's own digestive process. This eventually should result in lesser volume of excreta with lesser nutrients leading to animal friendly- and environmental friendly- and profitable animal production.

Feed enzymes for a superior vegetable protein

Vegetable protein supplements obtained from sunflower, groundnut, rapeseed, lupins etc., are rich in protein and cheaper although their protein is less digestible compared to the expensive soybean meal. The carbohydrate composition of these oilseed meals is relatively complex compared with cereals. The poor protein digestibility in such feeds is partly due to the presence of antinutritional factors such as arabinoxylans and pectins and can be improved by the addition of xylanases and pectinases, respectively at suitable dose.

Antinutritional factors

Feedstuff	Arabinoxylan index	Pectin index
Soybean meal	100	100
Sunflower seed meal	117	113
Rapeseed meal	130	156
Groundnut meal	71	137
Lupin seed meal	165	57

1. The higher the total content of antinutritional factors, the poorer is the protein digestibility.
2. Further, the presence of high concentration of antinutritional factors not only results in reduced feed performance when significant amount of sunflower seed meal are included in the diet, but can also provoke health and quality problems, including liquid faeces and dirty eggs.
3. The physical and chemical structure of antinutritional factors along with their anatomical arrangement within each specific raw material influences the accessibility of protein for digestion.
4. Protein and other mutrients are, to a greater or lesser degree, "imprisoned" inside the fibrous structures and unavailable for digestion by the birds' own proteases and other endogenous enzymes.
5. Feed enzyme complexes containing arabinases, xylanases and pectinases (pectin esterase, pectin lyase and polygalacturonase) break down the antinutritional factors at strategic points and liberate the protein. This action of feed enzymes not only improve the digestibility of protein, fat and starch in the diet, but also shift the site of digestion further upstream in the intestine, which is more efficient for growth and production. Thus feed enzymes (which

are not native to birds or mammals) complement the action of endogenous enzyme systems.

Inclusion of sunflower seed meal in poultry diets

1. Sunflower seed meal was increased from 5% to 16% in the diet of layers replacing 40% of the soybean meal content of maize-soya based diet without causing a drop in egg production or quality, or an increase in dirty eggs due to the incorporation of feed enzyme complex containing Pectinases (Grindazym GP 5000 from Danisco Ingredients at 0.5 kg/ton of feed).
2. Addition of the same enzyme complex to a barley-based diet containing 20% sunflower seed meal increased egg weight, reduced the percentage of dirty eggs, and improved faecal quality by preventing over-consumption of water.
3. Similarly studies in broilers indicated that sunflower meal can replace 43% of soybean meal without affecting growth or feed efficiency. Pectinases (including arabinases and xylanases) seem to convert sunflower meal into soybean meal in terms of nutritional value. Thus addition of feed enzymes facilitate the inclusion of economical vegetable protein supplements in poultry diets even in high viscosity cereal-based diets by incorporating the right mix of enzymes at optimum dose.

Enzyme supplementation to maize-soybean meal (SBM) diets
Reality of maize and SBM

Enzyme addition to diets based on low viscosity grains such as maize and sorghum and soybean meal is more recent concept. Maize and soybean meal (SBM) are the most preferred feeds for poultry. But they do have antinutritional factors. Soybean meal has ?-mannans in higher concentration than in other commonly used feedstuffs and it has about 22.7 % hemicellulose (Chesson, 1987), which are non-starch polysaccharides (NSP) virtually indigestible by monogastrics including poultry and pigs. The β-mannans (galactomannans) have several negative physiological effects on poultry and pigs apart from its poor digestibility. Even low concentrations of β-mannans have been shown to reduce the rate of glucose absorption from the intestine and consequently carbohydrate metabolism by interfering with insulin secretion and insulin-like growth factor (IGF) production (Nunes and Malmlof, 1992). Other negative effects include decreased nitrogen retention, fat absorption and amino acid uptake, as well as reduced water absorption which results in excess moisture in excreta (Kratzer et al., 1967).

Maize contains higher starch content (72.8%) and lower water insoluble cell walls (9.6%). Maize starch digestibility had been thought by many to be complete in poultry. However, recent ileal digestibility research proves that in some varieties of maize some of the starch may not be digested by the bird at all. Rather, it may be fermented by bacteria in the hindgut and may only be partly available as a source of energy. Further, starch granules are embedded in a protein matrix.

With reference to soluble sugars, maize has negligible amounts of arabinose (0.02%) and xylose (0.01%) and no mannose and galactose (Mathlouthi et al., 2003).

In contrast, SBM has lower content of starch (10.2%) and higher content of water insoluble cell walls (21.1%). A higher galactose (0.17%), arabinose (0.11%) and mannose (0.06%) and negligible level of xylose (0.01%) are reported. Rani et al.(2003) reported that maize and SBM contained 7.13% and 11.63% total non-starch polysaccharides (NSP), respectively. The insoluble NSP of maize and SBM were 4.6% and 10.1% while the soluble NSP were 2.5% and 1.5%, respectively. Classen (1996) reported a range of 4.2 - 8.1% NSP content in maize. This wide variation existing in NSP content and their digestibility among different cultivars of maize (Summers, 2001) may be responsible for conflicting reports on beneficial effects of NSP hydrolyzing enzymes in poultry diets.

While arabinoxylans, galactomannans and pectins are the major NSP in soybean meal, the structure of these NSP especially pectic polysaccharides appear unique and add to the antinutritive effect in the commercial maize-SBM diet (Chesson, 2001). Bedford (1995) reported an increase in viscosity in the small intestine due to high soluble molecular weight forms of, e.g., ?-glucans and arabinoxylans, which resulted in decreased diffusional rates of the nutrients. Edwards et al.(1988) reported a substantive impairement in mixing the contents of feed in the gut while Danicke et al.(1995) observed reduction in emulsification of fats as the intestinal viscosity increases. The high digesta viscosity alters the gut enterocyte turnover rates, endogenous enzyme synthesis rate and microflora populations (Choct et al., 1995).

What types of enzymes are needed?

A specific enzyme complex of xylanase, amylase and protease has been developed to target mainly the maize starch and protein content of maize and soya. This enzyme complex offers unique characteristics in enhancing the energy and protein value of even higher quality raw materials such as maize or sorghum - soya diets.

With reference to other feed ingredients, enzymes to breakdown fibre and phytic acid, and enzymes to increase the availability of starches, proteins, lipids and minerals that are enclosed within fibrous cell walls are needed. EES is also used to complement the endogenous enzyme production of young animals. The underdeveloped digestive system of young animals may not be able to make optimal use of the large storage proteins (glycinin and conglycinin) found in soybean meal. Enzymes thus play an increasingly important role in helping to create effective diets at a low price.

Relation between storage period and the nutritive value

There is a concern that feeding newly harvested cereal grain results in poor performance in poultry. Waters and Choct (1998) indicated that the nutritive value of cereal grains for poultry generally changes during storage, which was attributed to degradation of the viscous NSP. It was reported that the levels of beta-glucan of barley decreased with storage. Degradation of NSP (during storage) would lower digesta viscosity and result in an improvement in performance, similar to that experienced when diets are supplemented with NSP degrading enzymes (Bedford 1996). Excreta dry matter is an indication of the viscous nature of digesta, since high NSP diets are implicated in the production of wet droppings (Bedford 1996).

Digesta viscosity and metabolizable energy value of the diet

Increased digesta viscosity results in a proliferation of microflora in the small intestine (Langhout et al. 2000). High digesta viscosity may therefore increase the proportion of nutrients that are fermented within the lumen of the digestive tract, thus resulting in a higher heat increment of digestion and thus giving a reduced amount of metabolizable energy available for carcass energy retention. Muramatsu et al. (1994) showed that conventional chickens had an increased heat production relative to germ-free chickens because of their increased microbial proliferation.

Enzymes for breaking down carbohydrates

Not only do NSPs increase the viscosity of digesta, which means that the animal's own enzymes have a harder time locking onto nutrients and the absorption of these nutrients is reduced, but they also encapsulate nutrients, thus making them unavailable to the animal. The addition of NSP enzymes to animal diets allows the breakdown of these anti-nutritional factors and thus faster and more complete digestion of the feed, leading to improved nutritive value.

Xylanase with a carbohydrate-binding module (Fontes et al., 2004) is more efficacious in wheat- and rye-based diet, since it facilitates greater degree of hydrolysis of insoluble carbohydrates releasing encapsulated nutrients. Efficacy of exogenous xylanase was compromised by the presence of xylanase inhibitors. There is considerable variation in the concentration of xylanase inhibitors in wheat, which arises from genetic sources as well as environmental conditions during growth, and also harvesting and storage conditions (Bonnin et al., 2005). The variable concentration of xylanase inhibitors in wheat may contribute to variation in its apparent metabolizable energy.

Quality control of commercial NSP-hydrolyzing enzyme preparations

Commercially available NSP-hydrolyzing enzymes are products of microbial fermentation. Strains of Trichoderma, Aspergillus and Bacillus are the most commonly used microbial sources. They regularly produce mixtures of enzyme. The components of these mixtures have different biochemical properties, because of their nature and origin. This must be considered when choosing the conditions for determining their hydrolytic activity.

How to measure the potency of enzymes?

A variety of NSP enzyme preparations are commercially available for feed supplementation. The enzyme activity declared on the labels cannot be compared among different producers because the analytical methods differ substantially and often suffer from pronounced non-linearity with reaction time or enzyme concentration. Quality control of commercial NSP-hydrolyzing enzyme preparations includes measurement of their enzymatic activity. This is achieved by following their hydrolytic action on model substrates e.g. wheat arabinoxylan for xylanolytic activity, barley ?-

glucan for ?-glucanolytic activity and carboxymethylcellulase for cellulolytic activity. The specificity of the individual hydrolases enables determination of the activity of several enzymes in the same sample.

Enzymes for reducing the phosphorus burden on the environment

Apart from contributing to improving nutritive value, feed enzymes can also have a positive impact on the environment by allowing better use of natural resources and reducing pollution by nutrients. In areas with intensive livestock production, the phosphorus output is often very high. This can lead to environmental problems such as eutrophication. Most (50-80%) of the phosphorus contained in feedstuffs of plant origin exists as the storage form phytate (Table 1), or phytic acid, and is indigestible for non-ruminant animals such as poultry and pigs. They cannot digest the phosphorus contained within these complex phytate structures, since they lack the enzyme to break down the phytate and free the phosphorus. The phytase enzyme is essential for the release of phytate-bound phosphorus. Therefore, sufficient phytase needs to be added to the feed.

Table 1: Total and phytate phosphorus content of certain common feedstuffs*

Feedstuffs	Total phosphorus, %	Phytate phosphorus, % of total phosphorus
Maize	0.26	66
Barley	0.37	59
Oats	0.36	58
Wheat	0.33	66
Sorghum	0.32	68
Rice bran	1.50	85
Wheat bran	1.37	70
Soybean meal	0.66	58
Sunflower seed meal	0.89	77
Rapeseed meal	0.70	59
Cottonseed meal	0.84	70

*A.Arun Kumar and A.K.Panda, Livestock International: April, 2006, 18-22.

Phytate also forms complexes with proteins, digestive enzymes and minerals, and as such is considered to be an anti-nutritional factor. Phytase frees the phosphorus contained in cereals and oilseeds, and by breaking down the phytate structure also achieves the release of other minerals such as calcium and magnesium, as well as proteins and amino acids, which have become bound to the phytate. Thus, by releasing bound phosphorus in feed ingredients of vegetable origin, phytase makes more phosphorus available for bone growth, and reduces the amount excreted into the environment. Use of the enzyme also has the added benefit of helping to conserve natural resources by eliminating the need to supplement feeds with sources of digestible inorganic phosphorus.

Exogenous Fibrolytic Enzymes for ruminants

Forage digestibility continues to limit the intake of available energy by ruminants, and correspondingly, contributes to excessive nutrient excretion by livestock. The use of exogenous fibrolytic enzymes holds promise as a means of increasing forage utilization and improving the productive efficiency of ruminants. Recent studies have shown that adding exogenous fibrolytic enzymes to ruminant diets increases milk production. These increases in animal performance are due to increases in feed digestion. However, not all studies report improved animal performance due to the use of exogenous enzymes and viewed across a variety of enzyme products and experimental conditions the response to feed enzymes by ruminants has been variable (Beauchemin et al., 2003).

In addition to relatively pure sources of enzymes, crude fermentation products and some nonbacterial direct-fed microbials (DFM) are also marketed, at least partly or implicitly, based on their residual enzymic content. Most nonbacterial DFM consist of A. oryzae fermentation extract, Saccharomyces cerevisiae cultures, or both.

Research has demonstrated that supplementing dairy cow and feedlot cattle diets with fibre-degrading enzymes has significant potential to improve feed utilization and animal performance. Ruminant feed enzyme additives, primarily xylanases and cellulases, are concentrated extracts resulting from bacterial or fungal fermentations that have specific enzymatic activities. Improvements in animal performance due to the use of enzyme additives can be attributed mainly to improvements in ruminal fibre digestion resulting in increased digestible energy intake. Animal responses are greatest when fibre digestion is compromised and when energy is the first-limiting nutrient in the diet.

Variable response: When viewed across a variety of enzyme products and experimental conditions, the response to feed enzymes by ruminants has been variable. This variation can be attributed to experimental conditions in which energy is not the limiting nutrient, as well as to the activities and characteristics of the enzymes supplied, under- or over-supplementation of enzyme activity, and inappropriate method of providing the enzyme product to the animal. With increasing consumer concern about the use of growth promoters and antibiotics in livestock production, and the magnitude of increased animal performance obtainable using feed enzymes, there is no doubt that these products will play an increasingly important role in the future.

Method of providing enzyme to ruminant animals

Applying fibrolytic exogenous enzymes in a liquid form onto feeds prior to consumption can have a positive effect on animal performance.

Exogenous enzymes in the rumen are generally more stable than previously thought (Hristov et al., 1998; Morgavi et al., 2000b, 2001), particularly when applied to feed prior to ingestion (Beauchemin et al., 2003). Application of enzymes to feed enhances the binding of the enzyme with the substrate, which increases the resistance of the enzymes to proteolysis and prolongs their residence time within the rumen. In the rumen, the close association between digestive bacteria and feed particles concentrates digestive enzymes close to their specific substrates. However, some ensiled feeds contain compounds that are inhibitory to xylanases (Nsereko et al., 2000). Hence, applying enzymes to dry feeds decreases the variability in response.

Applying enzymes to feed also provides a slow-release mechanism for enzymes in the rumen (Beauchemin et al., 1999). Thus, the greater the proportion of the diet treated with enzymes, the greater the chances that enzymes endure in the rumen. Without this stable feed-enzyme complex, the enzymes are solubilized in ruminal fluid and flow rapidly from the rumen. There is evidence for preconsumptive effects of exogenous enzymes causing the release of soluble carbohydrates, and in some cases, partial solubilization of NDF and ADF. Nsereko et al. (2000) demonstrated that applying enzymes to feed causes structural changes to occur, thereby making feed more amenable to degradation. Cell wall hydrolysis in the rumen proceeds in an erosive manner (White et al., 1993), and it is well recognized that a major constraint to digestion is the limited colonization and penetration of cellulolytic microbes and their hydrolytic enzymes onto the exposed surfaces of feed particles.

It is most likely that the major portion of the positive production responses resulting from the use of enzyme additives is due to ruminal effects. Adding exogenous enzymes to the diet increases the hydrolytic capacity of the rumen mainly due to increased bacterial attachment (Yang et al., 1999, stimulation of rumen microbial populations (Nsereko et al., 2002), and synergistic effects with hydrolases of ruminal microorganisms (Morgavi et al., 2000). The net effect is increased enzymatic activity within the rumen, which enhances digestibility of the total diet fed. Thus, improvements in digestibility are not limited to the dietary component to which the enzymes are applied, which explains why fibrolytic enzymes can be effective when added to the concentrate portion of a diet. Increased hydrolytic capacity of the rumen can also lead to an increase in digestibility of the nonfibre carbohydrate fraction, in addition to increasing digestibility of the fibre components of a diet, which explains why fibrolytic enzymes can be effective in high-concentrate diets.

3

Effect of Exogenous Enzyme Supplementation on Broiler Performance

Maize and soybean meal (SBM) are the most preferred feeds for poultry. But they do have antinutritional factors. Use of cereal grains in animal diets creates a competitive conflict with human nutrition, and the use of soybean is expensive. Proprietary broiler chicken feeds contain cereals up to 70%. The choice among the cereals primarily depends upon their availability, price and nutritive value. Economically efficient broiler feeds must achieve a low feed conversion ratio (FCR) (kg feed eaten per kg of weight gain) but also allow the birds to maximize their rates of weight gain.

Enzymes for the feed industry

The commercial application of enzymes as a feed additive has a history of less than 20 years (Choct, 2006). During this period, the feed enzyme industry came into existence and it has gone through several phases of development. The first phase was the use of enzymes to enhance nutrient digestibility, focusing primarily on removing the anti-nutritive effects of NSP such as arabinoxylans and β-glucans, from poultry and pig diets based on viscous grains. During the early 1990s, the scope of enzyme application expanded to consider nutrients other than NSP and benefits other than digestibility enhancement. Phytase is an apt example, where not only was it used to increase the utilization of phytate P, but also to alleviate environmental burden by reducing P excretion in the excreta. The feed industry then started to advocate enzyme addition to poultry and pig diets based on non-viscous grains.

The next phase is the application of enzymes to non-cereal grain components of the diets. These vegetable protein sources are often high in NSP, which are poorly characterized in regard to their molecular structures. Characterization of the NSP is in progress. Research workers in feed industry and academic institutions have been striving hard to produce commercially viable products that consistently improve the digestibility of vegetable proteins.

Exogenous enzyme supplementation (EES) on broiler perfromance

Enzyme supplementation significant reduced the intestinal digesta viscosity and increased the DM content of excreta in broilers were reported (Balamurugan, 2004). With maize grain, Noy and Sklan (1994) indicated that ileal starch digestibility rarely exceeds 85% in broilers between 4 and 21 days of age. The addition of an amylase to broiler feed can help to expose the starch more rapidly to digestion in the small intestine. Much of the recent work on supplementation of amylase, xylanase and protease mixture to maize-SBM broiler diets suggested a 2-5% improvement in available energy (Summers, 2001).

Marsman et al. (1997) and Rama Rao et al. (2004) reported no improvement in growth in broilers fed maize-SBM based diets upon supplementation with NSP hydrolyzing enzymes and plausible reason cited was very low concentration of NSP in the maize. Supplementation of commercial enzyme preparations or formulated enzyme preparations to maize-SBM diet did not improve the weight gain, feed intake, feed/gain and dressing yield (Nageswara et al., 2003).

Studies in broiler chickens (Brenes et al., 1993) indicated that enzyme addition to the barley based diet reduced the relative size of the gastrointestinal tract, pancreas and liver. Ciftci et al. (2003) reported that enzyme supplementation increased relative liver weight, but not that of heart and pancreas and reduced the relative weight of total digestive tract in laying hens. On the contrary, Ramakrishna Roy (2001) and Chandra Reddy (2003) reported that enzyme supplementation did not influence dressing yield, abdominal fat and weights of gizzard, heart and liver.

Experiments conducted in broiler chicken fed on maize-soya diets showed that β-mannanase supplementation increased energy utilization (compensated for energy decreases of 143 kcl ME/kg diet) as demonstrated by improved feed conversion and growth (Mark Jackson, 2001). Kocher et al. (2002) reported no improvement due to addition of enzyme in AMEn values in broilers but observed improvement when the level of enzyme was increased by 5 fold or when the diet was low in energy and protein (Kocher et al., 2003).

Naveed et al. (1999) reported that xylanase (0.05g/kg), protease (0.2g/kg) and cellulase (0.5g/kg) enzymes in the diet increased amino acid digestibility though they did not influence the performance. The protein concentration in breast muscle was increased significantly with supplementation of NSP hydrolyzing enzymes to maize-SBM diets (Rama Rao et al. 2004).

Marsman et al. (1997), Nageswara et al. (2003) and Rama Rao et al. (2004) reported that exogenous enzyme supplementation to maize-SBM diets in broiler chicken did not affect growth and feed efficiency while Devegowda and Nagalakshmi (1992) found improvement in performance of broilers with dietary enzyme supplementation through better feed conversion ratio.

Multienzyme supplementation to maize-SBM broiler diets

An experiment was conducted in broiler chicks to study the effect of enzyme supplementation to maize-soybean meal diet (Table1) (Reddy et al., 2003) on weight gain, feed conversion ratio, protein efficiency ratio, energy utilization, certain digestive system traits, dressing percentage, breast muscle yield, blood glucose and triglycerides levels and organ weights.

Experimental procedures

The experimental broiler starter (0 to 3 weeks) and broiler finisher (4 to 6 weeks) diets (Table1) were formulated as per the specifications of BIS (IS 1374:1992, Fourth revision). The cocktail enzyme prepared for the maize-soybean meal diet by the Kemin Nutritional Technologies (India) Pvt Ltd was supplemented at the rate of 50g per 100kg Control-1diet (Treatment-1). One hundred and two day old commercial Cobb broiler chicks (51 male chicks and 51 female chicks) were divided randomly into eight groups of 12 (6 male+6 female) chicks minimum and placed on two diets (control-1 and treatment-1) in four replicates. The chicks in each replicate were housed (0.9m x 2.0m) in deep litter system in RCC building. Routine managemental practices were followed for brooding and vaccination. Feed and water were made available at all times.

Table 1. Ingredient and Chemical composition (%) of Broiler diets*

	Control-1		Treatment-1	
	Starter	**Finisher**	**Starter**	**Finisher**
Feedstuffs (%)				
Maize	54.00	62.70	54.00	62.70
Soybean meal	40.25	32.00	40.25	32.00
Oil	1.00	1.00	1.00	1.00
Dicalcium phosphate	2.00	2.00	2.00	2.00
Calcite	1.75	1.3	1.75	1.3
Salt	0.4	0.4	0.4	0.4
Methionine	0.14	0.04	0.14	0.04
Trace mineral mixture**	0.1	0.1	0.1	0.1
Choline chloride	0.1	0.1	0.1	0.1
Enzyme	---	----	0.05	0.05
Cost per 100 Kg, Rs	1024	974	1038	988
Calculated Values				
Crude protein, %	22.97	19.94	22.97	19.94
Metabolizable energy, Kcal/kg	2809	2910	2809	2910
Crude fibre, %	3.87	3.47	3.87	3.47
Chemical composition(% on DMB)				
Crude protein	24.81	21.44	24.81	21.44
Ether extract	2.82	3.64	2.82	3.64
Total ash	8.89	9.48	8.89	9.48
Crude fibre	3.25	3.99	3.25	3.99
Nitrogen free extract	60.23	61.45	60.23	61.45
Acid insoluble ash	1.56	1.87	1.56	1.87

*Other microingredients added: AB_2D_3K, 0.025; coccidiostat, 0.05; zinc bacitracin, 0.1; toxibind dry, 0.25 and endox dry, 0.0125%.

**Trace mineral mixture provides 5.4g manganese, 5.2g zinc, 2.0g iron, 0.2g iodine, 0.2g copper and 0.1g cobalt.

At the end of the fifth week, 6 birds of equal body weight were selected randomly per diet for metabolism study to calculate the apparent metabolizable energy (AME) and true metabolizable energy (TME) of the experimental diets. During the metabolism study the birds were kept individually in cages (44cm L × 32cm W × 45cm H) fixed to a stand of 3 feet height. Six unfed birds were used to calculate the metabolic and endogenous losses. All the birds (12 Nos) were starved for 24 hours to empty their digestive tract and 30g of the test diets (Sibbald, 1976) were force fed to each six birds. Initially the birds were allowed to feed voluntarily for 20 minutes and then the left over feed was force fed so as to ensure complete consumption. Starvation was continued for the six unfed birds for another 24 hours. For the quantitative estimation of excreta the bottom and sides of the cage was well covered with plastic sheet, which rested over the dropping tray of the cage. The excreta collections in fed and unfed birds were done for exactly 24 hours. Wholesome drinking water was made available throughout the experimental period.

The excreta was recovered completely from the plastic sheet for each bird after removing feathers and other extraneous material. After taking representative sample for nitrogen (N) estimation, the remaining was kept in hotair oven at 800C. Dry matter (DM) was estimated and DM of the sample used for N estimation was added to obtain the total DM of the excreta. The dried excreta samples of all the 12 fed birds and six unfed birds were packed individually in polythene covers and stored for gross energy estimation using Gallenkamp adiabatic bomb calorimeter.

At the end of the sixth week, 8 birds (4 males and 4 females) of equal body weight were selected randomly per diet and kept for fasting overnight before slaughter to estimate dressing percentage, breast muscle yield, organ weights and weight and size of digestive system. The full weight of total digestive tract (TDT) was recorded after cutting open the tract (including the crop, proventriculus and gizzard) and emptying. The length of TDT was measured after emptying the contents. The weight of contents of TDT was also recorded. Blood was collected from wing vein into centrifuge tubes and the serum was used to estimate glucose and triglycerides levels. Serum glucose was estimated by O-Toluidine method using Nice diagnostic kit while serum triglycerides were estimated by enzymatic kit method using Span Diagnostics Ltd. Statistical analysis of the data was carried out using't' test (Snedecor and Cochran, 1967).

Salient findings of the study

Male chicks gained higher weight in both control-1 and treatment-1 groups during starter period, finisher period and overall period. Enzyme supplementation did not affect weight gain of chicks during starter period although 4.9 % and 3.0 % increase was observed during finisher and overall period, respectively.

Enzyme supplementation had decreased the contents of total digestive tract (TDT) by 13% whether expressed on total weight of the bird or on relative weight (g/100g LW) (Reddy et al., 2003), which is in agreement with the increased DM content of excreta (Balamurugan, 2004). This implies that dietary nutrients are better digested and utilized for body weight gain and thus reduced the volume of excreta in the birds on enzyme supplemented maize-SBM diet.

Enzyme supplementation apparently increased marginally the ME values and metabolizability of the diets though the differences were not statistically significant (Reddy et al., 2003). This might possibly be due to the low level of enzyme and is in agreement with Kocher et al. (2002 and 2003).

Chicks on enzyme supplemented diet had higher breast muscle indicating that enzyme supplementation enhanced yield of breast muscle by 5.3%.

Nitrogen retention was enhanced by 26 per cent in the broilers fed on enzyme supplemented maize-SBM diet (Reddy et al., 2003) and this is reflected in laying down more lean muscle mass (breast muscle) in birds.

Exogenous enzyme supplementation marginally increased the weight gain of broiler chicks, specifically the breast muscle yield through better feed efficiency although statistically nonsignificant.

The use of NSP as energy sources

Large amounts of grain byproducts, such as brans, and non-conventional ingredients, such as palm kernel cake, sunflower meal, etc, are available for use in poultry and pig diets. But these feedstuffs are characterized by their very high contents of mostly insoluble NSP. Rice bran contains approximately 20-25% NSP, half of which is cellulose. Palm kernel cake contains high levels of mannans or galactomannans, with a total NSP level reaching 70%. World-wide grain and oilseed are used for biofuel production. The co-products such as distillers' dry grains (DDG), the dried residue of distillers' grains, and distillers' dry grain with solubles (DDGS; the DDG with syrups added) are available for animal feeding. DDG accounts for approximately 30% of dry grains for ethanol production, and it contains 25-28% protein, 8-9% fat, 5% ash and the remainder is believed to be NSP (Choct, 2006).

Currently DDG is used predominantly in ruminant feeds. The potential of using enzymes to DDGS for the release of ME for monogastric animals is enormous. However, the current enzymes are not designed to degrade NSP to monomeric sugars within the food transit time of the chicken and pre-treatment is necessary in order to yield a substantial amount of simple sugars. With development of highly sophisticated enzymes and fine-tuning of pre-treatment procedures, these NSP sources represent a large source of potential energy and prebiotics with specific functions for monogastrics (Choct, 2006).

Multienzyme supplementation to maize-SBM-DORB broiler diets

Maize and soybean meal are the most preferred feeds for poultry. High cost of these ingredients spurred the pursuit of alternate ingredients to reduce the cost of production. Deoiled rice bran (DORB), which has higher content of non-starch polysaccharides (NSP), is one such alternate ingredient. Exogenous enzyme supplementation helps in utilizing more economical feed ingredients high in NSP. An experiment was conducted in broiler chicks to study the effect of enzyme supplementation to maize-soybean meal-DORB diets (Reddy et al., 2003) on weight gain, feed conversion ratio, protein efficiency ratio, energy utilization, dressing percentage, breast muscle yield, blood glucose and triglycerides levels and organ weights.

The experimental broiler starter (0 to 3 weeks) and broiler finisher (4 to 6 weeks) diets (Table 2) were formulated to contain crude protein (CP) and metabolisable energy (ME) lesser (1 unit CP% and 100 Kcal ME) than BIS specifications. The cocktail enzyme prepared by the Kemin Nutritional Technologies (India) Pvt Ltd was supplemented at the rate of 50g to the control diet of 100kg (Treatment 2).

Table 2. Ingredient and Chemical composition (%) of Broiler diets*

	Control–2		Treatment–2	
	Starter	**Finisher**	**Starter**	**Finisher**
Feedstuffs (%)				
Maize	45.50	51.50	45.50	51.50
Soybean meal	36.50	28.00	36.50	28.00
Deoiled rice bran	12.00	14.00	12.00	14.00
Oil	1.00	1.50	1.00	1.50
Dicalcium phosphate	1.82	1.90	1.82	1.90
Calcite	1.90	1.50	1.90	1.50
Salt	0.4	0.4	0.4	0.4
Lysine	0.10	0.06	0.10	0.06
Methionine	0.15	0.04	0.15	0.04
Trace mineral mixture**	0.10	0.10	0.10	0.10
Choline chloride	0.10	0.10	0.10	0.10
Enzyme	---	----	0.05	0.05
Cost per 100 Kg, Rs	994	954	1005	964
Calculated Values				
Crude protein, %	22.20	19.13	22.20	19.13
Metabolisable energy, Kcal/kg	2703	2792	2703	2792
Crude fibre, %	5.09	4.94	5.09	4.94
Chemical composition(% on DMB)				
Crude protein	23.94	20.31	23.94	20.31
Ether extract	2.38	3.29	2.38	3.29
Total ash	10.29	10.66	10.29	10.66
Crude fibre	5.21	4.93	5.21	4.93
Nitrogen free extract	58.18	60.81	58.18	60.81
Acid insoluble ash	3.32	3.75	3.32	3.75

*Other microingredients added: AB_2D_3K, 0.025; coccidiostat, 0.05; zinc bacitracin, 0.1; toxibind dry, 0.25 and endox dry, 0.0125%.

**Trace mineral mixture provides 5.4g manganese, 5.2g zinc, 2.0g iron, 0.2g iodine, 0.2g copper and 0.1g cobalt.

Salient findings of the study

Male chicks attained higher weight gains irrespective of the diet and of age i.e. during starter, finisher or overall period. The weight gain of broiler chicks fed enzyme supplemented diet (Treatment 2) was not different from that of the chicks fed on control diet during starter, finisher or overall period.

Enzyme supplementation reduced (P < 0.10) the feed consumption of broiler chicks by 3.5% during starter period while in finisher period and overall period the trend was continued though it had not attained statistical significance (Reddy et al., 2003). The reduction in feed consumption observed in the present study during the starter period is in agreement with Devegowda and Nagalakshmi (1992), and Marsman et al. (1997), who reported that synergism among the enzymes supplemented was responsible for better performance of broilers. Similarly enzyme supplementation improved the feed conversion ratio during starter period and the same trend was observed during overall periods.

Broiler chicks fed enzyme supplemented diet tended to have higher (P > 0.10) blood glucose and triglycerides. Weights of heart, liver, pancreas and spleen were not statistically different between broiler chicks fed on enzyme supplemented diet and enzyme unsupplemented diet.

Enzyme supplementation increased the breast muscle by 8% (Reddy et al., 2003). The higher nitrogen retention (22%) in enzyme supplemented broilers (Reddy et al., 2003) may be related to increased amino acid digestibility due to the action of exogenous enzymes on the diet (Naveed et al., 1999). This higher nitrogen utilization is reflected in higher breast muscle yield in broilers fed enzyme supplemented maize-SBM-deoiled rice bran diet.

Enzyme supplementation to maize-SBM-DORB broiler diets reduced (P < 0.10) the feed consumption and increased the breast muscle yield implying that higher lean muscle mass was laid in the enzyme supplemented broiler chicks which is reflected in slightly better feed efficiency.

Benefits of exogenous enzyme supplementation

- Reduce the variability in nutritive value between feedstuffs: The soluble and insoluble fibre content of feeds vary considerably according to variety, climatic conditions, agronomic practices followed, and the soil as well as the period of storage before feeding. Variation in apparent metabolizable energy (AME) of wheat- or barley-based diets was significantly reduced with enzyme supplementation, indicating that low AME cereal grains generally benefit more from enzyme supplementation than high AME cereal grains.
- Contribute to clean environment by way of reduced manure volume (up to 20%), nitrogen excretion (up to 15% in pigs and 20% in poultry) and phosphorus excretion
- Improve the efficiency of utilization of nutrients: Enhances nutrient availability by digesting hither to indigestible nutrients; enhances the capability of animal enzymes by reducing viscosity of digesta thereby improving the feed efficiency.
- Releases bound minerals and other nutrients, thereby reducing the need for their supplementation. Increase the uniformity of flock, thus helping management and improve profitability
- Reduction of sticky droppings (lower risk of dirty eggs, hock burns and breast blisters) and improvement of litter quality in poultry; improve the general health status and well being of animals

- Improve the accuracy of feed formulations
- Overall, EES help improve the sustainability and reduce the costs of animal production.

Innovative applications of feed enzymes

- The feed/food enzyme industry is constantly searching for new areas of application. Recently published data indicated the role of glycanases (carbohydrate degrading enzymes) as an alternative to in-feed antibiotics.
- It is possible to produce enzymes tailored for the generation of specific low molecular weight carbohydrates **in vivo**, which, in turn, produce specific health benefits in birds (Choct, 2006). A specific range of oligomers can be produced from a given NSP source **in situ** with a particular enzyme. Some of these carbohydrates may be used to stimulate the growth of beneficial microflora in the gut (or reduce the load of pathogens in the gut) and have specific effects on the immune system. Thus enzymes may be used to generate certain end products for their secondary effects.

Production of xylo-oligosaccharides by the use of xylanases in wheat-based diets could be one way to encourage the development of a healthy gut microflora (Vahjen et al., 1998). Sinlae and Choct (2000) demonstrated that broilers fed a wheat-based diet with xylanase had a negligible number of *Clostridium perfringens* compared with the control birds. Further detailed study (Bedford and Apajalahti, 2001) showed that xylanase supplementation markedly reduced the coliforms, lactic acid bacteria, enterococci and the total bacterial count in the small intestine of birds.

Manno-oligosaccharides have been reported to boost immune system in poultry (Spring et al., 2000). Producing specific manno-oligomers from copra meal and palm kernel cake **in situ** is possible.

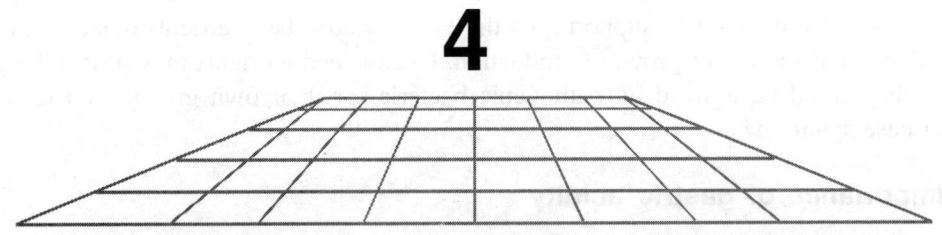

4

Importance of Gastric Acidity in enhancing the Livestock Productivity; Application of Acid Binding Capacity of Feedstuffs

INTRODUCTION

The gastrointestinal tract (GIT) provides a complete interface between the animal and its environment. GIT is the last line in the body's defence against the entry pathogens and against feed toxins. Though GIT is inside the animal body, the lumen of the GIT is outside the body of the animal. It has to cope with abrupt dietary changes at birth and weaning. The maintenance of gut health in the young weaned piglet is of paramount importance if the young animal is to achieve its full genetic potential for growth.

Healthy and functional GIT

The gastrointestinal tract is an important battle ground between potential pathogens and the immune system of the body. The lumen of the GIT has an enormous population of non-pathogenic organisms as well as pathogenic microorganisms, which frequently lead to high incidences of enteric diseases. Enteric diseases contribute to poor feed conversion rates and ultimately result in reduced efficiency of production. Thus in commercial / intensive animal production health problems have important animal welfare and economic consequences.

Animals must have a healthy and functional GIT where the growth of pathogenic microorganisms is discouraged and efficient digestion and absorption of nutrients occur, which only assures excellent feed efficiencies and growth.

The intestinal epithelium must be maintained with a very high physical integrity to prevent the bulk transport of pathogens into the body from the gut lumen. Even minor damage to the GIT by pathogens may cause poor feed efficiency and decreased growth rates.

The intestinal epithelium must also be sufficiently thin to actively transport nutrients into the body to support growth. It is only absorbed nutrients that are of any value to the animal for growth / production. Unabsorbed nutrients may pose a danger as they could be utilized by pathogenic bacteria for their own growth and lead to disease syndromes.

Importance of gastric acidity

Gastric acid, hydrochloric acid (HCl) is secreted in the stomach to lower the pH of the digesta. A low gastric pH is important for several reasons.

Protein digestion begins in the stomach with the action of pepsin, secreted as the enzyme precursors, pepsinogens by stomach mucosa. Conversion of pepsinogen to pepsin occurs rapidly at pH 2.0 but only slowly at pH 5.0 to 6.0. In turn, pepsin enzymes work best in an acidic environment, pH 2.0 to 3.5, and activity declines rapidly above this pH. If gastric pH remains high, protein breakdown in the stomach is impaired, which not only affects the digestibility and utilization of nitrogen, but also minerals. Under these circumstances undigested proteins reach the lower digestive tract. In the jejunum and colon, excessive protein fermentation may occur, leading to the formation of toxic biogenic amines.

Carbohydrate hydrolysis in the stomach occurs by the action of salivary amylase, which, in contrast to pepsin, is inactivated once pH falls to 3.5 (Yen 2001).

In the suckling pig, acid secretion is low and the principal source of acidity is bacterial fermentation of lactose from sow's milk to lactic acid (Kidder and Manners, 1978). A high level of lactate in the stomach tends to inhibit HCl secretion (Yen, 2001). Ingestion of solid feed reduces the level of lactic acid in the stomach (Yen, 2001) and stimulates HCl production (Cranwell, 1985) but, in practice, creep feed consumption is low and variable at least up to four weeks of age (Lawlor et al., 2002). At weaning, a combination of low acid secretion, lack of lactose substrate, and consumption of large meals at infrequent intervals can result in elevated pH, often to over 5.0 and it may remain high for several days (Kidder and Manners, 1978).

A low gastric pH is also essential to control the bacterial population in the stomach. The gut microflora comprises both commensals (Gram-positive) and enteropathogens (Gram-negative). In healthy animals, there is a balance between the Gram-positive and Gram-negative bacterial population. A healthy gut has a preponderance of Gram-positive bacteria. Proliferation of pathogenic bacteria such as *E.coli*, most *Salmonella spp.*, *Campylobacter jejuni* diminish in an acid environment, while beneficial Bifido and Lactobacilli bacteria species are more tolerant towards low pH values.

A high gastric pH will allow pathogens to survive and allow them greater opportunity to colonise the digestive tract (Bolduan et al., 1988; Yen, 2001).

Phasing out of antimicrobial growth promoters

Acceptance of antibiotic growth promoters (AGP) in animal production is rapidly disappearing because of the concerns about development of antimicrobial resistance. Government regulations and consumer preference are driving this change. Early concern about the development of antibiotic resistance in human pathogens and recommendations to ban sub-therapeutic use in animal feeds was discussed by Swann in a report to the British Parliament (1969). Indeed, evidence exists that antibiotic resistance genes can be and are transmitted from animal to human microbiota (Greko, 2001).

The World Health Organization (WHO) published a report on the medical impact of the use of antimicrobials in food animals suggesting a link between use of AGP in animal production and increasing infections of humans by antibiotic resistant microorganisms on an epidemiological basis (1997). WHO has issued a report entitled "Global Principles for the Containment of Antimicrobial Resistance in Animals Intended for Food" (World Health Organization, 2000). This report recommends, on precautionary grounds, that national governments adopt a proactive approach to reduce the need for antimicrobial use in animals and establish surveillance of antimicrobial usage and resistance. With respect to the use of antimicrobial growth promoters, WHO suggests that use of antimicrobial growth promoters that are in classes also used in humans be terminated or rapidly phased out.

On a global level, a joint workshop was held involving the WHO, the Food and Agriculture Organization of the United Nations (FAO) and the World Organization for Animal Health (OIE, Office International des Epizootis) on non-human antimicrobial usage and antimicrobial resistance (Geneva, Dec. 2003). The resulting report recommends implementation of the WHO global principles for the containment of antimicrobial resistance in animals intended for food (WHO, 2004). In addition, the report recommends the implementation on a national level of risk assessment studies and establishment of surveillance programmes to monitor AGP use and antimicrobial resistance in bacteria from food animals.

The ban on antibiotic growth promoters (AGPs) led to review of organic feed acids as feed additives in place of AGPs since feed acidification can promote a better growth performance. Organic feed acids are already in use as feed preservatives. Several trials were conducted between 1975 and 1995 on organic acids such as acetic acid, adipic acid, benzoic acid, butyric acid, citric acid, formic acid, fumaric acd, lactic acid, malic acid, propionic acid, sorbic acid, succinic acid, tartaric acid, etc. and their salts such as sodium formate, calcium formate, potassium diformate, etc. to study their effect on growth rate and feed conversion ratio in piglets and chicken. A realization has emerged that the benefits of feed acidification of a monogastric diet do not relate simply to a lowering of the dietary pH. But beyond doubt acidification reduces the diet's buffering capacity.

Acids can be divided into organic and inorganic acids.

Organic acids are also referred to as carboxylic acids, since they have the typical carboxyl group: R-C00H, which can easily split off an H+, which makes them react as an acid. Inorganic acids do not have this carboxyl group. They split into a cation and an anion, e.g. HCl giving H+ and Cl-, thereby lowering the pH value of the feed.

Mode of action of organic feed acids

Organic acids associated with specific antimicrobial activity are short chain acids and are either simple monocarboxylic acids (formic, acetic, propionic and butyric acids) or carboxylic acids bearing an hydroxyl group (lactic, malic, tartaric and citric acids).Salts of some of these acids also demonstrated performance benefits. Other acids such as sorbic and fumaric acids have some antifungal activity.

Antimicrobial activity: Organic acids are weak acids and are only partly dissociated at physiological pH ranges. Acid dissociation is measured by pKa, the pH at which the acid is half-dissociated. Organic acids with antimicrobial activity commonly used as dietary acidifiers for pigs and poultry have a pKa between 3 and 5 (Table 1). The magnitude of the antimicrobial effects varies from one acid to another and is dependent upon both concentration and pH. At low pH, more of the organic acid exists in the undissociated form. Undissociated organic acids are lipophilic and can diffuse across cell membranes, including those of bacteria and moulds. Once in the bacterial cell, the higher pH of its cytoplasm causes dissociation of the acid. The resulting reduction in pH of the cell contents disrupts enzymatic reactions and nutrient transport systems.

Table 1. Antimicrobial organic acids

Organic feed acid	pKa
Formic acid	3.75
Acetic acid	4.76
Propionic acid	4.88
Butyric acid	4.82
Lactic acid	3.83
Sorbic acid	4.76
Fumaric acid	3.02
Malic acid	3.40
Tartaric acid	2.93
Citric acid	3.13

This direct antimicrobial activity also is responsible for feed and food sanitation and preservative effects and explains the synergy between mineral acids such as hydrochloric acid and organic acids. The presence of HCl reduces the digesta pH, allowing more of the organic acid to be present in the undissociated form. After ingestion of organic acids direct antimicrobial activity is greatest in the foregut. This part of the digestive system includes the crop and gizzard of poultry and stomach of swine.

Reduce the subclinical infection of pathogenic organisms: A consequent reduction in subclinical *E. coli*, salmonella and campylobacter infections may contribute to a reduction in nutrient demand by the gut-associated immune tissue. The relatively low pH of the upper gut tends to favour not only the antimicrobial activity of organic acids but also their absorption by diffusion into the gut epithelium.

Reduce the pH of digesta: Organic acids reduce the pH of digesta in the gut lumen, particularly in the foregut. The magnitude of the reduction is at its maximum in the stomach, reaching 0.5-1.0 pH units. This helps to improve digestibility of protein and amino acids and reduction in ammonia and biogenic amines.

Another benefit of lower pH in the GIT is an improvement in microbial phytase activity. Microbial phytase has two pH optima - pH 2.5 and pH 4.5 to 5.7- and phytic acid is much more soluble at lower pH. These effects combine to give an improvement in phosphorus digestibility and retention.

Thaela (1998) reported that dietary supplementation with lactic acid stimulated pancreatic and bile secretion in weanling pigs. This effect is mediated by the acids diffusing into the cells in the undissociated form, and then dissociating in response to the higher pH of the cell cytoplasm.

Lower the microbial proliferation in the jejunum: The higher luminal pH in the lower gut would appear to favour the dissociated form of the organic acids, which would reduce uptake by diffusion. However, an acidic micro-environment exists at the gut epithelial surface and this permits the diffusion of the undissociated form into the bacteria and into the enterocytes themselves. Thus the antimicrobial activity of organic acids persists even in the jejunum and ileum. Lower microbial proliferation in the jejunum reduces the competition of the microflora with the host for nutrients. This reduction in competition may be one of the mechanisms responsible for improved digestibility of nutrients, which has been reported in both pigs and broilers.

Organic acids-slow-release acid effect

Dietary acids can be used singly or in combinations, and as feed additive products may be protected by encapsulation technology or put into a specific fatty acid or orthophospho-glucopeptide matrix. This protection is used as a delivery mechanism to obtain a slow release of the acids and to gain a wider activity throughout the digestive tract.

Unprotected acids can cause a fast drop in pH and, by dissociating quickly in the stomach or upper small intestine, may not be effective lower down the tract. Less acid product is needed when the acids can be released slowly, and in combination it covers a wider range of dissociation constants.

Another approach involves feeding an acid-salt that remains in a stable form until it reaches the digestive tract where the acid releases. BASF's **potassium diformate** (Formi[R]), the first non-antibiotic performance enhancer for pigs, remains stable until it reaches the pig's gut where it dissolves into formic acid, formate and potassium. Kinetic study showed that 85% of formate survives the stomach and appears in the duodenum. This means significant amounts are present to exert antimicrobial effects in the small intestine.

In microorganisms, organic acids have been implicated in the disruption of amino acid metabolism, of DNA synthesis and of energy metabolism. Acids may lower the intracellular pH and cause alterations in cell membrane permeability.

Organic acid salts as growth promoters

Monogastric animals: In monogastric animals organic acids are used as acidifiers and inhibitors of pathogenic microbes.

Ruminants: In ruminants they may act as rumen function 'enhancers' especially in intensively fed animals on high-concentrate (high in non-structural carbohydrates) diets which present a risk of acidosis. Various strains of Selenomonas ruminantium account for 22-51% of ruminal bacteria and they can use lactate as a substrate.

Certain C4 dicarboxylic acids, malic and fumaric, acts as key metabolites for some ruminal bacteria in the citric acid cycle. These acids affect microbes in two important ways: their dissociation capacity leading to acidification; their capacity to pass through the microbial cell wall undissociated and to modify metabolism or DNA synthesis inside the cell.

Conclusion

Thus organic feed acids are used for their antimicrobial effects on pathogenic bacteria, promotion of beneficial or probiotic bacteria and nutritional value, improved nonspecific immunity, stimulatory effect on pancreatic secretion, and increase gastric acidity. Variability in the beneficial effects due to organic feed acids has been reported. This lack of consistency in performance response may be due to several reasons that include buffering capacity of dietary ingredients, managemental practices, etc.

Acid: base value to the feed

It is important to consider the acid: base value of the feed while formulating a ration. This is because the use of alkaline feed can compromise the ability of the bird's digestive tract to maintain a level of acidity to support a healthy gut microflora. In poultry layers and breeders high calcium requirements are usually satisfied by adding limestone, which result in an alkaline feed and an 'alkaline gut'. This can create a gut environment that favours several potentially dangerous microbial species (Reddy, 2006).

By contrast, a digestive system at the correct pH minimizes the risk of pathogens. The use of gut acidifiers has been proven to be of immense help in maintaining the microbial balance of the gut. Acidifiers are acids that are included in the feed in order to lower the pH of the feed and gut and most of gut acidifiers consist of organic acids.

Buffering capacity / acid-binding capacity of feedstuffs

Buffering action is the ability of a solution to resist a change in pH through the addition of acid or loss of alkali. The intrinsic buffering capacity of a feedstuff was defined as the ability of a given amount of this feedstuff to resist a change in pH after the addition of either an acidic or a basic solution (Jasaitis et al., 1987; Bolduan et al., 1988). Buffering by ingredients is most often measured as their acid-binding capacity (ABC). Essentially the measurement is taken by preparing a suspension of the feed sample in water and checking how much of a standard acid must be added in order to reduce the pH to a target level.

Effects of acid-binding capacity (ABC) of feedstuffs

Effective antibiotic-free post-weaning pig diets require a sufficiently high level of organic acids and low acid-binding capacity. The greater the quantity of ABC in meq/kg, the more that feedstuff will be able to neutralize the digestive acid released by the gastric mucosa.

The high acid-binding/ buffering capacity of the feed (its ability to neutralise feed acid) helps to further raise the stomach pH (Jasaitis *et al.*, 1987; Bolduan *et al.*, 1988). Inclusion of whey or lactose in the starter diet ensures continuation of bacterial fermentation and some, though reduced, lactic acid production (Kidder and Manners, 1978). Development of HCl secretory capacity occurs more rapidly in the weaned pig than in the suckling pig (Cranwell and Moughan, 1989). Raised stomach pH after weaning results in reduced digestion of feed, which will then be fermented in the hind gut and may provoke diarrhoea.

The concept of manipulating stomach acidity by adding acid to feeds or using feeds of low acid-binding or buffering capacity (Jasaitis et al., 1987; Bolduan et al., 1988) has been around for a long time and addition of organic acids to piglet starter feeds is a common practice. However, there is little information on the acid-binding capacity (ABC) of ingredients that are used in formulation of complete feeds. The limited published sets of data have been compiled using methods with different titration-end points (e.g., pH = 3.0 or pH = 4.0) and hence the values are not comparable (Jasaitis et al., 1987; Bolduan et al., 1988; Giger-Reverdin et al., 2002).

Measurement of acid-binding capacity of feedstuffs

Lawlor et al. (2005) modified Jasaitis et al. (1987) procedure to determine pH and acid-binding capacity. A 0.5 g sample of ingredient / feed was suspended in 50 ml of distilled and de-ionised water and continuously stirred with a magnetic stirrer. Titrations were performed by addition of 0.1N HCl in increments of 0.1 to 10ml depending on the ingredient type and the stage of titration. Acid was added so that it would take approximately 10 separate additions of acid to reach pH 3.0. Initial pH and all further readings taken during the titration were recorded after equilibration for three minutes. ABC was calculated as the amount of acid in milliequivalents (meq) required to lower the pH of 1kg of sample to (a) pH 4.0 (ABC- 4) and (b) pH 3.0 (ABC-3).

The buffering capacity (BUF) was calculated by dividing the ABC by the total change in pH units [from initial pH to the final pH of (a) 4.0 (BUF- 4) and (b) 3.0 (BUF-3)]. BUF expresses the amount of acid required to produce a unit change in the pH of a feed ingredient / feed sample.

Feeds/ingredients with a pH less than 3 or 4 were titrated as above but against 0.1 N NaOH until pH 4.0 and/or pH 3.0 was reached. ABC and BUF values in these cases were given negative values.

Results showed that acid salts and minerals (zinc oxide, limestone, sodium bicarbonate) had the highest ABC and BUF values. Meat and fish meal, milk products, amino acids, root and pulp products and vegetable proteins were the categories of organic ingredients with the highest ABC and BUF values. Cereals had the lowest values among the organic ingredient categories. With regard to organic ingredients, their ABC values are positively correlated with their ash and protein contents (Jasaitis et al., 1987). It is reported that the geographic origin of an ingredient can affect its ABC because it influences the ion concentration of the ingredient and this may help to explain the variation in ABC values found for individual ingredients.

Of the ingredients, both inorganic and organic, the acids category had the lowest ABC and BUF values. Most ABC values for the individual acids were negative with orthophosphoric, fumaric, formic, malic and citric acids having the most negative values.

The use of these organic acids in starter diets offers the opportunity to lower the diet ABC without having to reduce dietary protein or mineral content and increase gastric acidity. However, the beneficial effects of organic acids on pig health are strongly dependent on the initial BUF value of the diet (Blank et al., 2001). 'Calprona P' (Verdugt company; a special acid calcium salt produced from combination of propionic, citric, formic and acetic acids) is reported to reduce the ABC value of the diet.

Conclusions

Some ingredients bind more acid in the stomach than others and for this reason their use in pig starter diets might result in a high gastric pH. A high gastric pH is detrimental to the pig because it allows the proliferation of deleterious microorganisms and inhibits protein digestion leading to inefficient growth and feed efficiency.

Diets can be formulated with low ABC values using the ABC values for ingredients. Such diets can be used when a high gastric pH is likely to be a problem (e.g., at weaning). These diets could also be employed as part of a strategy to reduce E. coli or Salmonella in older pigs.

Feed manufacturers and nutritionists can make use of the acid-binding capacity of feed ingredients and feed additives as well (hither to neglected area) apart from their nutritive value when formulating diets for livestock and poultry. In diets for ruminants and healthy, mature animals, diets of low ABC may not be especially important to overall animal performance. However, a low value in the feed offers a number of advantages. It may be especially advantageous in diets for young animals and animals under stress, where a low-ABC feed can help to improve growth performance and productivity.

5

Functional Amino Acids and Fatty Acids for Enhancing Production Performance of Pigs

Functional animal nutrition

Functional animal nutrition is aimed at supplying the nutrients to the animals matching their requirements to improve not only the animal physiology and health with better nutrient efficiency and lowered environmental pollution, but also the enrichment of their products (milk, meat and eggs) with omega fatty acids, antioxidants, trace minerals, etc for good health of the consumers.

Functional amino acids and fatty acids

Nutritional and physiological status of pregnant and lactating sows directly affects foetal and neonatal growth and health. Genetically improved modern sows are highly prolific and their progeny possess great potential for rapid growth. However, the current restricted feeding programme for pregnant sows limits nutrient availability for foetal growth especially during mid- to late-pregnancy (Ji er al., 2005; Kim et al., 2005). Additionally, low voluntary feed intake during lactation resulted in reduced provision of nutrients for milk production, thereby causing massive maternal tissue mobilization (Kim and Easter, 2003). The maternal catabolic conditions may impair the growth of the foetus and the neonate as well as increase their morbidity and mortality. It is implying that the availability of functional amino acids and fatty acids may be declined, though the underlying mechanisms are not fully understood.

Functional amino acids and fatty acids are essential not only for normal growth and maintenance of animals but also for the syntheses of many bioactive compounds (Wu and Self, 2005). Amino acids and fatty acids with special functions include arginine, branched-chain amino acids (alanine, valine, leucine, isoleucine, methionine, proline, cysteine), glutamate, glutamine, tryptophan, glycine, taurine, conjugated linoleic acid (CLA), docosahexaenoic acid (DHA), and eicosapentaenoic acid (EPA).

They can benefit pregnant and lactating sows under catabolic conditions with improved foetal growth, neonatal health, and lactation performance. Guoyao Wu, Sung Woo Kim and several of their coworkers did considerable work on dietary uses of functional amino acids and fatty acids to enhance reproductive performance and health of sows as well as the growth and immune status of their foetuses and neonates.

Functional amino acids

The biochemical properties and functions of amino acids (AA) differ remarkably because of variations in their side chains. Their concentrations also vary greatly in fetal fluids during pregnancy, in plasma of neonates during the first weeks of life, and in plasma of all animals under catabolic conditions. Glutamine is particularly abundant in sow's milk (3.5 mM at Day 28 of lactation), plasma (0.5 to 1 mM), skeletal muscle (5 to 20 mM), as well as amniotic fluid (2-3 mM) and allantoic fluid (3 to 25 mM during early pregnancy. Arginine and citrulline (precursor of arginine) are unusually rich in porcine allantoic fluid (4-6 mM) and ovine allantoic fluid (5-10 mM), respectively, during early gestation.

Over 300 amino acids occur in nature, but only 20 serve as building blocks of protein in animal cells (Table1). Recently, there has been growing interest in nonessential (NEAA) and conditionally essential amino acids because of their unique, versatile functions in metabolic regulation and physiology. Recent evidence shows that some amino acids can regulate intracellular protein synthesis and degradation. In addition, amino acids are substrates for the synthesis of many biologically active substances (including NO, polyamines, glutathione, nucleic acids, hormones, and neurotransmitters) that are essential to the life and productivity of

Table 1. Nutritionally essential and nonessential amino acids in animals

Monogastric mammals		Poultry	
EAA	NEAA	EAA	NEAA
Arginine1	Alanine	Arginine	Alanine
Histidine	Asparagine	Glycine	Asparagine
Isoleucine	Aspartate	Histidine	Aspartate
Leucine	Cysteine	Isoleucine	Cysteine
Lysine	Glutamate	Leucine	Glutamate
Methionine	Glutamate	Leucine	Glutamate
Methionine	Glutamine	Lysine	Glutamine
Phenylalanine	Glycine	Methionine	Serine
Threonine	Proline2	Phenylalanine	Tyrosine
Valine	Tyrosine	Threonine	
		Tryptophan	
		Valine	

1 Arginine may not be required in the diet to maintain nitrogen balance in most of adult mammals but its deficiency in the diet may result in metabolic, neurological or reproductive disorders.

2 Proline is an essential amino acid for young pigs.

animals (Table 2). Their abnormal metabolism negatively alters feed intake, disturb whole body homeostasis, impairs animal growth and development, and may even cause death (Wu and Self, 2005).

Table 2. Important nitrogenous products of amino acid metabolism in animals
(Sung Nor Kim et al., 2006)

Precursors	Products	Functions
Arginine	NO	Vasodilator; neurotransmitter, signaling molecule; angiogenesis; cell metabolism; apoptosis (programmed cell death); immune response
	Agmatine	Signaling molecule; inhibitor of NO synthase and ornithine decarboxylase; brain and renal functions
Cysteine	Taurine	Antioxidant; muscle contraction; bile acid conjugates; retinal function
Glutamate	γ-Aminobutyrate	Neurotransmitter; inhibitor of glutamatergic, serotonin and NEPN activities
Glutamine	Glucosamine	Glycoprotein and ganglioside formation; inhibitor of NO synthesis
	Ammonia	Renal regulation of acid-base balance; synthesis of carbamoylphosphate glutamate and glutamine
	Serine	One-carbon unit metabolism; ceramide and phosphatidylserine formation
Glycine	Heme	Heomoproteins (e.g. hemoglobin, myoglobin, catalase, and cytochrom C); roduction of carbon monoxide (CO, a signaling molecule)
	Histamine	Allergic reaction; vsodilator; gastric acid and central acetylcholine secretion
Hi.tidine	Homocysteine	Oxidant; inhibitor of NO synthesis; risk factor for cardiovascular disease
Methionine	Betaine	Methylation of homocysteine to methionine; one-carbon unit metabolism
	Choline	Synthesis of betaine, acetylcholine (neurotransmitter and vasodilator) and Phosphatidylcholine
	Cysteine	An important sulfur-containing amino acid; formation of disulfide bonds
	DCSAM	Methylation of proteins and DNA; polyamine synthesis; gene expression
	Tyrosine	A versatile aromatic amino acid containing a hydroxyl group
Phenylalanine	H_2O_2	Killing pathogens; intestinal integrity; a signaling molecule; immunity
Proline	P5C	Cellular redox state; DNA synthesis; cell proliferation; ornithine formation; bridging the urea cycle with Krebs cycle; gene expression; tumor growth
	Glycine	Antioxidant; bile acid conjugates; neurotransmitter; immunomodulator; one-carbon unit metabolism

Precursors	Products	Functions
Serine	Serotonin	Neurotransmitter; smooth muscle contraction, hemostasis; immunity
Tryptophan	Melatonin	Circadian and circannual rhythms, free radical scavenger; antioxidant
	Anthranilic acid	Inhibiting production of proinflammtory T-helper-1 cytokines; preventing autoimmune neuroinflammation; enhancing immunity
Tyrosine	Dopamine	Neurotransmitter; apoptosis; lymphatic constriction; control of behaviour
	EPN & NEPN	Neurotransmitters; smooth muscle contraction; CAMP production, glycogen and energy metabolism
	Melanin	Dark-color pigment; free radical scavenger; chelator of metals
	T_3 and T_4	Gene expression; tissue differentiation & development; cell metabolism
Arginine and Methionine	Polyamines	Gene expression, DNA and protein synthesis, ion channel function; apoptosis, signal transduction; antioxidants; cell function, proliferation & differentiation; spermatogenesis; viability of sperm cells
Glutamine, Asparagine and Glycine	Nucleic acids	Coding for genetic information; gene expression, cell cycle and function; protein and uric acid synthesis
Glutamine and Tryptophan	NAD(P)	Coenzymes for oxidoreductases; substrate of poly(ADP-ribose) polymerase
Arginine, Proline or Glutamine	Ornithine	Glutamate, glutamine and polyamine synthesis, mitochondrial integrity
Arginine, Methionine and Glycine	Creatine	Energy metabolism in muscle and nerve; antioxidant; antiviral; antitumor
Cysteine, Glutamine and Glycine	Glutathione	Free radical scanvenger; antioxidant; formation of leukotrienes, mercapturate, glutathionylspermidine, glutathione-NO adduct and gluthionylproteins; signal transduction; gene expression; apoptosis; spermatogenesis; sperm maturation; cellular redox state; immunity
Glutamine, Glutamate and Proline	Citrulline	Free radical scavenger, arginine synthesis; urea cycle
Lysine, Methionine and Serine	Carnitine	Transport of long-chain fatty acids into mitochondria for oxidation, storage of energy as acetylcarnitine

DCSAM = Decarboxylated S-adenosylmethionine; EPN; Epinephrine; NEPN = Norepinephrine; P5C = Pyrroline-5-carboxylate; T3 = Triiodothyronine; T4 = Thyroxine

Secretion of hormones and regulation of intermediary metabolism

Hormone secretion: Many polypeptide and low molecular-weight hormones are synthesized from specific amino acids (Table 2). For example, tyrosine (or phenylalanine) is the precursor for the synthesis of epinephrine, norepinephrine, and thyroid hormones. Amino acids are also potent regulators of secretion of hormones from endocrine cells (Newsholme et al., 2005). Arginine stimulates the secretion of insulin, growth hormone, prolactin, glucagon, and placental lactogen (Flynn et al., 2002). Glutamine and leucine also increase insulin release from the pancreatic β-cells. Interestingly, dietary supplementation with glutamine reduces the production of glucocorticoids in weanling pigs via yet an unkown mechanism (Zhou et al., 2006). These amino acids may partly mediate the effect of dietary protein on the metabolism of protein, lipids and glucose, fertility, growth and production performance, and health of animals.

Regulation of intermediary metabolism

In addition to their effect on plasma levels of hormone, amino acids directly participate in the regulation of intermediary metabolism and thus the efficiency of utilization of dietary nutrients.

1. Arginine is an allosteric activator of N-acetylglutamate synthase, a mitochondrial enzyme that uses glutamate and acetyl-CoA as substrates. Thus, arginine and glutamate maintain the urea cycle in an active state.

2. Alanine inhibits pyruvate kinase, thereby regulating gluconeogenesis and glycolysis to ensure net glucose production by hepatocytes during periods of food deprivation.

3. Glutamate and aspartate mediate the transfer of reducing equivalents across the mitochondrial membrane and thus regulate glycolysis and cellular redox state.

4. Arginine and phenylalanine up-regulates expression of GTP cyclohydrolase-I expression and activity, thereby increasing the availability of tetrahydrobiopterin for NO synthesis from arginine and for the hydroxylation of aromatic amino acids. The arginine-NO pathway can also be modulated by a number of other amino acids (including taurine, lysine, glutamate, and homocysteine) to exert their physiological and pathological effects.

5. Arginine or its metabolites up-regulate expression of key proteins and enzymes (e.g., AMP-activated protein kinase and peroxisome proliferators-activated receptor ? coactivator-1?) responsible for mitochondrial biogenesis and substrate oxidation, thereby reducing excess fat mass in obese animals.

6. Methionine, glycine, and serine play an important role in one-carbon metabolism and, thus, the methylation of proteins and DNA, thereby regulating gene expression and protein activity (Stead et al., 2006). Finally, coordination of amino acids metabolism among the liver, skeletal muscle, intestine, and immune cells maximizes glutamine availability for renal ammoniagenesis and therefore the regulation of acid-base balance in animals.

Immune functions
Glutamine, arginine, and cysteine

Protein deficiency has long been known to impair immune functions and increases the susceptibility to disease in animals. However, the underlying cellular and molecular mechanisms have begun to unfold from 1990. A dietary deficiency of protein reduces the availability of most amino acids in plasma, particularly glutamine, arginine, tryptophan, and cysteine. The roles of glutamine, arginine, and cysteine in enhancing the immune function have been well established.

Glutamine is a major fuel for lymphocytes and is essential for their proliferation and function. This amino acid also enhances the phagocytic activity of macrophages, cytokine production by T-lymphocytes, and antibody generation by B-lymphocytes. The availability of cysteine is a major factor that limits the synthesis of glutathione, the most abundant low-molecular weight thiol and a key antioxidant. Thus, dietary supplementation with N-acetylcysteine (a stable precursor of cysteine) is highly effective in enhancing immune functions under various disease states. A large amount of NO synthesized from the arginine by inducible NO synthase is cytotoxic to pathogenic microorganisms and virus. Therefore, this free radical is a key mediator of the immune response in animals. Dietary supplementation with the arginine enhances the immune status of milk-fed piglets (Kim et al., 2004) and pregnant sows (Kim et al., 2006).

Tryptophan and proline

There has been growing interest in recent years in the role of tryptophan and proline in immune functions. There is a progressive decline in plasma levels of tryptophan in pigs with chronic lung inflammation (Melchior et al., 2003). Catabolism of tryptophan appears to be critical for the functions of both macrophages and lymphocytes. Oral administration of tryptophan has been reported to enhance the innate immune response (Esteban et al., 2004). Interestingly, anthranilic acid (a metabolite of tryptophan via the indoleamine 2, 3 dioxygenase pathway) inhibits the production of proinflammatory T-helper-1 cytokines and prevents autoimmune neuroinflammation (Platten et al., 2005). Most recently, Ha et al. (2005) discovered that a lack of proline catabolism via proline oxidase due to a deficiency of the intestinal proline oxidase impairs gut immunity. The major mediator derived from proline oxidation is H2O2, which is cytotoxic to pathogenic bacteria and is also a signaling molecule. It can be conjectured that a high activity of proline oxidase in the porcine placenta (Wu et al., 2005) and the piglet small-intestine (Wu, 1997) may play a crucial role in protecting these organs from infections during the critical periods of fetal and neonatal development.

Functional fatty acids

One of the most interesting findings in recent lipid nutrition research is the role of omega-3 fatty acids (ω3 FA) in both humans and animals. Their potential benefits in improving health and preventing certain diseases have now been widely recognized. Compared to omega-6 fatty acids (ω6 FA), smaller amounts of ω3 FA are found in the typical grain-based animal feeds. Studies with livestock indicated that dietary supplementation with ω3 FA holds great promise in improving the productive performance of sows.

Nutritional characteristics of omega-3 and 6 fatty acids

Omega 3 FA and ω6 FA are polyunsaturated fatty acids (PUFA) and can be distinguished from each other based on the location of the first double bond from the methyl end. Among PUFA, α-linolenic acid (ALA; 18:3 n-3) and linoleic acid (LA; 18:2 n-6) are classified as nutritionally essential fatty acids (EFA) because mammals cannot synthesize them. ALA and LA are the precursors of other PUFA that are both nutritionally and physiologically important. ALA can be converted to EPA (20:5 n-3, also known as timnodonic acid) and DHA (22:6 n-3, also known as cervonic acid), whereas LA can be converted to arachidonic acid (ARA; 20:4 n-6) (Figure 1). Thus, animals can obtain DHA and EPA either directly from the diet or by *de novo* synthesis from dietary ALA.

LA and ALA can be obtained from grains and vegetable oils, whereas EPA and DHA are predominantly found in marine products. Both ω3 FA and ω6 FA are metabolically and functionally distinct, are not interchangeable, and may have opposing physiological functions. These PUFA give rise to different types of eicosanoids, which play important roles in the regulation of inflammatory reactions, blood pressure, and platelet aggregation. In addition, ω3 FA and ω6 FA are essential constituents of plasma membranes in the brain, central nervous system, and vascular systems, making them critical components during rapid tissue formation (i.e. gestation and foetal growth).

Omega-3 fatty acid in sow diets

Maternal omega-3 fatty acid intake and transfer to progeny: Several studies have shown that dietary fatty acid composition of sow affects the fatty acid content of its milk and its nursing piglets.

Feeding sows with diets containing cod liver oil from 107 d of gestation to weaning increased EPA and DHA contents in colostrum and milk (Taugbol et al. (1993). However, no differences were observed in piglet weight gain and overall morbidity. Dietary supplementation with fish oil to sows between d 4 before parturition and d 15 postpartum (Arbuckle and Innis (1993) increased milk DHA and EPA contents but had no effect on ARA. Other studies have also shown that maternal supplementation of ω3 FA reduced ARA content in the liver, but not in the brain of new-born piglets (Rooke et al., 2001c). Further, Bazinet et al. (2003) reported that high maternal intake of ALA (flax seed oil) increased both ALA and DHA content in sow's milk and neonatal tissues (including the brain, liver, and carcass). Similarly, Rooke et al. (1998) found that feeding sows with diets containing tuna oil during late gestation and during the first week of lactation increased ω3 FA but reduced ω6 FA content in new-born piglets. Omega 3 FA concentrations in colostrum and milk were also increased in response to the maternal dietary supplementation with tuna oil (Rooke et al., 1998).

Available evidence suggests that dietary supplementation with ω3 FA and ω6 FA is effective in increasing their availability in the porcine conceptus.

Rooke et al. (1999; 2000) noted an increase in plasma DHA in fetal umbilical cord at birth when sows were fed diets containing tuna oil. These results suggest that PUFA can cross the placenta into the fetal circulation. Also, other researchers (Brazle et al., 2005; Brazle et al., 2006) reported a marked increase in ?3 FA concentrations in the porcine conceptus during early gestation when maternal diets were supplemented with ω3 FA. Further, Fritsche et al. (1993) have demonstrated that inclusion of fish oil in sow's diets resulted in elevated levels of ω3 FA in milk as well as both maternal and neonatal plasma.

In contrast, some studies suggested that there was little or no transfer of fatty acids across the porcine placenta during late gestation (Thulin et al., 1989; Ramsay et al., 1991). However, this conclusion is solely based on the measurement of fatty

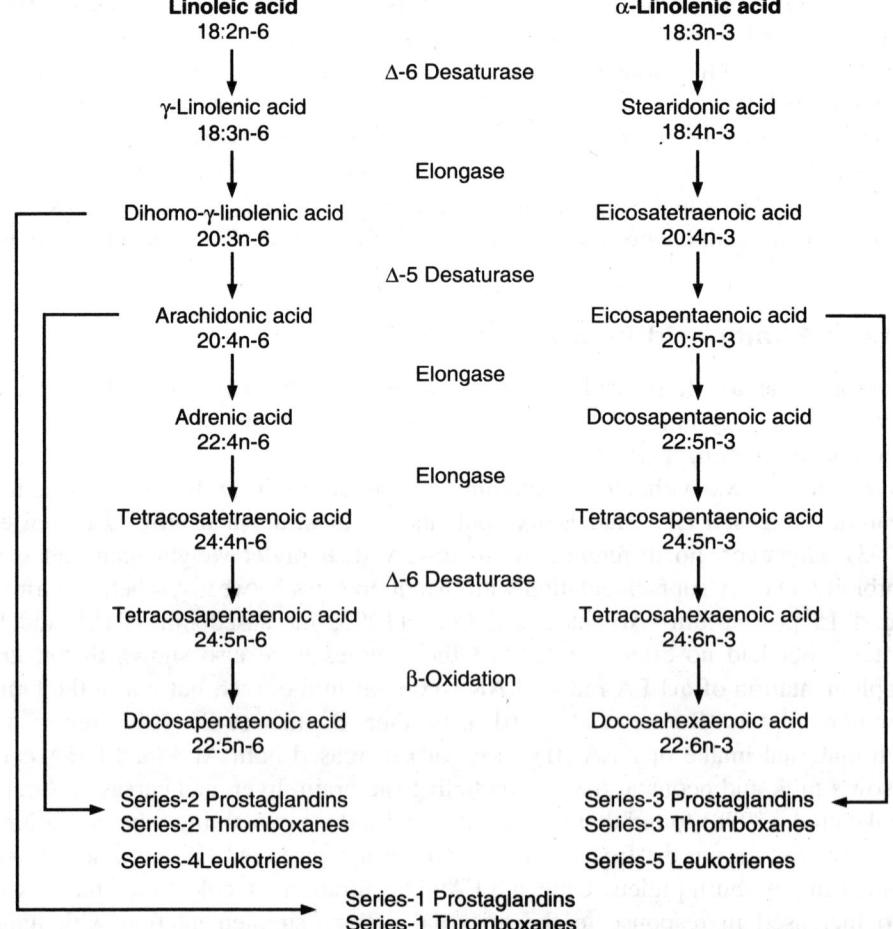

Figure1. Biosynthesis of long-chain polyunsaturated fatty acids and eicosanoids from essential fatty acids (Modified from Uauy and Castillo, 2003)

acid concentrations in plasma, which depends not only the entry of $\omega 3$ FA or $\omega 6$ FA into the umbilical vein but also their utilization and oxidation by the fetus. Rooke et al. (1998; 2000) have demonstrated the placental transfer of $\omega 3$ FA during late gestation in pigs and suggested that either the net transfer is small or there is a selective transfer of some EFA (i.e. DHA). Indeed, selective transfer of DHA from mother to fetus has been demonstrated by other investigators, such that maternal dietary intake of DHA can greatly influence DHA availability in the developing fetus (Innis and Elias, 2003).

Omega-3 fatty acids and eicosanoid production

As mentioned earlier, both ARA and EPA are precursors of eicosanoids (such as prostaglandins, thromboxanes, and leukotrienes), which play critical roles in inflammatory and immune responses (Figure 1). However, unlike those synthesized from EPA, eicosanoids derived from ARA are generally pro-inflammatory, potent platelet aggregators, and vasoconstrictors. Furthermore, competition occurs between ARA and EPA for eicosanoid synthesis at the cyclooxygenase and lipoxygenase levels (Simopoulos, 1991). Thus, the balance between $\omega 3$ FA and $\omega 6$ FA may determine the type of eicosanoids produced, and therefore the response of animals to eicosanoid synthesis.

Substituting menhaden fish oil for lard as a source of fat in sow's diets during late gestation and lactation substantially increased concentrations of $\omega 3$ FA (i.e. EPA) in immune cells of nursing pigs and reduced *in vitro* eicosanoid release by alveolar macrophages. Studies with humans and animals have also demonstrated that $\omega 3$ FA and $\omega 6$ FA modulate the production of pro-inflammatory cytokines. Compelling evidence shows highly beneficial effects of $\omega 3$ FA in improving the host immunity under a number of inflammatory conditions. Thus, the ability of EPA to competitively inhibit eicosanoid synthesis from ARA is an important factor for its anti-inflammatory effects. Studies have also suggested that $\omega 3$ FA intake may improve resistance to infectious disease by altering cytokine and/or eicosanoid synthesis. Finally, some findings suggest that $\omega 3$ FA delays the onset of parturition, thereby increasing gestation length in sows, possibly by reducing intrauterine production of prostaglandins such as $PGF_{2\alpha}$, an eicosanoid synthesized from ARA.

Omega-3 fatty acids and litter size

The original work of Webel et al. (2003) has led to growing interest in the role of w3 FA in improving pregnancy outcome in pigs. These researchers found that the inclusion of w3 FA in sow's diets during lactation and post-weaning period increased the litter size by 0.6 piglet in comparison with the control group. Most recently, Spencer et al. (2004) reported a similar increase in litter size when sows were fed diets supplemented with $\omega 3$ FA between d 30 prior to breeding and farrowing. The increase in litter size was associated with a decrease in the piglet birth weight (1.42 vs. 1.37 kg/pig; p<0.05; compared to the control group), without changes in the distribution of low-birth-weight piglets. Consistent with this finding, Rooke et al. (2001c) reported that sows fed diets supplemented with salmon oil produced lighter pigs at birth but these piglets had a higher pre-weaning survival rate than the control group. Additionally, a mechanism for the beneficial effect of supplementation with 03FA to sow's diets involves an increase in embryonic survival (Webel et al., 2003).

Omega-3 fatty acids and behavioural response

With the high $\omega3$ FA content of the brain, it is likely that these fatty acids have significant impacts on brain development and function and thus behaviour. DHA is especially important for the development and proper functioning of brain in neonates (Crawford, 2000). Rooke et al. (2001b) found that piglets from sows fed diets containing tuna oil had a more active suckling behaviour immediately after birth, which contributes to their enhanced growth during the entire lactation period. Further, fat composition in the diet had significant effects on piglet behaviour, which may result from a change in the metabolism of dopamines and other neurotransmitters (Delion et al., 1994; Zimmer et al., 2000). In support of this notion, piglets fed milk formula containing ALA and DHA had higher serotonin concentrations than piglets fed formula without ALA and DHA (Owens and Innis, 1998). Serotonin has also been implicated in a variety of neural functions, including feeding, sleep, and cognition (McEntee and Crook, 1991). However, further investigations are required to determine positive behavioural changes of piglets in response to maternal $\omega3$ FA supplementation.

Conclusion

Amino acids and fatty acids display remarkable metabolic and regulatory versatility. They serve as essential precursors for the synthesis of a variety of molecules with enormous importance, and also regulate metabolic pathways and processes vital to the health, growth, development, reproduction, and functional integrity of animals. Currently amino acids are provided for optimum protein synthesis. However, in view of the crucial regulatory roles of functional amino acids, their supplementation to the sow's diet can be highly beneficial for enhancing production performance.

Typical grain-based sow's diets contain low levels of $\omega3$ FA and high levels of w6 FA. This leads to a deficiency of $\omega3$ FA and an imbalance in the proportions of these EFA and their derivatives, thus negatively impacting piglet survival and immune functions. These findings underline the practical importance of an adequate supply and balance of EFA during gestation, lactation and piglet growth. Further research is required to provide accurate recommendations for formulating sow's diets with optimal amounts of functional amino acids and fatty acids.

6

Growth Potential of PIGS-Strategies for Feeding the Piglet

Growth potential of pigs

Dr. Campbell of Bunge Meat Industries in Australia (Pig International Dec 1997; P:15) has reported that an average weight gain of 700 g per day from birth to slaughter is possible with the latest production systems, which means a 100 kg pig can be produced in 143 days. In Table 1, he summarized the potential growth rate at each stage from a continuous flow type of production system, together with performance levels recorded and some realistic targets.

Table 1: Potential, commercial and realistic weights for age at different stages of production

Age (Days)	Potential		Commercial		Realistic target	
	Weight (kg)	Growth (g/d)	Weight (kg)	Growth (g/d)	Weight (kg)	Growth (g/d)
0	1.5		1.5		1.5	
25	10.2	350	7.5	240	7.0	360
45	22.7	625	13.0	275	14.2	360
65	38.7	800	25.0	600	27.8	680
110	87.7	1000	56.5	700	63.8	800
145	122.7	1000	86.3	850	95.3	950
Growth rate from birth		835		584		658

The gap between potential growth rate and that expressed commercially tends to decline with age and weight. Evidently biggest gap separating the pigs' inherent potential from the commercial growth data occur during 25 days and 45 days of age.

Obviously there are many reasons for this underperformance (gap between on-farm results and the genetic potential of the animal) and the nutritionists must consider how they can access more of the existing genetic potential through improved feeding. In fact the work of breeders and of nutritionists shows that lifetime lean tissue growth rates are determined by nutrition, virtually from the moment the pig is born. An insufficient energy intake during the early stages of life is one of the main factors limiting later growth performance.

Phase feeding helps the piglets to make rapid gains during early age.

Phase feeding certainly should be considered for the nutritional management of the weaned piglet (weaned at 3 weeks of age) so that the formulation meets the specific needs of the animal at that time. Between weaning and 15 weeks old, using as many as 5 diets can often be justified on the basis of cost-effectiveness and improved growth rate. For example, pig's requirement for amino acids changes very rapidly throughout the time from 63 to 110 days old. In fact the dietary lysine levels needed for near - maximal growth performance between 63-84 days of age actually depress the rate of weight gain in the 85-112 days period.

Breeders estimate that the lean tissue growth rate of genetically improved pigs is rising at a rate of between 1-2% per year. Proportionately the quantity of energy, protein, lysine, etc. to achieve its lean growth potential also rises. But the pig's total feed intake has not increased significantly in the last few years. It is a challenge to the nutritionists to use feeds with a higher nutrient density in order to match their escalating needs.

Ideal Protein Concept

Dietary protein has been supplied mainly for the lean growth of animals. To enhance lean growth and to spare costly protein with the advent of ideal amino acid profile, researchers have focused on the relationship between lean growth and amino acids rather than protein.

The benefit of an ideal protein concept in diet formulation is to set all essential amino acid (EAA) requirements on the basis of lysine. Ideal protein concept, therefore, is a statement of requirements in a proportional relationship to the requirement for lysine. Thus, the dietary percentage of lysine is set and the concentration of other EAAs is determined as a percentage of the lysine concentration according to the ideal amino acid balance (Owen et al., 1996). Amino acid requirements relative to lysine for various growth stages of pigs (NRC, 1998) are presented in Table-2. With the advent of segregated early weaning (SEW; weaning at 3 weeks age), there has been marked changes in amino acid nutrition for very young pigs (Tables 3 and 4).

Lysine Requirements

Daily lysine requirement of a growing pig has two components-requirement for body maintenance and that for protein accretion. Lysine is needed in a much larger proportion for the synthesis of new (lean) tissue than for maintenance. Dietary lysine requirements reduce as live weight of the pig increases reflecting the pattern of growth - earlier growth is more of lean tissue while later it is more of fat. The decline has been

Table 2: Ideal amino acid patterns for various growth stages of pigs (NRC 1998)

1	Lys	Arg	His	Trp	Ile	Leu	Val	Phe + Tyr	Met + Cys	Thr	Lys requi -rement (% to diet)
3-5	100	39	32	18	55	100	69	94 (60)	57 (27)	65	1.50
5-10	100	40	32	18	54	98	68	93 (59)	56 (26)	64	1.35
10-20	100	40	31	18	55	97	69	92 (59)	57 (26)	64	1.15
20-50	100	39	32	18	54	95	67	92 (58)	57 (26)	64	0.95
50-80	100	36	32	18	56	95	69	93 (59)	59 (27)	68	0.75
80-120	100	32	32	18	55	90	67	92 (57)	58 (27)	68	0.60

reported to vary between 0.05 - 0.12 percentage units as live weight rose from 23 kg to 27 kg while a weight increase from 64 kg to 68 kg would lower the requirement by 0.01 - 0.02 percentage points. Lysine requirement is influenced by the sex (gilt, board, barrow), genetics, health, season of the year and stocking density. As genetically lean pigs have higher lysine requirement, they do have greater *threonine* requirement.

Table 3: Recommended lysine levels for SEW Pigs

Body weight (kg)	Total lysine %	Digestible lysine, %
< 5	1.7–1.8	1.4–1.5
5 - 7	1.5–1.6	1.25–1.35
7 - 11	1.34–1.45	1.10–1.20
11 - 13	1.25–1.35	1.05–1.15

Table 4: Recommended level of amino acids relative to lysine for SEW Pigs

Amino acids	Ratio
Lysine	100
Isoleucine	60
Methionine	27.5
Met + Cys	55
Threonine	65
Tryptophan	18

Strategies for feeding the piglet

Aforementioned are the genetic potential of the modern pig and its nutrient requirements, which are to be translated into diets to exploit the inherent potential. Strategic feeding of the piglet should start even before it is born.

Feeding of fat to the pregnant sow

Studies in the literature indicate the importance of adding fat to sow diets to improve piglet survival. The optimum level appears to be between 7.5 and 15% to the sow's diet from day 100 of pregnancy to parturition (114 days). It was suggested that at least 1 kg of fat should be fed to the sow before furrowing. Feeding a diet with 10% added fat (using vegetable oil is easy for handling. But animal fats such as tallow are usually less expensive) for seven days before farrowing would achieve this goal.

Once it farrows it is not uncommon for her to support a gain in the live weight of her litter of 2.5 kg/d during the first three weeks of lactation. Over the last 40 years the age at weaning of piglets has been steadily reduced from eight to three weeks of age. It is common practice to offer feed to piglets while they are still with their dam in an area separated from the dam by a selective barrier, usually a low rail, known as the 'creep' area.

Enzyme secretary pattern in the piglet

Suckling baby pig secretes large amounts of pancreatic lipase, lactase, and several proteolytic enzymes. Lactase activity is high from birth to 25 days of age, while maltase and sucrase activity are poorly developed. Starch digestion is difficult for the baby pig because the amylolytic enzyme activity of the pancreas is trivial up to about 20 days of age. Hence the newborn pig is not physiologically prepared to utilize many of the feed ingredients that are economically attractive i.e. cereal-soya diets compared to milk products. Poor upper gastrointestinal tract digestion of carbohydrates in piglets may contribute to increased fermentation in the large intestine and subsequently to osmotic upset and diarrhoea.

Favourable ingredients for piglets

Piglets are fed starter diets at 3 weeks of weaning age. Feed ingredients for such piglets must be highly digestible and free of allergenic compounds or other nutritional inhibitors. These include skimmed milk powder, whey powder, allergen-free soyprotein, fish meal, protein products processed from blood such as spray-dried plasma and spray-dried whole blood.

Spray-dried whole blood has darker colour due to the high iron content in the red blood cells. This contributes darker colour to faeces. It can be fed up to 5% of a diet. Spray-dried (Blood) plasma is now fed to an estimated 30-35% of the world's pigs at an early stage of their life. In the United States it is in every feed for the first 7 days after weaning, while in Europe it is used primarily up to 14 days and from 14 days to 65 days little is used. Dried plasma has 100 different types of proteins, though albumin and immunoglobulins are the predominant ones. The product is available as spray dried powder and granulated plasma and the latter is specifically processed to ensure a uniformly high gamma-globulin inclusion.

Maize is an excellent source of energy for baby pigs that gives the nutritionlist few problems when formulating starter diets for piglets at 3 weeks of weaning. Medium grinding (600 µ particle size) is preferred for better nutrient utilization and to avoid health problems (gastric ulcer) and feeder bridging (in storage bins) when diets are fed in meal form. Alternative cereals are good quality wheat, low-tannin sorghum, naked oats, oat groats or white rice. Barley is unsuitable because of high beta-glucan content while rye and triticale are unsuitable because of higher pentosan concentration. Tallow or vegetable oil is also included at about 3% level.

Exogenous enzyme supplementation certainly makes several feedstuffs suitable for feeding the piglets. Refer the chapter on enzyme supplementation for further details. Similarly other feed additives are needed to be supplemented to improve nutritive efficiency.

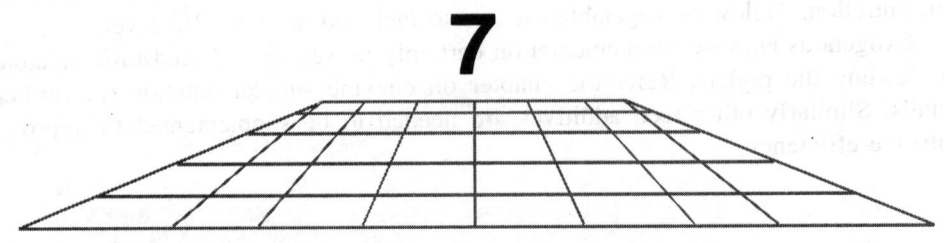

7

Environmental Sustainability and Social Desirability Issues in Pig Feeding

INTRODUCTION

The use of pigs as converters, rather than scavengers, to transform farm left-over or kitchen swill to favourable animal products not only provides organic fertilizer for crops, but is also beneficial for nutrient management. Pigs are traditionally kept in small herds. Pig rearing has rapidly industrialized (in Europe and in Americas) and changed from extensive to intensive due to greater demands for animal-derived food consumption. The increase in real incomes of consumers and in urbanization has led pork to be produced in intensive systems, thus lowering the cost of production through economies of scale. Pig husbandry has evolved into commercial pork production through the adoption of modern technologies of animal science, and knowledge of finance and commerce, to meet the consumption needs of urban consumers with high disposable incomes.

Fallout of intensive / industrial systems of pig production

- The concentration of large quantities of pig manure in small areas is hazardous to the environment. This problem is aggravated by the expansion of metropolitan areas, and the placing of production near large cities to allow good market access.
- High densities of animals in intensive production systems also impose a constant health threat for both animals and humans. Example is recent occurrence of swine influenza epidemic.
- The use of growth promoters and preventive medicines for higher efficiencies, such as in-feed antibiotics, also induces microbial resistance, and consequently affects human therapeutics through horizontal gene transfer or survival niche movement.

- Consumers are questioning the ethics of raising animals in intensive systems, and are increasingly willing to pay more for similar products with ethical as well as ecological values.

Environmental issues, animal welfare and safety are particularly important in the knowledge-based economy, and have moved animal production beyond the singular goal of providing animal products and maximizing profit (Yang, 2006). Therefore, feeding pigs is not only a consideration of economic traits such as growth rate, lean percent, feed efficiency and litter size, but also environmental traits (e.g. less excretion of N and P) and welfare traits (e.g. little stereotypies, maternity, fitness and disease resistance). Producers seeking a fair income for their current work and investment are facing challenges, because feeding pigs should not only be environmental friendly and biologically safe, but also be accommodate social ethics. These are achievable by feeding pigs in precision animal nutrition mode (Reddy, 2011).

Environmental Sustainability
Life cycle assessment

Feeding pigs involves two major sustainability issues: **eutrophication or acidification**, and **global warming or energy consumption**. The environmental impact of pig production can be described on the basis of life cycle assessment (Yang, 2006). A comprehensive set of programmmes focusing on sustainable pig production should employ the life cycle assessment (LCA) to promote production patterns. The fundamental principle of the LCA is to follow the product through its entire life cycle from extraction of raw materials to final disposal or recycling. LCA is a tool to assess the environmental impacts of product systems and services, accounting for the emissions and resource usage during the production, distribution, use and disposal of a product (ISO 14043, 2000). It also includes methods for grouping different emission based on the extent of the environment impact caused when released.

The environmental impact of pig production in a life cycle perspective has previously been described (Basset-Mens and van der Werf, 2005). High nitrogen utilization is generally agreed to be the most important measure for reducing hazards of acidification and eutrophication in a pig production system. The European Union's Nitrate Directive (91/676/EC), which permits a maximum of 170 kg N/ha to be applied to cultivated land each year to keep the N concentration of surface water below 50 mg nitrate/L, indicate that a manure surplus in N is considered as a threat to water quality. Reducing N loss from the farm must begin with proper animal feeding and management to reduce N excretion. A low-protein pig diet has been recommended to improve the environmental performance, and can be achieved by including a certain amount of synthetic amino acids.

Several general strategies of nutrition and feed management besides amino acid supplementation help to reduce nutrient excretions and odours from pig manure. Avoiding excessive amount of dietary P, balancing diets on the basis of available P, and use of phytase, are practical for reducing the level of P in manure. Use of reduced or organic forms of Cu, Zn, Fe and Mg decrease the excretion of these minerals in manure. Maintaining the proper acid-base balance and buffering in the diet can significantly lower odourous compounds. Additionally, adding acidifying Ca salts to the diet rather than CaCO3 could lower urinary pH, and consequently decrease ammonia emission by 26 to 53% (Sutton and Richert, 2004).

High electrical conductivity in effluents: Effluent from pig farms contains large quantities of electrolytes that create additional difficulties. A high electrical conductivity ranges from 2,000 to 6,000 µs/cm, depending on the amount of flush water used in cleaning, was recorded from a family-based small production unit. This level far exceeds the maximum limit of 750 µs/cm, 25oC for crop irrigation. Two periods of irrigation with maximum conductivity allowance generally build up a soil limit of 4,000 µs/cm, which can retard crop growth (Yu et al., 2005). Channeling the pig farm effluent into irrigation system is therefore detrimental to crop field, and paddy may be the most vulnerable crop due to continuous wetting.

Attempts to minimize electrolyte content in pig excreta to reduce conductivity by dietary modification have not been successful (Yang, 2006). Decreasing dietary protein content by 20%, and mineral supplements by 40%, (Ca, P and other salts) would reduce nutrients supply close to maintenance level of pigs. However, this level could only decrease waste water conductivity by 30%, leaving it well beyond the irrigation allowance (Yu et al., 2005). The conductivity is significant, especially in areas where pig feeding and crop growing often co-exist in integrated farming systems within a small close community. An independent watercourse is undoubtedly a burden if it becomes a prerequisite for feeding pigs.

Prebiotics lowered ammonia emission and reduced odour from pig farms.

Dietary carbohydrate (nonstarch polysaccharides, NSP) manipulations have recently attracted significant interest. They act as prebiotic (replace the in-feed antibiotics) and reduce environmental impact by lowering ammonia emission from manure. Including fermentable carbohydrates in diets has reduced the ratio between urinary N and faecal N, reducing emission because faecal N is less easily degraded to ammonia. Further, slurry pH is reduced, which decreases the potential for urease activity and ammonia volatilization (Nahm, 2003). A linear inverse relationship was found between the intake of dietary nonstarch polysaccharides (NSP) and ammonia emission.

Practically, the use of **raw potato starch** rather than maize starch in the diets of growing pigs lowered ammonia emission by 13% (Lenis and Jongbloed, 1999). Resistant potato starch also led to a dose-dependent reduction of **skatole** in the gut content from 134 µ/g dry matter (control) to 4.8 µ/g in the 40% group. Back fat skatole concentrations and belly fat skatole concentrations also followed the same trend (Losel and Claus, 2005) and significantly improved odour control from pig facilities (Willig et al., 2005). Furthermore, fermentable carbohydrates are showing considerable promise as dietary agents capable of increasing bacterial populations considered advantageous to host health or, alternatively, in suppressing those that may promote pathogenesis (Crittenden et al., 2002). Therefore, selecting appropriate carbohydrate sources is beneficial for both N emission and animal health, as well as for public health, because it reduces the use of in-feed antibiotics to manage colonic problems.

Actions to be taken on priority

If animal welfare is the major concern, then animals should have outdoor opportunities, be able to access to a paddock, and be raised in groups to avoid re-ranking and fighting. Strategic feeding is applied with diets diluted with forages to increase the feeding time. Mental enrichments by providing stimuli (e.g. bedding, toys) are also encouraging, and maternal traits are also important for selection and breeding. The management practice should be chosen to achieve high hygienic feed quality and a healthy physical environment for the herd. These animal welfare measures lead to the highest production cost because of larger space required to produce animals (Stern et al., 2005).

Eutrophication and acidification are important factors in a large production unit, so controlling the emission of N, P and other substances is the top priority. Thus, 'phase feeding of protein' and 'efficiently used slurry' should be adopted.

Social desirability

Removing antibiotics from pig rations is imperative to minimizing public health concerns associated with intensive pig farming.

Reducing antibiotic-resistance threats

Antibiotic use in intensive pig production has contributed to the development and persistence of multidrug-resistant bacteria. Subtherapeutic doses of in-feed antibiotics have been shown to select bacteria for resistance to high concentrations of antibiotics. Furthermore, antibiotic resistant genes have become highly mobile and their spread has occurred by all known bacterial gene transfer mechanism (Seveno et al., 2002). Multiple classes of antimicrobial compounds were detected in swine slurry lagoons, nearby surface soil, ground water samples, and pig farm dust (Compagnolo, 2002). The exposure pathway for transfer of resistant organisms from pigs to humans thus has become multiple. Inhalation of air at an intensive production site, and drinking nearby ground water has also become pathways. Removing antibiotics from pig rations is imperative to minimizing public health concerns associated with intensive pig farming.

Decreasing subtherapeutic antibiotic use is obligatory. However, producers have a difficult time finding consistently effective substitutes with acceptable costs. Producers have relied, since decades, on in-feed antibiotics to maintain health and growth of herds raised in sub-optimum sanitary environments. Consequently, many producers believe such antibiotics are a necessity. A sudden withdrawal of in-feed antibiotics typically causes an immediate production loss particularly in subtropical and tropical environments. A great loss in efficiency is primarily due to gastrointestinal problems in early weaned pigs even when supported by health management plans.

Alternative strategies of feeding to the use of in-feed subtherapeutic antibiotics

Numerous studies have shown that beneficial effects can be attained through diet modification, including supplementation with prebiotics, probiotics, synbiotics, minerals, organic acids, nutraceuticals and herbs. Feeding pigs with probiotics, or living microorganisms such as lactic acid producers (lactobacilli and bifidobacteria), streptococci, yeast and saccharomyces species, has shown that these microorganisms may be substituted for in-feed antibiotics in high-health nurseries (Kritas and Morrison, 2005).

Efficacy of probiotic feeding

Interest in probiotics has been fuelled in recent years by an increasing number of animal and human studies demonstrating the beneficial effects of probiotic cultures on numerous health conditions, including reduced atopic eczema symptoms and severity and duration of gastro-intestinal infections, particularly rotavirus infections (Doron and Gorbach, 2006). Probiotics may not be consistently successful. Well-known factors such as pH, temperature, and oxygen, variations in starter cultures, prebiotics, oxygen scavengers, water activity and sugar concentrations all dramatically influence probiotic survival during storage and feeding. Consequently, effectiveness can vary among farms, places and times and seasons.

Prebiotics

Inclusion of non-digestible or fermentable carbohydrates in pig diet is a practical approach for controlling ammonia and reducing nitrogen excretion as mentioned earlier. However, equally important, fermentable carbohydrates reportedly have significantly affected monogastric animals by encouraging proliferation of select groups of colonic microflora (Brown et al., 1997). A number of non-digestible oligosaccharides such as fructo-oligosaccharides (FOS) and galacto-oligosaccharides (GOS) are recognized as prebiotics. Prebiotics have been shown to selectively promote proliferation of bifidbacteria in the colon. Other prebiotics include gentio-oligasaccharides, isomalto-oligosaccharides, xilo-oligosaccharides, soybean oligosaccharides, in addition to lactulose, lactosucrose and inulin.

Prebiotics are fermented in the colon by endogenous bacteria and function as metabolic substrates with lactic and short-chain carboxylic acids as fermentation end-products. These metabolic products have emerged as important metabolic fuels for colonocytes and also have specific actions that increase normal colonic function (Wong et al., 2006). In early weaned pigs, supplementation with FOS and lactobacillus significantly improved weight gain and feed efficiency. When infected with Salmonella typhimurium, 2-day-old piglets did not develop diarrhoea upon feeding a diet containing 7.5 g/L FOS. The effectiveness of these prebiotics in monogastric animals depends on initial concentration of indigenous prebiotic species and intra-luminal pH (Duggan et al., 2002). Prebiotic oligosaccharides are currently utilized as functional food ingredients for human use and thus, their use in animal feed is cost-prohibitive.

Non-digestible carbohydrates, including resistant starches (RS) and fibre-like non-starch polysaccharides (NSP), which have also shown promise as prebiotics, beneficially modify intestinal function of weaning piglets and other monogastric animals. Resistant starches, named for their resistance to amylolysis, occur in many foods, e.g., whole grains and seeds, raw potatoes and green bananas.

Interest in RS as a prebiotic developed from the appreciation that consumption of large amounts of RS led to a time-dependent shift in faecal and large-bowel profiles of short-chain fatty acids (SCFA), primarily acetate, propionate and butyrate as end-products of colonic fermentation. Butyrate is the major energy source for colonocytes, whereas propionate is largely taken up by the liver and acetate enters peripheral circulation and metabolized by peripheral tissues. Specific SCFA may reduce risk of developing gastrointestinal disorders and it is likely that some or all of the effects of RS are through the actions of SCFA (Wong et al., 2006).

Interest is increasing regarding prebiotic potential: For example, in children with acute diarrhoea, adding amylase-resistant starch to glucose oral rehydration shortened diarrhoea duration compared with that achieved with a standard treatment (Raghupathy et al., 2006). In weaning piglets feeding a diet based on cooked rice (high in RS) supplemented with either animal or plant protein lowers the incidence and severity of diarrhoea with a consequent reduction in mortality (Montagne et al., 2004). This finding is of particular interest for pig producers in Far Eastern regions where low-cost locally grown rice is readily available (Yang, 2006). Suitably processed rice may be a useful feed option for pig herds in which post weaning colibacillosis is endemic and resistant strains of *E. coli* are present.

Synbiotics (probiotic with prebiotics)

Both FOS and RS raised faecal bifidobacteria numbers by roughly equal amounts when fed separately to pigs. In a human study, these increases are of a generally similar order to those reported for prebiotics such as FOS (Tuohy et al., 2001). When fed FOS and RS together, an increase exceeding individual increases suggests that they operate through different mechanisms. Furthermore, FOS and RS maintain colonies in pigs when probiotics supplementation ceases. Thus, when pigs were fed a control diet, faecal bifidobacteria numbers declined rapidly following probiotic withdrawal. However, this decline was much slower than that in those fed either FOS or RS. When FOS and RS were consumed together, no decline existed in faecal numbers (Brown et al., 1997). Maximal effectiveness may be achieved when preparations could be a mixture of FOS and RS, as these agents seem to have additive effects. Also, combining several probiotic bacteria will achieve stronger effects and this effect was the same as combing different prebiotics (oligosaccharides and RS).

Formulating synbiotics (probiotic with prebiotics): It can be likened to an art as different environments require different strategies. Availability or the source of RS, selection of probiotic strains, palatability considerations, manufacturing (pelleting), storage, etc., all render formulating a new generation of carbohydrate-manipulated diets complex. Moreover, fermentable carbohydrate in certain circumstances is detrimental rather than beneficial to pigs. For example, the incidence of pig dysentery can be largely reduced with a low NSP diet (Pluske et al., 1996, 1998). This reduction is simply because colonization by spirochaetes is highly related to dietary NSP concentrations, while incidence of dysentery was also reduced when diet included low RS (Durmic et al., 2002). Given the diverse nature of carbohydrate substrates and the SCFA patterns produced by their fermentation one should exercise caution in formulating synbiotics. Studies are also required to quantify the health benefits of prebiotics and synbiotics and their interactions in different feeding environments.

Importance of low gut pH

Luminal acidification as reflected by low faecal pH is a positive response to diet containing probiotics, prebiotics or synbiotics feeding. Additionally, maintaining intestinal luminal pH at approximately 4.5 is necessary to support proliferation of beneficial bacteria and exclude gut pathogenic. This low luminal pH is particularly important for weaning piglets as they suffer environmental and psychological stressors during transit and develop a high gastric pH when milk diet is replaced by dry feed and, thus, are at high risk of developing diarrhoea (Kim et al., 2005). Directly adding organic or inorganic acid to weaning diet or drinking water is an alternative approach to providing a favourable acid environment and it has been shown to improve feed efficiency and enhance growth performance in piglets (Franco et al., 2005). The practice of diet acidification by adding organic acids in excess of 2.7 kg per ton is becoming more popular as a method of reducing feed pH and controlling enteric pathogens in growing pigs.

However, at such high acid levels, palatability becomes a problem for weaning piglets. They are reluctant to eat dry feed and avoid acidified diets when given a choice. Adding 1.2% of potassium diformate to acidify piglet diet does not decrease feed intake or negatively affect piglet dietary preferences (Ettle et al., 2005). Notably, minimizing the addition of alkaline compounds such as calcium bicarbonate or protein from fish and milk products helps to optimize the benefits of diet acidification resulting from decreasing buffering effects (Hardly, 1999).

Botanicals and nutraceuticals

These have been proposed as alternatives to in-feed antibiotics, and, have generated promising results. Some herbs are valued for their medicinal properties, flavour or aroma. It has been suggested that many plant extracts and spices act as immuno-modulators when administered in low doses and show great promise as feed additives to replace current antimicrobial agents.

Antimicrobial peptides

Development of novel anti-infection agents to cope with the antibiotic-resistance threat is urgently needed in human and animal medicine. A source of compounds considered promising is the large number of gene-encoded antimicrobial peptides in animals and plants. These peptides are also termed bacteriocins and are constitutively produced or synthesized following infection or injury. Mammals have a large variety of antimicrobial peptides that function as natural innate barriers suppressing microbial infection, or, in some instances, they act as integral components in response to inflammation or microbial infection (Brogden et al., 2003). These peptides have broad-spectrum activity against a wide range of microorganisms, including Gram-positive and Gram-negative bacteria, protozoa, yeast, fungi and viruses. The so-called epithelial defensins that are produced by Toll receptors once the bacteria are recognized are actually comparable with antibiotics.

In pigs, more than a dozen distinct anti-microbial peptides have been identified, some of which include defensin. These peptides are naturally present in the gastrointestinal tract and act as a common mechanism of host defense (Zhang et al., 2000). High (20-200 ug/ml) concentrations of porcine ?-defensin are expressed in the dorsal tongue, and are synergistic with other porcine antimicrobial peptides against E. coli and multidrug-resistant salmonella. Some bacteriocins are in commercial production: for example, nisin is used to control bacterial spoilage in heat-processed, low-pH food worldwide; lactoferrin along with some probiotics is employed as health food supplement. However, use of purified or recombinant bacteriocins in animal rations is unlikely in the foreseeable future simply because these are not cost-effective. Immuno-modulation to enhance in vivo expression, synthesis and release of bacteriocins is likely a feasible approach.

Domesticated pigs are now used for pork production, as an animal model in biomedical research and for future xenotransplantation organs. Intensive pig production should adjust to conform to the social demands of environmentally and animal-friendly and to generate a high quality and safe product.

REFERENCES TO THE LITERATURE (PARTIAL LIST)

Blank, R., Sauer, W.C., Mosenthin, R., Zentek, J., Huang, S. and Roth, S. 2001. Effect of fumaric acid supplementation and dietary buffering capacity on the concentration of microbial metabolites in ileal digesta of young pigs. Canadian Journal of Animal Science 81: 345-353.

Bolduan, G., Jung, H., Schnabel, E. and Schneider, R. 1988. Recent advances in the nutrition of weaner pigs. Pig News and Information 9: 381-385.

Cranwell, P.D. 1985. The development of acid and pepsin secretory capacity in the pig. The effects of age and weaning. 1. Studies in anaesthetized pigs. British Journal of Nutrition 54: 305-320.

Cranwell, P.D. and Moughan, P.J. 1989. Biological limitations imposed by the digestive system to the growth performance of weaned pigs. In: Manipulating Pig Production 11, pp 140-159. Edited by J.L. Barnett and D.P. Hennessy. Werribee, Victoria, Australia: Australian Pig Science Association.

Giger-reverdin, S., duvaux-Ponter, C., Sauvant, D., Martin, O., Nunes do Prado, I. and Miller, R. 2002. Intrinsic buffering capacity of feedstuffs. Animal Feed Science and Technology 96: 83-102.

Jasaitis, D.K., Wohlt, J.E. and Evans, J.L. 1987. Influence of feed-ion content on buffering capacity of ruminant feedstuffs in vitro. Journal of Dairy Science 70: 1391-1403.

Kidder, D.E. and Manners M.J. 1978. Digestion in the Pig. Bristol: Scientechnica. Cited by Lawlor et al., (2005).

Lawlor, P.G., Lynch, P.B., Caffrey, P. J. and O' Doherty, J.V. 2002. Effect of pre- and post-weaning management on subsequent pig performance to slaughter and carcass quality. Animal Science 75: 245-256.

Lawlor, P.G., Lynch, P.B., Caffrey, P.J., O'Relly, J.J. and O'Connell, M.K. 2005. Measurements of the acid-binding capacity of ingredients used in pig diets. Irish Veterinary Journal 58: 477-452.

Thaela, M.J., Jensen, M.S., Pierzynowski, S.G., Jakob, S. and Jensen, B.B. 1998. Effect of lactic acid supplementation on pancreatic secretion in pigs after weaning. Journal of Animal and Feed Sciences 7 (supplement 1): 181-183.

Yen, J.T. 2001. Anatomy of the digestive system and nutritional physiology. In: Swine Nutrition. Second edition, pp 31-63. Edited by A.J. Lewis and L.L. Southern. Boca Raton: CRC Press.

Reddy, D.V. 2001. Growth potential of pigs - Strategies for feeding the piglet. Feed Trends, VII (5): 5-8.

Reddy, D.V., Elanchezhian, N. and Uma Maheswari, D. 2003. Final Report of Collaborative Research Work between Department of Animal Nutrition, RAGACOVAS, Pondicherry and Kemin Nutritional Technologies (India) Pvt Ltd on "To study the efficiency of different enzymes in broiler performance mainly on energy and protein utilization".

Reddy, D.V. 2006. Recent concepts in application of acid-binding capacity of feedstuffs in enhancing the livestock productivity Compendium for ICAR sponsored Summer School on "Recent advances in the feed additives for production of residue free livestock / poultry products" held at Department of Animal Nutrition, Madras Veterinary College (Tamil Nadu Veterinary and Animal Sciences University), Chennai, from 17-08-2006 to 06-09-2006, pp 57-63.

Reddy, D.V. (2011). Precision animal nutrition for pigs: A tool for economic and eco-friendly animal production. Textbook Chapter, the book is being edited by Dr. U.R. Mehra.

SECTION IV
Plant Feedstuffs and the associated Toxic & Antinutritional Factors and Mycotoxins

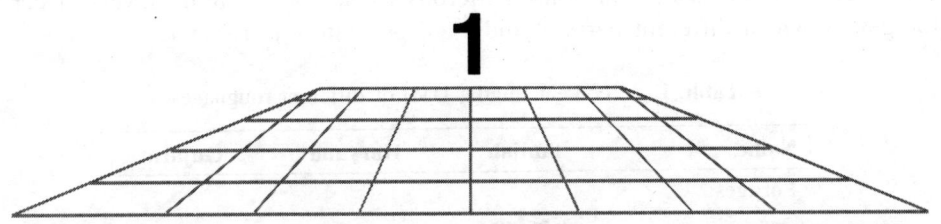

Toxic and Antinutritional Constituents present in Livestock Feedstuffs

Toxic Constituents in Plants

Selenium

Selenium (Se) is not an essential element for plant growth. But its concentration in animal feeds and fodders is important to animal and human health. The beneficial effects of selenium depend upon its concentration and other factors such as vitamin E, fatty acids, protein and sulphur. The minimum nutritional requirement of animals is about 0.05 to 0.10 ppm in dry fodder and feed. Dietary level of 0.1 to 1 ppm of Se seems to offer protection against some diseases like cancer and cardiovascular diseases. Toxic effects of Se may appear with exposure to dietary levels of more than 5 ppm.

Selenium content in soils

Concentration of Se in soils and forages varies considerably because of the origin of the soil material, climate and the vegetation. Selenium deficiency is generally found in intensively farmed lands that are heavily fertilized with commercial fertilizers. Selenium deficiency in domestic animals occurs over much larger areas of the world and these are more likely to occur when feeds are grown on acidic soils. Soils containing more than 0.5 ppm Se are considered to be toxic, because crop plants grown on such soils contain Se more than the maximum permissible limit for animal consumption (Dhillon et al., 1992).

Selenium content in plants

Plants growing on seleniferous soils may vary significantly in their ability to accumulate selenium. Most of the selenium in these plants occurs in water-soluble forms like selenate and several seleno-amino acids. Example: species of *Astragalus* plants. Ingestion of these plants at a rate providing about 10 to 15 mg Se / kg body weight can be lethal. However, these plants are generally not very palatable. Some grasses, small grains, etc. may contain 5 to 10 mg Se / kg. But these are more likely to be grazed because they are more palatable. Most of the plants contain less than 1 mg per kg when grown on nonseleniferous soils. The selenium levels of certain forages grown in different parts of India are presented in Table-1.

Table 1. Se content (mg/kg DM) of different roughages

Name	Punjab[1]	Haryana[2]	Gujarat[3]
Forages			
Oat	0.35-40.6	2.0	—
Sorghum	5.20-12.3	—	0.68
Lucerne	0.6-29.7	0.9-2.8	0.4-0.9
Sugarcane tops	7.3-14.5	—	—
Mustard tops	80.5-159.7	—	—
Natural grasses	Tr-0.36	—	0.23-0.45
Straws			
Rice straw	0.09-19.8	—	0.62
Wheat straw	0.13-57.5	—	0.59
Bajra straw	8.90	—	0.66

[1]Dhillon, K. S. and Dhillon, S. K., 1991. Intern. J. Environmental Studies, 37:15-24.
[2]Arora et al., 1975. Indian J. Dairy Sci., 28:249-253.
[3]Patel, C. A. and Mehta, B. V., 1970. Indian J. Agric. Sci., 40:389-399.

Effect of selenium in animals

Chronic selenosis has been reported in animals on daily consumption of diets containing 4 to 5 mg Se per kg and more (NAS-NRC, 1983). Rosenfeld and Beath (1964) observed two types of selenium toxicosis: acute (blind staggers) and chronic (alkali disease). The Degnala disease, which has been reported particularly from rice growing areas of Punjab, Haryana, Kerala and West Bengal, is believed to be associated with selenium intoxication. The rice straw contains 2.14 ppm Se as against 0.21 ppm in wheat straw. The research studies conducted in buffaloes at Punjab Agricultural University revealed that rice straw feeding in certain areas having alkaline soil with poor drainage resulted in degnala disease with typical symptoms of selenosis. The daily intake of selenium in the experimental group (n=6) was 8.56 mg. All the animals died within 7-8 weeks.

Selenium passes the placental and mammary barriers, so that the offsprings in seleniferous areas may be born with the typical deformed hooves or may develop them during the suckling period. The selenium concentrations in milk and eggs are particularly sensitive to high selenium intakes by cows and hens.

Symptoms of selenium poisoning

Symptoms, in general, are hooves become swollen and drop off in livestock, loss of mane and tail hair and sloughing of hooves in horses and loss of hair and nails in humans. The affected animals develop dark watery diarrhoea, fever and respiratory distress. Symptoms in case of chronic form include emaciation, dullness, and rough coat, loss of long hair at the base of tail or mane and soreness. In acute cases, the animal may become completely blind and develop paralysis, grinding of teeth, salivation and grunting. Death can occur due to respiratory failure.

The autopsy lesions were acute ulcerative and haemorrhagic, gangrenous syndrome, fibrous pericarditis, neurotic hepatitis along with the clinical symptoms of loosening hooves from the laminae followed by sloughing, necrotic skin, necrosis of tail and ear tips, swollen extremities, phimosis, alopecia, lameness and general debility.

Treatment

Treatment is done in three steps. First, remove the dietary source of selenium. Second, eliminate the selenium from the gut and body organs by using saline purgatives such as magnesium sulphate (@ 200-500 g / adult cattle) orally. Third, provide supportive therapy to alleviate the symptoms of selenosis; penta sulphate mixture (comprising magnesium sulphate, 100g; ferrous sulphate, 16.6g; copper sulphate, 2.4g; zinc sulphate, 7.5g and cobalt sulphate, 1.5g) has been reported to be effective in the treatment when administered at the rate of 15- 40g / day along with vitamin B_1 (10-20 mg / kg BW) and ascorbic acid; the affected animal should be fed on high protein diet.

Deficiency of selenium

Deficiency is becoming much more common than selenium toxicity because of its presence in glutathione peroxidase (GSH-PX), a selenoenzyme. Selenium is indispensable for protection of haemoglobin and the erythrocyte membrane. Erythrocyte glutathione peroxidase activity is an important indicator of the selenium status of livestock.

Oxalates

Oxalic acid is an organic acid occurring in a range of plant species commonly consumed by ruminants. It is toxicologically antagonistic to divalent cations such as calcium, magnesium, etc. The dietary intake of oxalic acid is dependant on the feeds and fodder ingested by the animals. For example, wheat straw contained negligible amount of total oxalate (0.17%) while paddy straw has 1.54%. This acid in ruminant diet has an adverse effect on calcium assimilation (Talapatra et al., 1948).

Oxalate poisoning in livestock occurs primarily from the ingestion of the oxalate-containing plants of the wood-sorrel family (Oxalidaceae) in Australia and of the chenopod or goosefoot family (Chenopodaceae) in North America (Greasewood plant) and in central Asia (Halogeton plant). The oxalate in the plants of Oxalis spp. and some species of Rumex exists chiefly as acid potassium oxalate while that in plants of Chenopodaceae, it exists chiefly as soluble sodium oxalate and insoluble calcium and magnesium oxalate. Grasses may have ammonium oxalate. Oxalic acid also forms on moist straw infected with the fungi, Aspergillus niger and A. flavus.

Oxalates present in certain tropical grasses such as those in the genera *Cenchrus*, *Setaria*, *Pennisetum*, *Digitaria* and *Brachiaria* may cause chronic renal failure in grazing ruminants due to formation of oxalate crystals and urinary calculi.

Oxalate content in green fodder

The oxalate content varied from 2.10 to 3.92% in both the hybrid napier cultivars (PBN-231, PBN-83).

Oxalate content %

Plant height (cm)	Oxalic acid Content %
144	2.78
155	2.70
182	2.62
210	2.52
230	2.52
242	2.41
290	2.30
300	1.93
330	1.03

Plant part	Bajra fodder	Napier grass	Bajra straw
Leaves	3.19	2.21	2.9
Stem	1.36	1.46	1.09
Whole plant (300 cm height)	1.93	1.60	1.88

In multi-cut grasses, total oxalate content increased linearly with the successive cut (Ahuja et al., 1998) and continuous feeding of such fodder could result in ruminal alkalosis. The oxalate content can be reduced by ensiling, since anaerobic microbes degrade oxalates to carbonates and finally to carbon dioxide which increase the silage pH. In single-cut grasses, total oxalates decreased with increasing age of plant (Middleton and Barry, 1978). Bajra fodder contained more amount of oxalate in the early stage than in the late stage of growth. Similarly leaves had higher amount of oxalate than the stem. Bajra fodder plant has 2.12% oxalic acid at preflowering stage. Soaking in water reduce the oxalic acid content (Parveen et al., 1988).

Ajaib Singh (2002) reported the seasonal variations in oxalate content of Napier Bajra Hybrid (PBN-233). The total oxalate contents increased linearly and varied from 2.20 to 3.60% during the successive cuts from April to August. The level of oxalate was significantly more in the month of June and July, which might be due to the peak growth in summer and rainy seasons. Roughly one third of the oxalates were found to be present in soluble form and the relative proportion of soluble and insoluble oxalate remained constant during this growth period. When the fodder was harvested at one and two metre heights, the total oxalate contents were found to be 2.80 and 2.30%, respectively. However, the proportion of soluble oxalates increased by 9.7% at two metre height.

Oxalate metabolism

The presence of oxalate degraders is widespread among the gastrointestinal tract of many species, including rodents, rabbits, guinea pigs, swine, horses, ruminants and human beings. However, not all individuals within a species possess oxalate-degrading bacteria. These bacteria, *Oxalobacter formigenes* are inhabitants of ovine and bovine rumens as well as the large intestine of human beings and other nonruminant animals. Adapted animals can tolerate levels of oxalates which would be lethal to nonadapted animals.

In ruminants, Talapatra et al. (1948) studied the dynamics of ruminal metabolism of oxalate using the plant *Halogeton glomeratus* (Halogeton is a branched annual herbaceous plant native to arid alkaline soils, barren soils. It contains high concentration of oxalate. Sheep die in a sleeping position, characteristic of the effect of hypocalcaemia due to halogeton poisoning). When oxalate is consumed by a ruminant animal, it may be degraded by certain rumen bacteria, *Oxalobacter formigenes* to a nontoxic form (formic acid and carbon dioxide), or it may combine with calcium or magnesium to form insoluble salt, or it may be absorbed from the rumen into the bloodstream where it may combine with calcium eventually to produce hypocalcaemia or oxalate may interfere with other body processes and / or be excreted.

Soluble oxalates are degraded in the rumen to carbonate and bicarbonate, which raises rumen pH (eventually leading to severe ruminal alkalosis) and slows down the microbial activity. Of course, this depends on the nutritional status of the animal and the functioning of the ruminal microflora. The insoluble oxalate salts may accumulate in various tissues, especially the rumen wall and kidneys. In certain cases calcium oxalates paralyse the brain. They may also cause destruction of the RBC. The studies of Panda and Sahu (2002) showed that soluble oxalates were completely degraded and about 50% of insoluble oxalates were broken down in the gastrointestinal tract of the bull. It can be concluded that the total oxalate intake at the level of 0.58% of the DM intake may be harmless with the calcium intake of 7.8 g/100kg body weight.

Oxalate intoxication

While delineating oxalate toxicosis, James (1972) attributed death of the animal to the following:
1. Hypocalcaemia
2. Uremia resulting from the damage of the kidneys by the oxalate crystals
3. Interference with energy metabolism since oxalate interferes with succinic dehydrogenase and lactic dehydrogenase enzymes.

Most oxalate-containing plants are palatable to livestock. Under normal grazing conditions, ruminants can consume large amounts of halogeton or greasewood without any harmful effect, if such plants are introduced gradually. If oxalate degraders are of sufficient numbers, the signs of toxicity are not seen. But when the animal eats too much of the plant too fast oxalate poisoning may occur because the rumen bacteria can not degrade oxalate to nontoxic form.

Symptoms: Oxalate poisoning is characterized by rapid and laboured respiration, depression, weakness, coma and death in case of sheep. Muscle tetany, renal failure and haemorrhagic gastroenteritis are also observed. In cattle, limbs become stiff, first in the front legs and then the hind legs. Rapid heart beat rate and rumenatonic hypocalcemia are also observed. In lactating animals, milk production is reduced due to depletion of calcium from stores.

Treatment: Once an animal has become intoxicated on oxalates, there is very little that can be done to save it. Force-feeding of water is the only treatment. Feeding dicalcium phosphate may be tried along with liberal feeding of green fodder, supplementing calcium, phosphorus and vitamin D in the ration. Calcium boroglucanate (25%) solution of 300-500 ml is also advocated in cattle and buffaloes via intravenous route.

Oxalate toxicity due to feeding overgrown napier grass

Cattle and buffaloes consumed the chaffed 6-18 month old napier grass *ad libitum* and fell sick (Sidhu et al., 1996). Overgrown napier bajra hybrid is rich in soluble oxalates and hence feeding ruminants with such fodder can cause rumen impaction which may lead to constipation and other side effects. The main toxic symptoms are dullness, dryness of muzzle, inappetance, dyspnoea, straining, constipation and decrease in rumen motility. Temperature was subnormal to normal. Treatment includes withdrawal of the napier grass, mixing of salt in drinking water, administration of linseed oil 1-1.5 L single dose orally on alternate days twice and calcium boroglucanate 450ml i/v for 5 alternate days. Blood clotting time reached normal (4 to 6 min) on 5th day. Calcium ions required for the release of neurotransmitters which control rumen motility and peristaltic activity of intestines. The thirst and straining may be due to alkalosis. It is reported that alkalosis is produced by soluble oxalates after detoxification into carbonates and bicarbonates in the rumen. Alkalosis also causes the inflammation of the alimentary tract which may lead to inappetance in the animals.

Nitrates

Existence of nitrate and its distribution

Nitrates are ubiquitous in feed, food and water and are essentially nontoxic. Nitrate (NO_3) becomes toxic when reduced to nitrite (NO_2) and can be a serious health hazard to ruminants grazing pastures or offered harvested feed and fodder, which contain nitrate in excess of one percent on DMB. Similarly drinking of water that contains 1500 ppm of nitrate can cause acute toxicity. Water from deep wells also contains higher levels of nitrate. National Academy of Sciences (Washington, D.C., 1974) recommended safe upper limits of nitrate and nitrite in drinking water as 100 and 10 ppm, respectively.

As plants mature, nitrate content rises until the prebloom stage, peaks and then begins to decline. The nitrate concentration has also been shown to increase during the first ten days of regrowth. The level of nitrate is highest in roots and stems, lower in leaves and almost negligible in flowers and seeds. Ensiled fodder usually contains less nitrate than fresh crop.

A number of plants are known to accumulate nitrates at potentially toxic levels under certain circumstances. For example, forage crops such as maize, kikuyu grass, johnson grass, oat hay, alfalfa hay. Nitrate is the principal inorganic nitrogen source for plants. Generally, only small quantities of nitrates accumulate because they are rapidly reduced (by nitrate reductase) and combined with carbohydrates to form amino acids.

Factors that favour accumulation of nitrates in plants

- The most common factors favouring accumulation of nitrates in plants include high nitrate content of soils, low intensity of light, drought, herbicide treatment with phenoxyacetic herbicides such as 2, 4-D., etc.
- Application of excessive nitrogen fertilizers may increase nitrate levels in some forages to toxic levels.
- Nitrate tends to accumulate in plants on cloudy days and in cool weather and at night. Cloudy weather may also inhibit reduction of nitrate to nitrite. So nitrate gets accumulated. Enough soil moisture may be present at night, even during drought, to allow uptake of nitrate and this gets accumulated because the activity of nitrate reductase is low during night.
- Hot, dry days may cause water loss and the wilting eventually leads to accumulation of nitrate.
- Use of crude sewage for irrigation is also credited with increasing nitrate content in plants. Seepage from highly fertile soil may increase nitrate content in deep well water to toxic levels.

Nitrate toxicity in livestock

Nitrate is not toxic by itself but becomes toxic when it is reduced to nitrite or hydroxylamine (NH_4OH), before being reduced to ammonia in the rumen. Accumulation of nitrite occurs in the rumen, when nitrate ingestion and reduction to nitrite exceeds that of nitrite reduction to ammonia due to different levels of reductive enzymes. Nitrate can be absorbed directly into the bloodstream and up to 27% is excreted in the urine within a few hours of dosing, although some can be recycled from the bloodstream into the gut through salivary and gastrointestinal secretions.

Nitrite toxicity occurs when nitrite oxidizes the ferrous iron of haemoglobin to ferric iron, producing a chocolate-coloured pigment called methaemoglobin that cannot carry oxygen to body tissues. Clinical signs of nitrite toxicosis appear when methaemoglobin concentration reaches 40% of total haemoglobin. Small amounts of methaemoglobin can be converted to haemoglobin by NADPH reductase.

Ruminants are particularly susceptible to nitrate poisoning because rumen microorganisms are responsible for reduction of nitrate to nitrite. Monogastric animals with significant microbial fermentation in the lower gastrointestinal tract (e.g., horses) are also more susceptible to nitrite poisoning than are monogastric animals such as pigs.

Ruminal pH is an important factor in nitrate reduction by rumen microflora. The optimum pH for nitrate reduction is 6.5 while 5.6 is required for nitrite reduction. When pH favoured nitrate reduction, nitrite appeared rapidly in the blood.

Among the ruminants, sheep are less susceptible to nitrate toxicity than are cattle. This kind of species susceptibility to methaemoglobinemia is related to the capacity to reduce methaemoglobin. The rate of methaemoglobin reduction in erythrocytes is highest in sheep and lowest in cattle among sheep, goats and cattle.

Haemoglobin from ruminants is more easily oxidized to methaemoglobin than from nonruminants. Swine showed the slowest rate of formation of methaemoglobin among the species studied namely man, goats, sheep, horses, cattle and swine.

Ruminants appear to adapt to continuing ingestion of sublethal levels of nitrate through the compensatory erythropoietic response of increasing haemoglobin levels, haematocrits and blood volumes.

Nitrate toxicity is influenced greatly by the diet of livestock. Adequate levels of readily fermentable carbohydrates increase nitrite disappearance in the rumen and protect the animal. Fasted animals are more susceptible to nitrite intoxication than are fully fed animals. It was reported that fasted animals eat more rapidly and may become intoxicated on forages grazed safely by fed animals.

Harvested forage fed to livestock may be more toxic due to a more rapid rate of nitrate ingestion.

Physical form of the feed can also influence toxicity. Nitrates are readily reduced in silages and moist hays.

Animals can adapt to relatively high nitrate levels in the diets if the level of nitrate incorporation is increased gradually. This adaptation is due to an increase in the rate of nitrite reduction in the rumen.

Rumen microbes for nitrite reduction

Fodders ingested by ruminants often contain high levels of nitrate and hence prevention of nitrite accumulation is particularly important. However nitrate reduction rate is much higher than nitrite reduction rate, which causes nitrite accumulation. High levels of nitrite might cause an acute intoxication to host animals. High levels also inhibit the growth of many kinds of ruminal microbes, especially cellulolytic bacteria, methanogenic bacteria and protozoa.

T. Hino and coworkers from Japan conducted several studies on these aspects and the relevant details are presented here. Addition of fumarate, lactate or formate to cultures of mixed ruminal microbes stimulated nitrate reduction and nitrite reduction also, to a greater extent. This stimulation is possible due to increased numbers of bacteria that reduce fumarate, nitrate and nitrite, such as *Selenomonas ruminantium*, *Veillonella parvula and Wolinella succinogenes*. The numbers of nitrate-reducing bacteria in the goat rumen were estimated by competitive polymerase chain reaction. The cell number of S. ruminantium was the largest of the three nitrate-reducing bacteria (107 cells / ml ruminal fluid) followed by V. parvula and W. succinogenes, which were less than 104 cells / ml. Therefore, S. ruminantium appears to be the most predominant in the rumen, but both the subspecies i.e., *ssp. lactilytica* and *ssp. ruminantium* are not able to reduce nitrate and nitrite equally. S. ruminantium ssp. lactilytica only is able to ferment lactate and glycerol while the other is unable to ferment them.

Studies of Yoshii et al. (2003) revealed that the cell number of S. ruminantium (*ssp. ruminantium*) that reduces nitrate and nitrite in the rumen was usually 8-10%

of the total number of *S. ruminantium* while the lactate-using *ssp. lactilytica* was less than 1% of the total number. The percentage was not affected by the roughage / concentrate ratio or nitrate content of the diet in 2 weeks. However feeding a high nitrate diet for 12 weeks increased the percentage. Nitrate reduction by *S. ruminantium* was enhanced by the coexistence of amylolytic bacteria (*Streptococcus bovis and Prevotella ruminicola*) in a medium containing starch and nitrite accumulation increased; nitrite might not be reduced because of exhaustion of starch. Coexistence of cellulolytic bacteria (*Ruminococcus albus* and *Fibrobacter succinogenes*) facilitated the growth of *S. ruminantium* in a medium containing cellulose and nitrite reduction increased. These results suggest that fibre digestion is important to decrease nitrite accumulation in the rumen, because fibre digestion may provide sugars and electron donors to nitrite-reducing bacteria after readily fermentable carbohydrate are exhausted. Hence it appears that measures followed to enhance fibre digestion may suppress nitrite accumulation in the rumen and save the ruminant animal from nitrate poisoning.

Symptoms of nitrate toxicity

Nitrate contained in forage may pose performance and health risks to ruminants. Nitrate risk to ruminants can be affected by various animal factors such as rumen microbes, age and condition of the animal, diet offered and the environmental stresses and water quality, as well as several plant factors including nutrient management, species, growth stage, environmental stresses, and nonstructural carbohydrate level. Forages containing less than 1000 mg NO_3-N/ kg (dry weight basis) usually pose no risk for cattle (Undersander et al., 1999). Low levels of ingested nitrate are reduced by rumen bacteria to nitrite and then ammonia (Cowley and Collings, 1977), and any excess ammonia absorbed by the blood stream is excreted in the urine as urea.

However, when high levels of nitrate are ingested, the capacity of the normal nitrate conversion process becomes overloaded and a portion of the nitrate is absorbed by the blood stream as nitrate and nitrite. Some of the nitrate that is absorbed recycles back to the rumen through saliva thereby adding again to the nitrate pool in the rumen. In contrast, absorbed nitrite inhibits the oxygen transporting capacity of red blood cells by oxidizing the ferrous iron of haemoglobin to ferric iron (methaemoglobin) leading to chronic animal performance problems including suppressed appetite, rate of weight gain, milk production (Undersander et al., 1999) and in severe cases, acute toxicity and possibly death. With timely and accurate assessment of nitrate concentration in forage and water sources, potential risks of livestock exposure to excessive nitrate intake may be properly managed or avoided.

Nitrate toxicity may be classified into acute and chronic type.

Acute toxicity: In acute type the affected animal may die within hours of ingestion of a lethal dose. Animal dies of hypoxia from lack of oxygen due to methaemoglobinemia. Ruminants develop a brownish discolouration of nonpigmented skin and vaginal membranes, and discolouration of the vaginal membranes in females is a reliable indicator before other clinical signs are visible. Staggered gait, accelerated pulse, frequent urination and laboured breathing, followed by collapse are the other symptoms. Lethal intoxications usually result in coma and death within two to three hours after the first appearance of symptoms. The blood is dark and red to coffee brown and clots poorly.

Chronic toxicity: Considerable controversy exists with regards to the symptoms of chronic nitrate ingestion. Symptoms are depressed appetite, reduction in weight gains, decreased milk production, abortion, vitamin A deficiency and hypothyroidism. Apart from nitrate to nitrite and eventual toxicity, the nitrate has a direct caustic action on stomach and intestinal mucosa and causes gastroenteritis. Fatal nitrite poisoning in pigs showed no external signs; postmortem shows discoloured tarry blood.

Diagnosis of nitrate poisoning

Analysis of nitrate content in feed and water is important to confirm the source of poisoning. A simple test 'diphenylamine blue test' is available for detecting nitrate in feed samples. Stock solution for test is prepared by dissolving 500 mg diphenylamine in 20 ml water and then adding sulphuric acid to make 100 ml volume. A working solution is made by mixing one part stock solution to one part 80% sulphuric acid. Both the solutions should be stored in brown glass bottles. Suspected feed materials are tested by placing a drop of working solution inside the cut stem at a node or joint. Development of deep blue colour within 10 seconds indicates 2% or more nitrate.

Treatment

Treatment involves conversion of methaemoglobin into oxyhaemoglobin by administration of suitable reducing agents such as methylene blue, thionin or ascorbic acid. Acute nitrate toxicity is treated with intravenous administration of methylene blue solution. Methylene blue apparently accepts electrons for NADPH reductase in the blood and acclerates the reconversion of methaemoglobin to functional haemogobin. The recommended dosage of methylene blue is 2 to 4 mg/kg to 15 mg/kg body weight (in severe methaemoglobinemia), intravenously in a one percent solution. The dosage should be repeated if clinical signs recur. Oral doses of mineral oil (one litre for adult cattle) or saline cathartics (sodium sulphate 500 g per adult cattle) are recommended as supportive treatment, which help in removing toxic materials from gastrointestinal tract.

To be at safer side, the fodder cut in the early part of regrowth may be fed mixed with other dry roughages to neutralize the nitrate concentration.

Nitrotoxins

Elevated concentrations of nitrates in feed and water can intoxicate an animal due to conversion to toxic nitrite. Studies of nitrate and nitrite metabolism with rumen microbes showed that ruminants are especially susceptible but can adapt if the initial levels of nitrate are below toxic levels.

Aliphatic nitro compounds such as 3-nitro-1-propanol (3NPOH), 3-nitropropionic acid (3NPA), miserotoxin (the β-glycodide of 3NPOH) are found in Astragalus species of plants that are important in the dietary of livestock. Out of these aliphatic compounds, 3NPA arises as a product of animal metabolism of 3NPOH as well as being a toxin within plants. When large amounts are consumed and absorbed, these produce clinical signs of motor weakness, dyspnea and death in ruminants.

Rumen microbes detoxify these 3NPA and 3NPOH to β-alanine and 3-amino-1-propanol. That is why, it is reported that nonruminants (toxicity is at 43 mg/kg body weight) are far more susceptible than ruminants (307 mg/kg body weight). Craig (1995) explained the dual role of rumen microbes in first producing the toxin and latter degrading them.

Cyanogenic glycosides

Most outbreak of HCN poisoning is caused by ingestion of plants, which contain cyanogenic glycosides [amygdalin (laetrile) and prunasin found in kernels of almonds, etc., dhurrin that occurs in sorghum species and linamarin that occurs in flax (linseed), cassava). The commonly found plants are sorghum, sudan grass, jhonson grass and linseed cake or meal. Cyanogenic glycoside content varies with the age of plant, environmental condition, nutritional status and genotype of the forage crop. Immature sorghum fodder contains a cyanogenic glycoside called "dhurrin" and this liberates hydrocyanic acid (HCN)/prussic acid on hydrolysis.

1. Cyanogenic glycoside $\xrightarrow{\beta-\text{gulcodidase}}$ sugar+ aglycone

2. Aglycone $\xrightarrow{\text{hydroxynitrile lyase}}$ HCN + aldehyde or ketone

The glycosides occur in vacuoles in plant tissue, while the enzymes are found in the cytosol. Damage to the plant from wilting, trampling, frost, drought, bruising (cassava), and so on results in the enzymes and glycosides coming together, causing HCN to be formed. These enzymes are also produced by rumen microorganisms. The optimum pH for the enzymes is near neutrality, so release of HCN is more rapid in the rumen than in the highly acid stomach of the nonruminant animal. That is the reason ruminants are more sensitive to cyanogens than the nonruminants.

Leaves of tender plants contain maximum poison. It is recommended that sorghum green fodder is harvested after 60 days of planting to avoid HCN poisoning. Rainfed crops contain more poison than those under irrigation. The glucoside content is highest when plants grow rapidly after a previous period of retardation. Thus wilted, frost bitten and young plants are likely to be more poisonous than the normal, mature plants.

HCN is readily absorbed and enters individual tissue cells. It inhibits cytochrome oxidase, the terminal step in electron transport. When cytochrome oxidase is blocked, ATP formation ceases, and the tissues suffer energy deprivation. Commonly HCN poisoning is always acute and affected animals rarely survive for more than 1-2 hours due to dysfunction of electron transport in the cytochrome system. The onset of signs is within 2-3 minutes and the signs may be delayed if the ingested materials are relatively indigestible.

Symptoms

The common clinical signs include dyspnea (difficult or laboured breathing), anxiety, restlessness, stumbling gait, tremor, moaning, recumbancy, convulsions with opisthotonus and sudden death. The blood of the affected animal becomes bright red due to suspended oxygen exchange and oxygen retention in blood. In prolonged course it becomes dark red colour. The odour of benzaldehyde or acetone may be detectable in the contents of the rumen if the dead animal is examined immediately. A level of HCN 0.63 ug/ml justifies a diagnosis of poisoning.

Treatment

Cyanide is readily detoxified, so acute toxicity occurs only when HCN levels are more.Liver, kidney, and thyroid tissue contain an enzyme called rhodanese (thiosulfate sulfurtransferse), which catalyses conversion of cyanide to thiocyanate. Thiocyanate is excreted in the urine. This reaction is employed in the treatment of cyanide toxicity. The standard treatment of intravenous injection of a mixture of sodium nitrite and sodium thiosulphate will give good recovery (5g sodium nitrite, 15 g sodium thiosulphate in 200ml water for cattle, 1g sodium nitrite, 3 g sodium thiosulphate in 50ml water for sheep). Sodium thiosulfate participates in the reaction, while nitrate converts haemoglobin to methaemoglobin. Sodium nitrite or sodium thiosulphate can be administered alone or together to produce low-level methaemoglobinemia.

Methaemoglobin has a strong affinity for cyanide and will bind the cyanide molecule and prevent inhibition of the cytochrome oxidation system. It was concluded that sodium thiosulphate without nitrite was an effective antidote for cyanide poisoning. Dosage is 660mg/kg body weight. Sodium thiosulphate should be given orally to fix the HCN in rumen at the dose of 30 g in cattle, 6 g in sheep and it is repeated at hourly intervals tills the signs disappear.

Differential diagnosis

Nitrite intoxication versus cyanosis (CO_2 poisoning) and cyanide poisoning

In acute cyanosis, the blood turns dark red to brownish because of a lack of oxyhaemoglobin. In cyanide poisoning (hydrocyanic or prussic acid poisoning) the blood turns cherry red because of an abundance of oxyhaemoglobin. Nitrite and cyanide have different modes of toxicological action.

Nitrite prevents oxygen transport to body tissues due to formation of methaemoglobin.

Cyanide prevents use of oxygen by the cytochrome system during oxidative phosphorylation.

Mimosine

Subabul (*Leucaena leucocephala*) contains a free amino acid, mimosine (Lucinol). It is found in leaves and seeds of tropical legumes of the genus Leucaena. Mimosine {β-N-(3-hydroxy-4-pyridone)-α-amino propionic acid} is a non-proteinaceous amino acid. It acts as an antimetabolite inhibiting the utilization of tyrosine needed for formation and growth of hair and wool. Mimosine is 3 to 5% of the dry matter and on feeding it may lead to goitre. Pregnant animals may produce weak offsprings with enlarged thyroid glands. The metal-chelating ability of the 3-hydroxy-4-oxo functional group of the pyridine ring in mimosine has been implicated in promoting deficiencies of mineral elements such as zinc and phosphorus and a poor blood amino acid profile. The metal-chelating trait of mimosine also impairs the activity of metal-containing enzymes.

It has been claimed that ruminants in some parts of the world (Indonesia and Hawaii) have microbes, which can alter mimosine to another compound, 3, 4 dihydroxy pyridone (DHP), which is then broken down further to non-toxic compounds. Introduction of rumen microbes that degrade DHP in ruminants has been successful experimentally in Australia (Jones and Megarrity, 1983). These ruminal microbial populations protect the host from leucaena toxicity. M.J.Allison and coworkers from USA isolated that gram-negative anaerobic bacterium and characterized the organism, *Synergistes jonesii*. This organism converted 3, 4-DHP to 2, 3-DHP and there are indications that acetate, propionate and ammonia are the products of 2, 3-DHP metabolism. Despite these reactions, considerable quantities of mimosine and DHP may escape metabolism to appear in the faeces. Further, conjugated forms of DHP may also appear in the faeces and urine, while mimosine may itself undergo decarboxylation within the tissues of the ruminant to yield mimosinamine, which is then excreted in the urine (D'Mello, 2000).

Akingbade et al. (2001, 2002) reported the presence of DHP-degrading rumen bacteria in South African goats. The DHP-degrading rumen bacteria played a beneficial role by carrying out complete biodegradation and detoxification of mimosine and its metabolites and thus overcame the chelating tendency of mimosine and its metabolites on haematological parameters.

The toxicity of mimosine can be overcome by restricting the proportion of subabul to 30% of DM intake in ruminants and 5 to 7% in pigs and rabbits. In poultry the maximum quantity of subabul leaf meal acceptable to layers is 2.5%.

Detoxification of mimosine

Plant cytogeneticists have evolved low-mimosine leucaena varieties like K-67 and K-29. It has been known that the enzyme necessary to convert mimosine to DHP is present in the subabul leaves and the conversion is initiated during maceration of leaves. The enzyme becomes inactive at pH 4 or below and also when dry heated suddenly. It has been reported that the mimosine content is reduced by sundrying to the extent of 10%. During ensiling mimosine is converted into DHP. Addition of ferrous sulphate prevents the absorption of mimosine (since it binds mimosine) and promotes its excretion through faeces. This is more useful for monogastric species.

Anti-nutritional factors in plants

The major anti-nutritional factors that may occur in different plant species is presented in Table 2. These substances may be divided into two categories: I. heat-labile group (e.g. lectins, proteinase inhibitors and cyanogens), which are sensitive to standard processing temperatures and II. heat-stable group (e.g. antigenic proteins, condensed tannins, quinolizidine alkaloids, glucosinolates, the non-protein amino acids S-methylcysteine sulphoxide and mimosine and phyto-oestrogens. It is generally accepted that the severity of adverse effects of anti-nutritional factors are greater in tropical legumes than in temperate legumes (Kumar and D'Mello, 1995).

Dietary antiprotozoal agents

Defaunation is difficult to achieve as there are no safe defaunation agents commercially available for use under practical conditions. Reduced fauna might also be beneficial as it increased milk yield and milk protein to fat ratio in dairy cows (Moate, 1989). Therefore, the use of dietary antiprotozoal agents with the potential to significantly reduce fauna might be more practical and effective in promoting animal productivity than the use of defaunating agents. e.g., dietary supplementation with bentonite (Ivan et al., 1992) and *Yucca shidigera* extract (Sarsaponin) (Hristov et al., 1999). Recently, there has been an increased interest in plant secondary metabolites for use as possible antiprotozoal agents. They function as a mechanism for defending their structure and reproductive elements from predation by animals and insects, apart from serving as nutrient resource. Foliage from a variety of different sub-tropical leguminous trees has been tested in vitro and in vivo for antiprotozoal acivity (Newbold et al., 1997; Teferedegne et al., 1999).

Table 2. An illustrative list of anti-nutritional factors in plants

Plant type	Plant species	Major anti-nutritional factors
Forage		
Legumes	*Medicago*	Phyto-oestrogens
		Saponins
	Trifolium	Phyto-oestrogens
	Lotus	Condensed tannins
Grasses	*Brachiaria decumbens*	Saponins
	Panicum	Saponins
Cruciferae	*Brassica*	Glucosinolates
		S-methylcysteine sulphoxide
		Erucic acid
Browse		
Legumes	*Acacia*	Condensed tannins
		Cyanogens
	Leucaena leucocephala	Mimosine
		Condensed tannins
Pine	*Pinus ponderosa*	Vasoactive lipids
Grain		
Legumes	Glycine max	Proteinase inhibitors
		Antigenic proteins
		Lectins
		Phyto-oestrogens
		Saponins
	Lupinus	Quinolizidine alkaloids
		Saponins

*Source: D'Mello, 2000

Newbold et al. (1997) suggested that saponins in the foliage were the antiprotozoal agent. From the trees tested, *Enterolobium cyclocarpum or Enterolobium timbova* foliage was identified as the one with best potential as a rumen antiprotozoal agent in sheep and goats (Leng et al., 1992; Chaudhary et al., 1997), but the population increased to the normal levels following withdrawal of the foliage supplement from the diet (Leng et al., 1992). However, the supplements in the above experiments were fed for only 7-8 days. Further, the rumen microbial population might adapt to the plant and degrade its antiprotozoal component (Teferedegne et al., 1999). They observed that feeding of *Sesbania sesban* foliage decreased the rumen protozoal population in sheep in Scotland, but not in Ethiopia, because the Ethiopian sheep might have been exposed to the plant previously. Hence Ivan et al. (2004) tested the antiprotozoal activity of *Enterolobium cyclocarpum* foliage in in vitro, using a technique that measures the breakdown of [^{14}C]-labelled *Selenomonas ruminantium*, and in vivo experiments for 41days.

Sun dried branches of the *E. cyclocarpum* tree were imported from Costa Rica. The foliage was removed from the branches and twigs by hand. The separated leaves were used in experiments with sheep (200 g dry leaves per sheep of 70±6 kg), while a part of the leaves were ground to pass through a 1 mm screen for use in an *in vitro* experiment. The in vitro assay showed a 20-95% decrease in the rate of breakdown of [14C]-labelled *Selenomonas ruminantium* by protozoa with increased amounts of *E. cyclocarpum* in the incubation media, ranging from 0.5 to 10 g/litre. The results of the in vivo experiment with sheep showed that the *E. cyclocarpum* supplement significantly reduced protozoal numbers during days 4-11 (by 49-75%), but the numbers gradually increased to the level of the control group by day 20. The reduction in the protozoal population was associated with a reduced concentration of ammonia-N in rumen fluid. pH and volatile fatty acid concentrations were not affected by the treatment. It was concluded that the antiprotozoal effect of the *E. cyclocarpum* foliage supplement was only transitory (up to 12 -14 days) and effective only the first time it was fed to the same animals.

Tannins

Trees and shrub foliage (leaves, pods, seeds) and agroindustrial byproducts are of importance in animal production because they do not compete with human food and can provide significant protein supplements, especially in the dry season. But, these feed resources are generally rich in antinutritional factors, particularly tannins. Tannins are polyphenolic substances with various molecular weights and a variable complexity. Tannin composition in plants is known to depend on soil fertility and environmental conditions. These are chemically not well-defined substances but rather a group of substances with the ability to bind proteins in aqueous solution. Their multiple phenolic hydroxyl groups lead to the formation of complexes primarily with proteins and to a lesser extent with metal ions, amino acids and polysaccharides.

Proteins and tannins

The protein content of forage tree legume leaves (12-30%) is usually high compared with that of mature grasses (3-10%). The proteins are digested in the rumen to provide ammonia and amino acids for microbial protein synthesis. Microbial cells then pass to the small intestine, providing the major source of absorbed amino acids for the ruminant. In some cases, feed proteins may escape digestion (bypass proteins) in the rumen and provide additional protein for absorption in the small intestine. The microbial population in the rumen requires a minimum level of ammonia (70 mg N/ l) to support optimum activity; lower values are associated with decreased microbial activity (digestion) and are indicative of nitrogen deficiency. Feeds containing less than 1.3% N (8% crude protein) are considered deficient as they cannot provide the minimum ammonia levels required.

All forage tree legumes have N contents higher than this value, and may be judged adequate in protein. However, tannins found in some tree legume leaves form complexes with plant proteins, which decrease their rate of digestion (degradability) in the rumen, thereby decreasing rumen ammonia concentrations and increasing the amount of plant protein bypassing the rumen. When the tannin-protein complexes are dissociated in the low pH of the abomasum, an additional source of protein is made available for absorption by the animal. In other cases, the tannins protect the proteins from digestion even in the small intestine. Tannins may therefore have a beneficial effect (increasing bypass protein or decreasing ammonia loss) or a detrimental effect (depressing palatability, decreasing rumen ammonia, decreasing post-ruminal protein absorption) on protein availability. It is clear that the interpretation of the nutritional value of protein in forage trees requires information on the nature and action of tannins.

The proteins in the leaves of species which do not have tannins (*Albizia lebbeck, Enterlobium cyclocarpum, Albizia saman* and *Sesbania* spp. have *in sacco* N degradability, respectively, of 78%, 96%, 90% and 96%.) will be rapidly degraded in the rumen, providing high levels of rumen ammonia, much of which will ultimately be wasted by excretion as urinary urea. Such feeds provide N in a similar way to urea. Species which contain some tannins will therefore provide both degradable and undegraded rumen N and will be more effective sources of supplemental N for ruminants. Nevertheless, the significance of tannins in tree legume forage is poorly understood, with low concentrations being beneficial and high concentrations detrimental.

Hydrolysable and Condensed tannins

Tannins decrease the palatability of forage due to astringency. Tannins are tentatively classified into two classes: hydrolysable and condensed tannins. Hydrolysable tannins are potentially toxic and cause poisoning in animals if sufficiently large amounts of tannin-containing plant material are consumed (Garg et al 1992). Condensed tannin are not toxic to ruminants, and when the concentration is below 4% of DM, they improve the nutritive value of herbage by binding to plant proteins and protecting them from excessive degradation in the rumen, besides preventing the establishment of parasitic nematodes (Barry and McNabb 1999). The amount of tannins that the tree and shrub foliage contain vary widely and largely unpredictably, and their effects on animals range from beneficial to toxicity and death (Makkar, 2003).

Condensed tannins

Condensed tannins are the most abundant type of tannins present in leguminous seeds and forages and certain cereal grains, particularly sorghum. On heating with strong acids, these polymerize further to yield small quantities of anthocyanidins, giving rise to the term' proanthocyanidins' as an alternative general name for condensed tannins (CTs). D'Mello (1992) reported that certain animals are capable of secreting proline-rich proteins (PRPs) in saliva, upon consumption of condensed tannins, which may constitute a first line of defence against ingested CTs. There are suggestions that the goat produces PRPs in significant amounts, whereas grazing ruminants lack these salivary proteins.

Goats are well recognized as mixed feeders, consuming appreciable quantities of CT-rich browse. Higher digestibility of fibre was reported in goats compared with sheep when both are offered leaves of *Acacia pendula* or *Prosopis cineraria*, whereas no species differences were observed with Lucerne as major feedstuff (Kumar and D'Mello, 1995). The two browse species, *A. pendula* and *P. cineraria* are known to contain CTs and if the synthesis of PRPs by goats is confirmed, this may account for the higher digestibility of fibre.

Condensed tannin (CT) concentration varies with cultivar and its accumulation is under genetic control. CT concentration is affected by the timing of fertilizer application, which can decrease its proportion relative to protein. Kamalak et al. (2004) determined the chemical composition including condensed tannin contents of leaves of some trees used for small ruminant animals and examined their relationships with *in vitro* gas production parameters. Total and soluble condensed tannins, NDF and ADF were negatively correlated with estimated parameters of gas production (Table 3) and *in vitro* dry matter digestibility. There was wide variation between tree species in terms of condensed tannins (TCT, BCT and SCT).

Table 3. The chemical composition of different tree leaves*

(%)	Juniperus communis	Quercus libari	Morus alba	Populus nigra	J. communis	Q. libari
DM	95.6	95.2	93.17	93.26	95.61	93.91
CP	5.7	8.9	14.00	14.11	5.62	8.65
NDF	57.2	38.5	42.33	43.11	56.98	46.13
ADF	39.2	27.2	25.35	24.92	34.22	28.30
EE	9.4	10.0	6.58	5.34	9.31	8.54
Ash	5.4	4.8	15.88	9.17	5.67	4.99
TCT	20.3	4.3	1.42	4.99	21.31	4.87
BCT	3.9	1.6	0.59	2.19	3.37	3.15
SCT	16.5	2.3	0.83	2.79	17.94	0.375
IVDMD	42.1	52.4	—	—	—	—

TCT: Total condensed Tannin, BCT: Bound Condensed Tannin, SCT: Soluble Condensed Tannin, IVDMD: in Vitro Dry Matter Digestibility

*Kamalak,A., Canbolat, O., Gurbuz, Y., Ozay, O., Ozkan, C. O. and Sakarya, M. 2004., Livestock Research for Rural Development 16, 6,

Condensed tannins (CT)-containing legumes are widely known for their beneficial or antinutritional effects when fed to ruminants. CT in birdsfoot trefoil (*Lotus corniculatus*) and sulla (*Hedysarum coronarium*) were estimated and their contents in fresh forage are 2.86 and 1.95 % in DM while in ensiled herbage are 2.90 and 1.87 % in DM. This suggests that total CT concentration is not affected by ensiling (Minnee et al., 2002/2003).

However, the amount of 'free' CTs (CTs not in complex with other molecules) was markedly reduced in the ensiled forages. Fresh forage had 67 % and ensiled herbage had only 11 % in birdsfoot trefoil while in sulla the respective contents were 88% and 8%. The remaining CTs were 'bound' to other molecules such as plant proteins or fibre. The binding capability of CT is significant to animal production, because those plant proteins bound to CTs are protected from microbial degradation in the rumen (Minnee et al., 2002/2003).

Condensed tannins (procyanidins or proanthocyanidins) form complexes containing proteins which protect the latter from rumen digestion and augment the bypass protein available for absorption in the small intestine. Condensed tannins bind strongly to proteins to form a pH-dependent complex that is not degradable at normal rumen pH (6.0-7.0), but dissociates at normal abomasal pH (2.5-3.5) with the protein absorbed from the small intestine. This seems to apply to species such as *Leucaena leucocephala*, *Gliricidia sepium* which often contain condensed tannins of the order of 2-5% and exhibit moderate protein degradability. On the other hand, high levels of CT are inimicable to intake and protein complexes may be protected from digestion even in the small intestine; *Calliandra calothymus* may contain 11% CT and have *in sacco* N degradability of only 30% (Ahn et al., 1989).

However, the results reported by Vitti et al. (2004) cast doubt on the generalisation that small amounts of condensed tannins (2.0-4.0%) produce beneficial effects or that high levels (>5.0%) are necessarily harmful. Rather it appears that tannins in some plants are either particularly beneficial or detrimental. Further, slight variations in the analytical method can also lead to variations in the tannin contents. In view of this, it may not be correct to predict beneficial or harmful nutritional effects from total tannin concentrations per se.

The polyphenolic compounds of certain tree leaves have been analysed in our laboratory (Table 4). The higher levels of polyphenolic compounds in cashew leaves reflected in their nutritive value in goats: DMI, kg/% BW was 1.44; DCP, 4.2% and TDN, 41.0% (Uma Maheswari, Elanchezhian and Reddy, 2008).

Tannins and PEG

Pritchard et al. (1988) showed that the feeding of polyethylene glycol (PEG) to sheep fed mulga markedly increased feed intake, weight gain and wool growth. Polyethylene glycol, a non-nutritive synthetic polymer having high affinity for condensed tannins, makes them inert by forming PEG- tannin complex. Polyvinylpyrrolidone (PVP) is also used as tannin-complexing agent. These tannin-complexing agents are also considered to break 'the already formed tannin-protein complexes' since their affinity for tannins is higher than for proteins. The affinity of PVPs for tannins was lower than of PEG. The PEG 6000 may be preferred for inactivation of tannins in feedstuffs as its binding to tannins was highest at near neutral pH values.

Table 4. Polyphenolic compounds in certain tree leaves*

Tree leaves/ Constituents	Total phenolics[1]	Non-tannin phenolics[1]	Total tannin phenolics[1]	Condensed tannins[2]
Acacia auriculiformis	13.44–14.68	0.48–0.51	12.96–14.17	12.29–13.62
Cashewnut	20.31–22.26	0.86–0.90	19.45–21.36	16.43–16.84
Gliricidia	5.63	0.35	5.28	3.44
Guava **	17.02	0.84	16.18	14.00
Jack	15.63	0.94	14.69	13.23
Sesbania grandiflora	9.38	0.74	8.64	5.71
Subabul	11.25	0.48	10.78	7.28
Yellow gold mohur	12.50	0.53	11.98	11.03

[1]as tannic acid equivalent, [2]as leucocyanidine equivalent.
* D.V.Reddy and N.Elanchezhian 2008, Livestock Research for Rural Development, 20, 5, 8 pages; ** N.Elanchezhian, D.Uma Maheswari and D.V.Reddy 2011, Indian Veterinary Journal, 88, 4 : 45–47.

The low quality of *mulga* is therefore related to its high content of condensed tannins and their capacity to bind feed proteins. These proteins are poorly digested in the rumen and appear also to be indigestible in the intestines. Consequently, sheep consuming *mulga* have low rumen ammonia and sulphur levels, which can be corrected by sulphur supplementation. The addition of PEG preferentially binds the tannins thereby making plant proteins more available for digestion. The increased digestion rate stimulates feed intake and changes *mulga* from a maintenance ration to one on which sheep can grow. Sulphur supplements to the drinking water are sufficient to produce this response. These findings are relevant to other Acacia species of low nutritive value.

Makkar (2003) advocated use of PEG both by farmers (give to animals through water, feed or spraying on tannin-rich feedstuffs) as well as by industry (incorporate PEG in a pelleted diet). The incorporation of PEG had beneficial effects for feedstuffs such as *Zizyphus nummularia* (Kumar and Vaithiyanathan, 1990) which are rich in tannins (condensed tannin content: 5-10%). On the otherhand, for *L. corniculatus*, the condensed tannin content of which varied from 2 to 4 %, addition of PEG decreased wool growth, weight gain, reproduction and milk yield. From these observations, it is clear that incorporation of PEG in diets containing high levels of condensed tannins is beneficial for ruminants.

Effect of tannins on the performance of animals

Feeding studies revealed that tannins could act as positive and negative effectors of digestion depending on concentration of tannin contained in the forage. Reed (1995) studied the nutritional toxicology of tannins and related polyphenols in forage legumes and reported that protein protection under the neutral conditions of the rumen was due to reversible protein-tannin binding which get reversed in the acidic conditions of the abomasum. However, tannins can complex with carbohydrates as well, so interactions may be more complex *in vivo*. Other studies suggested that somehow tannins increase passage rate through the rumen thereby decreasing the rumen residence time and thus proteolysis in the rumen.

High concentrations of CT in feed can result in poor digestibility but a little can be beneficial; a CT content of 2-4% of dry matter has been suggested to be needed for significant protein protection.

The presence of condensed tannins has had a bacteriostatic and bactericidal effect on pathogenic microorganisms, as well as inhibiting cellulose-digesting ruminal microbial enzymes.

Anti-nutritional effects

Tannins can produce toxic and antinutritional effects in monogastric and ruminant animals: reduced feed intake, lower nutrient digestibility and protein availability. Tree leaves did not exert any deleterious effect on the feed consumption and nutrient utilization with a total tannin content of up to 5.5 % and condensed tannin content of 3.4 % (Ally and Kunjikutty, 2003). The higher levels of total tannin phenolics in cashew leaves (Table 5) reflected in their low nutritive value in goats: DMI, kg/% BW was 1.44; DCP, 4.2% and TDN, 41.0% (Uma Maheswari, Elanchezhian and Reddy, 2008).

There is unequivocal evidence that sheep and cattle are sensitive to CTs. Adverse effects may be seen in sheep when CTs such as that in lotus (*Lotus pedunculatus* (*L.uliginosus; greater bird's foot trefoil*), *L.corniculatus; bird's foot trefoil*) or in browse legumes such as Acacia species (*A. nylotica, A. aneura, A. cyanophylla*) comprise a significant part of their diets (Kumar and D'Mello, 1995). Primary manifestations include impaired rumen function, resulting in depressed intake, wool growth and live weight gain. The deleterious effects on rumen function have been ascribed to complexing of CTs with microbial extracellular enzymes. High-tannin forages and browse may lead to an overall deficit of rumen-degradable N and this undersupply may reduce the digestibility of structural carbohydrates.

In the protein-tannin complex, protein is digested in the abomasum and the acid-stable CTs are not totally digested during passage through the gut and increase the tannin load on the land. The environmental impact of increasing forage CT is not known.

Beneficial effects

1. Aerts et al. (1999) reviewed the beneficial effects of proanthocyanidins in forages and stated that tannin has long been appreciated as a modulator of forage quality and tanniniferous species are believed to be beneficial in preventing bloat and parasite load.

2. Condensed tannins may confer protection from degradation of leaf protein in the rumen through reversible hydrogen bonding between them, which is stable between pH values of 4 and 7, but readily dissociates on either side of this range. The obvious implication is that CTs protect labile plant proteins in the rumen, thereby increasing the supply of high-quality protein (undegraded dietary protein, UDP) to the duodenum. However, it is not such

a straightforward thing, since the CTs of *P.cineraria* retain their capacity to precipitate pepsin at pH 2.0 and, consequently pepsin is not available for digestion.

3. Lower level of condensed tannin (2-4%) increased the bypass protein into the duodenum which increased both milk yield and protein content of milk in dairy animals. Avijit Dey et al (2008) reported that condensed tannins from *Ficus infectoria* leaves at 1.5% could be used as organic protectant of protein in the diet of ruminants. Lower condensed tannin content of *Lotus pedunculatus* increased the milk yield. In grazing sheep fed *Lotus corniculatus* in New Zealand, CT increased wool production by 10%, milk production of ewes by 15%, and promoted high rates of live weight gain in weaned lambs.

4. Condensed tannins from Lotus corniculatus reduced the rate of proteolysis and inhibited the growth of proteolytic rumen microorganisms.

5. CTs are able to increase transulphuration of methionine to cysteine, a major component of wool protein.

6. They are also implicated in bloat suppression in cattle. Bloat is often associated with low-tannin pasture legumes such as lucerne and clover, but sainfoin, lotus and tropical browse legumes are considered to confer protection by virtue of their content of CTs.

7. High-tannin legume, sulla (*Hedysarum coronarium*) reduced the gastrointestinal parasitism (nematode, *Trichostrongylus colubriformis*) in lambs. Sainfoin (*Onobrychis vicifolia*) also contains higher condensed tannins. There is a reduced need for anthelmintic drugs to control gastrointestinal parasites in grazing goats fed CT-containing foliages (Leucaena, Jackfruit and Cassava).

8. A number of tropical forages (*Acacia spp.*) are endowed with defaunation (particularly *Enterolobium* species) properties, possibly arising from the secondary compounds they contribute.

9. Tannins isolated from leaves of various multipurpose trees and browses have anticarcinogenic activity (Perchellet et al., 1996).

10. Tannins promote both elevation of faecal nitrogen and rumen microbial protein output in sheep (Beever and Siddons, 1986; Van Soest, 1994).

Phyto-oestrogens

The phytooestrogens are a diverse group of isoflavonoid compounds found primarily in legumes. It is well recognized that soybeans contain relatively high concentrations of the glycosides of the isoflavones, daidzein, genistein and glycitein. The oestrogens in *Trifolium spp.* are mainly isoflavones, whereas those in *Medicago spp.* are usually coumestans. The phyto-oestrogens occur in plant tissue as water-soluble glycosides. The isoflavones are synthesized by plants from phenylalanine, while the coumestans are synthesized from cinnamic acid.

Phytooestrogens are actively metabolized in the rumen but the activity of these substances in the plant depends upon the extent of microbial transformations in the rumen. For example, genistein is degraded to non-oestrogenic compounds.

Formononetin, however, is demethylated and reduced to the more oestrogenic compound, equol in the rumen. Rumen microbes may require up to 10 days adapting to phytooestrogens, so genistein may initially evoke oestrogenic effects. Equol is the major isoflavonoid in plasma of livestock and appears to be the oestrogenic agent in clover disease in sheep. Ewes grazing on oestrogenic pastures around the time of mating develop 'temporary infertility' characterized by low ovulation and conception rates. This form of infertility is reversed within 4-6 weeks of transfer of ewes to non-oestrogenic pasture. Prolonged consumption of oestrogenic pasture can induce permanent infertility in ewes.

Isoflavonoids may also impair male reproductive function by reducing testicular development and spermatogenesis.

Some plants are normally non-oestrogenic but upon fungal infection can produce high concentrations of coumestan. The consumption of oestrogenic forages causes severe infertility in sheep but not in cattle and post-natal deaths in lambs (McDonald et al., 2002). The excessive intake of lucerne and clover affects the reproductive functions in ruminants.

Steroid saponins

Steroid saponins also referred to as sarsaponin occur in yucca (*Yucca shidigera*). Yucca is sometimes grazed by cattle in New Mexico, in the U.S., particularly in times of drought and feed shortage. These saponins have favourable effects upon ruminant digestion and performance, especially microbial nitrogen metabolism. They control ammonia levels in poultry houses. Hence yucca shidigera extracts are popular feed additives.

Silica urinary calculi or urolithiasis

Silica can comprise up to 10% of grasses on a dry matter basis. It can substantially reduce forage digestibility at high level. Silica, particularly in association with low water intake, is also responsible for the development of silica kidney stones and the condition known as silica urinary calculi or urolithiasis. This malady occurs in both cattle and sheep, especially in castrated males. Silica stones collect in the urethra, thereby interfere with urine flow; in advanced stages the bladder may rupture and urine collect in the abdominal cavity, leading to an extended abdomen referred to as "watery belly". Other symptoms include tail twitching, uneasiness, kicking at abdomen and straining in an attempt to urinate.

Prevention includes encouraging high water intake for diluting silicic acid and other interacting minerals in the urine. Force feeding high levels of common salt will increase water intake. Ammonium chloride and phosphorus supplements aid in acidifying the urine and reducing the formation of silica stones.

Roots and Tubers
Roots

The most important root crops used in the feeding of farm animals are turnips, swedes, mangels and fodder beet. Swedes (Brassica napus) and turnips (Brassica campestris) are liable to taint milk if given to milch animals at the time of milking or just before milking. The volatile compound responsible for the taint is absorbed by the milk and is not passed through the milk.

Mangels, fodder beet and sugar beet are all members of the same species, Beta vulgaris (oxalate producing plant). Roots are characterized by high moisture content, low crude fibre content and low crude protein content. Most of the organic matter is sugars (glucose and fructose) and is of high digestibility.

Green tops: Mangel, fodder beet and sugar beet tops contain oxalic acid and its salts and other toxic ingredients, yet to be identified. Animals suffer from diarrhoea and the condition may lead to death, in extreme cases. The risk appears to be reduced by allowing the leaves to wilt. Swede and turnip tops may cause haemolytic anaemia in ruminants. All these green tops are excellent sources of β-carotene.

Tubers

The main tubers are potatoes, cassava and sweet potatoes. These contain either starch or fructan as the main storage carbohydrate unlike glucose or sucrose in root crops. Tubers have higher dry matter, lower crude fibre and lower crude protein.

Potatoes: Potatoes (*Solanum tuberosum*) have an alkaloid, solanidine, which occurs free and also in combination as the glyco-alkaloids, chaconine and solanine. Solanidine and its derivatives are toxic to animals and causes gastroenteritis. The alkaloid levels may be high in potatoes exposed to light due to the production of chlorophyll. That is why, green potatoes should be regarded as suspect. Young shoots are also likely to be rich in solanidine and these should be removed and discarded before feeding. Immature potatoes have been found to contain more solanidine than mature tubers. Cooking of tubers reduce the toxic risk. Ensiling also destroys some of the toxin. Ruminants are more resistant to toxicity than monogastric animals, possibly due to partial destruction of the toxin in the rumen.

Cassava: Cassava or manioc (*Manihot esculenta*) tubers are used for the production of tapioca starch for human consumption although the tuber is also given to livestock and poultry. Cassava plants and tubers contain varying proportions of two cyanogenetic glucosides, linamarin or phaseolunatin and lotaustralin. These are readily broken down to give hydrocyanic acid and hence are toxic to a certain degree. Boiling remove the glucosides.

Sweetpotato: Sweetpotato (*Ipomoea batatas*) is an important tropical plant. These are popularly grown for human consumption. Trypsin inhibitors are reported to be present in the tubers.

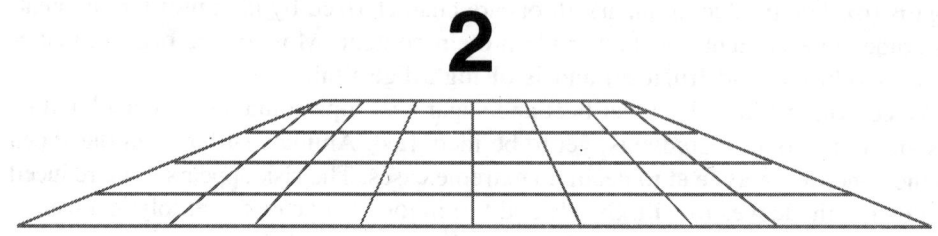

Mycotoxins Associated with Roughages Plant Poisoning in Animals

Mycotoxins associated with roughages

Dicoumarol

Dicoumarol is anti-metabolite of vitamin K. Fungal infestation of sweet clover plant produces dicoumarol and feeding of such fodder cause sweet clover poisoning or bleeding disease with internal haemorrhages. Coumarin (chemically the lactone form of coumaric acid) is found in sweet clover (Melilotus spp) as melilotoside, which is converted to dicoumarol by mould growth. Dicoumarol is the oxidation product of coumarin and it is responsible for poisoning.

Mouldy infestation of rice straw

Mouldy infestation of rice straw in winter season causes a disease which resembles clinically "chronic ergot poisoning" has been reported among cattle and buffaloes in rice growing regions of India. The outbreak is common in winter when 'rice straw' constitutes the major component of diet. Studies have indicated the presence of mycotoxins. Rice straw has oxalates. The affected animals exhibit the clinical symptoms within 5 to 14 days of eating the straw. Symptoms include lameness, disinclination to move and swelling of the legs particularly the fetlock region. Oedema and gangrene of the earlobes, tail and tip of the tongue are also observed. Milk production is reduced. The mortality rate in buffaloes is 20 percent. Treatment includes change of feed, administration of arsenical preparations and antiallergic drugs. Antibiotics to prevent secondary bacterial infection may also be used.

Ergovaline

Endophytes are symbiotic fungi and contaminate certain grasses and produce the mycotoxin, ergovaline, which is known to be toxic to livestock.

Zearalenone

It is a non-steroidal oestrogen produced by Fusarium sp. of fungi that are commonly found in pastures under hot, dry conditions and has been found to reduce reproductive performance (incidence of ovulation, fertilization rate, etc) in sheep if concentrations in the pasture exceed 1 mg/kg DM. Poplar leaf rust severely contaminated the poplar tree leaves and produces an unknown oestrogenic substance, similar to zearalenone. Ingestion of such mycotoxins produced by the fungal contaminate *Melampsora larici populina* (poplar leaf rust) or an associate fungus may also reduce ovulation rate.

Trichothecenes

Trichothecenes (nivalenol, deoxy-nivalenol) are a group of mycotoxins produced by Fusarium spp. that can cause a variety of human and animal toxicity. Trichothecenes may partly be responsible for animal 'ill-thrift' (failure to grow or produce) disorders.

Fungal tremorgens

Ryegrass staggers is a neuromuscular disorder affecting sheep and cattle grazing perennial ryegrass pastures. Ryegrass staggers generally occurs when the pasture is short. The toxic fungal toxins called tremorgens (verruculogen and paxilline) are produced by Penicillium spp. such as *P. paxilli*. It is believed that the predominant means by which livestock acquire the toxins is through ingestion of soil when grazing short pasture. The toxic pasture grass in general does not seem to contain the tremorgens. Apparently the presence of ryegrass is necessary for the growth of the Penicillium spp. in the soil, where it produces toxin. Heavy grazing intensity increases the likelihood that the grass supply will be depleted, causing close grazing that increase soil, and hence toxin ingestion. It is reported that the tremorgans can be absorbed by ryegrass plants from the soil and translocated to the leaves. It is also reported that an endophytic seed-borne fungus was associated with the occurrence of ryegrass staggers.

Paspalum staggers occurs in cattle, and occasionally in sheep and horses in several parts of the world where Paspalum spp. are grown as pasture grasses. The grass is frequently infected by ergot (Claviceps paspali), and for many years ergot was believed to be the causative agent of paspalum staggers. But it appears that paspalum staggers is caused by tremorgens produced by Claviceps paspali infection of Paspalum seed heads.

Fungal phomopsins

The growth of the Phomopsis (*Phomopsis leptostromiformis*) fungus on lupine may be weather related, with warm, wet, humid conditions favouring its growth. It infects the green lupine plant initially, but persists on the stubble. All lupine stubble is potentially toxic. Sheep and cattle, when graze on these stubbles, get this lupinosis (Cheeke and Shull, 1985) due to the ingestion of toxins (phomopsins) produced by the fungus. Lupinosis is characterized by severe liver damage. The first signs of development of lupinosis are a loss of appetite and a loss of weight and condition.

Liver and gall bladder are increased in size. Symptoms of jaundice appear. The membranes of the eye and mouth may be intensely yellow. In Australia, sheep exposed to lupinosis toxins may also consume pyrrolizidine alkaloids in such plants as *Heliotropium europaeum*. Because both have hepatoxic effects, it is likely that they could have additive or synergistic activity.

Sometimes cattle develop photosensitization in addition to liver damage. Generally, this condition occurs when new grass growth begins at the beginning of the pasture season. The udder is often affected, and the cow refuses to let the calf nurse. The photosensi-tization is probably a result of the increased chlorophyll intake when grass growth begins (Cheeke and Shull, 1985). The increased phylloerythrin load cannot be excreted by the damaged liver, and secondary photosensitization occurs.

Photosensitizing agents

- Photosensitization is caused by ingestion of buckwheat which contains photodynamic compound, fagopyrin.
- Photosentization is seldom fatal and disappears if the plant containing photodynamic agent is withdrawn. Light skinned animals are more susceptible.
- Photosensitization may also occur with other green grasses such as Panicum and Brachiaria (Negi, 1961).

Primary and secondary photosensitization

Photodynamic substances in the peripheral circulation may cause the development of photosensitization reaction i.e., animals become hypersensitive to light. It may be primary or secondary. Primary photosensitization is caused by ingestion of photodynamic agents, which are absorbed and react with light at the skin's surface and produce lesions. The symptoms consist of dermatitis, oedema, necrosis and peeling of skin.

The secondary photosensitizers are compounds that induce liver disfunction and obstruction of the bile duct. The liver toxin is not photodynamic by itself, but the liver damage prevents the normal excretion of phylloerythrin and bilirubin, degradation products of chlorophyll. Phylloerythrin is more photodynamic compared to bilirubin. Secondary photosensitization is caused by phylloerythrin, a metabolite of chlorophyll. It is normally excreted in the bile, but in cases of liver damage phylloerythrin enters general circulation and causes skin lesions when it reacts with ultraviolet light. The symptoms include icterus and anorexia (in addition to those of primary photosensitization) which may cause death of the animal.

Mouldy straw-induced photosensitization

Cheeke and Shull (1985) mentioned a photosensitization condition in cattle in Utah, USA which appears to be associated with the consumption of mouldy wheat straw during winter season in beef cattle. Affected cattle show the usual clinical signs of photosensitization, including ulcerated lesions in nonpigmented skin. The eyes and skin around the eyes are particularly affected, as are the muzzle, underside of the jaw, the teats, and the lower limbs. These areas have the shortest hair coat and receive both direct light and light reflected from snow. Evidences of liver damage are observed. The affected cattle recover when removed from access to the mouldy straw.

Plant Poisoning in Animals
Bracken fern (*Pteridium aquilinum*) poisoning

Bracken fern is poisonous to all classes of livestock. It is unpalatable and must be grazed over a long period of time before poisoning occurs. Livestock rarely graze bracken fern if good forage is available. Bracken fern contains an enzyme thiaminase, which causes a thiamine deficiency. Poisoning cases can be treated with thiamine. Bracken fern also contains a cyanogenic glycoside, prunasin and carcinogens.

Kikuyu poisoning

Kikuyu grass is a tropical forage species used extensively in pastures. In New Zealand, South Africa and Australia, kikuyu poisoning has been observed in cattle, sheep and horses. It was first reported in New Zealand. Signs of toxicity generally occur 24-48 h after animals consume the toxic pasture. Clinical signs include anorexia, depression, drooling, colic, grinding of teeth, cessation of ruminal and intestinal movement, and lack of faecal excretion. Muscle twitching, a high stepping gait, and occasionally convulsions are seen. A distinctive feature is 'sham drinking', cattle congregate at water tank/pond and even put their mouths into or onto the water, but fail to drink. The most striking lesion is an intensive necrosis of the rumen and omasum mucosa. Mortality of affected animals is about 80%. In some cases, kikuyu poisoning is associated with army worm infestation of the pasture; trichothecene mycotoxins are also involved.

Lantana poisoning in cattle

Lantana spp. are commonly grown as hedge plant and are seen in fallow land. *Lantana camara* is widely present in hilly regions of India, for example in Kangra valley of Himalchal Pradesh. They grow well during rainy season. Cattle occasionally graze on *Lantana camera leaves* when they are hungry leading to toxicosis. The problem has often been overlooked as it occurs sporadically in cattle. Triterpenes are stated to be the principal toxic agent. Lantadene A is reported to be most toxic of triterpenes. Consumption of L. camara leaves causes hepatotoxicity and photosensitization. It brings intrahepatic cholestasis leading to jaundice. This may be accompanied by kidney failure due to tubular degeneration and necrosis.

Symptoms: The common clinical signs are dullness, loss of appetite, jaundice, slow pulse, subnormal temperature and constipation in some cases. Some affected animals show signs of excitability for 2-3 days initially. Photosensitization dermatitis, especially on ear and perineum is also observed.

Treatment: Treatment includes parental administration of dextrose, pheneramine maleate and liver extract and oral administration of liver tonics. Recovery has been observed in 73% of cases.

Toxicity of Brassica forage crops

The important species of the genus *Brassica* are kales, cabbage, rapes, turnips and swedes. These are grown as forage, root or oilseed crops. All brassicas contain glucosinolates, S-methylcysteine sulphoxide (SMCO) and erucic acid. Glucosinolates are thioglucosides, which are of particular significance in brassica vegetables and forage crops. The most common breakdown products (by plant or microbial thioglucosidase or myrosinase) are isothiocyanates and nitriles and a number of other metabolites. Important examples are kale (*Brassica oleracea* var. *fruticose* & var. *acephala*), rape (*Brassica napus* / *Brassica campestris*), cabbage (*B. oleracea*, var. *capitata*).

A goitrogen present in brassicas has been identified as L-5-vinyl-2-oxarolidine-2-thione (goitrin). This inhibits the iodination of tyrosine and thus interferes with thyroxine synthesis. Therefore, it cannot be overcome by adding more iodine to the diet. Thiocyanate, another goitrogen is also present. Goitrogenic activity of the thiocyanate type is prevented by supplying adequate iodine in the diet. The goitrogenic substance present in the forage crops of the brassica is mainly the thiocyanate type and hence its effects can be overcome by increasing the iodine content of the diet. Goitrogens have been reported in milk of cows fed on goitrogenic plants. It has been suggested that drinking of such milk may cause goiter in children (McDonald et al., 1995; pp449). Pregnant ewes delivered either dead or deformed lambs.

Forage brassicas may also cause a haemolytic anaemia or kale anaemia in ruminants when the blood haemoglobin content falls to only one-third of the normal value and the haemoglobin of the rapidly destroyed red blood cells appears in the urine (haemoglobinuria). The condition is due to the presence of unusual amino acid, S-methylcysteine sulphoxide (SMCO), which is reduced to dimethyl disulphide in the rumen. The dimethyl disulphide is known to damage the red blood cells. A severe haemolytic anaemia develops within 1-3 weeks in animals fed mainly on Brassica forage. If the forage is withdrawn, blood chemistry is restored to normal within 3-4 weeks. This condition can be avoided by limiting the kale or rape not more than one-third of the animal's dry matter intake.

Oak (*Quercus incana*) leaf poisoning in cattle

Tannins, such as tannic acid and its phenolic acid constituent, gallic acid, are the causative agents. Poisoning of cattle occurs from consumption of oak buds, leaves, twigs, and acorns. The tannin content of leaves and other parts are high in the immature stages. Consumption of mature oak leaves does not normally cause the death of animals, though their consumption impairs production (Makkar, 2003). Rumen microbes are capable of degrading hydrolysable tannins. Poisoning from the consumption of oak leaves therefore, appears to be due to absorption of degraded products of hydrolysable tannins (in particular gallotannins) and higher load of phenols in the blood stream, which is beyond the capability of liver to detoxify them. Very high levels of tannin intake by animals can produce toxicity and can even cause death (Garg et al., 1992).

The condensed tannins are not absorbed into the blood stream and hence, are not likely to damage organs such as liver, kidney, spleen, etc., under normal physiological conditions. However, when intestinal damage occurred either due to consumption of high levels of tannins or other intestinal membrane irritants, condensed tannins may get absorbed into blood and can cause damage to organs similar to those observed for hydrolysable tannins.

The initial signs of oak poisoning include anorexia, depression, clear watery nasal discharge, rumen stasis, excessive thirst, and frequent urination. Initial constipation is follwed by the excretion of dark, thin, mucoid, and often bloody faeces. The principal lesions are gastritis and nephritis. The abomasum and small intestine are often inflamed and haemorrhagic.

Goats can utilize oak browse productively. Feeding high levels of immature gambel oak (*Quercus gamnelii*) to goats did not produce any toxicological reactions (Nastis and Malechek, 1981). It was concluded that feeding mature oak leaves contribute effectively to the nutrition of growing and lactating goats, while immature oak leaves had a low ME content and of low palatability but not toxic.

3

Natural Plant Toxicants in Milk

Naturally occurring toxins in feedstuffs

The U.S. Food and Drug Administration (FDA) is responsible for ensuring the safety of the human and animal food supply. Within the FDA, the Center for Veterinary Medicine (CVM) has the responsibility for ensuring that the animal feed supply is safe and wholesome. The CVM carries out this mission in part through the Feed Contaminants Program (FCP). The FCP provides guidance for the 1. Selected inspection of animal feed establishments, 2. Collection and analysis of animal feed samples for pesticides, industrial chemicals, heavy metals, mycotoxins and microbial agents and 3. Investigation into the causes of chemical and biological residues in meat and poultry reported to the FDA through the USDA's Contamination Response System (CRS). Based on the data during 1989-1992, the FDA analyzed on average 1,172 animal feed samples annually, of which 1,024 were surveillance samples and 148 were compliance samples.

Surveillance samples: Samples collected on an objective basis where there is no inspectional or other evidence of a problem with the product.

Compliance samples: Samples collected on a selective basis as the result of an inspection, complaint, or other evidence that there may be a problem with the product. Aflatoxins have been a significant problem since their discovery in the early 1960s. Hence about 40% of the time was spent on mycotoxin surveillance.

Gossypol: Gossypol is a yellow, polyphenolic pigment found primarily in the glands of cottonseed from the genus *Gossypium*. The gossypol content of cottonseed varies from approximately 0.002% (20 ppm) to 6.64% (66,400 ppm) and is believed to provide insect resistance to the plant. Cardiac, reproductive, pulmonary and hepatic lesions have been observed in animals poisoned by gossypol. Nonruminants and immature ruminants (functionally undeveloped rumen) are particularly susceptible to gossypol toxicity. However, there are cases of gossypol toxicity in mature dairy cows and deaths of cows have been reported. The finished feed of those cows contained approximately 1,800 ppm gossypol and the cottonseed in the diet contained approximately 13,000 ppm of gossypol. The CVM recommended that the liver and kidney from any dairy cow that died be discarded before rendering.

Glucosinolates and Erucic acid: Crambe meal and rapeseed meal / canola meal contain them.

Many natural plant toxicants (Table 1) are known to be present in milk of lactating animals that graze the plants containing them. Panter and James (1990) reviewed the various toxicants present in plants, their transfer to milk and their potential to humans and suckling animals.

Table 1: Plants and their toxicants

Name of the plant toxicant	Name of the plant
1. Tremetol or tremetone	White snakeroot (*Eupatorium rugosum*) Rayless goldenrod (*Hap opappus heterophyllus*)
2. Pyrrolizidine alkaloids	*Senecio spp.* *Crotalaria spp.* *Symphytum spp.* (comfrey) *Heliotropium spp.*
3. Piperidine alkaloids	*Conium maculatum* Cassia Prosopis
4. Quinolizidine alkaloids (anagyrine, thermopsine, cytisine)	Lupinus, Golden chain (*Laburnum anagyroides*)
5. Sesquiterpene lactones (Tenulen)	Bitterweed, Rubberweed, Sneezeweed
6. Glucosinolates	*Brassica* (Cabbage, broccoli, Kale, Rape, turnips) *Amoracia* (horseradish) *Limnanthes* (meadowfoam) *Raphanus* (radish)
7. Indolizidine alkaloids (Swainsonine, Slaframine)	Locoweeds (*Astragalus lentiginosus* and *Oxytropis serecia*) *Rhizoctonia leguminicola* (fungus)
8. Selenocompounds	Selenium accumulators Astragalus, Stanleya

Elimination of plant toxicants by lactating animals via milk is considered a minor route of excretion. Even then, the consumption of such milk can induce poisoning in humans or in suckling animals. Poisoning can be more severe in young suckling animals since they have less ability to eliminate or detoxify xenobiotics. The rate of elimination of toxins through milk is dependent on its concentration in the blood, its ability to diffuse across cell membranes, its affinity for certain constituents in the milk and efficiency of the major routes of detoxification and excretion (through liver, urine, faeces, etc.) to eliminate the toxin.

Glucosinolates

Glucosinolates and their derivatives can be transferred to the milk of lactating animals.

Consumption of such milk causes thyroid enlargement in young animals and in humans. Placental transfer of these compounds also may occur.

Quinolizidine alkaloids

Lupines are known to cause skeletal defects and cleft palate in calves when their dams ingested lupine plants during 40 to 70 days of gestation. Lupines contain the quinolizidine alkaloid, anagyrine. There are few reports of quinolizidine alkaloids in milk. Ortega and Lazerson (1987) reported a case of skeletal abnormalities in a child in California (USA) wherein the mother consumed milk (during pregnancy) from goats, which had grazed bush lupine plants. Several of the goats among the herd showed spontaneous abortion and the fetuses had skeletal defects. The alkaloid cytisine is found in golden chain (an ornamental tree) and in the leguminous weedy shrub (Cytisus). Cytisine is excreted through milk.

Indolizidine alkaloids

Locoweeds (*Astragalus lentiginosus* and *Oxytropis serecia*) contain swainsonine. It is an indolizidine alkaloid and may be transferred in the milk. James and Hartley (1977) fed milk from cows fed locoweed to calves, kittens and lambs and observed microscopic lesions of locoweed poisoning such as neurovisceral foamy cytoplasmic vacuolation. It seems likely that other indolizidine alkaloids such as slaframine, castanospermine may be eliminated via the milk.

Selenocompounds

Certain species of *Astragalus, Stanleya* and others may accumulate high levels of selenium. Most of these selenium-accumulating plants are unpalatable. In areas where soil selenium is high, grasses may accumulate enough to adversely affect livestock production. Selenium is present in cow's milk in concentrations in direct proportion to selenium intake. Human milk may contain selenium in concentrations twice as high as reported in cow's milk (National Academy of Science, 1976). Young animals are more susceptible than adults to the toxic effects of selenium.

Sesquiterpene lactones

The sesquiterpene lactones present in bitterweed, etc. impart a bitter flavour to the milk of lactating animals when such plants are consumed. The bitter principle in sneezeweed and bitterweed, tenulen make milk bitter even at 1 ppm level in the milk. Similarly when dairy animals eat onion, garlic (*Allium spp.*), the milk (and meat) may have a disagreeable taste.

Bracken fern

The toxin present in bracken fern is carcinogenic and milk from the cow fed bracken fern has induced urinary carcinomas in rats (Pamukcu et al., 1978).

It appears that majority of toxicants transferred into milk belong to the chemical class, alkaloids. Plant alkaloids frequently are quite basic and they tend to accumulate in the milk. Further, if the plant toxicant possesses a reasonable degree of lipophilicity, it may be irreversibly retained in the milk. Thus a combination of basicity and fat solubility may result in accumulation of the plant alkaloids in the milk and reduced excretion by normal processes.

4

Plant Secondary Metabolites – Detoxification by Rumen Microbes – Toxins Produced by Rumen Microbes

Secondary Plant Compounds (SPC)

Forage plants often contain antinutritive or secondary compounds that can seriously restrict their value as animal feeds. Plants contain lignin, cutin, suberin and biogenic silica and a far more diverse and active chemical defense arsenal of secondary plant compounds. They physically impede digestive enzymes or microorganisms and their effects can range from feeding deterrence to toxicity. They have been labeled "secondary" because few have primary metabolic functions within the plant and at one time they were viewed as end products of other metabolic systems.

Secondary Plant Compounds are antiherbivory chemicals. Although SPC are invariably viewed as antinutrients, some may have beneficial roles in animal nutrition. The three most prevalent groups of SPC are soluble phenolics, alkaloids and terpenoids. Soluble plant phenolics include flavonoids, isoflavonoids (phytoestrogens) and hydrolysable and condensed tannins. Certain of these substances such as estrogens and cyanides have more effect upon the animal and its metabolism than upon digestion process.

Detoxification by rumen microbes

The plant secondary metabolites are thought to have a defensive role that ensures survival of the plant, by protecting them against insect predation or by restricting grazing by herbivores. There are many examples of plants being toxic to nonruminant but not to ruminant animals, because ruminal microbial activity transforms or degrades these compounds into less toxic or harmless products (Hobson and Stewart, 1997; Mackie et al., 1997).

Apart from degrading polysaccharides, nitrogenous compounds, lipids and nucleic acids, the ruminal ecosystem has the ability to adapt and increase its capacity to metabolize minor components, such as plant secondary compounds. The best example of the commercial exploitation of ruminal detoxification for production purposes is the use of the ruminal bacterium *Synergistes jonesii* to detoxify the mimosine. Goats in Indonesia and Hawaii are adapted to Leucaena by degrading the mimosine to nontoxic products. Rumen liquor transfer from such animals to Australian ruminants successfully has provided the precedent for exploiting the diverse and dynamic population of rumen microorganisms as a solution to the antinutritive properties of many forages (see Table 1 for details). The ecology of *Synergistes jonesii* is remarkable and exceptional in that the organism appears to be transferable between cattle, sheep and goats and can establish in the rumen after being cultured in the laboratory.

Table 1: Rumen metabolism of toxins associated with fodder plants

Compound	Detoxification mechanism	Microorganisms involved
1. Nonprotein amino acid Mimosine	Ring cleavage of 3,4-dihydroxypyridine	*Synergistes jonesii*
2. Aliphatic nitro compounds 3-nitro-1-propionic acid (3NPA) 3-nitro-1-propanol 3NPOH)	Reduction of the nitro group and deamination to β-alanine Reduction to 3-amino-1-propanol	*Megasphaera elsdenii* *Coprococcus spp.*, *Selenomonas spp.*
3. Nitrate-nitrite	Reduction of nitrate to nitrite Reduction of nitrite to ammonia	*Selenomonas spp.* *No isolates identified*
4. Phenolics Hydrolysable tannin	Ester hydrolysis	*Selenomonas ruminantium* *Streptococcus spp.*
	Eubacterium Dehydroxylation	
Trihydroxybenzenoids (gallate)	Ring cleavage *Coprococcus spp.* Unknown Dehydroxylation	*oxidoreducens* *Streptococcus bovis* *Syntrophoccus bovis* *Selenomonas spp.*,
Ferulic and p-coumaric acid Flavonoid glycosides	Glycoside hydrolysis	*Butyrivibro spp.* *Peptococcus spp.*, *Eubacterium*
	Heterocyclic ring cleavage *oxidoreducens* *Butyrivibro spp.*	
Condensed and hydrolysable tannin	Tannin tolerance	*Streptococcus gallolyticus*, *Streptococcus bovis* *Clostridium spp.*, *Prevotella ruminicola*, *Selenomonas ruminantium*
5. Phytooestrogens Isoflavones Formononetin, daidzein, genestein, Biochanin, coumestrol	Demethylation Heterocyclic ring clevage	No isolates identified

Compound	Detoxification mechanism	Microorganisms involved
6. Oxalate	Metabolized to formate	*Oxalobacter formigenes*
7. Pyrrolizidine alkaloids Heliotrine	Ester hydrolysis of carbon side-chain; reduction of 1,2 double bond of the heterocyclic ring	*Peptococcus heliotrinereducens*
8. Mycotoxins, Tricothecenes	De-epoxidation	*Butyrivibrio fibrisolvens*
T-2 toxin, HT-2 toxin Deoxynivalenol, Diacetoxyscirpenol, ochratoxin	De-esterification Isovalerylde-esterification	*Selenomonas ruminantium*

Toxins produced by rumen microbes

Rumen microbes convert nontoxic compounds into toxic ones resulting in animal disease or death.

- Hydrolysis of cyanogenic glycosides to hydrogen cyanide causing sudden death due to lack of oxygen supply
- Metabolism of tryptophan to 3-methylindole resulting in acute bovine pulmonary edema and emphysema
- Reduction of nitrates to toxic nitrites
- Reduction of S-methylcysteine sulfoxide to dimethyl disulfide, and
- Ovine rumen microbial production of toxic sapogenins, epi-sarsasapogenin and epi-smilagenin from signal grass (*Brachiaria decumbens*). It appears only sheep rumen microbes produce toxins and not that of cattle.

SECTION V
Feed Technology

Dr. Harry B. Pfost and Feed Manufacturing Technology books

No person has contributed more to the technology of feed manufacturing or has had more influence in moving the industry from the state-of-the-art to the state-of-the science than Harry Pfost.

Dr. Harry B. Pfost, Professor in the Department of Grain Science and Industry at Kansas State University, USA, was responsible for publication of Feed Manufacturing Technology (FMT) books. As Editor-in-Chief, he brought out "Feed Production Handbook" in 1961. Subsequently, Dr. Pfost served as Technical Editor for AFMA publications "Feed Manufacturing Technology" I (1970) and II (1976) and was a major chapter contributor to both the editions. Later FMT III (1985) and FMT IV (1994) have been brought out. These have become popular books of feed manufacturing throughout the world.

The feed industry got its start in the United States primarily as an outlet or dumping ground for milling byproducts, first feed mill being built in 1875. Pelleting was introduced into Europe about 1920 and into the US feed industry in the late 1920's. Its popularity has grown steadily and currently about 80% of all feed in the US are pelleted.

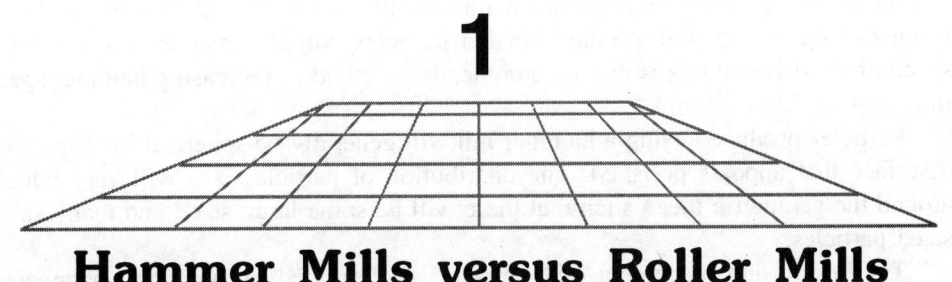

1

Hammer Mills versus Roller Mills

Effect of particle size on energy consumption and production rate

Work from Kansas State University demonstrated that hammer milling maize to mean particle sizes of 1,000, 800, 600 and 400 microns slightly increased milling energy from 2.7 to 3.8kWh/t as particle size decreased from 1,000 to 600 microns. However, the energy required to reduce particle size another 200 microns to 400 microns was more than twice (i.e., 8.1 kWh/t) the energy needed to mill maize to 600 microns. Production rate also decreased slightly as mean particle size decreased from 1,000 to 600 microns, but grinding to a smaller size drops the output to a lower volume fast (Dick Ziggers, Feed Tech, 5, 7, 9-12).

Degree of processing varies with the animal: Every animal has its own needs, which means that the degree of processing for various diets must also vary. Ruminants have rather long, complex digestive tracts and so require a less processed feed material. Pigs have a fairly short, simple digestive system (similar to humans) and, therefore, benefits from a more highly processed feed. Poultry have a short but rather complicated digestive system, and depending on the make up of the diet, can efficiently utilize feedstuffs less highly processed than pigs. The size and age of the animals also affect the dietary requirements concerning particle size. In general younger animals benefit more from a finer, more highly processed feed than older livestock that have a fully developed digestive tract.

Machines used: When it comes to particle size reduction there are two main machines used: the hammer mill and the roller mill. Both are capable of producing the desired particle size. However, there are advantages and disadvantages that must be considered to determine the best mill.

Hammer mills

Size reduction using a hammer mill is accomplished through the impact of a slow moving target, example a cereal grain, with a rapidly moving hammer. The target has little or no momentum, whereas the hammer tip is travelling at a minimum of 5,000 to 7,000m/min. The collision fractures the grain into many pieces. The size reduction is influenced by hammer tip speed, hammer design and placement, screen design and hole size, and the use of air. Impact is the primary force in a hammer mill to reduce particle size. Anything that increased the chance of a collision between a hammer and a target, increase the magnitude of the collision.

Increasing the rotor diameter in a hammer mill at a constant drive speed and with a constant screen size will produce smaller particles. Simply changing the rotational speed of the drive source is not a recommended method of increasing hammer speed in excess of 7,000 m/min.

Particles produced using a hammer mil will generally be spherical in shape with a surface that appears polished. The distribution of particle sizes will vary widely around the geometric mean such that there will be some large sized and many small sized particles.

The design and placement of hammers is determined by operating parameters such as rotor speed, motor horse power, and open area in the screen. Optimal hammer design and placement will provide maximum contact with the feed ingredient. Koch (1995) advised a hammer length of 25 cm, width of 6.35 cm and thickness of 6.4 mm when the rotor speed is approximately 1,800 rpm. One hammer for every 2.5 to 3.5 hp should be sufficient. For a rotor that runs at 3,600 rpm the hammer can be smaller: 15 to 20 cm long and 5 cm wide. Also one hammer for every 1 to 2 hp is advised. Hammers should be balanced and arranged on the rods so that they don't trail one another. The distance between hammer and screen should be 12 to 14 mm.

Screen of the hammer mill

What actually determines the sizing and grinding effect of the hammer mill is the screen. When the open area in the screen is not in line with the (horse) power of the hammer mill heat will generate. A temperature rise of the grinded material to 45oC may decrease the capacity by as much as 50 percent. A correct ratio of open screen to horsepower would be 55 square cm area per horsepower. If the open screen area is too small, particles will be swept along the face of the screen and will cause a fluidised bed of material. As these particles rub against the screen and each other, their size is continually reduced by abrasion, resulting in energy waste, heat production, restricted throughput, and particles become too small. A **correct ratio of screen opening to horsepower** in combination with a **proper distance between hammers and screen face** will ensure a timely exit of ground material of the required size from the mill.

To avoid this fluidised bed effect most hammer mills are designed with an air assist system that draws air into the hammer mill with the product to be ground. On the exit side of the screen reduced pressure disrupts the fluidised bed of material on the face of the screen. Also in full circle hammer mills the screen is in two pieces where on the upward arc of the hammers a larger hole size is used to further reduce the amount of material on the face of the screen.

Air assist systems in hammer mills

A properly designed and sized hammer mill provides the impact at the hammer tips required in either breaking or cutting the product being ground. Without proper air flow, this high speed rotation and its attendant grinding action will not only hold sized product in rotation, but create a heating action within the material being ground leading to many other problems (Jerry R. Olson, 1984).

The air assist system controls the environment of the grinding chamber in the hammer mill and provides the critical path of exit to aid in breaking the rotational pull of the hammers to efficiently move the sized product through the screen perforations. This rapid movement of material away from the grinding area avoids over-grinding of material to help maintain uniform particles size control. An air-assisted hammer mill uses a positive air fan and cyclone collector pulling through an air product conveyor. Some use a self-cleaning fabric filter to pull air through air product conveyor. A cross sectional view of the air-assisted hammer mill is shown in Fig. 1. Such air-assisted hammermilling system, will deliver maximum throughput at the lowest power cost, efficiently control particle sizing, eliminate, or reduce to a minimum, the product heating and control dusting and pressure buildup from the hammer mill. Air assisted milling systems will produce by 15 to 40% more than non-assisted hammer mills. Well designed air-assisted hammer milling systems are energy efficient, environmentally sound, high capacity uniform product producers, and economically feasible with a surprisingly fast return on investment.

Advantages

➢ Produce a wide range of particle sizes
➢ Work with any friable material and fibre
➢ Less initial purchase cost compared to roller mill
➢ Offer minimal expense for maintenance
➢ Generally feature uncomplicated operation
➢ Greater capacity per unit horsepower than roller mill

Disadvantages

➢ Provide less efficient use of energy compared to the roller mill
➢ May generate heat (energy loss)
➢ May create noise and dust pollution
➢ Produce greater particle size variability

To conclude, hammer mills have a greater capacity per unit of horsepower, and it is easy to change from grinding one grain to another by changing screens. However, a hammer mill requires more energy than a roller mill and will produce a higher percentage of fines and dust.

Roller mills

While hammer mills have been the most common grinder used in the feed industry, roller mills have also been used for many years. Roller mills have been used to perform a wide variety of tasks related to the production of animal feeds. There are several potential advantages of a roller mill grinder over a hammer mill, especially when grinding down to particle sizes typical of mash type feeds. The greatest advantage can be found in energy savings. Because of an efficient reduction action, roller mills will produce 15-40% more tonnes per hour at a given horsepower than full circle

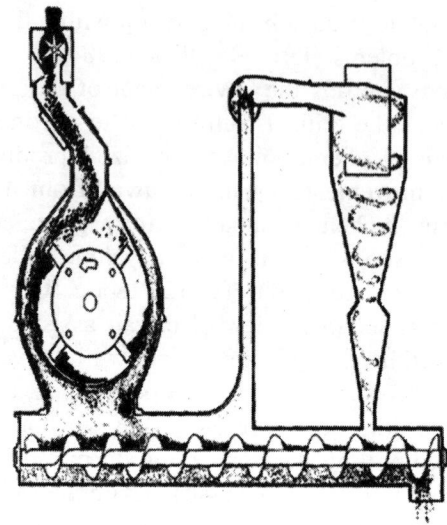

Figure 1. A cut away view showing air and material flow as they move through an Air Assisted Hammermilling System

hammer mills, when producing the same finished particle size.

Roll corrugations

In a roller mill one roll is fixed in the frame and the opposing roll can be adjusted to vary the clearance between the rolls. Roll corrugations (or roll cut or fluting) will vary depending on the material to be processed, initial and finished product sized, and the product quality desired. Coarse grooving will produce a coarse finished product at high capacities, while finer grooving produces a finer finished product at lower capacities. The corrugation helps to slice the grain kernels. Every grain type has its optimum number of corrugations per cm of roll, for example maize is best ground with 3 to 4 corrugations per cm of roll, for wheat, barley and oats 4 to 5 corrugations are optimum and for sorghum 5 to 6 corrugations/cm are best. The smaller the grain the more corrugations per cm are required to get the desired grind. The corrugations should have a 2.5 to 5 cm/m spiral to increase the shearing potential and to eliminate fines.

Different roll speeds

A roller mill set up to grind mash feeds requires a special configuration. The rolls will have relatively high peripheral speeds of 450 to 900 m/min and operate with a roll speed differential. This differential drive turns one roll in each pair faster than the opposite roll. This is often expressed in the form of a ratio with the slow roll expressed as one (1). The most common arrangement for a roller mill grinder is a differential ratio of 1.5:1 with the fast roll operating a 1000 rpm, which puts the slow roll at 667 rpm. Another option is that one roll counter rotates at the same speed as its partner roll.

Each pair of rolls in a roller mill has a limit to the size of particle it can produce based on the size of the particles going in. This grinding ratio varies on the material being processed but is approximately 4:1 for most feed ingredients. When a greater reduction of particle size is required more sets of rolls are needed in one configuration. Sizing of the material is dependent upon the gap between the rolls along their length. If this gap is not uniform it will lead to increased maintenance costs, reduced throughput, and overall increased operation costs.

Advantages of roller mills

> Energy efficient
> Uniform particle size reduction
> Little noise and dust generation
> More exact control of particle size
> Reduced moisture loss from the grain

Disadvantages of the roller mills

> Little or no effect on fibre
> Particles tend to be irregular in shape and dimension
> May have high initial cost
> Maintenance can be expensive
> Adjustment needed for each grain

By stacking pairs of rolls on top of one another (two or three high) it is possible to reduce particle size down to 500 microns, similar to the size reducing capability of a hammer mill for grains. For coarse reduction of grain, a roller mill may have a significant advantage (85%) over a hammer mill in terms of throughput/kWh of energy. For cereal grains processed to sizes of 600 to 900 microns the advantage is about 30 to 50 percent.

Different particle shape

A roller mill performs its particle size reduction by compressing the particles between the rolls while at the same time cutting and shearing them using the combination of corrugations and roll speed differential. These forces produce particles that have very rough, jagged shapes with many edges and corners. A **hammer mill** grinds by impacting the particle until it passes through a screen. These particles are more spherical and polished. Rough particles from a roller mill have more surface area exposed to the animal's digestive system than particles from a hammer mill, which tends to improve the overall feed efficiency.

Because the grind produced by a roller mill is very uniform, the finished products have a good physical appearance. The low level of fines and lack of oversized particles make a feedstuff with good flow and mixing characteristics. This is very important for mash or meal feeds where the flow from bins and feeders can be difficult to control, and where segregation and separation may occur during shipping and handling.

Product quality is affected by wear of the rolls. In a roller mill the roll corrugations will wear out over time. As these items wear, there will be changes in the size and consistency of the product. However, it is possible to compensate for the gradual changes in finished products that occur due to wear by adjusting the gap between the rolls. Some materials are naturally abrasive, such as 44% soybean meal, sunflower meal, canola meal (due to the hulls), and cocoa hulls. Little can be done to reduce the effects of processing materials with highly abrasive characteristics. Using the coarsest corrugations that will achieve an acceptable grind will produce the best results in terms of roll life.

Roller mills have many distinct advantages over hammer mills, but are also limited in their use. A roller mill cannot grind the same wide variety of materials that can be ground in a hammer mill. Roller mills have trouble in grinding fibrous materials such as hulls or straw. Also products with a high fat content can clog up the rolls.

2

Feed Pelleting Technology including Newer Developments

Benefits of the pelleting technology

The pelleting process is widely used because of both the physical and nutritional benefits it provides. The physical benefits include improved ease of handling, reduced ingredient segregation, less feed wastage in the form of dust, etc., and increased bulk density. Nutritional benefits have been   measured through animal feeding trials. Feeding pelleted feed improves animal performance and efficiency of feed utilization compared with feeding a meal form of a diet. The improvements in performance have been attributed to decreased feed wastage, reduced selective feeding, less time and energy expended for prehension, destruction of pathogenic organisms, thermal modification of starch (gelatinization, etc) and protein, improved palatability.

Herein described is an account of pelleting unit, newer developments in feed pelleting technology and factors affecting pelleting of feeds.

Definition

Pelleting can be defined as the agglomeration (process of molding into a mass) of small particles into larger particles by means of a mechanical process in combination with moisture, heat and pressure. Pelleted feeds are agglomerated feeds resulting from extruding either individual feed ingredient or feed mixture by compacting and forcing through die openings by any mechanical process and subsequent cooling.

Principle of pelleting

Feed is conditioned by addition of steam (heat and water). The conditioned feed, when sufficiently controlled compression is applied, forms a dough dense mass shaped to conform to the die against which it is pressed. When it is cooled, the pellet retains its shape and density, and is of such `toughness' as to withstand handling during transport without much breakage and has retained or enhanced its nutritive value. Properly ground and mixed feed is a prerequisite for pelleting of mixed feed.

Purpose of pelleting

Finely ground, sometimes dusty, unpalatable and difficult to handle feed material is made into larger particles by application of heat, moisture and pressure. These larger particles are easier to handle, more palatable and usually result in improved feed efficiency. The increment in bulk density consequent upon pelleting allows storing more feed. Flowability of feed is also improved.

Size and shape of pellets

Pellets have diameters from 10/64 inches to 48/64 inches (3.97 to 18.8 mm) and maximum diameter generally accepted is no greater than 16/64 to 24/64 inches (6.35 to 9.53 mm). Shape of pellet is cylindrical though large sized pellets [32/64 inches (12.5 mm) and above] may be triangular, square or oval in shape. Modern pellet mills (die holes) can have diameters ranging from 1 mm to over 20 mm depending on the material to be pelleted or the animal species to be fed. Also special forms (squares, biscuit, clover, etc.) are available, which are often used for producing pet foods.

Pellet quality

Pellet quality may be defined as a certain hardness or water stability, which assures efficient use without loss in handling on land or in water. Mean particle size, inherent binding capacity and fat content of the feed mixture play major roles in pellet durability.

Types of pellets

Hard type pellets and soft type pellets. Soft type pellets are those containing over 30% molasses.

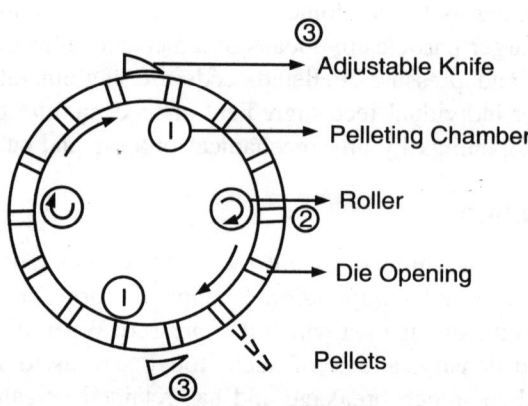

Figure 1. Hard Pellets

Hard type pellets

Mechanically, the process of pelleting involves forcing soft feed through holes in a die (Figure 1). Single or double rolls are mounted inside the die ring on a cam or eccentric. The die is driven by a motor and the rolls turn only as feed between rolls and die develops friction. The basic principle of the pellet mill is as follows.

- Blended and conditioned mash is introduced into a pelleting chamber and distributed by means of gravity, centrifugal force and mechanical deflectors.
- Pressure resulting from rotation of die and rollers forces feed through perforations in die, which compresses and forms the feed into pellets.
- Adjustable knives cut pellets into desired length.
- The pellets are then cooled and dried before bagging or binning.

Pelleting system

The pelleting system composed of different machines designed specially to accomplish the pelleting task. The component parts are as follows (Figure 2).

1. Storage bin (or) Supply bin
2. Pellet mill
3. Cooler
4. Crumbler
5. Elevating system
6. Pellet scalper (sifter or screen)
7. Steam supply

1. Storage bin or supply bin

Supply bins store mixed mash feed for pelleting in adequate quantity to ensure continuous operation of the pellet mill. This means a minimum of two bins each with a capacity of not less than one and half times the capacity of the batch mixer used to supply conditioned feed to the pellet mill.

2. Pellet mills

Pellet mills are available in a wide range of sizes: 20 to 40 horsepower to 700 horsepower. The inside diameter of the pellet die on the large mill is 37 inches (81.3 cm) versus 12 in. (30.5 cm) on the small mill. Working area on the large die is 804 sq. in. (5,190 cm2) while on the small die it is 90 sq.inches (581 cm^2). Now it is not uncommon to find a single pellet mill producing 60 tons per hour.

Pellet mills are being built with reliability and reduced maintenance in mind and are thus being designed much simpler and more rugged with prolonged longevity. Automatic lubrication systems are available with some pellet mills. By this method, grease can be supplied to the rolls and main shaft at regular intervals while the machine is running. This guarantees the right amount of lubricant to the bearings, thus avoiding excessive amounts being used which results in unnecessary costs. Excessive amounts of lubrication can also cause failure of bearings and seals.

Parts of a pellet mill

The conventional pellet mills comprise the following parts. 1. Feeder, 2. Conditioning chamber, 3. Pelleting device, 4. Speed reduction device, 5. Prime mover, and 6.Base. They are depicted in Figure 3.

Feeder

It is generally a screw type with some variation in flight arrangement such as single flight, double flight, full pitch or one half pitch to accommodate varying conditions. The feeder is equipped with some type of speed control such as a variable speed electric drive or a ratchet speed control device. The purpose of the feeder is to provide a constant controlled even flow of feed to the mixing and pelleting operation and any variation in flow results in poor conditioning and a variable product.

The component parts of a pelleting system are as follows

1. Pellet mill mash supply bin
2. Pellet mill
3. Vertical Cooler (could be horizontal)
4. Pellet Crumbler
5. Bucket elevator
6. Scalper
7. Cyclone Collector
8. Fines from cyclone returned either to mash supply bin or to pellet mill feeder
9. Overs top scalping screen flowed either to pellet bin or to crumbler for recrumbling (finished product)
10. Overs bottom scalping screen flowed either to crumble bin or to mash bin (finished product) or pellet mill feeder for repelleting
11. Fines returned either to mash supply bin or to pellet mill feeder for repelleting.

Conditioning chamber

Feed conditioning is accomplished by addition of controlled amounts of steam. Steam is preferred since it is cheap, easy to control and easy to introduce. Addition of steam supplies moisture for lubrication, liberates natural oils, and in some cases results in partial gelatinization of starches. A mixer, low speed (up to 125 rpm) or high speed (125 to 500 rpm) model, is provided in order to properly condition the feed. Further this mixer can be used for the addition of molasses up to 15% without special attachments and up to 30% when properly equipped. In some cases small amounts (1%) of fat and fish solubles can also be added.

The optimum conditions for pelleting are 13-17% moisture and 170-190°F (77-88°C) temperature as the feed enters the die. The normal moisture of mash is about 10%. It can be assumed with reasonable accuracy that 1% moisture will be added to the feed as the temperature is raised 20°F by steam addition.

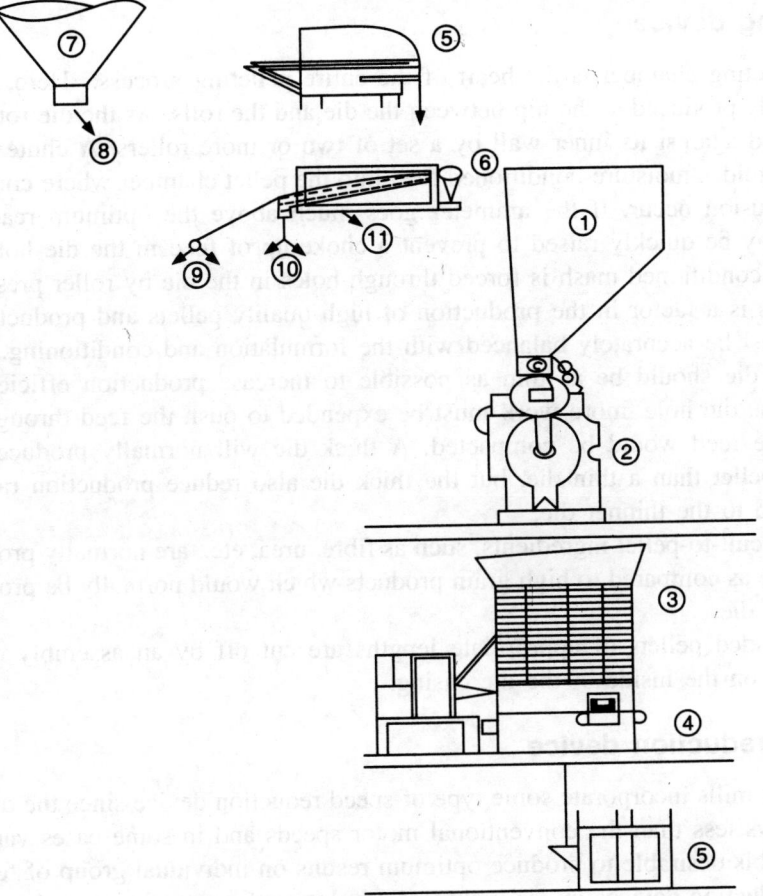

Figure 2. Typical flow chart using the cooler immediately below the pellet mill and a bucket elevator for handling the cold pellets

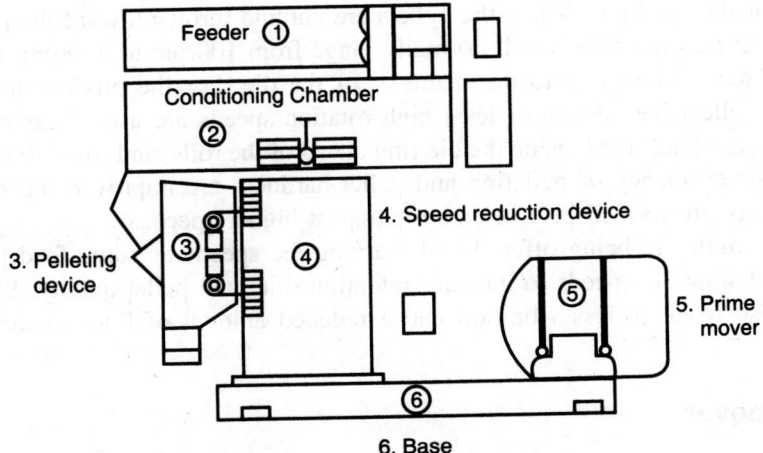

Figure 3. Parts of a Pellet Mill

Pelleting device

The pelleting chamber is the heart of the entire pelleting process. Here, the pellet is actually produced at the nip between the die and the rolls. As the die rotates, feed is pressed against its inner wall by a set of two or more rollers. A chute or funnel usually guides moisture-conditioned feed into the pellet chamber where compression and extrusion occur. If the ammeter goes much above the optimum reading, this chute may be quickly raised to prevent a choke-up of feed in the die holes.

The conditioned mash is forced through holes in the die by roller pressure. Die thickness is a factor in the production of high quality pellets and production rates. So it must be accurately balanced with the formulation and conditioning.

The die should be as thin as possible to increase production efficiency. The longer the die hole, more work must be expended to push the feed through the die and more feed would be compacted. A thick die will normally produce a better quality pellet than a thin die, but the thick die also reduce production rates when compared to the thinner die.

Difficult-to-pellet ingredients, such as fibre, urea, etc., are normally produced on a thin die as compared to high grain products which would normally be produced on a thicker die.

Extruded pellets of appropriate lengths are cut off by an assembly of knives mounted on the inside of the die casing.

Speed reduction device

All pellet mills incorporate some type of speed reduction device since the die speeds are always less than the conventional motor speeds and in some cases variation in die speed is desirable to produce optimum results on individual group of feeds. The speed reduction devices in use include direct coupled gear trains, V belts, cog belts and combination of belts and gear trains.

Pellet dies must turn fast enough to keep the feed in the pelleting chamber from plugging the mill but slow enough to keep the peripheral speed of the die from causing quality problems when the pellets are cut and thrown toward the pellet mill door. Pellet mill die speeds will normally range from 100rpm to 400rpm. RPM will have a direct relationship to the diameter of the die. For the production of small diameter pellets (i.e., 3 mm or less) high rotation speeds are used. This result in a thinner layer of soft feed inside the die ring ahead of the rolls, and for a given volume of feed the efficiency of pelleting and pellet hardness are improved. Feeds of low bulk density are formed best in dies rotating at higher speeds.

Pellet mills are being offered with varying die speeds as some feed plants are requesting slow die speeds to increase retention time and pellet quality. Slower die speeds also result in less vibration and a reduced amount of fines in the finished product.

Prime mover

Most pellet mills are installed with an electric motor as the prime mover. In some cases combustion engines are used.

An ammeter should be included as a part of the electrical system which will facilitate to allow the operator to adjust the feed rate to secure the maximum capacity of the mill without over loading the motor. It should be emphasized that the pellet mill operates most efficiently when the motor amperage use is optimum for the voltage available. It is important to watch the ammeter gauge frequently during pelleting.

Base

The pellet mill and motor are usually mounted on a common base to maintain alignment of the pellet mill and motor and to provide a rapid, simple and efficient method of installing the equipment.

3. Coolers

Pellets will leave the pellet mill at temperature as high as 190°F and as high as 17% moisture content. The moisture must be reduced to 10% and temperature to room temperature which is accomplished by passing a stream of air through a bed of pellets which evaporates excess moisture. Cooling is accomplished by a rather complex thermodynamic phenomenon combining evaporative cooling, conduction, convection and radiation.

Most of the coolers fell into 2 classes: Vertical and Horizontal. A third type of cooler known as a cylinder type has been used to a lesser extent.

Vertical cooler

The vertical cooler (Figure 4) is made up of two columns [approximately 9 inch (22.9 cm) wide] covered with wire mesh on the inside face and with louvers on the outside face. In operation, the pellets flow vertically by gravity through these columns. The flow of pellets is automatically controlled by means of a discharge gate which keeps the cooler full during operation. As the pellets flow through, they are exposed to high velocity air that cools and dries them, and air is drawn through pellets by a centrifugal fan which discharges into a dust collector for removal of fines.

Horizontal cooler

The horizontal cooler (Figure 5) is constructed using a wire mesh belt or perforated flexible metal tray mounted horizontally. A bed of pellets is carried on this belt and is made to flow through the bed by reducing the pressure in the chamber above the belt with a centrifugal fan discharging into a cyclone dust collector. Thickness of the pellet bed is controlled by the belt speed. It is a moving belt type cooler. Pellets remain stationary and this is best for fragile pellets and cubes.

Cooler that is to be preferred

The cooler type will often be determined by the plant layout and the product mix.
- Where floor space is limited, the vertical or cylinder type cooler is the most appropriate. Where height is limited, as in a basement location, the horizontal cooler is preferred.

- Vertical type coolers are normally best for small diameter pellets if the height is available for installation. Its design is simpler, with lesser maintenance and energy costs.
- The pellet discharge from a vertical cooler has a very smooth, constant flow rate that makes it ideal for feeding crumble rolls.
- Due to the configuration of the horizontal cooler, there are fewer tendencies to pull fines into the air stream than in a vertical cooler. The horizontal cooler is more complicated from a mechanical stand point; more moving parts mean higher maintenance costs. The tray type horizontal cooler has a surging (roll on like waves) discharging characteristic, which is not an ideal way to feed crumble rolls. Therefore, proper attention must be given to spouting, speed adjustment, and bed depths to achieve the best crumbler performance.
- Horizontal coolers are particularly used when very sticky   feeds are manufactured. Best for fragile pellets and cubes.

Parts of a vertical coller

1. Hopper and level sensing device to maintain a supply of pellets ahead of cooling columns
2. Cooling columns
3. Air chamber
4. Discharge drive gate motor and controls
5. Discharge gates
6. Centrifugal fan
7. Fan drive motor
8. Cyclone or dust collector

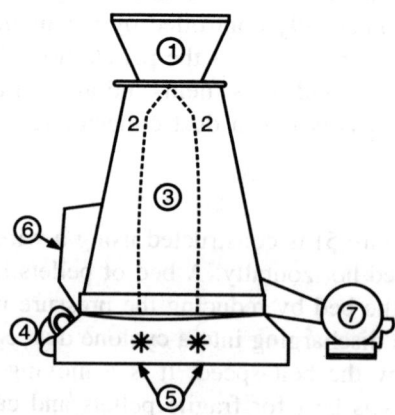

Figure 4. Vertical Pellet Cooler

Parts of a horizontal cooler

1. Oscillating feeder device
2. Product carrying belt

3. Air chamber
4. Air inlets
5. Cooling belt drive

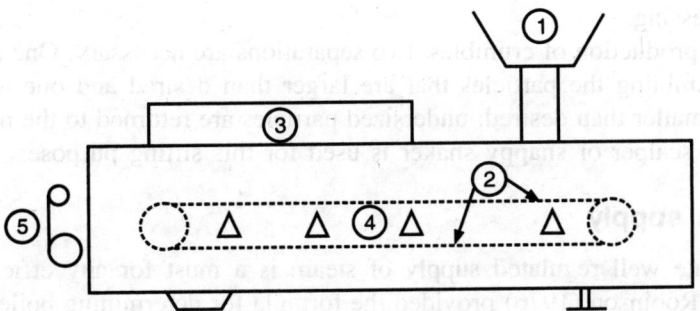

Figure 5. Horizontal Cooler

4. Crumbler

It is economical to produce 10/64 or 12/64 inch pellets and reduces to desired particle size by means of crumbling. The objective of crumbling is not merely to reduce the size of pellets but to control the reduction to a specific particle size with a minimum of fines. In this process pellets of 10/64 in. (3.97 mm) or 12/64 in. (4.76 mm) diameter are ground on corrugated rolls and the resultant product is graded by sifting over appropriate screen sizes.

Most crumbling mills consist of one pair of corrugated rolls mounted in a frame directly below the cooler. Crumbling rolls are up to 12 in. diameter and up to 72 in. length.

There are two basic types of roller corrugations, the Le page cut and the Twin-City cut. The Le Page cut has a fast roll that is cut longitudinally, acting as a feed roll and the slow roll has corrugations circumferentially around the roll. The Twin-City cut has both a fast and a slow roll with longitudinal corrugations.

Bypass valve of the crumbling mill diverts the pellets to the nip of the crumble rolls when crumbles are required and around them when crumbling is not required.

5. Pellet elevating systems

Pellets are usually elevated either by standard bucket elevators or by air. Bucket elevators are exclusively used for cold pellets as these are less expensive to install and operate and result in less product abrasion. Pneumatic conveyors are generally used for hot pellets.

Pellets are most vulnerable to damage before being cooled. Conveying equipment between the pellet mill and the cooler creates fines. Belt conveyors and drag conveyors will normally create less pellet damage than other types of conveyors when handling pellets after they leave the cooler or crumbler rolls. Conveying equipment should be operated as slowly as possible.

6. Sifting devices

Some type of sifting is necessary to remove fines produced during pelleting and crumbling and while passing through the cooler. Fines are returned to the pellet mill for reprocessing.

In the production of crumbles, two separations are necessary. One to remove for further crumbling the particles that are larger than desired and one to remove the particles smaller than desired; undersized particles are returned to the pellet mill. An oscillating scalper or snappy shaker is used for this sifting purpose.

7. Steam supply

An adequate well regulated supply of steam is a must for any efficient pelleting operation. Robinson (1976) provided the formula for determining boiler horsepower (HP) requirement for pellet production.

$$\text{Boiler H.P. required} = \frac{F \times M}{0.83 \times 34.5}$$

Where, F = Pounds of feed per hour

M = Per cent of moisture to be added by steam

0.83 = An approximate correction factor for make up water at 50°F (Leaver, 1980)

34.5 = The amount of water evaporated in one hour at 212°F which equals one boiler HP.

As general rule, 5% moisture is accepted as a maximum though in some cases this may be exceeded. For a pelleting system with an average capacity of 10 tons (1 ton=2000 lb) per hour, assuming a 5% moisture addition to the mash, the boiler HP would be 20000 × 0.05 ÷ 0.83 × 34.5 = 34.9.

Once the quantity of steam is determined it must be delivered to the pellet mill at a constant pressure and free of entrained water (steam quality of 97-100%). Any pressure variation will immediately result in variation in product quality and in pellet mill capacity.

High pressure steam is being used more and more since it provides good quality dry steam to the conditioner without risk of condensate build-up. High pressure steam has a higher BTU value which can add more heat to the product. High pressure steam also facilitates the use of smaller valves and piping thus making it a more economical installation than that using low pressure steam.

The pelleting process is very energy intensive demanding up to 50% of the total power required for feed manufacturing. Energy is the major recurring expenditure for the processing of feedstuffs in a feed processing unit, apart from the cost of the equipments. The electrical power consumption in a feed unit and proportional motor size and cost for feed milling is given in Table 1.

Factors affecting pelleting

There are many variables which affect the pelleting process. These are due to the machinery used, due to the feed materials being processed and due to the conditioning of the feed.

Table 1: Proportional motor size and cost for feed milling (% of total)

Unit/operation	Feed mill (2 ton/hr)	
	Motor size (%)	Unit cost (%)
Weighing	-	7
Elevators/augers	3	7
Holding bins	-	5
Grinding	34	13
Mixing	10	12
Pelleting	43	17
Steam production	1	11
Pellet cooling	9	11
Bag-off weigh	-	7
Electrical control system	-	10
Total	**100** (110 KW)	**100**

A. Ingredient characteristics

These can be determined by factors such as protein, fat, fibre, starch, density, texture and moisture. Starch, protein and fibre change physical or chemical structure during processing and can affect the final pellet quality. Each ingredient has a unique composition. Even the same ingredient has different composition depending upon the place of purchasing. The quality of the pelleted feed will be different as the ingredient composition changes. It is reported that wheat and wheat products, barley and mustard meal improve pellet quality because of their natural inherent binding capacity while maize and soybean meal have low inherent binding capacity. A good quality control programme is needed to keep the variance of the ingredient characteristics at a minimum.

Pellet binders include lignosulphonate, hemicellulose extract, bentonite, gelatin, while lignosulphonates are commonly used for pellet binding.

Feed formulae can be classified into six broad categories
1. Heat sensitive feeds

These feeds contain high percentages of dried milk, whey, or sugar. These materials will start to caramelize at about 140°F (60°C). This causes plugging of the pellet mill. Steam addition should be low to keep the meal temperature below 140°F. Thin dies that reduce frictional heat and fat added to the formula for lubrication can aid in reducing plug-ups.

2. Urea feeds

Little or no steam should be added to this group of feeds. Urea becomes more soluble as the temperature rises. Steam supplies the heat and moisture to dissolve the urea.

Meal would be wetter. The hot pellet temperature should be higher than 140°F. Thin dies that reduce frictional heat should be used to keep the temperature low, and fat added to the formula for lubrication will help. Too much steam causes plug-ups as well as severe bin hang-up problems.

3. Molasses feeds

Since molasses has approximately 26% water, the quantity of steam that can be added must be reduced otherwise the meal will become too wet. That condition will result in plug-ups due to roll slippage. Adding live steam into the molasses line will raise the molasses temperature to 200°F (93°C). Under those conditions, higher meal temperature can be achieved without exceeding the maximum moisture level.

4. High natural protein feeds

This group includes supplements, concentrates, and dairy feeds. Heat is more important than moisture to plasticize the protein. These feeds require more steam than the urea and heat sensitive feeds but less than high starch formulae.

5. High grain feeds (high starch)

High temperature (82°C/180°F) and high moisture (17-18%) are necessary to gelatinize the starches in the grain. The gelatinized material acts as a binder to produce tough pellets. The hotter the meal, the greater is the degree of gelatinization.

6. Complete dairy feeds

These contain 12 to 16% CP. They also contain large amounts of fluffy, roughage type ingredients and are low in grain content. These ingredients have a low ability to accept moisture. Steam addition should be low to keep the meal temperature below 140°F (60°C) and the maximum moisture level at 12 to 13%. If these levels are exceeded, the pellets expand and crack after leaving the die.

Fat

Some nutrients can change the pelletability of a formula even when present in small amounts. e.g., fat. Generally speaking addition of fat makes a pellet less durable. Usually it is more satisfactory to keep the fat content of the formula to be pelleted down around 1 to 2%. This will enable better pellets to be made and will simplify the die selection problem. The remaining fat necessary for the total formula can be sprayed on the pellets after they are made while they are hot. The fat easily penetrates into the pellets. However, it is difficult to cool and dry the pellet. Modern methods are used nowadays to add 6-8% fat, enzymes, etc.

The amount of moisture and heat that can be added will be influenced by the pellet mill die, rollers, and environmental conditions that exist. Therefore, it will require experimentation to determine optimal temperature and moisture for each category. Conditioning directly affects frictional heat, and frictional heat directly affects die wear.

B. Fineness of grind

The fineness of grind of the various ingredients will have an impact on pellet quality. The different feed ingredients used in a formula will normally be a mixture of different sized particles (3 to 10 mm).

It has been suggested that a variety of particle sizes in the formula will improve pellet quality and production rates when compared to a formula composed of ingredients 'all of the same grind'. The reason given is that small particles can fill the void between the large ones when pelleted. The elimination of air space or voids between individual particles improves particle contact surface area and the pelleting characteristics of the feed.

The size of the large particles must be kept in balance with the size of the pellet that is being produced. Large particle sizes cause fracture of pellets. Also, large particle sizes will tend to cause a grinding action on the face of the pellet mill die, which will increase die friction and lower production rates. Experience indicates that the best particle size for material to be pelleted would be that all material passes through a 7 mesh screen (Approximately hammer mill equivalent is 8/64 inches or 3.18 mm). Pellet durability decreases and fines increase as mean particle size of pellet increases. As a rule of thumb, when the desired pellet diameter is 4mm or less, the suggested maximum particle size should be one-third the diameter of the orifice-i.e, a maximum particle size of a little over 1300 μ for 4 mm pellets.

C. Conditioning of feed

Improved conditioning of feed prior to pelleting can result in increased production, improved pellet quality, longer die life, reduced energy consumption, and a more efficient ration resulting in a better feed conversion ratio.

Large conditioning chambers are being used more and more in order to increase the retention time and thoroughly condition the material to be pelleted.

Conditioners are now available that are completely insulated to prevent heat loss, reduce energy consumption and improve performance. Steam inlets into the conditioner are being designed to prevent condensate build-up which can cause choking of the die.

D. Pelleting Operation

After conditioning, the mash is ready to be agglomerated. In most pellet mills this is done by forcing or extruding the material through holes in a ring type die by pressure exerted by roller assembly.

Most important factors that affect the performance of pelleting operation

    (a) The physical and geometric characteristics of the die and rolls,
    (b) Adjustment of the roll to die clearances,
    (c) Proper speeds of rotation, and
    (d) Maintenance of the rolls and die.

Die: The die (or more precisely the holes in the die) is what make the pellets. It is the single piece of equipment that is responsible for the various forms of pellets in animal feed. Depending on the type of pellet mill, a die can be flat or have a ring shape. Most pelleting machines operate with ring shape dies. Most of the manufacturers use stainless steel forgings with high chrome content to protect the material against corrosion, heat and acids. The die holes are gun-drilled and gun-drilling leaves a smooth mirror like finish on the holes, which is subjected to a critical heat treating process under vacuum to ensure that holes keep their smooth surface and perfect round shape. This results in less friction, easier start-up, higher throughput and lower operating horsepower requirements **and less heat** is generated. The lower temperature makes the burning of feed in the holes less likely which is especially advantageous when pelleting heat sensitive mixtures such as those containing urea, milk powder, or sugar products.

The overall average life of dies is probably between 4000-8000 tons production while in many installations particularly on easy to pellet formulae the die life of 15000-20000 tons is not unusual. The alloy of die can be varied to produce maximum life. A variety of stainless steels are used for pelleting formulations with corrosive ingredients. Special case hardened carbon steel dies are used now (which contain higher alloy content) for increased hardness and abrasion resistance.

The longer the die hole (Fig. 6), the more work must be expended to push the feed through the die. The die must be of sufficient thickness to furnish the amount of compaction required to agglomerate since the die should be as thin as possible to increase production efficiency.

The size of the pellet being produced affects die thickness. An important consideration in this respect is the ratio of die thickness to diameter of hole. As a rule of thumb the ratio of hole length (die thickness) to hole diameter is from 7 to 10, to 1 for many feed materials.

Variations in die Relief

The variations in die relief are shown in Figure 7.

    (1) Standard die with no counter bore or relief

    (2) Standard relieved die has all holes relieved to an equal depth. The primary purpose is to add strength to the die while maintaining desired effective length.

    (3) Outside rows relieved die: Only a few of the outside rows relieved. The primary purpose is to keep the outside rows from plugging when pelleting certain products that have a tendency to squeeze out to the side of the die.

    (4) Variable relief die: There are variations in the depth of relief. Serves the same basic function as an outside rows relieved die, but represents the variations some times needed for special applications.

Rolls: In order to reduce the energy costs and make pellet mills more efficient, manufacturers are incorporating the largest diameter rolls possible within a given die cavity. By keeping the die cavity clear of as many obstacles as possible, this area becomes more sanitary with less chance of feed contamination. The two significant factors in roller assemblies are adequate bearing capacity to withstand stresses in the pelleting operation and proper roll surface to give maximum traction, thus keeping the roll from slipping.

There are 3 basic types of roll shells

1. Tungsten carbide roll shell: That is a rough surface composed of tungsten carbide particles embedded in a weld matrix. They are long wearing with excellent traction characteristics.
2. Corrugated shells: There are two types: the open end corrugation and a modified version with the ends closed to reduce side slippage. The greatest advantage of that type of shell is resistance to plugging.
3. Indented Roller shells: These have indentations drilled on the surface which fill with feed and produce a friction surface for traction.

Of the different types of rolls used with pellet dies, the closed end corrugated roll is probably the most practical as it does not allow the material to squeeze out of the edges; thus ensuring that even the outermost row of holes in the die continue to produce pellets. These type of rolls produce a rougher pad of material between the die and the rolls, creating a better driving force, caused by the deep corrugations in the roll surface. Rolls having dimpled and tungsten carbide surfaces are generally only used in special applications.

Small hole die

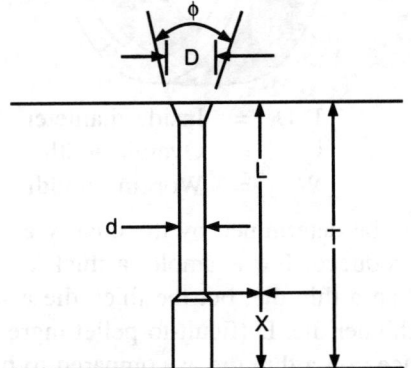

Figure 6. Significant parts of a pellet mill die

d = Pellet diameter. Normally range from 0.125 in. (3.18 mm.) to 0.75 in. (19.05 mm).

L = Effective length or diameter. That is the length of die, which is actually performing work on the material.

T = Total thickness (overall thickness). The overall thickness of a die relates to the stresses on the die during the pelleting operation. The thicker the die, the stronger it is. Normal die thickness increments vary by a quarter inch between 1.25 in. (3.175 cm) and 5 in. (12.70 cm) thick.

X = Counter bore depth (T-L). A die is counter bored by taking a large drill and
    drilling in from
  the outside of the die, thereby relieving the pressure of the die on the material.

D = Inlet diameter. Most dies have a tapered inlet to ease the flow of material
    into the hole. That taper also begins to compress material as it enters the
    hole, thereby doing work on the material.

    Compression ratio = D/d (a relationship of inlet area to pellet cross sectional
          area). For smaller pellets, it is normally 1.56 to 1.

Φ = the inlet angle. That is normally a 30 degree included angle on small hole
    dies and is designed to ease the feed into the hole. A die will eventually
    wear to its own angle after it has been in production, so the taper is provided
    to start the flow.

L/d = Performance ratio (a relationship of effective thickness of a die to the diameter
    of the pellet i.e., hole length to hole diameter). Pellet mill die

Pellet mill die

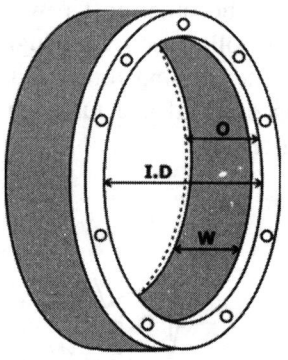

I. D.	=	Inside diameter
O	=	Overall width
W	=	Working width

Die thickness should be determined by the quality and production rates desired for the product being produced. For example, a thick die will normally produce a better quality product than a thin die, but the thick die also reduce production rates when compared to the thinner die. Difficult-to-pellet ingredients, such as fibre, urea, etc., are normally produced on a thin die as compared to high grain products, which would normally be produced on a thicker die.

E. Coolers

Horizontal coolers in more width are now available. These compact coolers operate on the counter-flow cooling principle, where the coldest air is drawn in at the bottom, at a point where the pellets are nearly completely cooled down. The air then travels upwards through the pellet beds as the pellets are descending down toward the bottom. Thus, as the air passes through the pellet beds, it gets progressively warmer and the temperature difference between air and the pellets is very little, which results in a gentle cooling effect.

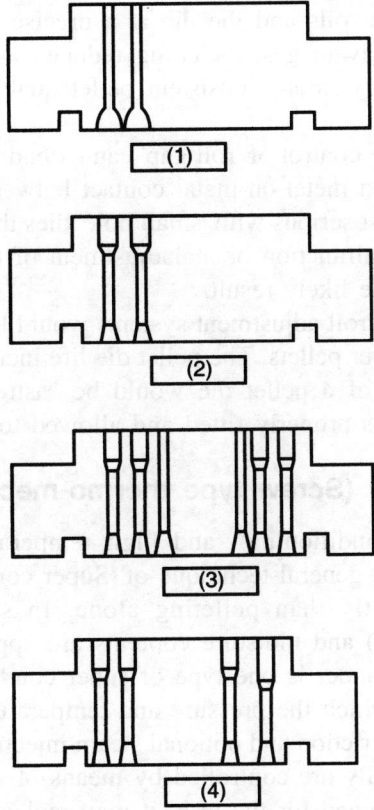

Figure 7. Variations in die Relief

As the air gets warmer, the relative humidity of the air decreases so that condensation within the cooler is minimized.

Another advantage of this type of counter-flow cooling is that the hot pellets entering the cooler will be exposed to preheated air, which prevents thermal tension within the pellets themselves. When hot pellets are exposed to cold air, as in the case of vertical and single deck horizontal coolers, only the surface of the pellets become cool and the centre remains warm which creates the thermal tension. This results in cracking and breakage which generates poor quality and fines.

There are vertical coolers that have moving baffles and these are recommended for handling pellets containing molasses in order to prevent the pellets sticking together and causing major blockages.

Newer Developments in Feed Pelleting Technology

Feed pelleting technology made rapid strides in 1990s incorporating advances upstream in super-conditioning as well as downstream in post-conditioning, cooling and micro liquid application. The modern pellet press, as well, has been benefited from many refinements and improvements in design, metallurgy and manufacturing techniques. Systems for the automatic or remote adjustment of the pelleting rolls or 'rollers' can be considered as a major advance. These systems seek to maintain the 'bed' or layer of feed mash between the rolls and the die at a precise and constant depth, such technology offers many advantages, including reduced labour requirements, faster start-ups, increased capacity, more consistent pellet quality and improved die and roller life.

Automated and remote control of 'roll gap' can extend the useful life of dies and rolls by reducing unwanted metal-on-metal contact between them. The problem of poor roll adjustment is most serious with 'small hole' dies that are in the range of 2.5-3.0 mm hole size. Any malfunction or maladjustment of the rolls can damage and a cracked die would be the likely result.

Automatic and remote roll adjustment systems would have a quicker payback in production of small diameter pellets. The pellet die life increase on average probably around 10-12%. The life of a pellet die would be "astronomical", if it could be properly mounted and rolls properly fitted and allowed to run their full lives.

Expander Technology (Screw type thermo-mechanical expander)

'Expanding', 'pressure conditioning', and high temperature short time (HTST) conditioning all describe a general technique of 'Super conditioning' which can kill salmonella more efficiently than pelleting alone. In super conditioning, high temperatures (above 90°C) and moisture contents are applied (for 15-20 seconds) prior to pelleting. An expander is one type of super conditioner that is a specially designed screw press in which the pressure and temperature of a feedstuff or feed mixture increases through friction and optional steam injection. Pressure, temperature and production rate typically are controlled by means of an adjustable die outlet.

If an expander is designed for the task, it may replace the conventional steam conditioner or both the conditioner and the pellet press in the production process. Usually, however, an expander is installed as an extra processing step between the steam conditioner and the pellet press. The expander is now common equipment in northern Europe - primarily in order to satisfy demands for better pellet durability and for greater flexibility in the inclusion of liquids and difficult-to-pellet ingredients. It is, moreover, a method of ensuring manufactured feed contains very little salmonella or other pathogenic microorganisms.

Now many feed millers have begun to use the expander as the sole thermal processing equipment to produce finished products called 'expandate' and 'expanded crumbles'. These are products that have been processed through the expander, but not pelleted. Such mills have feed storage bin, expander, expandate crusher, horizontal cooler, pre-crumbling screener and crumbler. The advantages of expander-only processing are less expensive machinery and lower production cost of expanded crumbles. Production costs can even be reduced further by using cheaper raw materials, which is possible because of the expander's higher processing temperatures and liquids addition capabilities.

The most serious challenges of expander-only processing: Expanded crumbles do have a lower bulk density and different flow behaviour. These characteristics may result in higher transportation costs.

As the expandate or expanded crumbles do not possess the high density of a pelleted feed, they are less suitable for broiler or turkey finisher feed. Nonetheless, the expanded products are used in feeding regimes of pigs, complete feeds for dairy animals, poultry feeds. Feed manufactures in northern Europe have been producing expanded but unpelleted products since 1990.

'Micro time' conditioning and pelleting or Pellet-cooker technology

This pellet-cooker was designed by Wenger Manufacturing Company, USA to exceed the performance and versatility of the expander pelleting system. Feed is subjected to a very high temperature of 125-150° C for only 3-4 seconds to minimize the destruction of valuable nutrients while feed gets pasteurized. The feed is formed into dense pellets rather than expanded chunks.

Pellet sizes are in the range of 2-18 mm and changeovers are made by quick and easy replacement of the pelleting head, which is comparatively light in weight. Changeover down time is less than 15 minutes. A rotary cutter on the pellet head cuts pellets to a specified length, depending on its adjustable rotation speed. Faster rotation produces shorter pellets - up to the speed at which the cutter produces feed 'crumbles'. This flexibility eliminates the need for crumble rolls to produce crumbled feed.

3

Pellet Quality–Pellet Durability Tests
Factors Influencing Pellet Quality

Pelleting was introduced into Europe about 1920 and into the U.S. feed industry in the late 1920's (Schoeff, 1994). Its popularity has grown steadily until about 80% of all feed in the U.S. are currently pelleted. Today, the process is widely used because of both the physical and the nutritional benefits it provides.

Effect of pellet quality on the performance of pigs

Stark (1994) conducted swine feeding experiments demonstrating that feed containing a high quality pellet (no fines) resulted in greater efficiency of gain than feed containing 30% fines. Gill and Oldfield (1965) and Tribble et al. (1979) reported poor animal performance when the feed contained significant levels of fines. However, when pellet quality was improved by changing the pelleting operation (i.e. thicker dies), animal performance was improved.

Effect of pellet quality on the performance of poultry

Pelleted broiler diets improve growth performance and feed conversion. Hussar and Robblee (1962) reported that reground pellets did not affect early bird performance. However, as the birds matured, birds fed whole pellets had better growth and feed conversion. Hull et al. (1968) reported birds fed pelleted diets had a 5% better feed conversion, but regrinding the pellets resulted in lower feed conversion than the meal diet.

Turkeys appear to be more sensitive to pellet quality and fines than broilers. Several studies indicate pellet fines decrease turkey performance. Proudfoot and Hulan (1982) reported pelleted diets improved feed conversions. However, as pellet fines increased from 0% to 60%, performance decreased. Moran (1989) showed a decrease in growth and performance when re-ground pellets were fed. This may explain why feed manufacturers place pellet quality as a high priority.

Pellet quality

Feed pelleting consists of a series of unit operations, including grinding, mixing, conditioning with moisture, addition of heat of both thermal and mechanical origin, expander treatment, pelleting and subsequent cooling of the product (Thomas et al., 1997). Technically pellet quality is controlled by the operations at the feed mill, by the raw material quality and addition of binders (Wood, 1987; Thomas et al., 1999). Optimisation of feed processing requires methods to measure the mechanical properties and the technical quality of the feed. The Holmen durability test and the Kahl hardness test are frequently used for this purpose (Thomas & van der Poel, 1996). Knowledge of technical pellet quality is also important relative to transportation and handling of the product. It is known that pellets can be damaged during transportation, but it is desirable that the product retains its structure during handling and conveying, until eaten by the animal (Behnke, 1996).

Feed pellets are heterogeneous agglomerate materials that contain water and ingredients with a variable particle size distribution. Pelleting and extrusion may cause expansion of the feed such that voids of different sizes are generated in the material. Thus, **pellets are three-phase materials** composed of solid particles, liquid and gas (Thomas & van der Poel, 1996). The strength of agglomerates can be estimated as the sum of the tensile yield stresses of the individual inter-particle bonds (Rumpf, 1962 in Knight, 2001). These bonds are due to liquid necking, adhesive and cohesive forces between the particles (Thomas & van der Poel, 1996). According to Knight (2001), the Rumpf theory is concordant with experimental results with wet granules, which show some plastic yield behaviour.

Pre-gelatinised starch: Wood (1987) revealed that the output rate of the pellet press increased with the pre-gelatinised starch content, and he suggests that gelatinised starch could have a lubricating effect in the die. Moreover, gelatinization of raw starch depends on the water content, heat, shear and time (Thomas et al., 1999). The physical quality of pellets made of pre-gelatinised starch is superior relative to feeds produced from native starch (Wood, 1987).

Pellet Durability: Quick and Simple 'State-of-the-art' Testing

Although fully automated 'on-line' pellet testing systems are available now, they represent a significant new investment in the pelleting line. Hence, at a much lower investment, the operator can test pellets for durability 'off-line' but quickly enough to adjust the pellet press before it produces a large amount of sub-standard pellets.

'Tumbling can' technique: In 1963, Dr. Harris Pfost, a feed science professor at Kansas State University in the USA, developed the 'tumbling can' technique to test pellet durability. The test is simple and inexpensive – tumbling a weighed sample in an airtight, baffled metal container at set rate and time period, then screening and weighing the surviving pellets.

The weight of the surviving pellets divided by the weight of the original sample yielded the **'Pellet durability index'** (PDI). Many feed compounders currently use tumbling cans of their own design and construction as well as their own testing procedures.

Holmen pellet tester: The next major improvement in testing technology came with the introduction of the Holmen pellet tester, developed by John Payne of England. This device uses forced air to circulate a sample of pellets through tubing such that the pellets strike against the tube's 90o angles, causing less durable pellets to fracture.

The sample size is 100g (one-fifth the size of the standard sample used in the tumbling can) and the test is much faster, 30 to 120 seconds, depending upon the size of the pellets.

Ligno Tester (Borregaard Ligno Tech of Norway): This pellet tester, also developed by Mr. Payne, further reduces the time required to test pellet durability. The device also used forced air to circulate 100g of pellets around a pyramidal, perforated chamber for 30 seconds and fines are removed continuously during the 'blow cycle' so there is no need to screen the pellets. At the end of this cycle, pellets can be dumped directly onto a balance to give an immediate reading of pellet durablity.

The unit includes a built-in-gauge to insure that air pressure (60 millibar) remains constant. Higher pressure can be used for extremely hard pellets or pellets larger than 6 mm. It is reported that this tester is faster than the tumbling can or the Holmen tester. It requires 3 minutes for the complete procedure (collecting pellets from the running pelleting press, cooling the sample, weighting the sample, loading the tester, conducting the test, discharging and weighing) under normal operating conditions. With almost immediate access to PDI data, a pellet mill operator may be able to improve pellet quality during the pelleting process. However, good planning is necessary at this fast pace of 'near on-line' analysis. Collection of more PDI information helps the feed compounders to tighten quality standards. Feed compounders can make adjustments to the pellet mills to get better quality while the feed is still running.

Mechanism of Adhesion in pellets: Different theories

Adhesion is the process by which materials are held together by a physical to chemical interaction of the material. This is accomplished by joining the surfaces of the material by melting the materials together or by applying an adhesive between them. An adhesive is defined as a material which, when applied to surfaces, can join them together and resist separation (Wake, 1976). In pelleting, however, we do try, through temperature and moisture control, to activate the natural adhesives that are typically found in the feed ingredients.

Several theories on the mechanism of adhesion at the interface between particles have been proposed (K.C. Behnke, 2001, Feed Tech 5, 4, 19 -- 22). The theories with application in the pelleting process include

- Mechanical interlocking
- Diffusion
- Adsorption

Kinlock (1987) described the basic concepts of each theory and the mechanisms by which adhesion occurs. **Mechanical interlocking** is based on the fact that adhesives flow into rough surfaces, become rigid, and hold the materials together. The theory also suggests that rough surfaces will improve the contact area and thus improve bond strength. The **diffusion theory** is based on the diffusion of polymers at the interface between material surfaces. Diffusion occurs when materials are heated and allowed to diffuse across the interface between materials. This phenomenon can occur only when the temperature of the polymer is above the **glass transition temperature of the polymer. Adsorption adhesion** occurs due to inter-atomic and intermolecular forces established between atoms and/or molecules at the surface of the adhesive and the substrate. The attractive forces are ionic, covalent, hydrogen bonding dipole interactions, and Van der Waal forces.

Rheological characteristics of feed ingredients

The rheological and functional characteristics of feed ingredients vary depending on their physical structure (crystalline vs amorphous) and chemical composition. Materials that are heated go through either **a first or second order glass transition or a combination of first and second order transitions.** First order transitions involve the melting of crystals, whereas second order transitions are a relaxation of polymers. Crystalline materials (e.g. sugar) go only through a first order transition. Amorphous materials (e.g. cellulose, lignin) exhibit only a second order transition.

Glass transition temperature: The temperature at which the amorphous regions of a polymer begin to relax or become mobile is defined as the glass transition temperature. Glass transition temperatures have been reported for starch, wheat gluten and for maize gluten. Glass transition temperature is inversely related to moisture content. **As the moisture in the system is increased**, the temperature at which the material becomes mobile decreases. Feed ingredients have glass transition temperatures below the temperature normally associated with the conditioning process (70-90oC) when the moisture content is between 15 and 18%. This suggests that feed ingredients begin to flow during the conditioning and pelleting process, and the amount and location of material flow depends on the temperature and location of the water (surface or intra-particle).

The level of total pellet starch gelatinisation and starch damage has been reported to be negatively correlated with pellet quality (Lopez, 1993). Starch damage was found to be greater at the outer surface of the pellet at lower conditioning temperatures. However, starch damage decreased as the conditioning temperature increased, indicating that the damage was primarily due to mechanical shear between the die surface and the starch and not due to hydrothermal elevation alone.

Functional role of starch and protein in the pelleting process: Woods (1987) examined the functional role of starch and protein in the pelleting process. The addition of raw soybean flakes increased pellet quality as compared to heat treated denatured soybean meal. In addition, pre-gelatinised starch improved pellet quality compared to native starch. Woods concluded that protein had a greater influence on pellet quality than starch. The data suggested that the level of starch gelatinisation may not be as important as the location of the gelatinised starch. It is apparent that the gelatinisation at the surface of the feed particles is critical to the formation of intra-particle bonds necessary for the formation of strong, durable pellets. Starch gelatinisation at the particle interface in conjunction with protein plasticisation would result in polymer diffusion between starch granules and protein molecules, resulting in adhesion to the particles.

Effect of diet formulation on pellet quality

Effect of addition of fat, protein and fibre: Least-cost diet formulation is designed to meet the nutritional parameters required by the target animal. However, the effect of formulation on processing, specifically pelleting, is seldom considered by most nutritionists. The addition of fat to the mash pre-pellet usually results in decreased pellet quality. However, the addition of protein and fibrous materials increase pellet quality. Fahrenholz (1989) reported an increase in the pellet durability of swine diet pellets when the level of wheat middlings increased from 0 to 45%. McKee (1988) increased pellet quality and water stability of catfish diets by increasing the level of wheat gluten from 0% to 10%. Lopez (1993) also reported that addition of wheat gluten resulted in a positive effect on pellet quality and water stability, but the addition of cassava meal had a negative effect. Lawton (1989) reported a linear increase in tensile strength as the amount of protein in a tablet increased at the expense of starch.

Maize versus wheat: Studies by Stevens (1987) and Winowiski (1998) have compared the pellet durability of diets containing maize with those where some or all of the maize was replaced with wheat. In both instances, pellet durability was higher for the diets containing wheat. It can be reasoned that this is due to the higher crude protein content of wheat (13%) as compared to maize (9%). This finding is in agreement with a study conducted by Briggs et al. (1999) which found that increasing the protein content in a poultry diet from 16.3% to 21% increased the average pellet durability from 75.8 to 88.8%.

Effect of particle size on pellet quality

Decreasing the particle size of ingredients resulted in a greater surface area to volume ratio. Smaller particles will have a greater number of contact points within a pellet matrix as compared to larger particles. Penetration of heat and moisture to the core of a particle can be achieved in a shorter amount of time with small particles and a large surface area per unit of weight. MacBain (1966) indicated that a variation in particle size produces a better pellet than a homogeneous particle size. Stevens (1987) reported no difference in pellet quality when the mean particle size of maize and wheat was reduced from 1023 to 551 microns (μ) and from 802 to 365μ, respectively. However, Wondra et al (1995) reported an increase in pellet durability as particle size was reduced from 1000 to 400μ.

The aquaculture feed industry grind ingredients to less than 250μ particle size for greater pellet water stability. Decreasing particle size from a coarse to a fine grind exposes more surface area per unit volume for absorption of condensing steam and increases the surface area available for bonding. The combination of small particle size and long term, high temperature conditioning produces pellets that have the greatest water stability.

Effect of conditioning on pellet quality

The importance of steam conditioning was quantified by Skoch et al (1981) in an experiment comparing dry pelleting with pelleting using steam conditioning. The results of the study indicated that steam conditioning improved pellet durability and production rates and decreased the amount of fines generated and energy consumption. It was concluded that steam acted as a lubricant to reduce friction during pelleting.

The nutritional, as well as physical properties of a wide variety of ingredients present in the mash feed have an effect on conditioning and eventual pellet quality.

Pellet quality is proportionally dependent on the following factors (Reimer 1992)

40% diet formulation, 20% particle size, 20% conditioning, 15% die specifications, and 5% cooling and drying. If this is correct, 60% of pellet quality is determined before the mash enters the conditioner. This increases to 80% after conditioning, but before mash has even entered the die chamber of a pellet mill. It can be concluded that there is still a great deal of art in the science of pelleting.

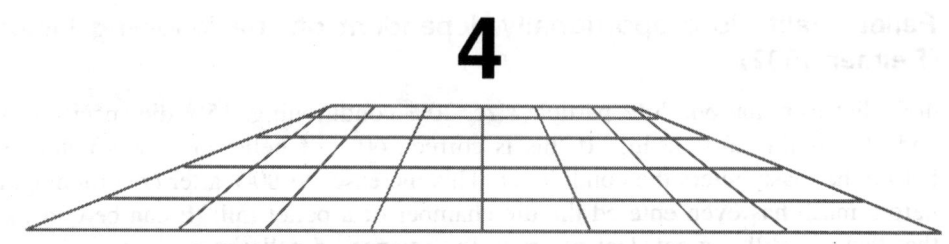

4

Power Consumption in Pelleting Feeds

Energy efficiency in feed mills has increased significantly since the mid-1980s due to improved electric motors and steam generating units. In feed mill design and equipment, there has been much greater attention on energy management. Equipment manufacturers and feed mill designers have made better use of process heat in space heating and conductive heating in the plant. Heat management in feed mills has also improved greatly. For example, the insulation of heated liquid storage - typically for fat and molasses - has improved, especially in temperate climates. There has been improvements in thermal processing equipment, particularly in conventional steam conditioners and systems to control steam quality, downstream from pelleting - in counterflow 'post-conditioning' and pellet cooling technology - heat used to process the product also has been used to cool and dry it. The net result is a reduction in total energy consumption per tonne, even with more energy - intensive feed processing.

Steam energy

Steam is usually generated in the mill from fossil, such as oil and gas. It is reported that a Kilowatt of steam energy is less costlier than a Kilowatt of electric energy. More steam energy is used per tonne of feed in Mash conditioning.

Super conditioners - such as expanders and other high-temperature-short- time (HTST) conditioning equipment - have become standard equipment in retrofits and new feed mills in Europe and North America in order to produce a sterile or atleast pathogen - free feed, to increase pelleting capacity, to incorporate a wider range of raw materials, to add more liquids and to improve pellet quality.

The super conditioning systems, including expanders and double pelleting systems increase pelleting capacity by 20-90% but pelleting energy consumption rises only 5-35% compared to a conventional, steam conditioning, single pelleting system.

Energy consumption of feed processing machinery

Based on a survey of 21 feed mills in France during 1985-1995, energy consumption of feed mills has been evaluated (Table1). There was a 9% drop in energy required to operate electrical machinery to produce 1 ton of feed and a 19% drop in energy required for steam production.

Energy costs of feed compounding
(a) Type of the ingredients in the formula

- Grinding of oil seed meals - sunflower, soybean, groundnut and rapeseed meals: 3.5 to 7.0 kwh per ton.
- Grinding of cereals - barley, wheat, maize: 7.0 to 15.0 kwh/t
- Byproducts of the food industry are increasingly used as feedstuffs and such materials often require more energy to pellet.

Table 1. Energy consumption of feed mills

Energy	Electricity kwh/t	%	Steam kwh	%
Pre-pelleting	13	28	0	0
Pelleting	26.8	60	26.1	83
Post-pelleting	5.7	12	5.4	17
Total	45.5	100	31.5	100

(b) Degree of processing used to manufacture finished feed

Amount of steam conditioning applied prior to pelleting is variable for different species depending upon the feed formulae.

A decrease in the proportion of cereals in feed formulations reduces the energy cost since cereals require more extensive steam conditioning. Higher the cereals greater the amount of steam required to gelatinize starch, and particle cohesion e.g., poultry & pig diets. High fat content also needs more steam.

Feeds with low cereal content, and high molasses and fibre levels (e.g. feeds for cattle, rabbits) receive lower levels of steam energy input but require higher levels of electric energy at the pellet die to generate friction and compression for pelleting.

Major factors affecting electricity consumption of the pellet press

(a) Type of the ingredients in the formula
(b) Degree of steam conditioning and compression in the die

It is possible to pellet some feeds without steam conditioning, which normally is in the range of 2-4.5% addition. Such feeds would contain no cereals, but would have a high moisture content and require much more friction - compression energy in the die.

Pellet die lubricant: Added fat or vegetable oil also is an effective pellet die lubricant, but usually reduces compression in the die as particles become coated with a water repellent film that inhibits natural binding. It results in the typical lower pellet quality.

Lubricating effect of steam: Soluble vegetable gums now are available as additives to provide pellet die lubrication without interfering with binding between feed particles. Steam used to condition feed materials does have a lubricating effect in most formulas. In maize-soybean diets, it was found that by increasing steam conditioned mash temperatures it was possible to reduce the energy required for pelleting.

That is how expanders and other super conditioners increase pelleting capacity since pellet press did less work per ton of feed (due to the lubricating effect of steam).

(c) Role of pellet binders

Certain pellet binders can also reduce the energy required for pelleting. For example, calcium aluminate provides both binding effect and lubricating effect. Hence, materials pass through the pellet die with less resistance, which reduces electric energy required for pelleting. Calcium aluminate is approved for use in animal feeds (0.8%) as a pelleting aid in the EU and the USA. The 'lubricating action' of calcium aluminate has been attributed to small particle size (less than 100 microns) and large hydration capacity, which reportedly increases steam absorption by the feed. Supplier data suggests that the calcium aluminate binder may improve pelleting energy efficiency as much as 20% in some feeds.

Pelleting feeds without chemical binders

Some diehard purists in feed industry swear they will never use a chemical binder. They stand by their super conditioners, computer controlled presses and high-tech coolers to explain that the new equipment can gelatinise starch, plasticise protein and atomise fat. It makes pellets as hard and clean as bullets. If there still is a problem with pellet quality, the diehards are confident to reformulate the diet with more wheat. Wheat is a pellet friendly ingredient. Residual pellet quality of feeds made out of wheat is quite high without the addition of pellet binders because wheat contains various glutens that act as natural binders.

Thus, pellet quality depends on type of ingredient and its quantity, equipments used for conditioning, pelleting and cooling. When pellet quality targets are not achieved, the options available are either the introduction of expensive pelleting constraints such as restricting fat, raising the cereal content and reducing high fibre raw materials, or by addition of a low inclusion pellet binder. The latter choice very often is financially the better solution.

In Europe the introduction of double pelleting and the use of conditioning expanders has sharply reduced the volume of pellet binder used in feeds.

Modern feed mills must do much more than in the past to keep higher standards of feed hygiene, safety and quality. These requirements often mean using more energy intensive processing. Hence feed mills must become more energy efficient to keep down the costs.

5

Expanded Structurized Feed

INTRODUCTION

Expanded structurized feed is produced with an expander, without using a pellet press (Dick Ziggers, 2003, Feed Tech 7, 6, 8-11). Such a granulate can considerably increase the value of meal feed and can in many cases replace pelleted meal. Thermal treatment in the expander improves the physical product qualities such as flow behaviour, structure and particle size. At the same time important ingredients such as starch, crude protein, fat and crude fibre are improved with respect to digestibility.

Production process for expanded structurized feed

The manufacturing process with the applied process parameters: temperature, product moisture, and energy input (kWh/t) is shown in Figure1. A mixing conditioner is used with a conditioning time of 0.5 to 2 minutes - depending on the granular size of the feed - for preconditioning the product by adding steam, water, and other liquids such as molasses or fat. Then the product goes through the expander for hydrothermal pressure treatment and for agglomerating of the feed to larger product lumps. A structurizing machine with screen inserts follows the expander. Screen perforation and speed determine the granular size.

For subsequent cooling a modified belt cooler is used, which is designed to suit the high specific surface of the expanded and structurized feed. For example, 5 mm pellets have a specific surface of 450 m2/m3 whereas expanded and structurized feed has a specific surface, which is more than seven fold (3250 m2/m3). A screening machine followed by a crumbler determines the final structure of the product. Equipment manufacturer Amandus Khal in Germany identifies the product as 'Expandat.'

Physical properties of 'expandat'

'Expandat' has some different characteristics compared to pellets.
*   The bulk density is reduced by 10 to 20% depending on the treatment intensity (average around 500 g/l). This must be taken into account when

designing and operating feeding plants. Pigs need to adjust their feeding behaviour since they have not been fed expandat from weaning. Despite the decreased bulk density the flow characteristics of expandat are similar to pellets and are 'easy flowing'.

- Compared with coarse feed meals the percentage of fines has been reduced considerably. The particle size spectrum is "narrower", i.e. the percentage of particles having the same size is higher. Typical particle sizes for a coarse meal would be between 100 um and 1,900 m, whereas an expanded structurized feed would have particle sizes between 500 um and 2,100 m.
- Expanding also creates an almost pathogen free product. The thermal treatment (up to 110°C) reduces total aerobic bacteria count by almost 50% and fully eliminates pathogens such as coliform bacteria, E.coli bacteria and moulds.

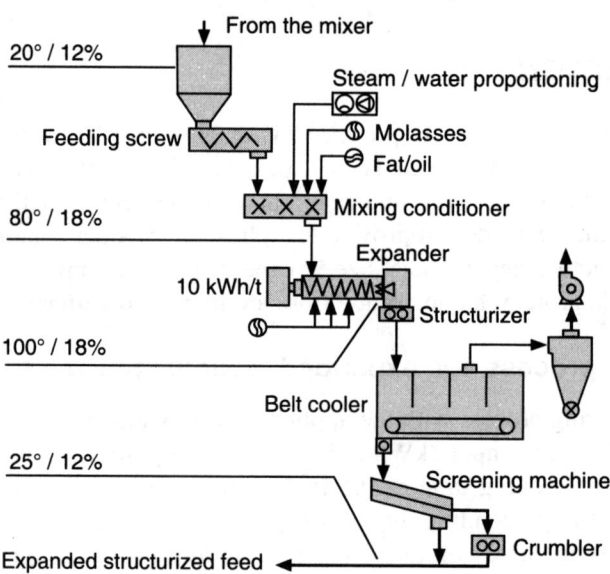

Figure 1. Production process for expanded structurized feed

Nutritional effects of 'expandat'

In pig feeding starch modification is desirable to improve pig performance. Gelatinisation in the raw materials (after grinding) averages around 10-12%. After passing through a conditioner this figure increases approximately to 25% and after pelleting around 40-42% of the starch is gelatinised. With expanding – depending on the treatment intensity – a starch modification of 50-60% can be achieved. When used in liquid feeding systems the expanded structurized feed dissolves faster and 50% better than a mealy or granulated feed, not only in water but also in other liquid ingredients such as whey, for example.

Expander treatment leads to an increase of the digestibility of the components, particularly of the fat and crude fibre fraction, and thus to an increase of the metabolisable energy. Research in Denmark showed that expanded structurized feed reduces the susceptibility of pigs to parakeratosis and gastric ulcers by 50%.

Environmental effect

In practice it has turned out that the quantity of liquid manure per pig is reduced if they are fed expanded feed. During tests carried out by the Kansas State University, USA, a lower water demand of the pigs was observed during the feeding of expanded feed (Hancock J.D. et al., 2000). A test with expanded piglet feed also shows reduced quantities of urine and faeces (Peisker, M., 1993). The reduced production of faeces reduces the cost of manure storage and distribution.

The improved crude fibre digestibility of expanded feed causes a reduction of the nitrogen content of the liquid manure. Due to the increased fermentation of the crude fibre, the nitrogen content in the faeces is slightly increased, but it is significantly reduced in the urine. On the whole the quantity of urine and the quantity of nitrogen excreted with the urine is lower if an expanded product is fed. The result is a lower ammonia load in the pig house, in the environment, and during storage and distribution of the liquid manure.

Expanded feed for young piglets

The digestive system of young piglets has a low enzyme activity and therefore has difficulties digesting other nutrients than from milk. For this reason piglet feed mainly contains milk products (skim milk, whey powder) and starch, which must be modified for replacing or supporting the enzymatic degradation. The most important criterion for the expansion of feed containing milk powder is the avoidance of the Maillard reaction, which a degradation of proteins through heat. On the other hand a high degree of starch modification is essential. This requires a two phase feed production. Firstly a separate modification of the starch of the grain components in the mixture by means of the expander and secondly expansion and – if necessary – pelleting of the complete mixture. If the product is pelleted additionally, the expander temperatures must be reduced by 10°C.

Starch modification of the grain components and production of the complete feed can be performed one after the other on the same machine. The starch modification of the grain components is comparable with steam-treated flakes or products modified by means of the extruder.

Benefits of expander technology in pig feeding

➢ Improvement of digestibility and feed value
➢ Low water consumption
➢ Improvement of the fattening results and shortening of the fattening period
➢ Lowered nitrogen excretion in urine and ammonia load in the environment

6

Aquafeeds Manufacture: Which process is preferable–Pelleting or Extrusion?

Good aquafeed requires minimum degradation or dissolution of the feed in water. Too rapid dissolution or break-up of the feed pellet before it is consumed, get decomposed. Any feed decomposition in the aquaculture environment inevitably reduce the level of dissolved oxygen (DO) and increase the biochemical/biological oxygen demand (BOD). A high BOD level can trigger an acute oxygen depletion of the water, causing very rapid and extensive mortality.

Early experiments demonstrated that diets for catfish and carp fed in meal forms were not as efficiently utilized as pelleted forms. When large fish are fed small - particle feeds or feeds containing significant amounts of poorly ground ingredients, the smaller particles may not be ingested, resulting in lowered feed conversion efficiency. Further, the unconsumed feed particles cause eutrophication of the culture system, which usually results in decreased dissolved oxygen levels and a buildup of waste matabolites. To minimise these undesirable effects on water quality and feed efficiency, aquafeeds are processed into water-stable particles of size and texture commensurate with the feeding preferences of the cultured aqua species.

The aquafeed manufacturer must design the physical size, shape and texture of feeds to accommodate the anatomical organs of the animal for seizing, swallowing, or otherwise ingesting food (Tables 1 and 2).

Shrimp are 'particle feeders' - unable to ingest an entire pellet at once - they typically require a very finely ground feed. There is much discussion and research on methods of preparing shrimp feeds to prevent wastage and the loss of water-

Table 1. Recommended feed particle sizes for channel catfish (Warmwater fish) fry

Weight of fish (g)	Feed size (mm)
0.02 – 0.25	0.42 – 0.84
0.25 – 1.5	0.85 – 1.4
1.5 – 5.0	1.4 – 2.8
5.0 – 20.0	2.8 – 4.0

soluble nutrients. Some commercial feeds can remain 'water stable' for more than 24 hours. Aquafarmers prefer a dry, durable, pelleted product.

Low density feeds or floating feeds Vs sinking feeds or high density feeds

The floating feeds may pose a problem when the fish fills its stomach before consuming enough nutrients for maximum growth. However, floating feeds generally have superior water stability, so the pellet does not dissolve before the fish have had an opportunity to eat. Any pellet that dissolves before it can be consumed represents a waste of money and can accelerate the depletion of dissolved oxygen. In addition, unconsumed feed particles offer surfaces for the colonisation of baceteria and fungi. Disease may be encouraged in culture systems that have a buildup of waste feed particles.

Table 2. Typical feed types and sizes for rainbow trout (Coldwater fish) in Japan

Fish size (g)	Feed type	Feed size (mm)
Fry < 0.5	Crumble	0.3 – 0.5 (300 to 500 microns)
0.5 – 1.5	Crumble	0.5 – 0.9
Fingerling		
1.5 – 5.0	Crumble	1.0 – 1.4
5.0 – 10.0	Crumble	1.5 – 2.5
Adult		
10 – 15	Pellet	2.4
15 – 40	Pellet	3.2
40 – 200	Pellet	4.4
200 – 400	Pellet	6.0
> 400	Pellet	8.0

Extruded versus pelleted products

Steam pelleting	Extruding
Steam pelleting, through compression, produces a dense pellet that sinks rapidly in water.	Extrusion is a process through which the feed material is moistened, precooked, expanded.
Steam pelleting is less expensive and generally costs 10 to 12% less than extruded fish feeds.	Extruded feeds float on the water surface and are very popular with catfish farmers. About 90% of the feeds for catfish are extruded.
Pelleting involves the use of moisture, heat and pressure to agglomerate ingredients into larger, homogenous particles. The steam added to the mash gelatinizes starch, and increase moisture and temperature to about 16% and 85°C,	Extrusion requires higher levels of moisture, heat and pressure than pelleting. Usually, the mash is conditioned with steam or water, and precooked before entering the extruder. The mash which contains 25% moisture, is compacted and heated from 135°C to 175°C

respectively, before passing through the pellet die. However, ingredient composition will influence these conditions.

Pellet binders are added to reduce fines and increase water stability.

under high pressure. As extruded pellets are coming out of the barrel, part of the water in superheated dough immediately vapourises and causes expansion.

Extruded feeds are more firmly bound, due to the almost complete gelatinization of the starch, and result in less fines than pellets.

Hilton et al. (1981) compared extrusion and steam pelleting as aquafeed processing techniques. These workers studied the effect of extrusion and steam pelleting of aquaculture diets on pellet durability, pellet water absorption and performance of rainbow trout (Table 3 and 4).

Table 3. Water - uptake of extruded and steam pellets*

Time of immersion (seconds)	Processing Method	
	Extruded	Pelleted
10	47.4[a]	23.7[b]
60	54.9[a]	38.9[b]
180	76.9[a]	50.0[b]

*Water-uptake of 100 g of feed after 10, 60 and 180 seconds immersion *in 15°C water.*

Pellet durability tests indicated that extruded pellets were more durable than steam pellets as measured by the amount remaining on various sieves. However, extruded pellets absorbed more water at a higher rate than did steam pellets as shown by the significantly higher water uptake by the extruded product. It was also found that extruded pellets maintained their shape during water immersion but were wet and soft to the core after 1 minute immersion. Steam pellets generally deteriorated after 1 minute immersion with the outer shell becoming extremely soft and wet.

Rainbow trout raised on a steam pelleted diet had gained significantly more weight during a 13-week growth trial, but with a lower feed efficiency than the trout reared on the extruded diet (Table 4). Liver:body weight ratios and percent liver glycogen were significantly higher in trout fed the extruded diet, while percent liver lipid and protein were significantly higher in trout fed the pelleted diet.

Table 4. Performance of rainbow trout fed the extruded and steam pelleted diets for 12 weeks.

	Processing Method	
	Extruded	Pelleted
Gain (kg/100 fish)	3.5[a]	4.0[b]
Feed: Gain	0.9	1.2
Mortality	3.7[a]	3.3[a]

Initial body weight of fish 2.9±0.1g; Mortality: Number of mortalities per 10,000 fish-days.

Kearns (1989) made a comparison chart for shrimp feed formulations that are typical for the individual process - extrusion and pelleting. Extrusion process facilitates least cost formulations (Table 5). Further, studies of Akimoto and colleagues (1992) revealed that extrusion process improved the nutritional value of brown fish meal as compared to conventional steam pelleting (Table 6).

Table 5. Comparison chart for shrimp feed formulations - extruded versus pelleted feeds

Ingredients	% CP	% in formulation Extruded	Pelleted
Soybean meal	44.0	34	12
Cottonseed meal	44.0	5	–
Fish meal (menhaden)	60.0	18	40
Meat bone meal	50.0	3	–
Fish soluble	32.7	3	–
Shrimp meal	40.0	10	6
Squid meal	70.0	5	4
Wheat middlings	15.5	10	4
Rice bran	12.7	5	–
Wheat gluten	80.0	–	3
Wheat flour (brown)	12.0	–	27
Brewers yeast	43.8	2	–
Fish oil	–	2	1
Vitamins & Minerals	–	3	3
Total		100	100
CP %		40.7	40.7

Making compound feeds for larval fish**

Extruded or steam pelleted growout rations provide improved rates of gain and feed efficiency for many popular aquaculture species. However, producing complete feeds in the diameter range of 200-500 m for fish less than 6 mm in length requires a 'quantum shift' from the manufacture of extruded or steam pelleted products. The aquafeed industry has been moving toward 'miniaturised' compound feeds, but may be about to make a 'quantum jump'.

The early commercial larval feeds were steam pelleted crumbles, which tended to have low palatability and poor water stability. More advanced extruded products reduced the fines and improved water quality through better stability. The latest generation of commercial larval feeds is in the form of a crumbled cake that is based on high quality fish meal and krill meal with zein protein as a binder. However, these products cost higher.

Table 6. Processing type versus nutrient composition of experimental diets for rainbow trout

Ingredient	Extruded	Pelleted
	%	
Brown fish meal	60.0	60.0
Starch	7.5	7.5
Wheat flour	15.0	15.0
Cellulose	5.0	5.0
Mineral premix	5.0	5.0
Vitamin premix	1.0	1.0
Choline chloride	0.4	0.4
Vitamin E	0.1	0.1
$Cr_2 O_3$	1.0	1.0
Pollack liver oil	5.0	5.0
Nutrient content on DMB (%)		
Crude protein	45.4	44.9
Crude lipid	16.0	15.5
Crude starch	20.0	19.8
Crude ash	12.5	12.5
Moisture	8.3	7.0
Gross energy (Kcal/g)	5.04	4.94
Digestible energy (Kcal/g)	4.24	3.95

**Source: Mian Nadeem Raiz (1997). Feed International, March 1997, PP 22-28.

Micro-extrusion marumerisation (the terms 'marumeriser' and 'marumerisation' come from the Japanese maru for circle or sphere) or MEM process

The U.S. Fish and Wildlife Service Bozeman Fish Technology Centre in Montana tested various larval feed production methods, trying to improve palatability and water stability while keeping production costs down. Some of the equipment is adopted from human food and pharmaceutical industries.

First, all dry ingredients are dry mixed, then the fish oil is added, then 32% of the batch weight is added as water. In the lab, 2-5 kg batches were used. The wet feet mash is the complete, compound larval feed, but it is not yet formed into discrete feed 'particles' of the necessary size, shape and density.

The wet feed mash is fed directly into a special low pressure, radial - discharge twin screw extruder model. The extruder normally operates at a screw speed of 19 rpm and discharges from the side, rather than the end of the barrel. It forces the extrudate through a die with 500 m holes to form wet 'noodles'. Then these noodles are transferred into the 'marumeriser'. This machine consists of a cylindrical chamber with a rotating plate on the bottom. The plate is grooved so that when it rotates the ridges strike the noodles. This energy fractures the noodles into the particles, then reshapes the particles. The 'marumeriser' can operate in the range of 300-1210 rpm.

The marumeriser also smooths particle edges, reducing the diameter slightly while increasing density of the particles. Production of fines is very low, because the formula encourages agglomeration while the marumerising action keeps the agglomerations from getting too big.

For this larval walleye formula (based on Krill meal, egg solid, herring meal), the marumeriser was operated at 1060 rpm for 10 seconds, followed by at 500 rpm for 90 seconds. The complete feed particles become spherical or ellipsoidal in shape with diameters in the range of 250-700 m.

The feed particles are dried in a forced air dryer to room temperature and to less than 10% moisture. The feed particles are separated into two size categories - 250-400 m for the first stage of larval growth from 1 day old for 7 days, and 400-700 m for the second stage of growth, usually three weeks to fingerling size. The finished feed is vacuum-packed in nitrogen-flushed plastic bags.

Product yield from the MEM process using the 500 m screen is 3 to 8% (by adjusting moisture content of the mash and marumeriser speed) in the 250-400 m range and 97% in the 400-700 m range. The MEM process has been tested in the lab and with feeding trials for more than seven years. In the case of larval walleye, this technique has eliminated the need to feed live artemia.

Particle - assisted rotational agglomeration or PARA process

The PARA process makes use of the marumeriser, but not the specialised extruder. It is particularly useful in making feeds smaller than 400 m because it produces a higher yield of smaller particles : 35-45% of 250-400 m particles and 20-25% less than 250 m.

Both MEM and PARA processes are sensitive to diet formulation, for example, the binding characteristics of the ingredients are important for either the method to work well, but particularly for the PARA method. The PARA process opens up a new frontier in 'micro compound' feeds.

Now we have to over supplement key nutrients in larval aquafeeds, such as vitamins and amino acids, in order to be sure leaching and oxidation do not degrade the product before it is consumed. This is especially a problem with larval fish feeds because the surface area-to-volume ratio is very high. Nutrients leach very quickly.

But with PARA method, it is reported that there is the potential to develop 'micro capsules' of individual ingredients 1–2µm diameter. These then may be proportioned correctly inside a larger 'micro sphere' perhaps 100-200 m in diameter. Each micro sphere would contain the complete diet, enclosed in a highly palatable coating designed to leach into the water as an attractant. With today's technology for fine grinding of feedstuffs PARA can produce complete larval fish feeds from 50 m onwards.

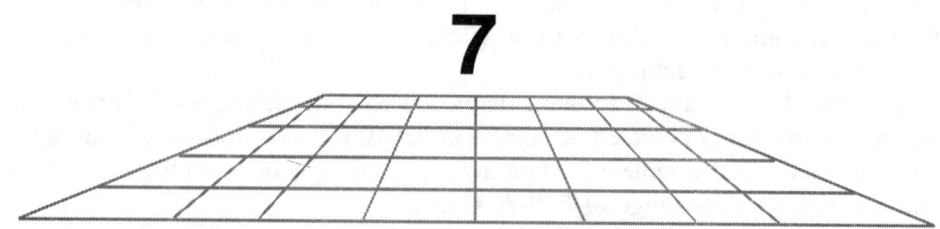

7

The importance of the Product Density in the Production of Fish Feed

Unlike land-living animals, fish have a very short digestive system, e.g. ten times shorter than the specific intestinal length of pigs, and therefore they need an easy to digest feedstuff. The feed has to be highly digestible so that the volume of faeces is as low as possible and water pollution due to faeces is the most minimum. Form and size of the feedstuff have to be adapted to the size of the fish, i.e. the mealy feed mixture has to be transformed into pellets. The sinking and floating properties (product density) have to correspond to the animal's natural way of feed consumption. Thus water pollution by feedstuff which is not consumed is avoided, and feed utilisation (kg feedstuff/fish) is improved (Hans Walter Lucht, Feed Tech, 5, 1, 31-33).

Feed utilisation has been steadily improved in the recent years. The water pollution due to feedstuff that has not been consumed could be drastically reduced. The increased digestibility of the feedstuff led to a remarkable reduction of the P and N emissions.

Requirements on fish feed quality

Corresponding to their original **feeding habits**, fish are **carnivores** (salmon, trout), **omnivores** (tilapia, carp), or **herbivores** (grass carp). The ingredients of the formulae have to be adapted to these requirements. The sinkability and floatability as well as the water stability of the feedstuff have to meet different requirements for cold water fish or predatory fish (salt-water or fresh water), such as salmon and trout, and warm water fish (fresh water or brackish water) such as tilapia and carp.

There is a further classification according to their feeding behaviour and habit

1. Groundfish usually consume feed on **the bottom** of the pond, e.g. carps or tilapia. As these warm water fish feed six times slower than predatory fish, the feedstuff has to be water stable. Or a floating feedstuff is fed in order to control the feed consumption. In this case, however, the surface of the pond has to be protected from birds by means of a wire screen. This is common in the rearing of catfish in the USA, for example.

2. Predatory fish "catch" the feedstuff while it is slowly sinking in the water, such as salmon, trout, or perch. Normally, these fish do not consume the feed on the ground.
3. Shrimps and other crustaceans are **"sleepers"**, they only eat at the bottom of the pond. Therefore the pellets have to be water stable for some hours.

The more intensive the type of breeding (the higher the number of fish respectively their size per m3 of water or per ha of pond surface) is, the higher the requirements on the form and on the digestibility of the feedstuff are in order to minimise water pollution by feed residues and excrement.

Types of fish feed

The following requirements have to be met with regards to the product density

- floating feedstuff for warm water fish (fresh water or brackish water) such as tilapia and carp
- slowly sinking feedstuff for cold water predatory fish (salt-water or fresh water), such as salmon and trout
- waterstable, sinking feedstuff for warm water fish
- sinking and extremely waterstable feedstuff for shrimps and other crustaceans

Structure and the particle size of the feedstuff: Important factors for the feeding method are the structure and the particle size of the feedstuff.

- Land-living animals such as pigs and poultry need only two feedstuff sizes in all their life.
- Fish may need up to 12 different particle sizes from 0.05 mm to 12 mm. A particular size of crumbles or pellets belongs to the different stages in the life of fish of each size. If the feedstuff is too big or too small, the fish will not eat it. The refused feedstuff sinks to the ground, rots, and pollutes the water, thus reducing its oxygen level. Therefore pellets have to be stable and free of fines.

Processes for the production

The density or specific weight of a pellet influences its sinkability or floatability. Floating pellets have a specific weight of 900 - 1000 g/dm3, whereas sinking pellets have a specific weight ranging from 1000 - 1200 g/dm3. In practice, this measurement is too complicated, so that the sinking or floating properties of a product are usually determined via the bulk density in g/l. This value, however, is slightly influenced by the pellet size as well as by porosity and inclusions of air. For estimations, the specific weight is considered to be about twice as high as the bulk density.

Before being transformed into pellets in the pelleting press or extruder, the feedstuff has to be conditioned using water and steam. This treatment takes place in a separate conditioner. The conditioning temperature is 80 - 90°C, the water content prior to the pelleting press is 15 - 16%, 18 - 20% if an expander is used, and 25 - 30% if an extruder is used.

The processes used in the fish feed industry for the production of pelleted feed

1. Pelleting using a pelleting press

During this process, the feedstuff is pressed through perforated dies by means of pan grinder rollers. The pellets are not expanded and there is no starch modification. The product density is constantly higher than 1000g/dm3, i.e. sinking pellets are produced. Furthermore, they contain 1-3% fines (in spite of screening), which are not desired by the consumer. Hence, the production of pelleted feedstuff is declining.

2. Expander with following pelleting press

In case of this process the pelleting press is preceded by an expander (Figure 1). The expander is defined as a single shaft extruder equipped with stop screws in order to provide the required kneading and shearing forces for the product. Furthermore the stop screws exert an additional mixing effect.

Just like the extruder, the expander works according to the HTST (High-Temperature-Short - Time) principle. The processing parameters such as moisture, temperature, pressure, and electromechanical energy input in the expander influence the physical characteristics and the nutritional value of the feed. As a variable pressure inside the expander is produced via the hydraulically adjustable outlet, the pellet density is influenced. However, the pressure is not enough to produce floating pellets. But the abrasion of the pellets is much lower than in the case of traditional pelleting.

3. Extruder or expander with perforated die

In order to avoid the disadvantages due to the functioning of traditional pelleting presses and the combination expander with pelleting press, the expander has been equipped with a die outlet. The die is movable and mounted on a hydraulic cylinder, thus offering more flexibility and operating safety than traditional single-shaft extruders. The expander/extruder with perforated die is equipped with a heating or cooling section in order to influence the expansion and thus the pellet density by means of the product temperature.

- A prerequisite for a high digestibility of the feedstuff and a high degree of starch modification is fine grinding of the feedstuff.
- The sinking speed of fish feed pellets for salmon, trout, or perch is to be as low as possible so that there is enough time for feed consumption. A comparison of the different processes shows that **extruded feedstuff** sinks only half as fast as **pelleted feedstuff.**

The bulk density and thus the product density depend on the starch content of the formula and on the degree of modification of starch. The starch content in salmon or trout feed is very low. These fish do not need any starch, it is used only as a binder and to influence the density.

- An important factor influencing the product density is the speed of the extruder / expander.

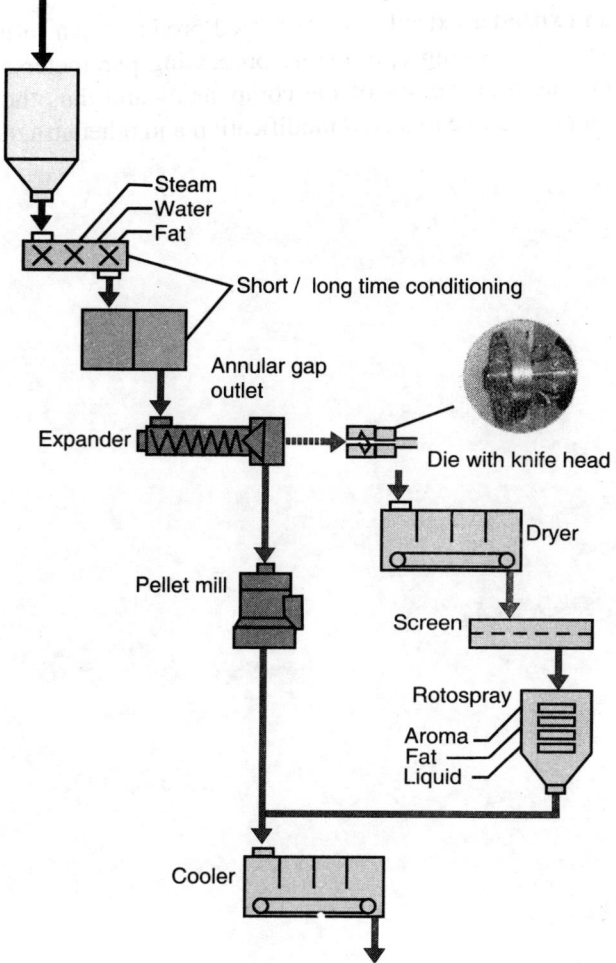

Figure 1. Flow scheme for the production of expanded pellets

- The density can also be modified by means of the oil addition. The added oil decelerates the starch modification by means of its sliding effect.

So there are possibilities of influencing the sinking and floating properties. With the same formula the bulk density can be varied between 430 and 550 g/l. The extruder is operated in dependence on the bulk density which is easy to measure. By selecting the required speed or oil addition, feedstuff for salmon or trout is produced as close as possible to the limit of floatability in order to obtain a slowly sinking pellet.

Conclusions

The adaptation of the product density to the feeding behaviour of the different types of fish is a prerequisite for successful fish farming. An appropriate adaptation reduces the losses as there is a lower water pollution caused by feed that has not been consumed and as there are no fines.

By using an expander/extruder the fish feed producer can influence the product density by means of choosing appropriate processing parameters.

Furthermore, the digestibility of the components and thus the nutritional value of the feed are improved due to starch modification and other structural modifications in the product.

8

Effects of Expander Processing on Macro- and Micro-ingredients

The expander - or, 'screw type, high-temperature short-time, shear conditioner' has been useful for feed manufacturers. Using the expander, we can sterilise feed, increase digestibility, add more liquids and use a wider range of ingredients, including more crop residues and food byproducts. Moreover, we can improve pellet quality, increase pelleting capacity, extend pellet die life and even eliminate the pelleting line itself.

What are the effects of the expander and other thermo-mechanical 'super conditioners' on individual ingredients and mixed feeds?

Macro ingredients

It is known that over-aggressive use of the expander can cause negative effects such as maillard reactions, formation of lysinoalanine and D-amino acids and ionic metal oxidation. However, feed mixture itself has inherent protective nature. Typical expander temperatures - 90–130°C - do not damage macro ingredients in mixed feed as severely as those ingredients processed individually. Protein molecules, for example, appear to bind physically with starch into a 'continuous phase matrix', which protects the protein from heat denaturation. Moreover, expander processing of a mixed feed decreases the tendency of protein to disperse upon heating, which may enhance the protective properties of the 'expanded' starch-protein matrix.

Micro ingredients

The Wageningen Feed Processing centre, University of Wageningen in the Netherlands, is a unique research institute dedicated to engineering, process development and evaluation of processing effects. Most investigators consider steam pelleting at best to be neutral toward feed additives - but it also can be destructive. However, different types of feed additives vary in their sensitivity to heat and moisture. With experience, feed manufacturers adjust the 'dosage safety margins' of sensitive feed additives to ensure that adequate concentrations survive processing. The same trial

- and - error adjustment is being done now with expanders with vitamins, anticoccidials and antibiotics, direct - fed microbial or enzymes.

Dr. van der Poel has estimated the feed additive stability in a range of feeds produced in feed plants in a variety of situations.

Vitamins

Many vitamins are essentially stable during expander processing, except vitamin A, vitamin K_3 (MSB) and vitamin C (Crystalline ascorbic acid). Stabilised formulations of vitamin A are available which offer protection against aggressive feed processive conditions, while other products dissolve at 40°C.

Anticoccidials and antibiotics

Most of these are relatively resistant to high temperature and moisture, with only small losses during the expanding process (100-130°C) and subsequent pelleting. e.g. salinomycin, lasalocid, avoparcin. Expander processing did cause losses of virginiamycin up to 40%.

A popular antibiotic that may be affected by expander processing is bacitracin. It is suggested that a protective formulation of the active compound may result in better stability in pelleted and expanded feeds. Dr. van der Poel himself recently demonstrated that the granular formulation of robenidine - HCl was more stable than the powder form in an expander processed broiler feed.

Enzymes

Expander processing is probably most destructive to feed enzymes. These complex proteins have specific, functional chemical structures that heat and moisture can inactivate or irreversibly modify. The critical temperature for these enzymes is less (e.g., 70°C for phytase, 80°C for carbohydrases) compared to expander operating temperatures. Most enzyme preparations are supplied in dry and liquid forms and a variety 'downstream' (i.e. post-expander) micro proportioning application systems are available. Liquid enzymes may be allergenic and hence safety of workers has to be kept in mind.

Direct-fed microbial products

These may be more sensitive to expander processing than the enzymes. However, some such 'probiotics' are available in heat protected forms or as spore forming organisms that can withstand the relatively high temperatures of steam pelleting in a dormant state. As with enzyme products, however, post processing application may be the most economical means to ensure dispersion of a 'live' product in an expanded feed.

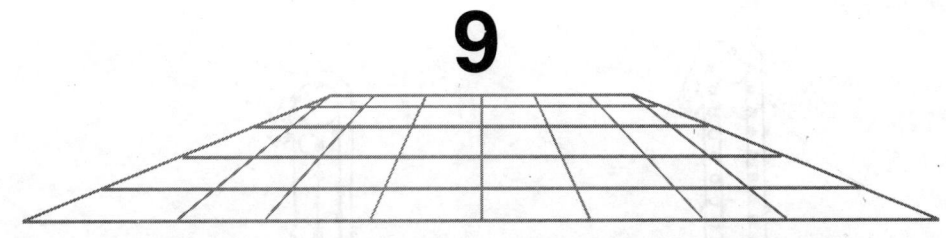

9

Commonly used Conveying Systems in Feed Mills

Different types

Conveyers are used to transport the material generally in horizontal direction, but with some modifications in vertical direction.

1. Screw conveyors
2. Drag conveyors: Two types a. Paddle type b. Bar type
3. Oscillating conveyors
4. Vibratory conveyors
5. Belt conveyors (Figure 1)

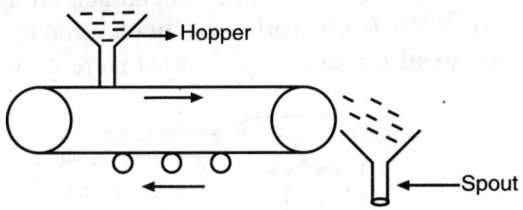

Figure 1. Belt Conveyor

6. Bucket elevators (figures 2, 3, 4, and 5)
7. Pneumatic conveyors (figure 6)

Bucket Elevators

An important feature of any feed manufacturing facility is the bucket elevator. Bucket elevators (legs) are the most efficient means of elevating grain, and other ingredients, pelleted feeds, mash finished feeds, and most materials except sticky material that will not discharge from the buckets. They consist of a belt or chain running in a vertical direction to which buckets are attached. Bucket elevators of the **centrifugal discharge type** (Figure 2) are normally used in the feed industry and most are of the belt type. Pellets might best be handled in **continuous bucket elevators** (Figure 3) that operate at slow speeds and are adapted for handling friable material. The buckets are discharged by gravity reducing breakage caused by the centrifugal force discharge of a centrifugal elevator.

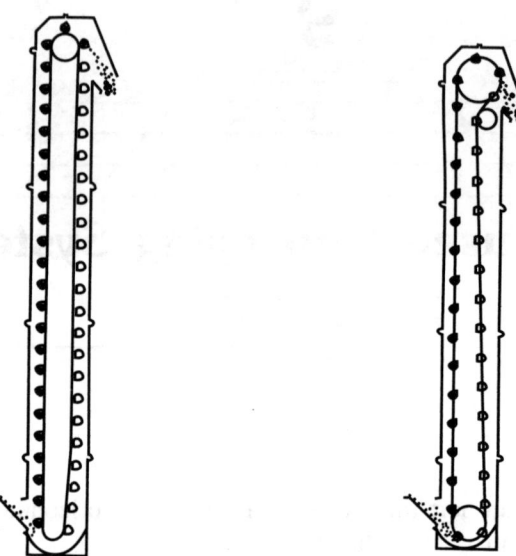

Figure 2. Centrifugal discharge bucket elevator

Figure 3. Continuous bucket elevator

Bucket elevators usually require the least amount of horsepower for vertical conveying of any conveying system. The buckets and belt are normally enclosed in a housing consisting of three major parts: **the boot** (product loading), **trunking** (product elevating), and **head** (product discharge) (Figure 4 and 5). This enclosure

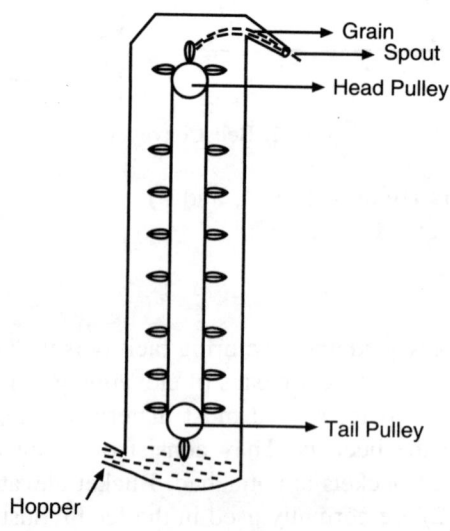

Figure 4. Bucket Elevator

keeps the conveyed material inside the leg, contains the dust, and can be weathertight for outside installation.

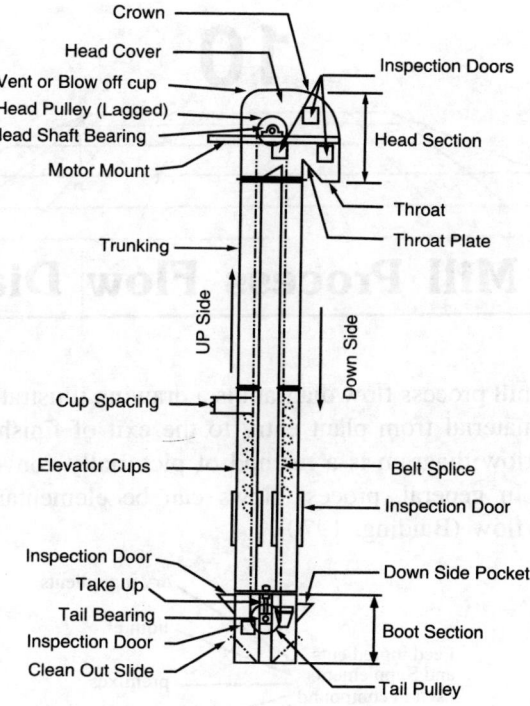

Figure 5. Bucket elevator components

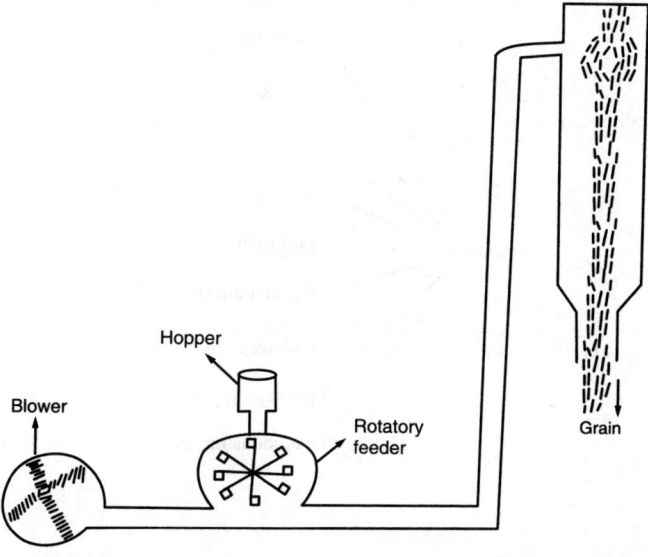

Figure 6. Pneumatic Conveyor

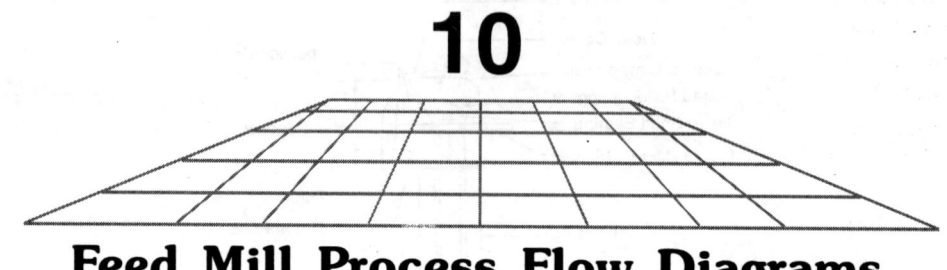

10

Feed Mill Process Flow Diagrams

A complete feed mill process flow diagram is a drawing illustrating all mill processes and the flow of material from plant entry to the exit of finished product from the plant. A process flow diagram is a method of pictorially conveying information of plant operations. In general, process flows can be elementary process flow and symbolic process flow (Balding, 1970).

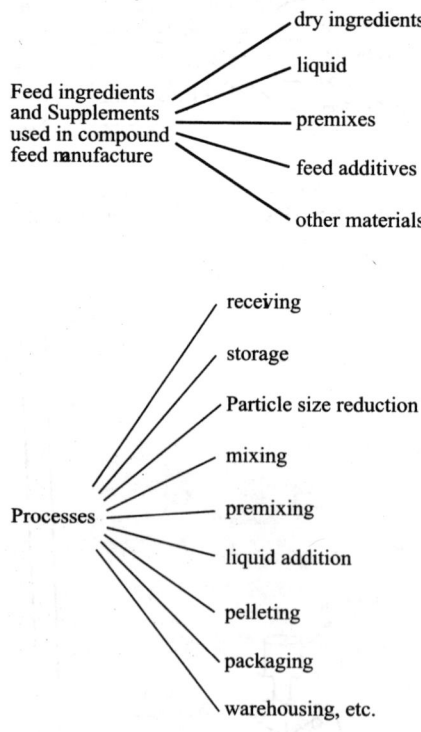

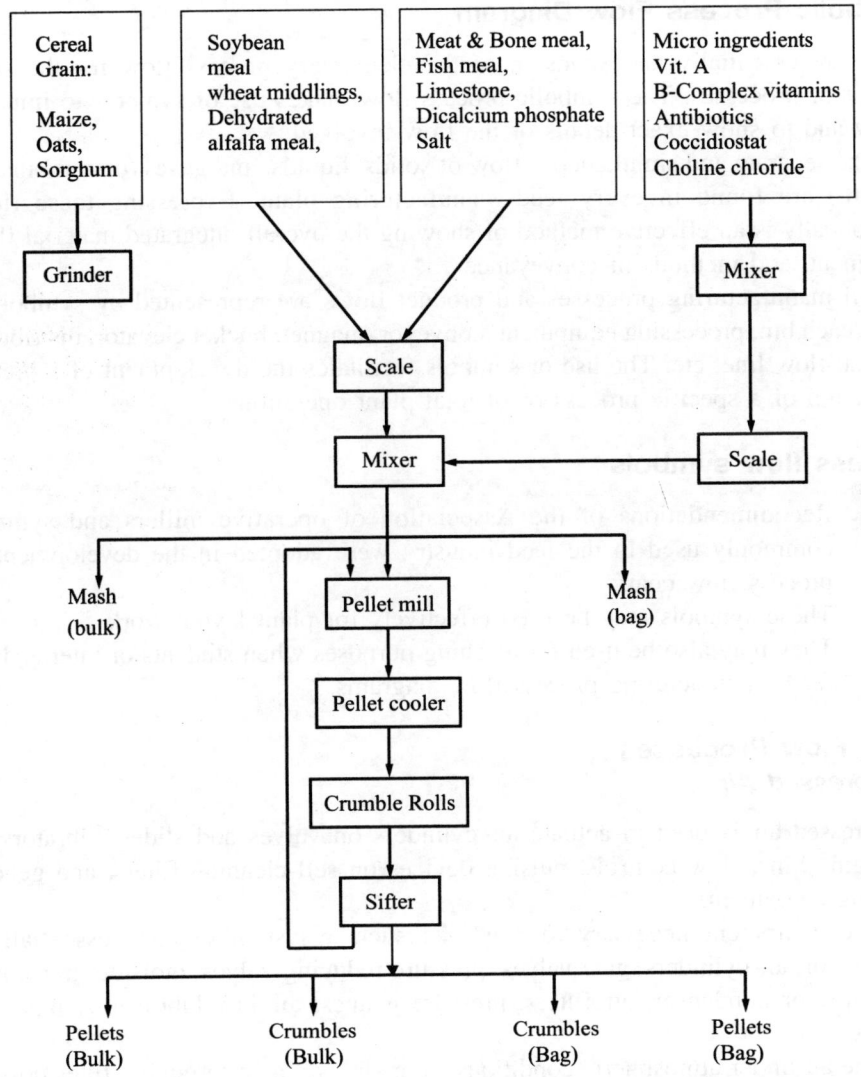

Figure 1. Elementary process flow for manufacture of complete poultry feed (Adapted from J.L.Balding (1970) Feed Manufacturing Technology)

Elementary Process Flow Diagram

An elementary process flow is a simple drawing that generally consists of a block diagram depicting the various processes and connecting lines to indicate flow of materials (Fig. 1). This type of process flow diagram can be effective in improving the understanding of existing plant operations or as an aid in preliminary planning of new plant design or remodelling projects.

It does not require a great deal of drafting skill to prepare and can easily be changed to incorporate desired plant features.

Symbolic Process Flow Diagram

These are essentially an expansion of the elementary process flow for the same process or processes. The symbolic process flow makes use of symbols to improve clarity and to show exact details of the flow involved.

The separate and simultaneous flow of solids, liquids, and **gases** (or combination of both) are found in every feed manufacturing plant. Expressing these flows symbolically is an effective method of showing the overall integrated material flow, equipment, and methods of conveyance.

All manufacturing processes and product flows are represented by symbols to depict each bin, processing equipment, conveyor, magnet, bucket elevator, distributor, material flow line, etc. The use of symbols facilitates the development of a precise illustration of a specific process or of total plant operations.

Process flow symbols

- Recommendations of the Association of operative millers and symbols commonly used in the feed industry were adopted in the development of process flow chart.
- These symbols may be used effectively for plant layout work.
- They may also be used for teaching purposes when students or interns draw feed manufacturing process flow diagrams.

Fluid Flow Processes
Compressed Air

Compressed air is used to actuate air cylinders on valves and slides, vibrators on packaging bins, flow controls, pulsing devices on self-cleaning filters, and general cleaning equipment.

The equipment necessary to construct such a system requires essentially a compressor, air cylinders, gate valves, pressure reducing valves, moisture traps, heat exchanger or condenser, air filters, pressure gauges, air line lubricators, pipe and fittings.

The air under atmospheric conditions (free air) is drawn through a filter prior to entering the compressor. This removes much of the dust prior to compression. Compression results in an increase in temperature and a decrease in volume. The hot air leaving the one - or two - stage compressor is forced through a heat exchanger (condenser) where it is cooled. Cooling of the compressed air to a temperature equal to or below its dew point condenses most of the moisture from the original air-water vapour mixture. From the heat exchanger the air is often passed through another filter to remove more of the dust particles before entering the compressed air tank. The air tank is a steel cylinder equipped with a pressure gauge and a moisture drain. This is necessary since further condensation in the air tank can occur and any accumulated sludge must be removed. Just beyond the compressed air tank, in the main distribution line, another large filter - condensate combination unit will generally be installed. Following this, a pressure regulator to overcome the lag and lead of the compressor and thus maintain a constant mainline pressure, is usually installed.

Molasses, with its high viscosity, presents handling problems, particularly at low temperatures. The fact that the viscosity and density of molasses decrease with increasing fluid temperature enhances its ability to be pumped satisfactorily from one location to another if it is heated. These characteristics combined with adverse environmental conditions will generally required that the molasses be preheated prior to leaving tank cars, storage tanks, or before entering the actual process. This requires a heat exchanger to improve the flow properties of molasses.

A heat exchanger is a device for transferring energy from a hot fluid (hot water or steam) to a cold fluid without mixing. This is attained by the transfer of energy across a tube wall separating the two fluids. A temperature-sensing device in the exit stream of the fluid being heated may actuate, in turn, a flow control device for increasing or decreasing the flow rate of the heating medium. Heat exchangers are classified in a number of ways: parallel-flow, counter-flow, cross-flow, single-pass, multipass, concentric tube, shell-and-tube type, and others.

Water and Steam

Water is used as cold water, hot water or steam would be primarily in heat exchangers, steam conditioning at pellet mills, grain steamers and grain cookers. Boiler water should be demineralized prior to heating. Otherwise mineral precipitation (scaling) will occur in the boiler, and other heat exchanger tubes.

Molasses handling system

Feed manufacturing processes often utilize liquid flow and heat transfer equipment for handling liquid and gaseous materials. These processes commonly involve the flow of air, molasses, fat, water and steam.

The equipment necessary for a molasses handling system in feed manufacturing will include a storage tank, work tanks, pumps, gate valves, globe valves, pressure relief valves, pressure gauges, flow meters, spray nozzles, check valves, pipe, fittings, heat exchangers and other related equipment.

Use of Process Flow Diagrams

1. These are generally recognized as useful aids in planning new feed mill design or remodelling projects.
2. These can be utilized to improve overall plant performance.
3. These are useful tools for training new employees to understand a specific plant operation. Diagrams will assist in explaining all the processes involved.
4. Plant quality control practices and procedures can be made more effective through the use of process flow diagrams. Equipment of particular concern would include mixers, surge bins, bucket elevators, distributors and bulk bins.
5. Plant safety can also be improved through the use of process flow diagrams during employee training activities. Use of process flow diagrams for employee training can greatly improve employee knowledge of safety responsibilities.

11

Grain dust–As a feed ingredient

Grain dust can be collected and compressed into pellets or wafers for use as an animal feed, a fuel or a fetilizer. Grain dust has attracted a great deal of attention because of its potential as a feed ingredient and also its potential as a safety hazard. Data through 1978 (Graziano, 1980) suggests the number of grain dust explosions and their severity have been increasing. No specific causes for the trend have been identified but contributory factors might include the quantity and rate at which grain is moved, facility design, government regulations and operating procedures (K.C.Behnke, 1982).

Environmental regulations in USA prevent grain dust from being vented to the atmosphere, hence the amount of grain dust being collected has increased significantly. The once common practice of returning grain dust to the grain or loadout (recycling) is losing favour with the recommendation by USDA that the practice not be allowed. These factors have led to a rather significant amount of grain dust being made available to the feed industry as an ingredient. It is anticipated that this trend will accelerate and certainly continue.

Variability: With any ingredient, there is a certain amount of variability in quality. This is particularly true for grain dust. Several factors have been identified that contribute to nutrient variability in grain dust (Behnke et al., 1979). Among them are: (1) dust system design (2) grain type handled (3) collection point in the marketing system and (4) season of the year. Perhaps the most important of the above factors are grain type and point in the marketing system. As a general rule, the nutritional profile of grain dust reflects the grain from which it originated. However, the nearer the collection point is to the point of harvest, the greater the amount of soil contamination and, therefore, the greater the ash content. This is particularly true of soybean dust.

Nutrient quality and composition: Even though grain dust has become a fairly common feed ingredient, there is no typical analysis listed in ingredient tables. Wade et al. (1979) surveyed grain dust properties at four large grain terminals to determine air concentration, particle size, and chemical composition at several locations within each terminal. A moisture range of 6.4 to 8.4 percent was found indicating that the grain dust was, generally, drier than the parent grain. Starch content varied from 50 to 65 percent except where soybeans were being handled. In that case, starch content was found to be 20 to 30 percent. The protein content of the grain dust was 6.5 to 11.6 percent where wheat and corn were the primary grains moved while soybean dust had 12.2 to 16.4 percent. Ash content was usually in the 10 to 12 percent range except for soybean dust which contained nearly 40% ash.

Lai et al. (1981) at the USDA grain Marketing Research Laboratory found that the protein content of the grain dust was comparable to the whole grain. However, the grain dust ash content was often found to be 8 to 19 times higher than the whole grain. Only nutritionally significant minerals were assayed. It was assumed that the additional major components were silica and aluminimum.

Amino acid composition of grain dust

Of particular interest to nutritionists is for lysine, usually the first limiting amino acid in grains. Only grain sorghum dust was found to be higher in lysine than the grain from which it came (Hubbard et al., 1982). The lysine content relative to total protein content was found to be higher in each grain dust than its parent with the exception of soybean dust. This was thought to be due to the fact that the protein in the outer layers of the kernel are higher in basic amino acid content than the whole kernel. The outer portion of the kernel is the most likely portion to be abraded off during handling. The authors concluded that mixing of grain dusts would not greatly change the amino acid profile of the grain dust protein because of the uniformity found in the samples assayed.

Behnke and Clark (1979) conducted a study in which mixed grain dust was collected at several inland terminals for the years 1976 through 1979. It was concluded that, while year to year variation did exist at each terminal, there was no specific trend evident. There was as much variation noted within yearly samples as between yearly samples.

Nutritional Utilization: After examining the nutritional data available, it might be concluded that grain dust from either a single source or mixed grain dust would be an acceptable feed ingredient in the diets of many animals. Most nutritionists and formulation experts are reluctant to use any ingredient unless controlled feeding trials are conducted to know its nutritive value. Factors such as potential toxicity, available energy and palatability are of great concern and need to be identified in order that an ingredient can be used with some degree of confidence.

Several feeding trials have been conducted with various classes of livestock and poultry. Pelleted and crumbled grain dust/mixed grain dust has been used in the place of grains. The results indicate that grain dust is a viable feed ingredient for both ruminants and nonruminants alike. In nearly all cases, a producer should be willing to accept slightly reduced performance from animals fed grain dust. The use of grain dust should, probably, be limited to 25% replacement of the grain portion of the diet except where economics might dictate a higher inclusion level.

Summary: Grain dust as an acceptable feed ingredient has been substantially addressed both from an analytical perspective and from an animal performance stand point. It appears that a reasonable level of grain dust could be included in many feeds without adversely affecting the performance of the feed.

A word of caution might be in order, however. The primary reason that substantial quantities of grain dust are being made available to the feed industry is due to the fact that the grain trade is attempting to "clean house." However, grain dust is at times, an attractive ingredient, it is extremely dangerous and difficult to handle in the unprocessed form. If a feed mill is to consider handling grain dust as an ingredient, physical modifications should be made to insure that it can be handled safety and property.

They are several processors currently pelleting grain dust and providing a safe and easily handled ingredient to the feed industry. Those considering the use of grain dust in feeds, should consider this product as an alternative.

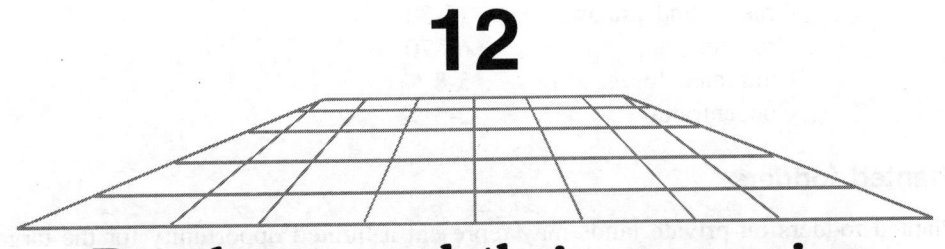

12

Roughages and their processing
N. Krishna

Roughages are feedstuffs of plant origin including pasture and agricultural byproducts containing more than 18% crude fibre or 35% cell-wall constituents or neutral detergent fibre (NDF) on dry matter (DM) basis. Roughages may be grouped into high quality and low quality types. High quality roughage is one that is usually low in lignin, high in protein and highly digestible. Low quality roughages are those which are usually low in protein, high in lignin and poorly digestible.

Roughages include green or dry forages, conserved forages, fibrous crop residues and agro-industrial byproducts of conventional or unconventional origin. Crop residues consisting parts of stem, leaves, seed coats etc. are available in the proportion of 1 to 3 times the yield of grains or seeds from cereals, legumes, millets and other crops, after harvesting.

Poor quality roughages generally constrained with less than 7.0-7.5 MJ of metabolizable energy (ME) per kg DM. These are the primary feed resources for feeding large and small ruminants in majority of the developing countries including India. They are generally fed in the form of grazed or harvested forages from cultivable or uncultivable land, forest areas, canal or tank bunds and stubbles left over after harvesting of cereal crops. The value of these low quality roughages as animal feed becomes more important to the Indian sub-continent.

A number of reports reveal that feed and fodder scarcity to be the major constraint to the growth of livestock sector, although actual deficit estimations vary among different sources. Countrywide survey, made by the 'National Institute of Animal Nutrition and Physiology (NIANP), Bangalore made during 2001 reveals a deficiency of 12, 34 and 64% in crop residues, green fodder and concentrates, respectively. Availability of balanced and quality feed and feed shortages in drier years is still the major limiting factor in increasing livestock productivity in the country.

Role of green forages

It is a common practice in India that the animals are allowed to forage during the day time on roadside grasses, community grazing lands, tree leaves, or cut grasses. In the evening they are fed straw in corrals or stalls. A survey conducted in India (Ranjhan, 1997), showed the following ranges in percentage of feed components in rations varying according to agro-climatic region, season and stage of the production cycle:

Grasses and grazing	15-30 %
Crop residues	66-70 %
Cultivated forages	5-8 %
Concentrates	2-5 %

Planted fodders

Planted fodders on private lands may represent a limited opportunity for the target group farmers. The Indian Grassland and Forage Research Institute (IGFRI) at Jhansi and others are carrying out a notable work with a wide range of fodder crops. There are few farmers currently allocating small areas of land to fodder crops such as berseem and lucerne. However, these interventions are mostly suitable for irrigated areas, which are largely under the control of the wealthier community groups. The NDDB is also testing a wide range of fodders through their milk unions that demonstrate newer varieties and invite co-operative members to visit fodder plots at the milk collection and processing plants.

Another alternative sometimes promoted is to grow forages on bunds between crops. Adoption of *Stylosanthes* spp. has been shown to be successful in a number of niches in India, particularly in tree plantations where it acts as a weed suppresser and provides nitrogen through 'N' fixation. Other successful initiatives of IGFRI station at Dharwad included a project where *Brachiaria, Cenchrus* and a Napier hybrid have been successfully established on more than 3000 farms on bunds in a DFID funded project operated by the BAIF. Generally that the areas where prospects for adoption are high would be where there is good access to milk markets and where there are breeds able to convert improved feed and fodder into a salable product.

Dual purpose crops and use of hybrids

There are clearly a number of issues to take into account when considering the potential for improved, dual purpose varieties of food crops such as sorghum, millet, maize and groundnut for small and marginal farmers that are growing subsistence crops in rain fed areas. A common experience of individuals working in the field is that the poor rely almost exclusively on saved seed from previous crops. These crops already have relatively high fodder yields and the inputs are restricted to manure from livestock that they own. Even farmers that grow grain for commercial purposes are observed to reserve a portion of the land for the local variety. It is likely that success will only occur where there is introduction of improved varieties, with high grain and fodder yields and perform well under existing farmer management regimes.

Management of common property resources (CPR) and water sheds

Institutions regulating the use of CPR earlier have since vanished and CPRs have declined or are being encroached upon. There has also been considerable decline in the quality of grasses in the CPRs and they turn into waste-land due to over-grazing, lack of management, and erratic rain fall. At the same time it is most often the poorest sections of the community, landless and small farmers who rely heavily on CPRs, community grazing lands, waste- lands and forest areas to supply the fodder needs of their livestock.

Change in cropping patterns

Cropping patterns are changing in many directions across India as a result of different forces. In Kerala farmers are moving from paddy to plantation as labour cost become a major constraint, resulting in an overall decrease in fodder supply from the land. In other states introduction of irrigation results in changes to cash crops providing limited fodder. For example, oil seeds replacing coarse grains; rice replacing a more varied range of crops including traditional legumes which provides high quality feed. Improvement of watersheds can increase area of land for cropping but at the cost of community grazing lands on which landless and marginal farmers rely to feed their livestock.

Researchable options for forage production

A number of researchable issues are identified that include:

> Participatory selection and evaluation of forage species and forage-based technologies
> Participatory selection and evaluation of different tree + grass + legume combinations on bunds and forage groundnuts in partially moist areas
> Performance of tree and grass species in silvi-pastoral systems without fertilizer
> Annual forage production systems for shifting cultivation.

In the development of CPRs as forage resource and their management, the following areas are researchable:

- Management of pasture / silvi-pasture and shrub density
- On- farm verification of grasses, legumes and nutrient cycling
- Faster growing vegetable hedges, with some economic value, for protecting common property lands
- Evaluation of different grazing management systems and optimal grazing pressure.

How to solve the fodder problem?

- There is a need to assess the feeding habits of animals. For instance, hill goats eat different types of grasses
- Participatory selection of fodder crops that need less water or care and management. Natural grasses with green fodder potential may provide more nutrients.
- Community action by social agro-forestry approach needs to be followed. Joint forest management and community fencing may be undertaken.

- To develop pastures in phases to cope with grazing demand in the crop season
- Community fodder banks can be established at village level.
- Dry fodder can be stored and shared among the village community. Such committees may be made at village, block and district levels.
- Involving government and local bodies in community action since the land belongs to the government and enrolling higher officials for advocacy and creating awareness.
- Involving local NGOs with interest in fodder development for implementation
- Encouraging crop insurance policies
- To develop local irrigation capacity for growing better crops that increase straw yield and grow forages where farmers may opt for them
- Fodder spaces can be grown around water harvest structures.
- Co-operatives need to be encouraged to collect milk from villages that are not linked with roads.

Nutritional parameters associated with poor quality roughages

It is an established fact that poor quality roughages are less palatable with low nutritional status than the cultivated grasses, cereal fodders or legumes and hence vast scope exists to improve their nutritional quality.

The major constraints associated with the use of crop residues such as straws as ruminant feed are low nutrient density and poor digestibility, which lead to low nutrient intake and reduced animal performance. The low nitrogen, energy and mineral profile, along with their high lignin and silica levels influence their nutrient digestibility. Consequently straw based rations hardly meet the maintenance needs of even non-producing ruminants.

Cellulose and hemicellulose are potential sources of energy for ruminants and these are in plenty in straws and other roughages. But their association with lignin and silica affects the extent of microbial fermentation in the rumen and thus cereal straws remain as poor sources of energy. There is a negative correlation between lignin and cellulose and digestible dry matter. Silica has more profound effect in reducing the nutrient digestibilities compared to lignin content of roughages.

Chemical and physical bonding of lignin and silica with hemicellulose and cellulose prevents sufficient swelling of fibrous feed resources thus blocking penetration by fibre digesting enzymes. Hence, the association of lignin and silica with cell-wall constituents influences the ability of microbial enzymes to digest these components and in turn limiting the nutrient availability to ruminants. As the cell-wall constituents increase above 50% of DM, voluntary feed intake declines (Van Soest, 1983). Low voluntary intake of lignocellulosic crop residues is due to their lower digestibility and longer retention time in the gastrointestinal tract of ruminants.

Importance of roughages in ruminant rations

Roughages are added to the rations not only to supply energy, but also to impart certain physical properties such as bulk to the rations which make them more acceptable to the animal. Some amount of roughages appears to be necessary in the rations in order to maintain proper rumen function and optimum health of the ruminant. In case of dairy cows, roughages are necessary in the rations in order to maintain satisfactory butter fat levels in the milk.

Mechanical processing of crop residues

Mechanical processing of crop residues leads to three major advantages such as increased voluntary intake, improvement in nutritive value and facilitation in the preparation of complete feeds. The aim of mechanical processing is to reduce the particle size of lignocellulosic crop residues thereby increase in the surface area exposed for enzymatic degradation. Bulk density of crop residues is very low as compared to cereal grains and oil meals. However, the bulk density of crop residues can be increased markedly by chaffing, grinding and pelleting. Particle size reduction generally improves the intake of roughages, the improvement being substantial with poor quality roughages.

Processing of roughages

Several methods of dry and wet processing are used in making better use of roughages for animal feeding. Dry processing methods include baling, chopping, grinding, pelleting, cubing and dehydration. Wet processing methods include chopping greens and conversion into high moisture silage and low moisture silage.

Roughages are subjected to various processing techniques such as physical, physico-chemical, chemical and biological methods.

Physical processing methods

Physical processing takes into account soaking, chopping, grinding, pelleting, extrusion, steam treatment under pressure and gamma irradiation. Strategic supplementation of deficient nutrients at rumen level and at host animal level works well in improving the nutritive value of roughages. Some of the most popular processing methods employed in India are briefly discussed below.

Soaking

Soaking in water overnight reduces dustiness, a problem with fine chaffed or ground residues even though the results are not always consistent. It affords an easy way to add urea in solution, with reduced risks of urea poisoning.

Chopping /Chaffing

It enhances ease of handling, facilitates mixing with other ingredients, reduces wastage, increases DMI and rate of eating and decreases the amount of chewing (Hadjigeorgiou et al., 2003). Chaffing is a less severe processing method that aimed to reduce the size of feed particles. Reduction in long stems of crops like straws / stovers has the advantage of easy handling, preventing selection of highly nutritive tender parts by the animals and easiness while blending with other concentrate feedstuffs. However, this method of physical processing has little effect on intake and rate of digestion.

Grinding

Grinding exposes the internal cell material to immediate microbial attack in the rumen, thus speeding up digestion and increasing the feed intake. Scope for selection by the animal is reduced thus ensuring increased use of the residue. Fine grinding is expensive and needs sophisticated machinery. Grinding in a hammer mill with the screen removed is suggested.

The digestibilities of NDF and ADF were reported to be lower through grinding compared to chopping due to faster rate of passage from reticulo-rumen of sheep and goats (Reddy and Reddy, 1992). To derive the maximum benefits of grinding on the DMI, improved nutritive value and to maintain milk fat level at a minimum processing cost for incorporation in complete diets, optimum particle size is required.

Grinding decreases the particle size, increases the surface area and enhances the bulk density of leaf and stem fractions of forages. Ground roughages often are further processed by pelleting or cubing before being fed. Benefits derived from pelleting include a further increase in bulk density, decreased dustiness and increased ease of handling. Grinding and pelleting of low-quality roughages increase the feed intake, daily gains and feed efficiency.

Grinding does not improve the digestibility of fibre fractions of crop residues but sometimes reduces their digestibility as compared to chaffing due to faster rate of passage from the reticulorumen. Digestibility of ground and pelleted roughages is generally depressed relative to that of the parent materials fed in either long or chopped form. The decrease in the digestibility of ground and pelleted forages is primarily due to reduced fibre digestion.

Grinding of either mixed grass hay or cotton straw through 8 mm sieve and pelleting through 9 mm die did not affect the milk fat percentage in crossbred cows or buffaloes. It is advantageous to retain large particle size for forage within the maximal limits for thorough mixing. The maximum required length of the particles should be about 10-20 mm. Finely ground roughages may be better utilized as a feed energy source in growing animals, though severe processing increases the cost of ration.

Pelleting

The beneficial effects of pelleting over chopped or ground roughages are further increase in voluntary feed intake, bulk density, nutrient digestibilities, reduced dustiness and ease in handling. It also brings about changes in the rumen VFA profile, produces more propionic acid and less acidic acid (Le Liboux and Peyroud, 1998).

Fine grinding and pelleting of forages dramatically reduces the time that ruminants spend on chewing and ruminating and consequently saliva production is reduced significantly. As a result of the decreased buffering capacity, the ruminal pH is also decreased. Low ruminal pH and increased rate of digesta passage result in decreased cell-wall carbohydrate fermentation in animals consuming processed forages. Acetate to propionate ratio is often reduced with these processed forages. Grinding and pelleting of roughages does not enhance the utilization of nutrients by ruminants. However, such processing increases the animal performance primarily due to increased digestible energy.

Chemical processing

There is considerable opportunity to improve the feeding value of roughages through chemical treatment in terms of increased feed intake and digestibility. Chemical processing hydrolyses the chemical bonds between lignin and hemicelluloses. Mild alkalis solubilize some of the cell-wall hemi-cellulose and non-core lignin. The chemicals employed are mostly sodium hydroxide, calcium hydroxide, ammonium hydroxide, anhydrous ammonia, urea ammoniation, sulphur dioxide, hydrogen peroxide, and ozone. Among several alkalies tried NaOH is the most potent alkali used for enriching the straws with 10-20% improvement in the OM digestibility. Alkali level of 2-5% has been found to be effective in reducing the amount of ADF and NDF in the treated straws. NaOH is caustic and can ulcerate the animal's mouth and pollute the soil via excretion in faeces and urine.

Ammonia, in the form of anhydrous NH_3, aqueous NH_3 or urea hydrolysed by food-borne bacteria is widely used (Sundstol, 1984). Ammonia is generally applied at the rate of 4kg/100 kg straw DM. At the ambient temperature the straw needs to be allowed for 7 days for effective fermentation or up to 21 days if it is used in the form of urea (Elangovan *et al.*, 2001).The beneficial effects of the treatment include increased fibre digestibility by 5-15% through solubilization of hemicelluloses, weakening of cell-wall and promoting the colonization by rumen bacteria and enhanced intake of digestible DM.

Physico-chemical processing methods include chopping and chemical treatment, chemical treatment and pelleting and chemical treatment and steaming.

Biological processing

A substantial portion of the energy from fibrous crop residues and coarse roughages is unavailable to the ruminants. The white rot fungi have the capacity to attack lignin polymers, besides opening aromatic rings to release low molecular weight fragments. The two-stage Karnal process developed for biological treatment of straws involved treatment of straw with urea during the 1st stage of 25 days followed by inoculation with *Coprinus fimetarius* spawn for a period of 5 days (Gupta 1986). Application of urea during the first stage results in breaking of lignocellulosic bonds besides providing a conducive alkaline pH for inhibiting the growth of undesirable microbes favouring growth of inoculated fungus. Increase in amino acid levels in the treated straw indicate that the fungus is capable of utilizing (free) ammonia generated during the 1st stage for synthesizing amino acids during the 2nd stage.

Subsequently, the process was further refined by Singh and Gupta (1994). In the modified method, the roughage source is first treated with anhydrous ammonia instead of urea and the treatment period is reduced from 30 to 7 days during the 1st stage. This is followed by 5-day period for the activity of fungal inoculation during the 2nd stage. The advantage of the modified method is that it is much faster without adversely affecting the nutritive value of roughage.

Fungal treated straw contains higher protein compared to urea treated straw but has the disadvantage of reduction in DM digestibility with lower TDN value. A combination of 4 % NaOH treatment plus 1hr steaming before inoculation with

Aspergillus terreus A$_2$ gives maximum increase in CP content (20%) in submerged fermentation under laboratory studies.

Enzyme treatment

Rumen microorganisms do not possess enzyme system for breakdown of lignin which prevents the utilization of other structural carbohydrates such as cellulose and hemi-celluloses which are associated with it in the plant cell-wall. The use of enzymes for upgrading of roughages is the upcoming area of research in the recent past. The main advantage of enzyme treatment is much greater control on the end products formed after treatment with little or no potential environmental pollution. The two main approaches to the use of enzymes recently examined have been related to the use of polysacharidases and ligninase enzymes with varying degrees of success.

Future methods of treatment are likely to involve bio-degradable materials such as enzymes. However, materials for on-farm use must be cheap, easily available, safe (both to handle and to feed) and conveniently transportable.

Complete diets

Complete diets provide all the nutrients required by the ruminants except water. All feed ingredients including roughages are processed and mixed into a uniform blend, which is available free choice to the animals ensuring supply of all the nutrients. The concentrate and roughage levels may vary from diet to diet so as to meet the optimum nutrient requirement of animals for different physiological purposes and levels of production. Complete feed contains minimum amount of 40% forage dry matter as hay or silage or 30% as straw in a total ration. Certain unconventional feeds such as sunflower heads/stalks, cotton straw, tree leaves, forest grasses, etc could be successfully incorporated in a complete feed after coarse grinding.

The desirable roughage component of complete diets is 40-50% for growing animals and 70-80% for dry animals. The roughage portion could preferably be a legume hay while the other ingredients would vary. These diets can be processed into mash, briquettes, blocks or pellets. The complete feed concept has the potential for utilizing existing feed resources more effectively for economic animal production.

Beneficial aspects of complete diets

- In India, where ruminants subsist on crop residues, poor quality roughages and agro-industrial byproducts, the complete diet system helps in utilizing these feed resources more efficiently.
- It also ensures the supply of ready-made balanced low cost feed for cattle, buffaloes, sheep and goats.
- It offers greater spread of consumption compared to the conventional system of feeding.
- More frequent feeding ensures steady state and optimum conditions in the rumen and thus enhances the utilization of NPN substances and absorption of nutrients in general.

- Rumen pH is more conducive for the activity of cellulolytic bacteria and thus fibre digestibility is increased.
- Dry matter intake of the animals is increased because of lesser digestive upsets on complete diet feeding.
- When large amounts of concentrates are fed separately from that of roughages rumen acidity is encountered.
- Milk production is increased through accurate balancing of ration and proper supply of nutrients to the animal for better utilization.
- Rumen contents are less acidic with acetic and propionic acids in the ratio of 3:1, which favour normal butter fat content.
- It allows better use of feed ingredients having low palatability since uniform blending helps to mask the offensive odours and bitter taste of feed ingredients.

Production of complete diets: mash feeds and expander-extruder feeds

Pioneering work has been undertaken on formulation and evaluation of complete feeds at ANGRAU, Hyderabad and BAIF Development Research Foundation, Uruli Kanchan under "Net Work Programme on Agricultural By-products as Animal Feeds as Complete Feeds". The complete diet system can be applied in two ways for feeding of livestock: mash feeds and expander-extruder feeds.

Mash feeds

These feeds are constituted by simple mixing of roughages (either dry or green) with concentrates in a proper proportion and are offered as wholesome feed to the ruminants in the name of 'Total Mixed Ration' (TMR). Individual dairy farmers and groups of small farmers can use the crop residues (chaffed) available with them to mix with either compound feed or individual feed resources such as oilcakes, grains, brans and minerals in appropriate proportion and produce balanced feeds. Such rations are cheaper and help in the optimum utilization of home grown forages and crop residues.

Expander-extruder technology for complete feeds

The expander-extrusion process involves pushing an extrudate through an opening to produce predefined shape. It is the process by which starchy and/or proteinous materials are partly cooked and plasticized in a tube by a combination of moisture, pressure, temperature and mechanical shear. This results in increased product temperature within the tube, gelatinization of starchy components and restructuring of tactile components and exothermic expansion of extrudate. The compound feed industry can adopt this technology to produce complete feed either in pellet form or block form.

Processing of complete feed as mash

The ingredients required for grinding are ground in a hammer mill. The ground ingredients are driven to a mixer through screw conveyer/bucket elevator and hopper above the mixer. The ingredients that do not require grinding are directly added to the mixer. Molasses is pumped from the storage tank to a heating tank where it is heated up to 70°C. The heated molasses is sent to the mixer through a dosage tank as per the formula. The micro-ingredients such as vitamins, minerals and antibiotics are made into a premix by diluting with the ground grain or bran and the required quantity of premix is added to a mixer directly. Subsequently, all the ingredients are mixed for about 10 minutes and collected into sacs and stored.

Pelleted feed

The mash from the mixer is conveyed into a hopper over the pellet mill. The mash is conveyed into conditioning chamber of the pellet mill through a screw conveyor. The rate of flow of the feed into the conditioning chamber is controlled by wheel valve. The required quantity of steam with 97-98°C temperature is added into the conditioning chamber through the control valve. The conditioned mash at 90-92°C temperature along with 16-17% moisture is conveyed to the pellet mill and extruded with a ring die of 9mm hole diameter. The pellets with 9mm diameter having 83-85°C temperature and 14-15% moisture are dropped from the pellet mill into the vertical cooler below the pellet mill. The cooled pellets are collected into sacs.

Expander-extruder processing

This is a system which combines the features of expanding (application of moisture, pressure and temperature to gelatinize the starch portion) and extruding (pressing the feed through constrictions under pressure). The mash at 12-13% moisture and room temperature is reconstituted with required quantity of water to get 17-18% moisture into the mixer itself. The material is then sent to the hopper above the expander-extruder from which it passes through a screw in which it attains a temperature of 90-95°C by the time it comes out of the die openings. Otherwise, the mash without reconstitution can be sent to the hopper and steam added to get required moisture while the feed is passed through the screw of expander-extruder. The pellets coming out of the expander-extruder are cooled and collected into sacs.

Densification of roughages

Densification is achieved by bailing, pelleting, briquetting and block making (Kundu and Veena Mani, 2009). Bailing is commonly applied on roughages and the volume reduction is comparatively quite less (bulk density 140-170kg/m3). Degree of densification is very high ($500-700kg/m^3$) in the pelleting process. But it is an energy intensive process because of chopping and grinding involved with roughages.

The briquetting process densifies the residues by 7 to 10 times by the application of pressure and heat. However, these pelleting and briquetting machines cannot handle feed mixture having larger particle size of straws and high proportion of crop residues. Densification through complete feed block preparation is comparatively a new concept in India and it offers several advantages over the former processes.

Development of block making machine

The densified feed blocks are made with an electrically operated hydraulic press machine (Nand Kishore and Lohan, 2009). The machine has two jackets of the dimensions of 23.5 × 23.5 × 23.5 cm each and two blocks can be made simultaneously each weighing about 3.5 kg.

The machine has a hydraulic jacket and a pressure gauge (0 to 420 kg/cm^2) to measure the pressure to be applied. The applied pressure can be kept for a fixed period of time (dwell time). The jackets are covered on the top with lids and are filled with material to be densified. The pressure is then applied and the densified material is taken out from the jacket in the form of a feed block.

The material to be densified is thoroughly mixed and required quantity filled in the jackets of the press machine. The optimum levels of molasses and moisture required are 15 and 15 to 17%, respectively to make more compact and durable blocks. The optimum dwell time is about 5 minutes. Berseem is an ideal legume source to be added to the blocks after 96 h of wilting. The complete feed blocks can be stored in godowns under natural climatic conditions for about one year without deterioration in quality.

Animal feed block formation machines

The machines for molding animal feed into blocks using a whole range of crop residues, feed supplements and suitable binders have been developed at IARI, New Delhi. It can form compressed blocks in the sizes appropriate and economical for handling, transportation and storage of large volumes of animal feed under Indian conditions.

A prototype machine for compaction of biomaterials using hydraulic cylinders for application of compaction pressure up to 6000 PSI has been designed, fabricated and extensively tested. The machine is powered with 25 HP electric motor to run its hydraulic system. It is very simple to operate and a single person can regulate the entire operation of the machine. The output capacity of the machine is 200-250 kg/h. It can compact all kinds of feed materials to a square shape (20 cm x 20 cm) blocks of desired thickness and weight. The bulk density of the roughage based feed blocks from this machine can be enhanced up to 4 to 5 times to that of the original feed material.

High capacity feed block formation machine (1 tonne/h) has also been developed to meet the industrial requirement. It forms feed blocks of 37 x 37 x 32 cm weighing 18-20 kg for commercial scale application. Similarly, a low capacity feed block making machine (40kg / h) has been developed for small ruminants such as sheep and goats and laboratory animals like rabbits to produce 0.5 to 1kg blocks.

Benefits of densified feed block

- The technique has the advantage of reducing the cost of transportation and minimizing the risks involved in the operation of voluminous sized of trucks while carrying the materials during trading.

- Densified products require much less storage space, which is a major limitation in and around cities and urban areas.
- Feeding of balanced complete feed blocks saves time and labour besides reducing the problem of nutrient deficiency and wastage of feeds.
- Selection by the animal is also lowered to a maximum extent.
- Feed blocks are comparatively cheaper as there is no need to grind the roughage portion as is the case with pelleting.
- Feed blocks are more palatable and digestible compared to pelleted feeds as well as to conventional feeding of straws and concentrates fed separately.
- The technology is helpful particularly in solving the problem of feeding livestock during natural calamities such as floods, droughts and cyclones.
- Feed blocks may be used as carrier of several chemicals such as feed additives and anti-helmenthic medicines with dual advantage.

REFERENCES TO THE LITERATURE (PARTIAL LIST)

Elangovan, A.V., Kishan, J. and Sahoo, A. 2001. Fate of lingo-cellulosic components and urea-nitrogen in urea-ammoniated wheat straw. Animal Nutrition and Feed Technology,1:61-68.

Gupta, B.N. 1986. Microbial treatment of lingo-cellulosic materials. Proc.Vth Animal Nutrition Research Workers Conference. M. L.Sukhadia University, Udaipur. July 14-17.p 94.

Hadjigeorgiou, I.E. Gordon, I. J. and Milne, J.A. 2003. Intake, digestion and selection of roughage with different staple lenghths by sheep and goats. Small Ruminal Research, 47:117-132.

Kundu, S S and Veena Mani. 2009. Densification of roughages and nutritional evaluation of feed blocks. In Proc.Satellite Symposium on Fodder Technology under ILDEX 2009, New Delhi. Pp 35-47.

Le Liboux, S. and Peyroud, J. L. 1998. Effects of forage particle size and intake level on fermentation patterns and sites and extent of digestion in dairy cows fed mixed diets. Animal Feed Science and Technology, 73: 131-150.

Ranjhan, S.K. 1997. Animal Nutrition in the Tropics. Fourth revised edition. Vikas Publishing House, New Delhi.

Reddy, M, R. and Reddy, G.V.N. 1992. Effect of processing on the nutritive value of eight crop residues and two forest grasses in goats and sheep. Australian Journal of Agricultural Science, 5: 295-301.

Reddy, D.V. 2004. Feed Pelleting Technology including newer developments. Proc. of Workshop on "Design and Development of Indigenous Equipments for Feeding, Manufacturing, Preservation and Package of Animal Feed" held at College of Veterinary Science & AH (Deen Dayal Upadhyaya Pashu Chikitsa Vigyan ViswaVidyalya Evam Gau Anusandhan Sansthan), Mathura, Uttar Pradesh, during April 16-17, 2004, pp 52-67. New subject matter is added.

Singh,G P. and Gupta, B N.1994. Evaluation of fungal treated cereal straw and further modification of Karnal process. Indian Journal of Animal Sciences, 64: 857-862.

Sundstol, F. 1984. Ammonia treatment of straw: methods for treatment and feeding experience in Norway. Animal Feed Science and Technology, 10: 173-187.

Thomas, M. and van der Poel, A.F.B. 1996. Physical quality of pelleted animal feed. 1. Criteria for pellet quality. Animal Feed Science and Technology, 61: 89-112.

Thomas, M., van Zuilichem, D.J. and van der Poel, A.F.B. 1997. Physical quality of pelleted animal feed. 2. Contribution of processes and its conditions. Animal Feed Science and Technology, 64: 173-192.

Thomas, M., Huijnen, P.T.H.J., van Vliet, T., van Zuilichem, D.J. and van der Poel, A.F.B. 1999. Effects of process conditions during expander processing and pelleting on starch modification and pellet quality of tapioca. Journal of the Science of Food and Agriculture, 79: 1481-1494.

van Soast, P.J. 1983. Nutritional ecology of ruminants. O and B books Inc; 1215. NW Kline Place, Corvallis, Oregon, USA.

Wood, J.F. 1987. The functional properties of feed raw materials and their effect on the production and quality of feed pellets. Animal Feed Science and Technology, 18:1-17.

SECTION VI
Feed Plant Management

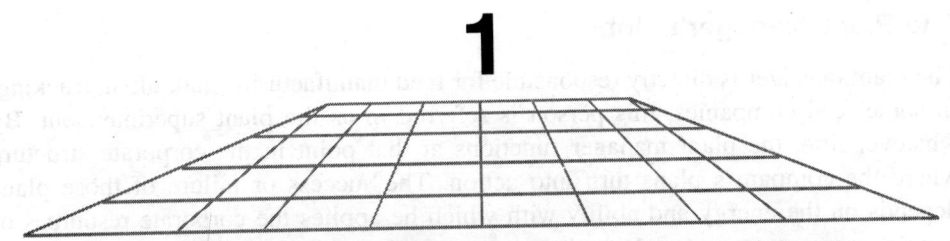

Feed Plant Management—Plant Manager's Responsibilities and Functions

Plant Management: The management of a feed manufacturing plant is not so different from the management of any manufacturing facility in any industry. Basically, a plant manager is responsible for the three P's - People, Product and Plant; The list of P's goes on to include Profits, Planning, Public, Productivity, Policies and Practices, Pride, Philosophy of management, and many others that are part and parcel of effective plant management (McEllhiney, 1985).

People/Personnel: It is the job of the plant manager to put his employee relationships on a business like basis with the overall goals of the company in mind (Becker, 1974). People responsibilities include the selection, training, treatment, and utilization of personnel to promote productivity, pride and peace in the work force.

Product/Production: The most obvious responsibilities of plant management evolve around producing a quality product on time at the lowest cost, safely and with good employee relations.

Physical Plant/Property: The capacity, effectiveness, quality, and reliability of the plants physical equipment are fundamental factors in the achievement of its manufacturing goals. The company expects plant management to husband its physical assets, to maintain and improve them, and to turn them over to the next generation of management in better condition than they found them.

Profits/Profitability: No responsibility of plant management is more important than that of contributing to the profitability of the business enterprise.

Planning/Projecting: Planning for the short term or long term (strategic) is critical to effective plant management from the planning of a production schedule to planning a budget to planning for capital improvements. The execution of plans is also a prime responsibility of plant management.

Public: The responsibilities of plant management to the public range from conforming to public laws and regulations to maintaining and promoting the company image in the community in which the plant is located. And, since some segments of the public are the patrons or customers of the plant, there is no higher order than to please them by providing products and services in a timely fashion at a price that is competitive.

The Plant Manager's Job

The Plant manager is directly responsible for feed manufacturing and, often, trucking. In some feed companies, this person is referred to as the plant superintendent. By whatever title, the plant manager functions at that point in the corporate structure where the company's plans turn into action. The success or failure of those plans depends on the energy and ability with which he applies the corporate resources of people, money, raw materials, and equipment to the task of producing the company's products and services (Becker, 1974).

The demands on the plant manager in his use of these resources grow heavier as the complexity and pace of the economy increase. Corporate management, caught in the profit squeeze, requires closer compliance to the budget and expects cost reductions to be achieved on a preplanned basis. New plant processes require more complicated equipment and tighter quality controls. The community and regulatory agencies at all governmental levels expect the plant to reduce noise, air and water pollution to lower levels. Paper work in the form of reports, analyses, computer printouts, correspondence, and so on flowing both to and from the plant seems overwhelming.

Manufacturing functions

The job of the production or manufacturing department of a feed company may be defined as, "to make a quality product on time at the lowest possible cost, safely and with good employee relations". But this definition falls short of the expectations and demands of companies today.

Product quality

The Plant must not only produce the products in required quantities on time to meet the demands of its customers but also it must play a larger role in the overall marketing scheme of the company than once might have been the case. The plant manager is expected to communicate knowledge developed in his operation, which may lead to new products or to improving old ones, and to guard the company against obsolescence by responding quickly to meet changes in markets, technology, and the intensity of competition. Manufacturing is not a stand-along function.

Cost Economics

The Plant manager is expected not only to produce quality products at the lowest possible cost but also to make prudent and profitable application of capital funds. The company looks for wise use of money in the purchase and installation of equipment that is labour-saving, maintenance-free, reliable, and offering flexibility for future developments.

The company must rely on the manufacturing people to protect its investment by proper maintenance, good house keeping, and the physical protection of plant property.

The company also expects the manufacturing group to help gain a competitive edge by continuously finding ways of reducing costs while improving products and customer service.

Social contacts

Maintaining good employee relationships is no longer considered a fringe activity by any serious plant manager. A low incidence of employee grievances or strikes is not just enough. It may require the active development of good relationships with the entire community in which the plant is located including neighbours, civic authorities, the business and professional community, minority groups, and those concerned with the environment as well as the company's employees.

Plant Manager's Responsibilities

Whatever is the size of the plant or nature of the corporate structure, the plant manager (PM) is expected to produce results in six basic areas: production, quality, costs, safety, house keeping and employee relationships.

Production

Manufacturing the required quantity of finished products in time to meet customer demands is a fundamental demand on the plant manager. The late arrivals of raw materials, absenteeism, bad weather, power failure / shortages, equipment breakdown, late orders etc are the obstacles that prevent his reaching the goal.

The plant manager must use his greatest powers of leadership to foresee and overcome the obstacles to meeting production schedules and to motivate his people to get the work out in spite of the difficulties. Failure to supply in time means driving away the valued customers. He accomplishes this by setting an example of refusing to yield to obstacles and exhibiting a tough minded approach in fighting for the way to get production out on time no matter what the difficulties.

The plant manager has to accurately determine the production capacity of the plant so that the company can make profitable decisions regarding sales and marketing strategies. Misleading the management can result in erroneous marketing decisions. In estimating production capacities, time allowances must be made for equipment downtime, cleaning, preventive maintenance, and other nonproductive plant hours. The plant manager must also communicate any additional capacity that might be obtained by increasing shifts or days worked in a week.

Quality

The plant manager must establish an attitude in his organization that reaches well beyond the passing of laboratory tests. He has to establish a programme of product integrity that commits the entire organization to manufacturing the products according to standard process instructions, each time, without shortcuts or individual deviation.

The plant manager should instill respect for total quality. In the quest for quality, the plant manager can't lose sight of his profit responsibilities. If the company's moisture standard for finished mash-type feed is 10.5 - 11.5%, it is a costly error to turn out a product at 9% moisture. It amounts to giving away more than 1 kg of feed for every 100 kg sold.

Costs

- The requirement to produce at lowest possible costs or within budgetary guidelines is the primary responsibility.
- The plant manager is to prepare or to be actively involved in the preparation of annual operating budgets for all plant functions such as production, maintenance and trucking, then to control expenses within the limits of those budgets throughout the year. He has to create a cost and value consciousness throughout his organisation.
- Company management expects the plant manager to set up result-producing, continuing programmes rather than following once-a-year crash programme for cost reductions.
- The Plant manager must participate in the company's capital expenditure programme. He makes recommedations for new plants and equipment to expand production, to reduce costs, to improve quality and service, to meet regulatory agency requirements, and so on. He has the responsibility to protect investments in existing facilities with sound maintenance practices.

Safety

The plant manager must do whatever he can to prevent the injury or death of his employees from a humanitarian standpoint.

House Keeping

The plant manager's responsibility for good housekeeping is critical, especially in the feed and other grain processing and handling industries. Product quality is threatened by dirty surroundings. The morale and efficiency of the work force are lowered if the plant is not clean. Housekeeping has to be an on-going activity to keep the plant clean throughout.

The plant manager has a responsibility to the community in which his plant is located to maintain a facility that does credit to the company and is a not a blemish on the community or a hazard or nuisance to its neighbours.

Employee relationships

It is not the job of the plant manager to keep every body happy. It is the job to put his employee relationships on a business-like basis with the overall goals of the company in mind. Becker (1974) stated that there are four result areas (3 of them measurable) on which to judge the plant manager's performance in his conduct of employee relationships:

1. Plant operations are not interrupted by events arising from poor employee relationships.
2. The prevailing atmosphere in the plant is not one of laxness (negligence) but of sense of purpose (subjective evaluation)

3. When company-employee relationships are put to the test by complaint or grievance procedure, the plant manager will have been found to have taken sound positions.
4. Absenteeism, tardiness, and accident frequency are all at low levels.

Special assignment
Engineering

Whether it is a small company where he may constitute the entire in-house engineering capability or it is a large corporation with a central engineering department, the engineering responsibilities of the plant manager fall into one or more of these categories.

1. **Plant engineering & maintenance:** The PM is always expected to take responsibility for keeping the buildings, grounds, and equipment in good condition.
2. **Process engineering:** The PM or someone working under his control should troubleshoot bottlenecks and problem areas in the manufacturing process.
3. **Project engineering:** In many companies, it is the responsibility of the local plant manager to oversee the project (adding new equipment, or replace old equipment), maintain the job cost records, prepare necessary reports, and control costs within the approved capital allocation.

Purchasing

In some small companies, the PM is the purchasing agent. In some large companies, the purchasing agent reports to him. In others, the purchasing function does not report to the plant manager but is performed in one or more corporate departments. If the PM is in charge of the purchasing function, he is expected to:

1. Assure the company of a continuing supply of raw materials and supplies of acceptable quality.
2. Arrange for the delivery of materials 'in time' to meet production requirements.
3. Reduce the cost of buying, transporting, and storing raw materials and supplies.

If he is not responsible for the purchasing function, the plant manager's responsibilities shift to the area of communication - keeping the purchasing department fully informed of inventory levels, changes in projected requirements, demurrage, late deliveries, or substandard quality. Close cooperation is required to avoid out-of-stock conditions while holding inventories at the lowest practicable level to avoid excessive working capital costs.

Traffic and Transportation

The PM is expected to provide for movement of the incoming and outgoing shipments by rail, truck or ship on time and at the lowest possible cost. Like purchasing, the traffic function offers many opportunities for cost reduction ranging from the selection of less costly routings to company ownership of its own means of transportation.

Traffic activities include scheduling shipments, selecting routes, choosing the mode of transportation, reviewing bills and charges, handling damage and other claims, keeping demurrage records, and maintaining transit records if rail shipments are made from the plant.

Community Relations

The PM is expected to maintain good relations with the communities in which the plant is located with the long range interests of the company in mind.

Relationships with other Department

Becker (1974) stated that the company cannot survive unless its divisions and departments form a smooth working team. The company's customers do not care whether production gets along well with engineering or sales with accounting - they want quality products delivered on time and will make no allowance for internal bickering.

Within the company, the interests and objectives of the various departments differ so much that sometimes conflict seems inevitable.

Sales

- In nearly every sales manager's office, there is a sign that says, "Nothing happens until a sale is made".
- Similarly there should also be a sign in the plant manager's office as "We make every sale after the first one". That means, repeat sales are the result of customer satisfaction with the product quality and service received. By the same taken, customer dissatisfaction with quality or service is very likely to result in lost sales.
- Close cooperation between the sales and production departments is obviously critical to the success of a company.
- The plant manager must keep the sales department advised of actual or potential interruptions of production, delays in delivery, or problems that might affect quality. The plant manager and his employees must strive to meet the requirement of sales department's commitment to the customers. The customer views the company as one unit and is not interested in its internal communications.
- The sales departments, for its part, must maintain contact with its accounts, avoiding "rush" deliveries and manufacturing surprises. The sales department should never make promises to customers without first checking with manufacturing.

Accounting

- The points of contact between the accounting and manufacturing departments lie in the areas of cost reporting and cost control.
- Manufacturing expects the accounting department to develop cost reporting systems that allow manufacturing managers to make the optimum financial

decisions in day-to-day operations. It also expects accounting to issue cost reports promptly.

- The accounting department expects to find a climate of cost consciousness in the manufacturing operation and a willingness to cooperate in cost control projects. To render prompt reports, it should get production reports, payroll records, receiving and shipping documents, inventory reports, and so on from production department.

Engineering

The engineering department's projects usually deal with the installation or modification of production facilities. Therefore, the relationship between these departments is a close and continuing one.

Manufacturing looks for engineering to

(a) Design equipment and installations with operating conditions in mind - ease of maintenance, convenient access to equipment and housekeeping, as well as production rates and product quality.

(b) Make use of the experience acquired by the manufacturing department with present plant and equipment.

(c) Submit preliminary plans and specifications to manufacturing for review and comment.

The engineering department should expect manufacturing to

(a) Supply complete and accurate data on the performance of existing equipment.

(b) Review plans and specifications promptly.

(c) Keep in mind engineering's responsibility for the cost of the project.

(d) Participate in the post-completion audit to determine whether the project is generating the cost savings or profit for which it was designed.

Financial justification or payback of engineering projects can fall to either department.

Science of Management

"Management is getting things done through other people".

"Management is a clearly defined set of activities and that the techniques used in its practice can be defined, described and learned".

Lawrence Appley, Past-President of the American Management Association, defined management as : "............ the guiding of human and physical resources into dynamic organization units which achieve their objectives to the satisfaction of those served and with a high degree of morale and sense of attainment on the part of those performing the service".

Practice of management consists of three essential activities - Planning, Organizing and Controlling.

Planning

Planning is the first step taken by a manager as he approaches a task assigned to him. He develops his plan by developing the objective that is to be reached and its time schedule and he determines exactly what activities must be carried out and by whom to reach the objective. A well defined plan must include costs, manpower requirements in numbers and skills, the machinery or tools and materials needed, and the order in which components of the plan will be executed.

Organizing

Organizing is the management process by which groups of people are assigned to the planned activities.

Controlling

Controlling may be the most important and, certainly, the most obvious of the essential activities of management. In this step the manager evaluates the progress of the organization toward its goal. He takes corrective action in time if he finds any problems.

Leadership Techniques

The basic driving force that gets things done is the leadership provided by the organization's leader or manager.

There are basically two parts to the plant manager's job.

1. In the first part, he responds to forces outside his control: customer order, employee grievances, assignments from superiors, equipment breakdowns, *inclement* weather, regulatory agencies, and many more. Successful completion of this part will only earn him a reputation for competence.

2. The second part of the plant manager's job consists of the work that he assigns to himself. It consists of the improvements he makes and the programme he carries out that are not required by outside forces. The work that he does on his own initiative is the work that sets him apart from the competent caretaker and establishes him as a leader in the eyes of his subordinates and his superiors.

The plant manager sets the tone of the work climate in the plant by the example he sets in the energy applied to the job, the determination to reach objectives, and the wisdom and ability to plan, organize and control events. If he expects high standards of performance from his subordinates, he must set even higher standards for himself. "Do as I say and not as I do" is not the motto of a successful plant manager.

Finally, the successful plant manager exhibits his leadership ability by the way the delegates work. If employees are to feel that, they are growing and developing in their jobs, they need to take on more challenging assignments. As these are successfully completed, their self-confidence and sense of participation increase. The manager who develops such subordinates not only has a stronger team working for him, but he opens up valuable blocks of time in which to pursue the initiative on his own job.

Keeping up with the times

There are three areas in which the feed plant manager needs to keep abreast of the times: the technical field of feed manufacturing, the field of management science, and social and economic trends.

- The successful manager is a student of the industry in which he works and so he never stops learning.
- The successful plant manager will avail himself of the opportunities - seminars, short courses, industry trade shows, trade publications and magazines for self improvement and urge his subordinates to do likewise.
- The feed industry is a dynamic industry as are most manufacturing industries. Progress in machinery, procedures, and techniques is continual and "the state of the art" is rapidly changing to "the state of the science".

Feed mill manager can turn inefficient and unprofitable feed milling operation into a more efficient and more profitable. Feed plant manager should follow the dictum mentioned below.

"If you want things to prosper, look after them yourself"

Production Planning and Scheduling

Production planning and scheduling (PPS) is the single most important function of feed plant management. Logistical, mechanical and human resources must be coordinated so that quality feed will be produced efficiently. Good production planning and scheduling will optimize capital use for ingredients and finished feed inventory as well as investment in plant and equipment. The plant operates at competitive efficiency.

Production planning and scheduling for a plant

The following description of a production planning and scheduling system is typical in the feed industry for a full product line plant producing meal, pelleted, bulk and bagged feeds. The production planning system consists of the following six steps:

1. Product is requested - Customer requests are communicated to the plant in person or by telephone.
2. Recap customer requests - A production planning worksheet is prepared.
3. Determine feed required - Consider present inventory, present demand and planned inventory.
4. Manufacturing schedule - A Production Record is prepared.
5. Manufacture - Operating personnel actually make feed.
6. Fill customer's request - Feed is loaded on company or customer vehicles.

To facilitate efficiency in operations feed orders should be received 2 days in advance of the date of despatch. Normally, this will allow the production planner to maximize plant efficiency by sequencing production runs, minimizing changeovers, and promote efficient truck dispatching.

2

Planning and Budgeting

INTRODUCTION

Every successful business must plan and budget in advance of execution. In some companies, the planning process is very complex and time consuming, while in others it is less complicated. But the purposes and procedures are essentially the same. In all cases, the purpose is to project the business year or years as accurately as possible. The reason for annual or strategic (long range) planning is to make a forecast of the company's profits or losses and to use that forecast as a basis for the management decisions that must be made.

All business activities produce results. Those results should be matched carefully to well-conceived goals that aim toward organizational objectives. One of the most important purposes of management's control function is to evaluate the progress being made toward organizational goals.

Strategic Planning

Strategic planning can be defined as forward thinking about courses of action based on full understanding of all factors involved and directed at specific objectives.

Strategic (long range) planning is practiced by most successful companies in one form or another and has been referred to as "road map". The analogy is appropriate. To use a road map, a person should know where he is at a given time and where he is going. Usually there are several routes that will get him there. Some routes are shorter than others, some have good roads and some do not, some involve certain known hazards while others appear to be reasonably safe, and some are more interesting and scenic than others. Planning ahead makes good sense and helps the traveler or businessman avoids surprises (Robert R. McEllhiney, 1985).

Other strategic planners compare the process to a military campaign in which the general or planner must understand the strengths and weaknesses of his own army as well as those of the enemy or competition. Success favours those organizations that are prepared and it is undeniable that aimlessness produces unpredictable results.

Mascarenhas (1977) said that the amateur hour for operational management is over. Managing the short term (from crisis to crisis) and firefighting the great part of the day (quite often the wrong fires) is frustrating, unproductive, and just wastes resources. The time has come to move from firefighting to fire protection, and for professional management to use the disciplined tools of strategic thinking and analysis to convert problems into opportunities and give companies a fighting chance to survive.

While strategic planning must involve all departments or functions of a company, this chapter will deal primarily with the manufacturing or production function and those responsibilities usually associated with it in the feed industry.

The procedural steps for strategic planning are shown in a logical sequence (McEllhiney, 1985).

1. Looking around -   environmental analysis
2. Looking within -   our present situation
3. Looking ahead -   identify and analyse
4. Developing objectives
5. Developing strategies
6. Identifying strategic resources - human, physical and financial

1. Looking Around (Environmental Analysis)

This phase of strategic planning involves a review of existing, favourable trends in the business environment and existing, unfavourable trends.

Existing favourable trends might be

- Increasing size of animal feeding units in the area
- A relaxation of regulatory agency activities or new, more reasonable, regulations
- A pull back of competition in the area(s)
- Changes in laws and other regulations affecting trucking operations
- Improvements in processing, materials handling, and control equipment for feed manufacturing
- Increased availability of local grains and other feed ingredients
- An improved labour climate in the plant or communities, changes in animal feeding operations in the area(s) that positively affect manufacturing and/or trucking costs

Existing unfavourable trends might be

- Increasing, repressive regulatory agency activities
- A deterioration of rail, truck, etc. service
- Intensified competition - new or remodeled plants
- Labour unrest or keener competition for skilled labour in the area(s)
- Increasing costs for energy, services and supplies
- Higher wage rates
- Changes in the types and forms of products required by customers: eg premixes or supplements instead of complete feeds

- Changes in animal feeding operations in the area that negatively affect manufacturing

2. Looking within (Situation analysis)

Manufacturing managers must have the capability of self-diagnosis and be able to articulate the results of that diagnosis to top management indicating major strengths compared to competition, major weaknesses, and a plan for correcting the weakness.

Major strengths may include

Lower manufacturing and/or trucking costs
Plant location(s)
Available production capacity
Trained, capable work force (people)
Product quality
Capability of manufacturing new product lines
Availability of ingredients at advantageous prices

Major weaknesses may include

Higher manufacturing and/or trucking costs
Plant location(s)
Lack of available production capacity for increased volume or new product lines
Lack of a trained, capable work force in the company
Poor product quality
Ingredients not available locally and are at higher prices
Having identified the major strengths and weaknesses compared to competition, manufacturing managers must *identify and list the improvement* the projects needed to correct the perceived weaknesses and *provide them* to top management showing priorities, costs and the payment for each project.

3. Looking Ahead (Planning Assumptions)

Management must be able to look ahead and identify favourable and unfavourable trends. These may be extentions of existing trends or they may involve totally new, anticipated activities in the business environment.

Favourable future trends might be

- Announced or anticipated increases in size and number of animal feeding operations in the area(s)
- Announced or anticipated withdrawals of competition from the area(s)
- New manufacturing machinery or transporting equipment now in the prototype stage which hold promise of improving efficiency, quality and costs

Unfavourable future trends might be

- Announced or anticipated further urbanization in the area of the **Plant** site(s)
- Abandonment of the rail road servicing the plant(s)

4. Developing objectives

The next step in strategic planning is to gauge the strengths, weaknesses, and trends and to develop objectives to take advantage of them.

1. Objectives should be stated as specifically as possible and they should be actionable.
2. Objectives should be aggressive and require hard work and dedication to be achieved.
3. Objectives are to be set not only for sales or profit targets and market shares but also for innovation, productivity and personal development.

5. Developing Strategies

Objectives can be merely wishful thinking or nebulous goals unless strategic programmmes are developed that will cause the objectives to be met. A strategy is the deployment of resources to meet the objectives.

Strategic programmes will usually include, but are not restricted to

• Commitments to capital investment on a programmed basis to maintain and modernize existing manufacturing and transportation facilities and equipment, to improve efficiency / productivity, or to increase the capacity of the business.
• Plans to acquire or dispose of business, facilities, equipment, etc. to achieve the stated objectives.
• Plans and commitments to identify, hire and / or train personnel to implement the programmes.

6. Strategic Resources

The success of a strategic plan ultimately depends on the availability and use of three resources: human, physical and financial.

Human resources: Planning group, implementers and monitors

Physical resources: They are the hardware of the business, now and for the future - plants, offices, distribution facilities, trucking equipment, etc. and their maintenance, improvement and modernisation, or acquisition and devestments.

Financial resources: The identification of financial resources by the planning team is a key element of any strategic plan. The necessary funds are to be raised for execution of the plans.

Planning strategically for the future growth and success of a company is an absolute necessity in today's business economy; but plans can fail.

McEllhiney (1983) described why strategic plans will sometimes fail

• Managers' lack of commitment to planning, preferably to fight fire and meet crises for the simple reason that doing so is more interesting, more fun, and gives a greater feeling of accomplishment.
• Lack of clear, actionable, attainable, and verifiable objectives or goals. It is impossible to plan effectively without knowing precisely what end results are sought.

- Neglecting or underestimating the importance of planning premises or assumptions. Unless people know and follow planning premises, their planning decisions will not be coordinated. Premises and assumptions include economic and market forecasts and anticipated changes in the technological, political, social, or ethical environment.
- Failure to place strategies within the total scope of plans. Unless strategies are seen as one of the major types of plans, it is easy to regard them as isolated directional decisions unrelated to other kinds of plans.
- Failure to develop clear policies. Without clear policies, plans tend to be random and inconsistent.
- Not keeping in mind the time span that should be involved. Long-range planning is not planning for future decisions, but planning the future impact of present decisions.
- Inability of some people to diagnose a situation in the light of critical or limiting factors.

A strategy is the art of devising or employing plans toward a goal (Webster, 1983).

The Strategic Model

Here objectives, opportunities and resources are brought together into a strategy.

A strategy that is implemented must be monitored and reviewed to measure its degree of success. In the review process, the strategic resources - human, physical and financial - are constantly employed to monitor and fine tune the implemented strategy.

Annual Planning and budgeting

An effective manufacturing operation must be budgeted. In most companies, planning and budgeting are an annual exercise.

Quantitative

All projections or forecasts are important to the annual planning and budgetary process. But the sales forecast must be developed first because of the impact that volume, types and forms of products, customer location, seasonal variation, etc. will have on the manufacturing and trucking plans.

This sales projection will assist manufacturing in the development of their overall plan and budget. Similarly cost increase is also to be considered. Given a reasonably accurate sales projection, the development of a manufacturing and/or trucking plan becomes a rather simple process. With it the *manufacturing manager* can quantitatively project his manpower and capital requirements and, more specially, his operating costs for the budget period.

Qualitative considerations

There are also qualitative considerations that must be part of budget development.
- **Concensus:** In concensus, knowledgeable people who are associated with the business are asked for their opinion about a particular factor.
- **Intuition and Experience:** Success lies in the ability of the manager to generalize past experience into a future setting.
- **Logic:** Another technique is logic or the combination of fact, induction, and deduction with or without the aid of colleagues. Logic must be fortified by pertinent information and data to be successful.
- **Scenerios:** Scenerios are a series of flexible possibilities. Those possibilities may vary according to such things as (sales) volume, economic conditions, labour settlements, etc. This technique can be most helpful, but the manager must be careful not to use the flexible situation as a crutch to avoid making decisions.

Many organizations develop budgets simply by taking last year's figures and adding or subtracting a fairly arbitrary amount. This may be better than no budget at all. But on the input side it fails to provide the flexibility and the recognition of change agents that are critical to dynamic, successful organizations.

The company's plans and budgets for next year's business must involve more than just plant and fleet management (manufacturing and trucking cost budgets). The planners must consider:

Sales and marketing
Purchasing, transportation and nutrition
Human resources
Capital plans

In the preparation of operating budgets, planners must take into account the impact of capital expenditures on the fixed costs of manufacturing and trucking - depreciation, interest on investments, taxes and insurance.

The planning and budgeting process is just an exercise unless a system of monitoring and controlling is established to keep all parties advised regarding the status of actual performance against budgeted performance.

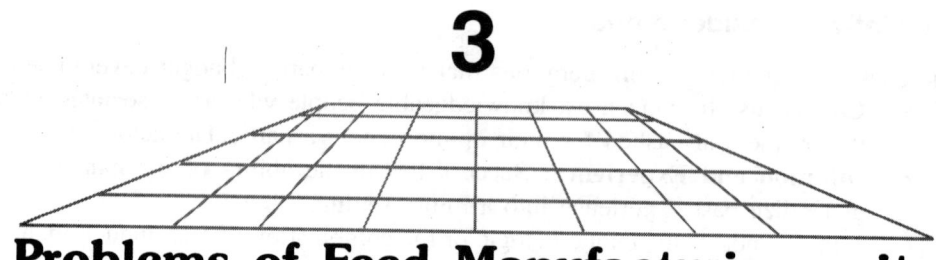

3

Problems of Feed Manufacturing units and Control Measures

The technical aspects of monitoring and control in the manufacture of compound feed present two problems (J.L. Vahl, 1984). The first is indirect measurement. To measure a certain magnitude one measures another and "computes" the required magnitude from it. The standard example is when one wants to know the mass, one measures volume.

The second problem is time delay. This is best explained with the aid of a diagram (Figure 1). A process has an input and an output. If we check the process for efficiency at the output, then we usually have to correct for discrepancies at the input. If the process is stable it does not matter much if intervention is delayed somewhat. Nothing much is going to change. If the process undergoes rapid changes, or is of long duration, or if the measurement takes a long time, we can regulate nothing.

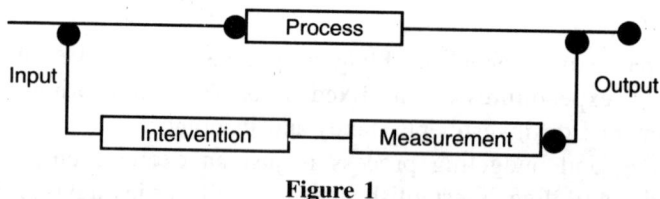

Figure 1

The result of feed analysis may be seen as an example of this. Most feeds are already in the customers' hands before the analysis has been completed. In this case we rely on the process having run through properly and the output is less accurate than it can, or should be. We are checking, therefore, the raw materials and the process, but not the result, at least not in adequate time.

Raw materials: Problems arising from measurements in the grain trade have been known from time immemorial. When it comes to ascertaining the soundness of the material, still more problems arise in connection with sampling, analytical accuracy and what additional analyses have to be made; mycotoxins e.g. cause considerable problems. Nowadays the quantity of the material is fairly accurately determined. But there will always be certain problems of quality. Many raw materials differ even within a single consignment.

Production: The classical measuring problem is stock-taking in the mill. We try to measure the volume of material in a silo and then multiply the answer with the density, which often has an inaccuracy of 15% (Figure 2). Thus, one sees that the monthly inventory will reveal discrepancies ranging from 0 to 5%, but the annual figure will be correct. One never knows, therefore, whether one is making mistakes or not. It is better to use a process control computer and to check at the time when the quantity of a certain material in certain silo is low or zero. The errors in the weighing machines are in tenths of one percent.

When stock is low or at zero, we know exactly when the product cycle is in agreement. When weighing, we must take care that the quantity is compatible with the machine used. It is customary to weigh e.g. calcium carbonate in quantities ranging from 250 to 400 kg on 1000 kg machines for laying hen feed. When one has to weigh 10kg for another type of feed this cannot be done accurately enough. One should then take a smaller weighing machine and use either a second metering screw or even a second silo. Such considerations have to be made regularly for all components.

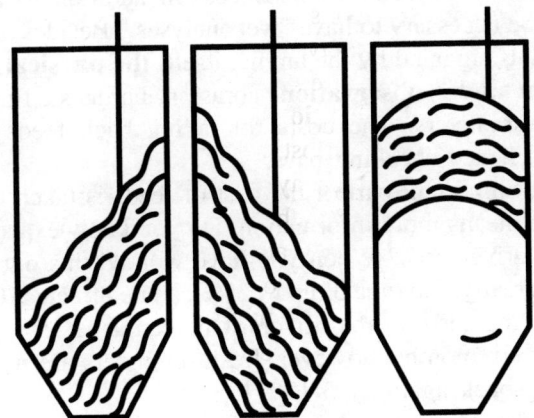

Figure 2. How many tonnes of feeds are there in a bin/silo?

Fluids are usually metered by volume. If the liquid is metered into the main mixer we again have an indirect measurement in addition to its inherent inaccuracy (1-2%). In extreme cases there can be a 10% difference in the density of liquids. These differences are not often recognized. One must measure not only the quantity but also the density. There are also metering procedures which measure time. Volume flow × Time × Density is Mass! Here everything is inaccurate. The situation becomes even worse when a volume proportionality is required, as is the case in the metering of molasses in continuous mixing. It would be better to exercise control via mass/volume proportionality.

The process control computer enables us to save on costs. The computer knows when certain conveyors and machines need not be used. For instance, a by-pass pipe can be fitted to the molasses mixer, so that it can be cut if feed is made without molasses, thus saving power. In a plant manufacturing 100,000 tons of 40% molassed feed, per annum power savings can be made through less wear to the mixer.

Monitoring during machine maintenance: With present day complicated machinery, a small defect often means the shut down of an entire factory. To avoid major breakdowns, we must work more preventively than ever before. Monitoring must help to do this. Here are some examples:

- Supervising rotational speed of elevators, chain conveyors and screws
- Monitoring ball-bearing temperatures in (e.g.) hammer mills
- Analysis of lubricating oil and grease (oil suppliers)
- Monitoring shock on ball-bearings
- Ultrasonic measurements of wall-thickness
- Pressure differential of filtering plants
- Air velocity in suction ducts

Monitoring the final product: Besides the nutritional value of the feed, the accurate addition of minerals and micro components also is important and should be checked. We all know how difficult it is to produce sheep feed with less than 15 ppm copper (sheep are susceptible to copper toxicity), and to ensure that no improper drugs get into feed. We need rapid and simple means of determining the presence/ absence and limit values of certain substances. In addition to the near infra-red analysis, it will also be necessary to have "wet analyses." Besides errors in nutritional value and contaminants signaled by the animal itself, **the physical properties of the feed have to be kept under observation:** abrasion, hardness, fineness of the flour and normal check parameters. The costs for taking back feeds from dissatisfied customers are rising, hence checking pays.

Forwarding: An important part of the cost of feeds is taken up by forwarding. Here, too monitoring means more information. Do you know exactly how much fuel each truck and each driver uses? When you have worked this out you will see that driving styles differ greatly. Savings of up to 25% can be affected. One can save only if this is pointed out regularly to the drivers. One can save 15% in fuel simply by word and deed: after six months, however, fresh reminders are necessary otherwise the savings will drop back again by 5-10%.

Training: A modern 'feed mixing plant' has need of personnel who can install, maintain and operate the facilities of modern technology. You must be open-minded about this. Training is very necessary. If people are motivated and given knowledge, they will use it. With monitoring one has a continuous insight into what is happening. Add knowledge and you know what you are doing.

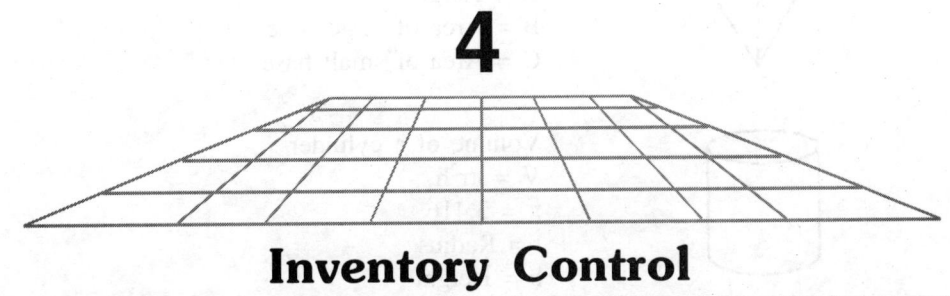

4

Inventory Control

Inventory is detailed list of household goods, stocks, etc. The proper management of inventories has a great impact on a company's profits. A well planned and effectively administered inventory control system is of paramount importance in any modern business operation and provides for proper coordination of sales and production.

Storage Space

Anderson (1976) stated that for new feed plant design, storage space provided should be equal to three times daily usage or one and one half times the shipment size for each bulk ingredient.

Inventory Practices and Procedures

Bin and Tank Calibration

Each bulk ingredient, in-process, and finished product bin or tank must be carefully calibrated to accurately determine the amount of material that is in each bin or tank at any given time. For dry material bins, standard practice is to determine the cubic feed of capacity of each storage bin in 1-foot increments and to physically inventory each bin for measuring the empty space with 'a drop line' that is itself calibrated in inches and feet. Calibration chart for that specific bin may be referred to determine cubic feet of material in the bin which provides the pounds of material when multiplied by the density of the material. The bins must be calibrated and calibration charts should be developed and used.

Liquid tanks are normally calibrated to provide gallons per inch and are measured for inventory purposes by reporting the depth of the liquid rather than the empty space, which then can be converted to weight.

Volume Computation

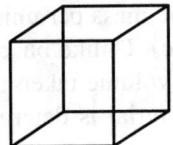

Volume of a square / rectangular tank

$V = W \times L \times H$ (width $\times$ length $\times$ height)

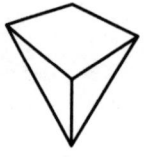

Volume of the frustrum of a pyramid
$V = 1/3H (B + b + \sqrt{Bb})$
H = Height
B = Area of large base
C = Area of small base

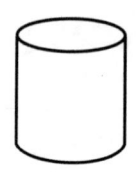

Volume of a cylinder
$V = \pi r^2 h$
$\pi = 3.416$
r = Radius
h = Height

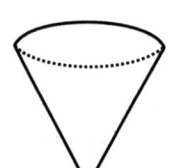

Volume of the frustrum of a cone
$V = 1/3h (r^2 + R^2 + rR)$
$\pi = 3.1416$
r = Radius of Small Base
R = Radius of Large Base

Physical properties of feed ingredients

Physical properties of feed ingredients are important to the design as well as the daily operation of feed plants. Some of the more important physical properties include: bulk density, compaction, specific density, coefficient of friction and angle of repose (Walter B. Appel, 1986).

Bulk density: The bulk density of a material is the mass per unit volume of that material. Density is easily measured by weighing the amount of material needed to fill a specific volume. The common units of bulk density are pounds per cubic foot (lb/ft3) and kilograms per cubic meter (kg/m3).

Procedure

1. Fill the cubic foot box to heaping
2. Lift it approximately 6 inches and drop it
3. Repeat step 2
4. Level the box with a straight edge and
5. Weigh and record the net weight of the material
   (weight of box + material – weight of box)

The density of a material varies significantly with particle size and compaction of the material. Even different lots of the same material may have different densities. Therefore, when accuracy is needed, it is best to measure the density (Table1) of a material than to use a value from a table. Dry and liquid materials will vary in their weight per cubic foot therefore, the density of each material must be known.

Specific density: Specific density, like bulk density, is the mass per unit volume of a material and is given in grams per cubic centimeter (g/cc). Unlike bulk density, specific density is the true density of a material because the volume taken up by air in the material is not included. The specific density of a material is determined by measuring the specific gravity of the material and converting it to a density. This is done by taking the specific gravity of the material and dividing by 0.99823.

$$\text{Density} = \frac{\text{Specific Gravity}}{0.99823}$$

Coefficients of friction: In the movement of materials, the force of friction plays an important role. **There are two different frictional forces that deal with the movement of materials: static and dynamic.** The static friction force is the force needed to start movement of a material. The dynamic frictional force is the force needed to stop the movement of a material. The coefficient of friction increases slightly with an increase in moisture content of the feedstuffs. The dynamic coefficient of friction is approximately 20% less than the static coefficient friction. The coefficient of friction decreases slightly with an increase in temperature (Kososki, 1976).

Table 1. Density of feeds*

Feedstuff	(kg/dm³)
Rice grains	0.72
Rice bran	0.30
Wheat	0.73
Wheat bran	0.24
Maize	0.68
Flaked Maize	0.21
G.N. Cake	0.60
Meat meal	0.64
Blood meal	0.43
Bone meal	0.83
Fish meal	0.56
Molasses	1.33
Ground limestone	1.14
Water	1.00

*Tropical feeds - F.A.O of the U.N. Rome, 1981; dm-decimeter

Bulk Density conversions: 1 kg = 2.2046226 lbs; Cubic feet to cubic meters = multiply by 0.028316847; Cubic meters to cubic feet = 35.314667;
Eg: 1.16 kg/cft = 2.55736 lb/cft = 40.92 kg/m³

The angles of repose: Angle of repose can be simply defined as the maximum angle (α) in degrees at which a pile of material retains its slope. As the moisture content of a material increases, the angle of repose also increased nearly linearly.

Compaction: Grains and other feed ingredients compact (pack) in bulk storage. Compaction of bulk materials in storage is known to occur but the degree of compaction can only be estimated. Compaction charts (Table 2; this chart is indicative of the intensity of compaction as bin diameter increases) are developed and used by the warehouse division and others. Such charts may be used as a guide, but there are many factors other than bin diameter that affect material compaction:

- The material, itself - its bulk density, texture, moisture content, particle size and shape, etc
- Depth of the bin or the depth of materials in the bin

382

- Bin wall material and /or condition - rough concrete, smooth concrete, wood, smooth steel, corrugated steel, etc
- Location of the bin in relation to seismic occurrences - for example, materials in a bin located near the main line or switch yard of a railroad will experience more settling (compaction) than in one where there are no ground tremors.
- Time in storage
- Relative amount of foreign matter in grain

Table 2. Compaction Chart

		Bushels per foot	
Bin diameter (feet)	% Compaction	No Compaction	With Compaction
10	4.85	62.83	65.9
12	5.00	90.47	94.9
14	5.30	123.15	129.6
16	5.50	160.84	169.6
18	6.00	203.57	215.2
20	6.70	251.32	268.1

Weights and weight control

An inventory control system is incomplete without accurate scales for receiving and shipping. It is critical to inventory management.

Physical inventories

Any good inventory control programme must include an examination of the condition of the product and the bin in which it is stored.

Packaged ingredients, suppliers and products

The best procedure for taking physical inventories in the warehouse involves a three-man inventory team of selected, literate employees. Two persons serve as counters and will give their count and the item to the third member who repeats the count and item, then records the inventory. An orderly warehouse makes inventory easier and more accurate.

- Employees must be trained and instructed that items must be stacked with a consistent number in each stack.
- Space should be provided around each stack or tier to facilitate inventory.

Bulk Storage bins: A two-man team should be used for inventorying bulk ingredient, in-process, and finished product bins. One person handles the 'drop line' and the other records the empty space measurement. The team should be provided with a bin chart, a bin measuring tape and plumb bob, an OSHA approved drop light, an OSHA approved flash light and a measuring stick for liquids.

One center hole for dry material bins of up to 8 ft in diameter and for liquid tanks is usually adequate for 'drop line' or measuring stick measurement and for visual inspection of the bin or tank. However, in larger diameter bins there should be multiple openings for more accurate drop line measurements.

Since stored dry materials tend to peak, cone, or rat hole in bins, employees must be trained to use calculated judgement in the bin level measurement that they report. One inch of shelled maize in a 20-ft diameter round bin will weigh nearly 1200 pounds. So missing the average measurement of such a bin can affect the reported inventory by tons. A good method to avoid such errors or to maintain a reasonably consistent error factor is to have the same person perform bin measurements for all inventories. Surprisingly, that person will become quite accurate.

Bin cleanout reports and records

It is good procedure to inspect bins when they are reported empty to determine whether there are material hang ups, signs of insect infestation, moisture build up (ground and flaked grain bins, for example) and the general condition of the bin walls, etc.

Conclusion

Inventory control is a way of doing business and is the responsibility of nearly every other function in a company: from the maintenance foreman who order maintenance supplies to the clerk who buys office supplies, to the purchasing department and commodity buyer, to the traffic manager, to the production staff, to the accounting department, to the trucking department, to the sales department, and so on. The economics of inventory control are the economics of doing business (McEllhiney, 1981)

5

Dangerous Atmospheres in Storage Bins—A silent killer

Grain storage bin atmosphere

The normal sounds of the feed mill are silent as you are lowered into the grain bin. As the manhole cover recedes overhead, you begin to feel drowsy as the 'bosum's chair' gently swings downward. Your thoughts begin to wander and you wonder why you are being lowered into the bin. Your ears begin to ring and breathing is somewhat difficult. You ignore the breathing difficulty, however, because you feel absolutely euphoric. You have a strong feeling of well being. As the 'bosum's chair' nears the bin floor and a mat of rotting grain, you slip into unconsciousness. Your coworkers at the top of the bin who are operating your hoist don't see you slump loosely in the chair. A few moments later you are dead (Frank Zaworski, 1985).

Life ceases quickly without oxygen

The atmosphere inside of grain or grain product bins, tanks, or silos can become dangerous and often deadly. Potentially dangerous atmospheres (toxic, oxygen-deficient, or combustible) may occur within grain or **grain product** bins usually as the result of either adding something to the bin such as pesticides, or by having the grain or grain product in the bin ferment, decompose or mould.

The fumigation of bins to kill pests may create particularly dangerous atmospheres. Fumigants, in addition to creating toxic atmospheres, may create a combustible atmosphere depending on what type of fumigant is used. Further, the fumigant may displace the normal oxygen in the bin resulting in an oxygen deficient atmosphere.

Consequences of storing of high moisture grain

Grain or grain products that are stored having a high moisture content (usually over 30 percent) and are not transferred for drying, processing, or packaging within a desirable time frame, can begin to naturally decay or ferment. This can cause the release of nitrogen dioxide, carbon dioxide, and in some cases, hydrogen sulfide.

According to the Grain Industry Safety and Health Center (GISHC) in Minneapolis (USA), products in advanced stages of decomposition may also give off methane gas.

Mill employees should always be on the alert for indications that something is amiss in product bins. For example, any unusual odour (nitrogen dioxide smells like bleach and hydrogen sulfide like rotten eggs) that can be detected at the opening of the grain bin should be considered a warning to test the atmosphere.

Mouldy grain can be particularly dangerous. Generally, mould growth occurs on the upper layer of stored, wet grain. In the wet growing condition, mould may not be very dangerous. The mould becomes dangerous when it begins to dry and the grain product is handled. This allows the mould spores to become airborne creating a respiratory hazard. If you need to enter a bin where adequate ventilation is not or cannot be provided, test for the presence of carbon dioxide, nitrogen dioxide, and oxygen deficiency. If grain has rotted, test for combustible methane gas.

Spouting and crusting or other unusual conditions in the grain may also be a warning signal that a dangerous atmosphere exists. Grain or grain products stored under improper conditions for an extended period of time may decompose to the extent that spontaneous combustion could occur, though it may be highly improbable. A fire, due to lack of air flow, is highly improbable. However, the oxygen in a bin can be used up by the smoldering grain and carbon monoxide may be created. Bins that contain products that are suspected to be smoldering (high temperature, smoky odour) should be tested for oxygen content and carbon monoxide.

Tests to be performed

Tests for oxygen deficiency, flammability and toxicity are recommended before and during each entry into a confined space. Testing equipment is generally available and easy to operate.

Detector tubes: Detector tubes are a simple method of determining the presence of combustible or toxic gases. However, they may not provide a precise quantitative measurement of concentrations.

Direct reading instruments: Direct reading instruments offer the user many distinct advantages. They provide an immediate readout of atmospheric levels, can continuously monitor these levels, provide alarms and activate hazard controls to correct the situation. Direct reading instruments are available in two basic types. One type indicates a hazard by a light and alarm. Another type has a continuous scale providing readings that indicate hazard levels. Such direct reading instruments are the only available method for determining oxygen deficient atmospheres.

Both detector tubes and direct reading instruments can be used to detect the presence of combustible gases. The most widely used type of portable combustible gas analyzer is sensitive to the heat of combustion.

Atmospheres containing less than 19.5 percent oxygen constitute a hazard to personnel. Normal atmospheres (fresh air) have an oxygen content of 20.9 percent. If entrance to a bin with an oxygen content of less than 19.5 percent is required, steps must be taken to ventilate the confined space. Alternatives include natural ventilation, forced ventilation, or use of appropriate respiratory equipment.

Safe bin and tank entry
What are some of the potential hazards of bin and tank entry?

These spaces (bins and tanks) come in a variety of shapes and sizes including elevator bins, concrete silos, steel storage tanks, bulk flour bins, feed trucks, liquid feed tanks, railroad cars, and even manholes or scale pits. Whatever size or shape the space, each presents its own unique set of **potential hazards** which may include insufficient oxygen within the space, bridging, dust conditions, faulty equipment, improper training or in some cases no training at all, lack of adequate rescue equipment, poisonous gases, violation of safety rules and practices, or failure to consider an alternative which would be a safer, easier way so that entry into the space would not be necessary.

How can the job be done safely?

Entry permit: The first procedure necessary to safeguard entry into a confined space is a properly executed entry permit. In order that everyone be informed as to what is going on no person should enter a confined space without written permission from his supervisor or management. This entry permit states who is going to enter the place, which space it is, when it will be entered, and for what purpose. It also specifies all requirements necessary to get the job done safely.

Supervisor must first look for **adequate ventilation**. A tank or bin open only on top will not allow easy dispersal of heavier than air gases. Opening up the bottom or side will allow air to circulate more freely or the use of a blower for forced ventilation is a good idea as the blower will speed up dispersal of harmful gases. So this requirement is marked on the entry permit.

Next, he requires a **watchman** since no one should ever enter a confined space alone without an observer and he names the watchman on the permit. The watchman must keep the lifeline properly snubbed with very little slack.

The requirement for a **harness and lifeline** since all persons entering a confined space from above should wear a safety harness connected to a substantial life line (a safety belt may be adequate for side entry).

The next consideration is the method to be used for entry into the space. Top entry should be made through an opening sufficiently large enough to permit easy access and egress. A good strong ladder may be used to lower the man into the bin, or the use of a sling or Boatswain's chair in which case the use of some form of reliable hoisting equipment, whether it be a portable type or a more permanent installation is required. If the entry is to be made through a bottom hatch, it is very important to inspect overhead areas to be sure that no hazard exists from products hung up in the bin.

One of the most important requirements for safe entry into a space is the **oxygen test** which determines whether or not there is sufficient oxygen to support life. Certain conditions, such as a musty smell with a wheat bin or a sour mash odour from a mould or fermented product, warn against entry due to oxygen deficiency. Reliable approved instruments are available for analyzing the air. Also, an anode can be slowly lowered into a bin to give a cross section of the available oxygen all the way to the bottom of the bin. If the oxygen content is low, the supervisor might specify the use of breathable air from compressed breathable air tanks. This air is used through long, quick-connect hoses fitted to a mask with a demand air regulator. Often however, if the oxygen content in the bin is low, the supervisor may abandon the planned entry and reventilate the space until the permissible oxygen level is obtained.

6

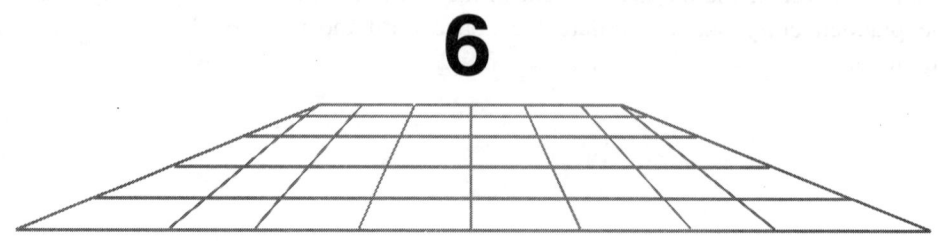

Bulk Solids Handling,
Freeing and preventing hung-up
material in confined spaces

Have you ever noticed the odd dimpled look of the bottoms and sides of metal bins in some feed mills? This phenomenon results from the impact of the head of a 3.5kg mallet on the bin. Such blows are occasionally applied by the hands of frustrated production supervisors who have just seen their mill come to a standstill because "the ground grain is hung-up in the bin."

The bridging (doming or arching) or funneling (piping or rat-holing) often cause bulk solids to fail to flow out of a bin by gravity (see figures 1 and 2). When such stoppage of flow occurs it becomes necessary to manually dislodge the hung-up material if mechanical devices for such purposes are either ineffective or unavailable. Whenever hung-up materials must be dislodged in bins, tanks, and silos, precautions must be taken to ensure the safety of personnel and equipment. Employees should never enter or work below hung-up or bridged material. Many injuries and deaths have occurred as a result of hung-up bridged material collapsing. Elevator, feed mill, and on-farm storage bins all too often make the news as sites of tragic accidents.

If material is hung-up, every effort should be made to dislodge the material from a safe location outside the confined space. Rapping the bottom or side of the bins with some type of tool is not recommended as a positive solution but such action can create vibrations that may work to free built-up or hung-up materials. If such persuasion is employed, a weighted rubber or soft metal mallet is suggested.

Long handled spuds or scrapers (non-ferrous to prevent sparks) at times can be used to knock down the hung-up material from the top bin opening. The employee attempting the dislodging should never physically enter the bin without proper precautions.

Some bins, particularly those that store materials that are noted for their tendency to hang-up can be equipped with vibrating bin bottoms that mechanically cause the bin bottom, sometimes the walls and often the material to vibrate, which can shake free the hung-up material.

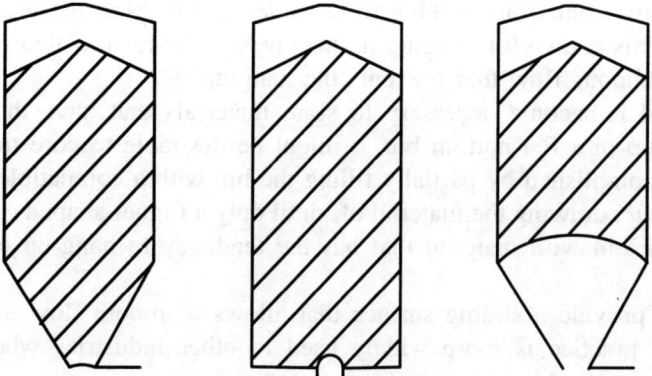

Figure1. Three cases of doming

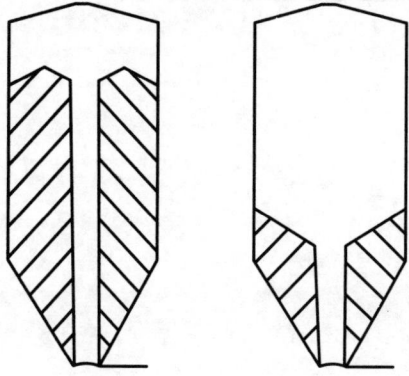

Figure 2. Example of piping

If it becomes necessary to enter a confined space to manually dislodge bridged or cored materials, safety procedures for confined spaces must be followed. Check for adequate oxygen in the bin. Use natural or forced ventilation to increase the oxygen level or use appropriate respiratory equipment. The employee entering a bin, tank, or silo should always be a member of a team. Never enter a confined space without the support of at least two persons remaining at the confined space entry point. Prior to entry, ensure that all loading and load out equipment is shut down and locked out. The employee entering the bin should always be attached to a lifeline of proven strength and condition. Wire rope is generally stronger than fiber rope. Whenever a bin or tank is entered through the top without a ladder requiring lowering of the entry team by a rope or cable, a reliable hoisting apparatus should be used to lower and lift the entry team safely.

How to deal with hung-up materials in bins?

The best method for dealing with hung-up material in confined spaces is the practice of prevention.

- Slick, smooth surfaces with a low coefficient of friction may help prevent some material from sticking to the sides and starting the hang-up.
- Materials known for hanging-up may need to be recirculated so that there is a continuous flow that prevents the hang-up.
- Should it become necessary to store materials that have the tendency to hang-up in a flat-bottom bin, it might be desirable to core the bin first.

This is accomplished by partially filling the bin with a compatible material that does not hang-up, drawing the material off until only a funnel-shaped core is left, and then filling the bin with material that has the tendency to hang-up or stick to the sides.

This may provide a sliding surface that allows a smooth flow of the problem material. This practice is more widely used in other industries where ingredient integrity is less critical.

Finally, materials that have a tendency to hang-up should be stored for only short periods to minimize the effects of temperature, pressure, air and moisture on the stored material in bins, tanks and silos.

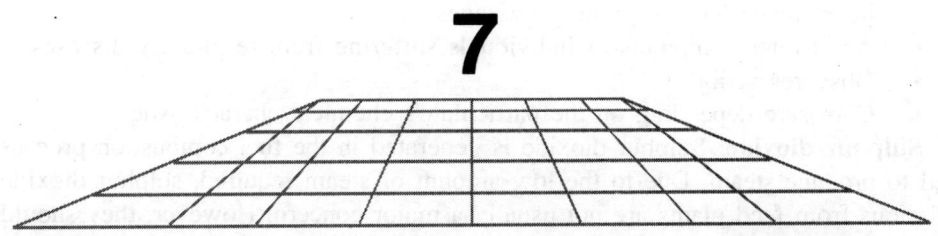

7

Environmental Management related to Feed Industry

Between 1970 and 1980 several environmental legislations were passed in U.S. These laws resulted from a growing public environmental awareness, a need to improve deteriorating water and air quality, a need to protect human health and welfare, and a need to preserve the country's natural resources (K.V. Lensmeyer, 1985). These include National Environmental Policy Act, Clean Air Act, Clean Water Act, Toxic Substances Control Act, Occupational Safety and Health Act (OSHA), Safe Drinking Water Act, Noise Control Act.

Benefits of sound environmental practices to the feed industry

1. Sound air pollution control practices result in lower ingredient losses and therefore, greater product recovery and productivity.
2. Effective waste water management results in reduced water use, which will minimise water charges.
3. Proper handling of hazardous materials and waste ensures worker safety and the integrity of the community through proper and effective storage and disposal techniques.
4. Effective spill control measures will reduce material leakage and loss through spill prevention and will eliminate or minimise costs in the event of a spill incident.

Air pollutants in feed manufacturing: Dust and sulphur dioxide

In feed manufacturing, the primary air pollutant is particulate matter, i.e., dust, while the secondary pollutant is sulfur dioxide. Particulate matter, i.e., dust is generated when ingredients or finished products are flowing in mass with or without the assistance of mechanical systems.

Dust: The handling of grain, starting with receiving and ending with shipping, generates particulates. Generation of particulates can, in certain circumstances and under certain conditions, have deleterious effects including, but not limited to, the following (G.J.Boresi):

- 'Precursor to dust explosions in confined areas
- Toxic to man and animals via the respiratory system as a result of physical interference with respiratory passages
- Aggravates symptoms of individuals suffering from respiratory diseases
- Obscures visibility
- Corrosive depending on the particulate's chemical characteristics

Sulphur dioxide: Sulphur dioxide is generated in the fuel combustion process used to produce steam. Due to the low amount of steam required, sulphur dioxide emissions from feed plants are not usually a major concern. However, they should not be dismissed. Sulphur dioxide can constrict respiratory passages that aggravate the symptoms of individuals suffering from heart and lung disease, be toxic to plants' foliage, be precursor to acid rain and obscure visibility. Acceptable sulphur dioxide emission rates can usually be achieved by using low sulphur content fuels.

Dust Collection Systems
Objectives of dust collecting systems

The objective of a dust collection system is to
1. Prevent outside contaminants from entering the processing area.
2. Prevent dusts from escaping from the processing equipment into the surrounding areas.
3. Reclaim the air-suspended materials which do escape into the area surrounding the process.

Perfection in all three of the above areas is difficult, since even the better filters are not efficient for collecting particles in the sub-micron range.

Advantages of dust collection systems

A dust collection system serves many purposes.
- Dust collection system prevents dust explosions in elevators and feed plants.
- Good housekeeping in conjunction with proper dust control will reduce insect and rodent problems and other hazardous contaminants.
- Good housekeeping could also result in a lower insurance rate. If a plant has an adequate dust control system, housekeeping will be accomplished with less effort and fewer man hours spent. Some insurance companies will not insure facilities that don't have pneumatic dust control systems that meet their standards (G.L. McDaniel, 1985).
- Dust control can reduce loss or shrinkage. Captured dust can be returned to the stock handling system. Reduced shrinkage can add to the profit of a company.

Dust Collection System suitable for grain industry

Basically, there are four types of dust collection systems: 1. high-efficiency cyclones, 2. wet scrubbers, 3. fabric filters, and 4. electronic precipitators. Most of these methods have some restrictions when dealing with the grain and feed industries.
- The high-efficiency cyclone induces a spinning action in a stream of air and

particles are thrown out of the airstream and collected. It is not effective on fine or very light particles.

- The wet scrubber, which removes particles from the air by scrubbing it with water, is useful on a wide range of operations, but as particle size declines, efficiency declines. It cannot be operated outdoors or in cold climates, which limits its use in the grain and feed industry.

- An electrostatic precipitator uses high voltage to attract electronically charged particles to the collecting surfaces. The design of such a unit produces sparking and cannot be used in industries where fire or explosions are a problem.

- **The fabric filter, is best suited for the grain industry** because it offers high efficiencies and widely varied size capacities. Initial costs are several times higher than the cyclone dust collector, and filters must be carefully maintained and operated to retain the design performance. The filter bags are tubular, cylindrical or envelope type.

Fabric filter and pneumatic dust collection system

The pneumatic dust collection system has four main parts - hoods and other enclosures, duct work, filter bags and the fan. It forces dusty air to pass through the filter fabric, and a mat of dust builds up on the dirty side of the fabric. As a mat builds up, there is increasing resistance to air flow. This resistance must be alleviated by removing the dust - through shaking or vibrating the fabric or by use of air in reverse flow, pulse-clean or pulse-jet systems. The dislodged dust falls into the lower chamber or hopper and is discharged through the air lock.

Evaluation of fabric filter

The fabric must efficiently release dust accumulations, not allow small-size particles to pass through and must be economical. Filter bags for pulse-clean collectors are available in a variety of fabric constructions. *Polyester and polypropylene needlefelts* with and without scrim reinforcement, singed or glazed surface finishes, innovative membrane surface laminates and more recently the development of seamless tube Beane Bag filter fabrics are used in the grain industry.

Polyester needlefelt bags with scrim reinforcement have been used for years, and continue to be the standard by which others are judged. As the polyester's efficiency rating increases, prices for the bags increase. In addition, worn polyester fabric cannot maintain under pressure as do needlefelt fabrics. The holes in the filtration fabric in needlefelt fabric are several times smaller than the polyester bags. This allows greater airflow and greater filteration.

Although the needlefelt bags are effective and efficient, dust is much more difficult to remove during cleaning, which in turn causes reduced air flow and increased energy usage. It is recommended that buyers try singed or glazed needlefelts. This surface treatment inhibits dust penetration into the fabric. Very fine particles can still penetrate glazed fabrics and as this happens, the filters must be replaced because laundering will not remove the particles. The Beane Bag filter is a circular knitted fabric with high air permeability with excellent filtration.

Control of pollutants: Excluding boilers, the control of air pollutants at a plant is limited to dust control. Cyclone separators, vent filters and baghouses are used to control dust.

Cyclone separators: These are the most commonly used air pollution control devices in feed manufacturing. Cyclones employ inertial separation as the removal mechanism. Centrifugal force separates the particulates from the air. The dirty gas is forced to rotate within the cyclone. The heavier particles impact the cyclone wall and fall to the bottom of the unit while the clean gas reverses its downward spiral and exits at the top of the unit. Cyclone separators are used to remove particles 10 to 20 microns in size and larger. The efficiency of cyclones in plant applications ranges from 80 to 95% depending on the dust stream and the type of cyclone employed. Cyclone applications in feed mills include pneumatic conveyors, storage bins, ventilating hoods, receiving systems, and processing units.

Vent filters: Storage bins without dust control can emit dust plumes that can completely obstruct visibility. Dust plumes emitted from storage bins and surge hoppers can be effectively controlled by fitting the vent with a filter consisting of a cloth sack or bag securely fastened to the vent. Cotton sateen is a common filter cloth material.

Baghouses are used in lieu of cyclones when greater removal efficiency is required. Baghouses or fabric filters can achieve removal efficiencies of 95 to 99.9%. However, they are more operation and maintenance intensive than cyclones.

What causes a dust explosion?

A grain dust explosion occurs if four factors co-exist: oxygen, an ignition source, a confined volume and suspended dust. Eliminating any one of the factors will eliminate the possibility of explosion. However this is easier said than done. Since the first three are somewhat uncontrollable, dust is to be controlled to lower the chances of dust explosion.

Dust Producing Points: These are receiving areas, hammermills, rollermills and crimpers, mixing system, elevator legs and distributors, screw and drag conveyors, belt conveyors, pellet scalpers, baggers and loadout areas.

Dust collecting devices

There are several basic types of dust control systems.

1. **A negative pressure system** includes all components handling dust ladened air under negative pressure.

   Advantages: Any air leakage of dust-ladened air from old or damaged ducting does not produce a dust emission point. One fan drives the entire system, which normally reduces installation, equipment and energy costs.

   Disadvantages: It can be disadvantageous where systems are large and pulling air from many points through the plant. All must operate if any are needed.

2. **Negative-positive pressure combination system:** This system utilizes negative pressure to capture the dust-ladened air at the pickup hood and into

the ducting but then passes through the fan and is blown by positive pressure into the filter.

Advantages: 1. System is adaptable where multiple pickup points are required with intermittent operations. **2.** This method lends itself to the future expansion of a dust system into existing bag houses.

Disadvantages: 1. Installation and equipments costs are greater. 2. Maintenance cost is higher.

Fans: Typical dust control equipment includes fans, cyclones and baghouse filters. Two styles of fans: 1.Backward inclined fan 2. Straight bladed fan

1. Backward inclined fan with wheels must be used in a clean air stream limiting it to a negative pressure system. It is more energy efficient fan style, as it will move more cfm of air per hp than does the straight bladed fan.

2. Straight bladed fans with wheels are capable of operating in a dust-ladened air stream because of their self-cleaning tendencies. Because of these wheels self-clean, they do not (under normal operating conditions) develop an uneven dust build-up on the fan wheel to cause an out-of-balance condition.

Baghouse filters

These are units in which dust is removed from the air stream by retention in or on a porous fabric filter bag through which the air flows. Fabric filters have the advantage of being a positive collector. That is, the filter media is positioned between the dust ladened air and the clean air plenum and forms a barrier to prevent the escape of dust. Because of this arrangement and with the proper filter media selection, efficiencies of 99.8% can be achieved.

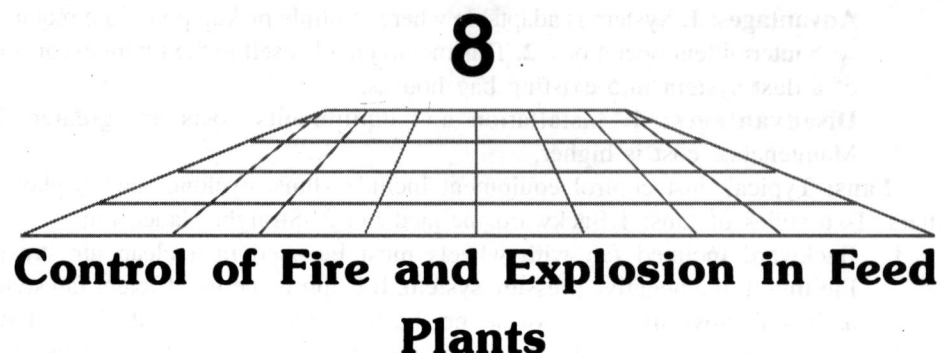

8

Control of Fire and Explosion in Feed Plants

The consequences of a fire or explosion in a feed plant can be devastating, resulting in human suffering, loss of life, property damage, and loss of business. Although the possibility exists for fire or explosion in a production facility that handles grain products, there are measures that can be taken to minimize the chance of such occurrences (Steven Jukes, 1985).

Grain dust rule

In 1979 Kansas State University and Grain Elevator and Processing Society organised a symposium on grain dust explosions. Science and Education Administration (SEA) of USDA also involved. Charles R. Martin found that maize dust contains more combustible material than dust from wheat, sorghum and soybeans, in descending order. The most noncombustible dust - dirt and silica - was confined to the fine particles and that coarse dust consisted largely of protein, fat and starch.

Fang S. Lal studied bench scale explosions using the Hartmann bomb to determine the explosive capability of dusts of feedstuffs. Mineral oil was applied to grains to inhibit dust. A dose of 1/200th of a percent oil mixture has been found to be adequate. But in 1987 it was reported that application of oil on wheat has had a negative effect on milling and flour quality. Poor yields and lower capacities of plants were reported. A general lowering of the flour colour score was observed. Mechanical problems like choking of the sifter at the soft wheat mill were observed.

The Occupational Safety & Health Administration (OSHA) formulated grain dust rule. The final rule says that dust can't accumulate to a depth of an eighth-inch anywhere within 35 ft. of an inside bucket elevator or other areas of potential ignition. But this requirement is difficult to meet. Grain handling industry and National Grain & Feed Association (NGFA), which have done considerable amount of research into the question of dust explosions, dispute OSHA's claim.

Grain dust fires and explosions

Grain dust fires and explosions had been reviewed for the 21-year period of 1958 to

1978 by the USDA Task Force. 250 dust explosions were reported in U.S. grain elevators and feed mills. At least 165 deaths and 609 injuries resulted. The problem of grain dust fires and explosions can largely be eliminated. The USDA Task Force has made several key recommendations. Among them:

1. Remove grain dust from handling facilities and prohibit its return to the grain stream.
2. Each grain handling facility is required to develop a dust control programme which would include mechanical dust collection, housekeeping and other control measures.
3. Study possible incentives including tax relief, direct subsidy and low interest loans which could be used to promote better dust control.
4. The development of standard operation plans are required which include programmes for maintenance, housekeeping, safety and security.
5. Establish better coordination between industry, government and professional organizations in the development of consensus standards for grain handling facilities.
6. Develop standard design and construction guidelines for all new grain handling facilities. These should include requirements to isolate hazardous processes and areas, dissipate explosion effects through relief venting and contain fire and explosions.
7. Develop specific handling techniques to deal with the problem of maize and its need for artificial design.

Elements responsible for dust explosion

Elements that must simultaneously exist for an explosion to occur are

1. Combustible dust in suspension
2. Oxygen
3. An ignition source
4. Confinement of the dust in suspension

Primary explosion: Typically, the sequence of events that results in a damaging explosion begins with a small primary explosion in a piece of equipment such as an elevator leg. The force of the initial explosion causes static dust, on or in equipment and structural members, to be thrown into suspension. That dust is the fuel for much stronger secondary explosions.

Secondary explosion: Secondary explosions are usually many times more powerful than the initial explosion and are usually the cause of major damage. Those explosions may occur many seconds after the primary explosion and can propagate throughout the facility in a series of secondary explosions.

Research has shown that even a layer of static dust less than 0.01 inch thick is sufficient to support a strong secondary explosion when it has been thrown into suspension by the primary explosion. A hot ember from the initial explosion is the ignition source for secondary explosions. This phenomenon explains how a small explosion in a piece of equipment can cause a larger explosion rupturing the equipment, then causing a third, even more violent explosion, inside the building.

The explosive hazard created by **agricultural dust** depends on its ease of ignition and the severity of the resulting explosion. The ease of ignition is related to the ignition temperature, the particle size, the minimum energy required for ignition, and the minimum explosive concentration (lower explosive limit). The severity of the explosion depends on the explosive pressure and the rate of rise of the pressure.

The U.S. Bureau of Mines has conducted tests on the explosibility of most types of dusts that would be utilized in a feed plant. They have developed empirical indices of explosibility using Pittsburgh coal dust as the standard for comparison. For any dust, the smaller the particle size the higher the explosibility index.

Explosibility Index = Ignition sensitivity × Explosion severity

The average particle diameter is related to both the minimum energy required for ignition and the rate of pressure rise. The explosibility index is not a constant for a given type of dust, such as ground maize. The method of preparation, aging, and treatment can cause differences among samples from various sources.

Primary areas of exposure in a feed plant

Combustible dust in potentially explosive quantities may be generated and maintained in suspension throughout many areas of a feed production facility. Therefore, it is of critical importance to identify and control the potential sources of ignition. The primary areas of exposure are bucket elevators (see page No. 337 for components of bucket elevator), grinders and hammermills, dust collection/pneumatic handling systems, storage bins, electricity equipment, improperly maintained areas, and areas of human activity.

Prevention and control

The most effective way to address the fire and explosion hazards in a feed plant is to eliminate or minimize their potential during the design and construction of a new facility or by modifying an existing facility.

General arrangement

The general layout and arrangement of the feed plant should attempt to segregate as much as possible the different operations. Those operations include raw material receiving, grain storage, feed production, finished product warehousing, and auxiliary areas (boilers, maintenance areas, grain dryers, and forklift battery recharging areas). Segregation can be achieved by physical separation or by providing fire barriers.

Construction

The predominant types of construction materials used in feed plants today are fire resistive and noncombustible (Steven Jukes, 1985). Due to the inherent fire hazards of wood, that type of construction should be avoided. Fire resistive construction is usually achieved by the use of masonry materials such as reinforced concrete, or specially designed concrete block walls. Yet, those types of construction are extremely susceptible to damage from the force of an explosion. Every effort should be made to provide maximum explosion relief by installing windows or blowout panels in the areas of a feed plant where an explosion potential exists.

Noncombustible construction usually consists of a metal or other type of noncombustible skin on a steel structure. While that type of lighter construction is less susceptible to damage from the force of an explosion, it will quickly deform and fail when exposed to heat generated by a fire.

Process equipment arrangement and controls

1. Elevator Legs

The bucket elevator is considered to be the most frequent source of an explosion in grain handling and processing facilities. Possible ignition sources in an elevator leg include slippage on the head pulley due to overloading or choking of the leg, overheating of the head or tail bearings, misalignment of the belt, and shifting of the pulley. Therefore, every effort should be made to prevent an explosion from occurring and to minimize the damage if an explosion occurs. That can be accomplished by providing elevator legs with features such as motion monitoring devices, bearing monitoring systems, belt alignment monitoring system, and careful leg location. Freeing the choked elevator leg to prevent fire and dust explosion is described in the following.

Freeing the choked elevator leg to prevent fire and dust explosions

Failure to properly operate and maintain the bucket elevator can result in an increased chance of fire and explosion. Poor operation and maintenance can also result in a reduced capacity due to poor performance, costly downtime and premature equipment failure. The majority of explosions which have occurred in grain handling systems in recent years have been the result of improperly maintained, operated or designed legs.

Two major reasons for choking: A common problem with elevator legs that could lead to a dangerous buildup of heat is choking. When a leg chokes, something has caused the belt to slow down and stop. The leg can choke for a variety of reasons. Two major reasons for choking are improperly designed input conveying to the elevator and backlegging. A conveying system bringing grain or other materials to the boot of an elevator whose bucket capacity is inadequate to handle the incoming material can cause the leg to choke. An elevator that is choking on a regular basis should be examined to insure that it is sized properly to the rate of flow of the incoming material. A blocked discharge spout on a leg can cause backlegging that could result in a choked leg. Plug switches can be installed on a discharge spout to detect obstruction of the spout.

When a leg chokes, something has caused the belt to slow down or stop. It is important that the operator shut down the operations and follow proper procedures to clear the choke and inspect for damage. The leg should never be jogged to clear it as such a procedure can cause the head pulley to move without moving the belt. Sufficient amounts of heat from friction can be created to ignite grain dust suspended in the air inside the leg casing.

When a leg choke condition exists, grain flow to the leg should be shut off

The first step to freeing the leg is the opening of the leg boot and removal of all accumulated grain. If the leg was shut off under load, the bucket conveyor should be allowed to back leg, dumping the grain from the loaded buckets. With all product or grain removed from the elevator, attempt to determine what caused the choke to develop. A first step is to check the discharge point to see if the spout or some downstream point is clogged. Inspect the alignment of the head and tail pulleys and the belt. Check for damaged buckets. Damaged buckets will not carry their rated capacity and could be causing the problem. The belt splice should also be inspected for damage.

When the cause of the choke has been determined and rectified, an attempt can be made to restart the leg. Someone should be posted to monitor the leg belt. This person should have the direct communication with the person operating the leg. When the leg is restarted, it should be monitored for a time to insure that it is operating normally. As a final measure, steps should be taken to avoid leg chokes from the same cause in the future.

Tips to follow when operating and maintaining the leg

Grain should feed evenly into the boot to avoid forcing the belt to either one side or the other. When the boot is loaded to one side it is difficult to get the belt to track properly. Installing a choke gate feed or spout baffle will insure the grain is fed evenly.

Occasionally a pulley can work loose on the shaft. Taper locks and screws should be tight on the pulley. When tightening locks and screws, make sure that the pulley is spaced properly in the boot section. This can be done by opening the inspection door and measuring the distance between the pulley and the casting. Record this measurement for comparison during future inspections. If this distance changes, the pulley is either moving on the shaft or the shaft is moving the bearings.

If the material has built up on the face of the boot pulley, poor traction can result along with misalignment and possibly damage to the belt and buckets. Clean off any built-up material immediately.

A build-up of materials on the pulley is likely to occur if the throat of the leg head funnels grain back to the down side of the leg. This causes back-legging grain to pass between the approaching down belt and the boot pulley. As the material builds up on the pulley, the belt is forced off centre and rubbing results.

Another bad result of material build-up on the pulley is rapid deterioration of the belt cover by the oil produced as grain is crushed between the belt and the pulley.

To solve this problem, back-legging grain should be funneled to the up-side leg casing. A winged type, self-cleaning boot pulley can be used to help clean grain from the face of the pulley. Automatic sensing switches are available that shut down a leg if any sustained misalignment is detected.

2. Dust Collection/Pneumatic Handling Systems

The primary exposure for fire or explosion with dust collection/pneumatic handling systems is when they are interconnected with a process machine, such as a grinder or hammermill. Sparks from tramp metal or burning embers can be conveyed to the dust collector. Therefore, consideration should be given to providing explosion venting and isolating the dust collector from the remainder of the plant, either by enclosing it in a separate room or locating it outside.

It should be noted that the high moisture content of the airstream in the cyclone and collectors used with pelleted and flaked grain cooling systems do not normally contain explosible levels of dust. Further, the dust collection system or phenumatic handling system should be properly grounded to avoid the generation of static electricity.

3. Grinders

Grinder and hammermills, including various type of roller mills, are machines with inherent fire hazards, due largely to the possibility of tramp metal being contained in the stock. Pieces of iron may be heated to the melting point in the grinding operation and conveyed to a bin where they are likely to start a smoldering fire and not break into active flame for several hours. Removal of tramp iron is accomplished by the installation of **magnetic separators** in the spouts leading to grinders.

Magnetic separators are relatively ineffective in spouts inclined at an angle greater than 45°. Hence, a means must be provided to regulate the thickness of the stream of stock passing over the magnet. Magnetic separators should be readily accessible for routine cleaning and the removal of accumulated metal.

4. Boilers

While boilers do not represent a dust explosion hazard, they should be provided with adequate safety combustion controls to minimize the potential for gas explosion or fuel fires and be separated from the remainder of the plant by locating them in a room with walls having a minimum one-hour fire rating (Steven Jukes, 1985).

National Fire Protection Association (NEPA, USA) issued guidelines of fire protection from time-to-time to be followed scrupulously. These include provision of portable fire extinguishers, automatic sprinkler system.

Explosion venting

There is an ever-increasing awareness of industrial explosion hazards from flammable dusts and all the concerned are sharing the latest developments and advancements in explosion protection technology. Indeed the state of the art is continually improving, but at the same time, there seems to be an alarming increase in the occurrence of industrial dust explosions. As a result, industry is seeking a practical solution. In many cases that practical solution may be explosion ventings (Bob DeGood, 1982).

Understanding explosions is a complex science, but in principle an explosion may be thought of as a fast fire. After ignition, a fire ball expands spherically. As the fireball expands spherically, a pressure wave develops ahead of the flame front and pressures inside the vessel increase. When the pressure wave reaches the wall of the vessel, it becomes reflected causing internal pressure to rise exponentially. Technically, these explosions are termed deflagrations, which are propagating reactions where the velocity of the reactions is subsonic within the reactant.

Five basic solutions

When explosions do occur in industrial equipment, the primary concern is avoiding the catastrophic bursting of the vessel. Once the hazard is recognized, there are five basic solutions which may be considered.
1. Design the system to minimize the possibility of an explosion,
2. Containment of the maximum explosive pressure within the process vessel,
3. Explosion suppression,
4. Explosion venting,
5. Some combination of items 1-4.

Designing the system to minimize the possibility of an explosion is always essential. This may include controlling the dust concentration below the lower explosive limit, operating under a purge of inert gas, or attempting to limit potential ignition sources. These attempts at controlling the process are subject to failure. Hence, the possibility of an explosion is only reduced, but not eliminated. Perhaps it is good to remember that the experts who study the remains of industrial explosions say 80-90% of all industrial explosions occur during start-up, shut-down, or an upset condition.

Designing and manufacturing process equipment to contain the maximum pressures developed by dust explosions is seldom a practical solution. Generally, maximum pressures developed in dust explosions range from 80 psi to 130 psi (See Table 1 for data).

An explosion suppression system is designed to stop the explosion after its ignition. Pressure rise is detected by a network of pressure sensors which send signals to a control unit. If conditions indicate activation of the suppression system is required, the control unit opens a valve flooding the equipment with the suppression agent, (e.g. typically Halon 1301 or 1011). One important thing to understand about explosion suppression systems is they are active systems. All of the elements must take an action in order for the system to function properly.

Explosion venting is a passive means of overpressure protection. The concept involves providing an opening large enough for the expanding gases to escape without overpressuring the equipment. The opening is covered by a "venting" device which is pushed open as the pressure develops. This represents a passive system.

Combining these methods of explosion protection has often provided workable solutions. Designing the system to minimize the possibility of an explosion is always essential. Although containment of the maximum explosive pressure is not always practical, increasing the confinement capability of the equipment will allow less explosion relief area to be used. Many users wish to utilize explosion venting as a method to limit explosive over-pressures after considering all options. There are many factors which influence the amount of relief area required. In general the magnitude of internal pressures during venting varies inversely with respect to the amount of vent area provided.

The severity of explosion hazards varies dramatically as illustrated by the maximum rate of pressure rise (Table 1). These values were established by the Bureau of Mines by testing each dust in the Hartmann Test Bomb, a 75 cubic inch cylinder. Even within the explosibility testing there are many variables which affect the test results such as particle size and dust concentration, but the primary objective is to identify the maximum rate of pressure rise in a worst case situation.

Table 1. Explosion characteristics of various agricultural dusts*

Food / feed	Maximum explosion pressure psig	Max. rate pressure rise psi/sec	Minimum explosion conc. oz./cu ft.
Alfalfa meal	66	1,100	0.105
Cellulose	130	4,500	0.055
Cereal grass	65	400	0.20
Maize	113	6,000	0.055
Maize cob grit	127	3,700	0.045
Cottonseed meal	104	2,200	0.055
Grain dust, winter wheat, maize, oats	131	7,000	0.055
Groundnut hull	116	8,000	0.045
Rice	47	700	0.085
Rice bran	61	1,300	0.045
Rice hull	109	4,000	0.055
Safflower meal	90	2,400	0.055
Soy flour	94	800	0.06
Soy protein	98	6,500	0.05
Wheat flour	97	2,800	0.05
Wheat gluten, gum	--	--	0.05
Wheat starch, edible	100	6,500	0.045
Wheat starch, allyl chloride treated	117	6,500	0.025
Wheat straw	117	6,500	0.055

*Data from the U.S. Department of Interior, Bureau of Mines, Report No.5753

9

Shrink Control in Feed Manufacturing

Shrink

Shrink is universally experienced in all feed manufacturing, flour milling and other grain processing and handling operations. Shrink is that loss of materials that occurs during manufacturing and materials handling processes. Losses may be in the form of dust, moisture, spoilage, theft, pest damage, or other forms. Shrink has been called "invisible loss" (McEllhiney, 1985).

Shrink = [Beginning inventory + receipts] − [Ending Inventory + Shipments]

Shrink by Weight

$$\text{Shrink \%} = \frac{\text{Shrink by Weight}}{\text{Shipments by Weight}} \times 100$$

The opposite of shrink is gain. It is possible to experience a gain in some processing operations under certain climatic conditions or during certain seasons of the year. U.S. feed manufacturers experienced an average shrink of 0.74% in 1976. Feed industry survey, 1982 showed an average shrink of 0.81%

Where does shrink occur?

Rank	Department
1	Receiving department
2	Warehouse
3	Packaging department
4	Pelleting system
5	Grain processing
6	Loadout
7	Mixing system
8	Delivery

What causes Shrink?

Department of Cost Center	Rank	Description of Loss
Receiving (bulk ingredients)	1	Dust loss during unloading
	2	Weighing errors
	3	Loss in transit (leaks, moisture)
	4	Spillage while unloading
	5	Railcar/truck/ship cleanout
	6	Shipper practices (water, foreign materials
Receiving (bagged ingredients)	1	Broken bags
	2	Underweight bags
	3	Count errors
Grain processing (grinding and cracking)	1	Dust loss
	2	Moisture loss
	3	Spills and leaks
	4	Spoilage (mould, etc.)
Grain Processing (flaking and rolling)	1	Moisture loss
	2	Dust loss
	3	Spoilage (mould)
	4	Spills and leaks
Batch Mixing	1	Moisture loss
	2	Scale accuracy
	3	Bin mixups
	4	Rework due to mixing errors
	5	Dust loss
	6	Spills and leaks
	7	Cleanout material
Continuous (in line) Mixing	1	Moisture loss
	2	Feeder Accuracy
	3	Rework due to operator error
	4	Spills and leaks
	5	Cleanout material
Pelleting	1	Moisture loss
	2	Dust loss
	3	Off-grade pellets
	4	Spills and leaks
	5	Cleanout material
Packaging	1	Overfill
	2	Scale accuracy
	3	Rework from setbacks, cleanout, and errors
	4	Broken or damaged bags
	5	Loss of packaging materials (bags, twine, tape, etc.)
Warehousing	1	Broken or damaged bags

	2	Moisture loss in bags
	3	Theft
	4	Damage due to dust, water, insects, rodents, and birds
	5	Rework due to poor inventory control and obsolete products
	6	Inventory errors
Bulk Feed Loadout (shipping)	1	Dust (wind) loss
	2	Spills and leaks
	3	Weather (rain, snow, etc.)
	4	Weighing errors
	5	Moisture loss
	6	Theft
	7	Cleanout material
Bagged Feed Loadout (Shipping)	1	Count errors
	2	Theft
	3	Broken bags
	4	Spills, sweepings
	5	Damage in railcar or truck
	6	Loading errors (wrong product)
Feed Delivery (trucking)	1	In-transit leaks or damage
	2	Theft
	3	Damage while unloading
	4	Dust loss or spills while unloading

Source: R.R.McEllhiney (1985) Shrink Control in Feed Manufacturing, pp 522-527.

Table 2. Moisture losses from grinding maize *

		Average Moisture (%)		
Plant	No. of Tests	Whole maize	Ground maize	% Shrink
# 1	24	14.96	14.07	0.89
# 2	22	14.25	13.23	1.02
# 3	32	14.38	13.35	1.03
# 4	37	15.13	14.29	0.84
# 5	32	14.78	13.83	0.95
Total (Average)	147	14.73	14.32	0.95 **

* Samples taken at discharge from the storage bin above the grinder and at the entry to the ground grain storage bin. ** Whole maize with a moisture content of 15% or more averaged 1.20% shrink. Whole maize with a moisture content of 14% or less averaged 0.81% shrink.

Moisture losses: Moisture losses from the receiving system to the outloading of feeds is a major cause of weight shrinkage in feed manufacturing. Wolfe (1982) studied moisture losses during the unloading of bulk feed ingredients over a 4-month period. The moisture content losses were found to be 0.095%, 0.23% and 0.18%, for maize grain, soybean meal and brewers' grain, respectively. Remen (1976) studied the effect of hammer mill grinding on the moisture content of ground grain. The study was conducted in five plant locations (Table 2).

Wolfe (1982) compared moisture losses in grinding over a 4-month period using two hammer mill screen sizes (Table 3). The effect of grinder system design on moisture loss during the hammer mill grinding process has been studied (Remen, 1976). The results are presented in Table 4.

Table 3. Moisture losses in fine and coarse grinding of maize*

Month	Fine Grinding[1] Moisture Content %)		Shrink (%)	Coarse Grinding[2] Moisture Content (%)		Shrink (%)
	Whole maize	Ground maize		Whole maize	Ground maize	
November	14.45	13.32	1.22	14.62	13.50	1.12
December	14.40	13.28	1.12	14.60	13.52	1.08
January	14.42	13.46	0.96	14.46	13.62	1.01
February	14.26	13.17	1.09	14.75	13.76	0.99
Averages	14.41	13.31	1.10	14.65	13.60	1.05

*Samples taken at discharge from the storage bin above the grinder and at the entry to the ground grain storage bin. 1. Used 1/8" screen with mechanical handling; 2. Used 3/16" screen with mechanical handling

Table 4. Moisture loss by Grinder System Design

Design	Av. moisture loss (%)
Bin over bin (no elevation)	0.10
Mechanical handling of ground materials	0.22
Pneumatic (air) handling of ground materials	0.95

Effect of pelleting on moisture losses

Pelleting has been identified as a cause of shrink in feed manufacturing operations and some share of that shrink is the result of moisture losses between the mash feed to the pellet mill and the cooler discharge (W.A. Wolfe, 1982; Table 5).

Ambient air temperature and the water holding capacity of air has a direct effect on the level of shrink occurring in the feed manufacturing processes. Wolfe (1982) reported that air has the ability to double its water-holding capabilities for every 20°F rise in temperature. It is exactly this air heating process that enables the feed manufacturer to dry pellets in a pellet cooler even on high humidity days. Hot pellets rise the air temperature enabling the air to pick up more moisture.

As an example, air at 70°F and 70% relative humidity (RH) has 0.011 lbs of water vapour per lb of dry air, air at 70°F and 100% RH has 0.016 lbs of water vapour per lb of dry air, while air at 90°F and 100% RH has 0.030 lbs of water vapour per lb of dry air.

Moisture control during feed manufacturing processes is a key to reducing shrink. Therefore moisture testing equipment should be provided and used for testing inbound ingredients, in-process materials and finished products.

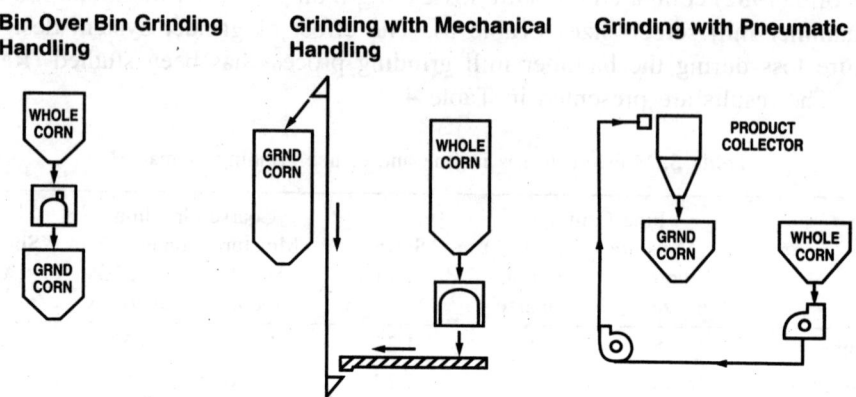

Bin Over Bin Grinding Handling

Grinding with Mechanical Handling

Grinding with Pneumatic

Table 5. Pelleting Moisture Losses

Sample Location	Moisture (%)	
	Dairy with 2½% molasses	Dairy with 1% molasses & urea
Feeder inlet	12.80	13.30
Conditioning chamber with molasses & steam *	16.37	16.61
Die discharge	16.67	16.81
Cooler discharge	12.62	12.70
Moisture loss	0.18	0.60

*Molasses added at conditioner

Effects of weather conditions

Midgley (1976) studied the effect of storage time, temperature and RH on weight loss or gain in sacked pelleted feeds. He found weight losses of up to 4.0% during hot, dry months and gains of as much as 3.0% during the cooler, wetter months.

Suggested methods of shrink control
Inbound materials

- Correct weight recording
- Routinely check the moisture and foreign matter content

Outbound finished products

- Weigh all trucks, empty and loaded, as they enter and leave the plant.
- Date code all products and sell the older stock first
- Return damaged or broken bags

Dust Control

- Check all dust collection and control equipment to be sure that they function well.

- Replace or repair leaking spouts, elevator legs, conveyors to control all sources of dust emission.
- Study the feasibility and economics of using tallow, mineral oil, water, or some other dust depressant to reduce emissions and losses.
- Enclose receiving and shipping areas to reduce losses caused by wind and rain.

Plant Security

Control theft by outsiders and/or employees

Inventory practices

- Accurate calibration of all bins, tanks and silos
- Keep a record of bulk densities of ingredients
- Instruct employees on proper inventory procedures and provide them with the necessary drop lines, lighting, calibration charts, forms and instructions.

Pest Control

- Establish baiting, trapping etc. to eradicate & control rodents
- Establish fumigation procedures to control insect infestation
- Keep birds out of the plant
- Keep the house neat and clean to eliminate pest harborages

Conclusion

The effect of shrink include reduction of profits, higher feed prices, increased cost of feeding animals, and higher food costs for everyone. Hence, shrink is a multimillion dollar problem for the feed industry and a great monetary loss to the producer.

10

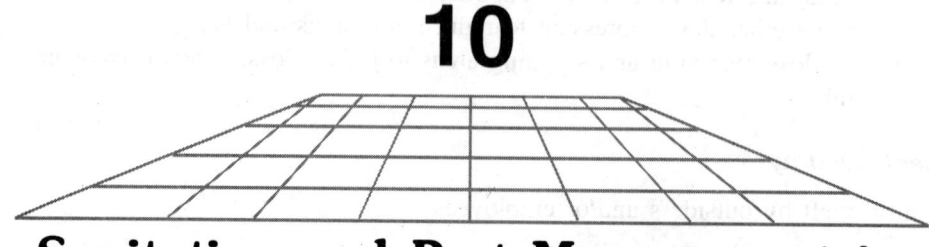

Sanitation and Pest Management in relation to Feed Plants

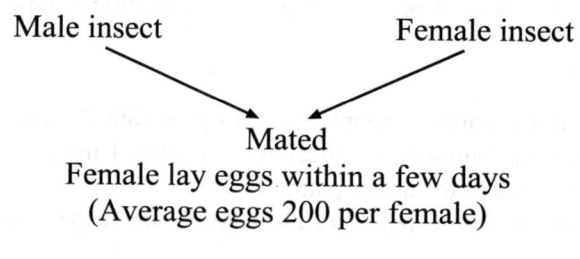

Male insect   Female insect

Mated
Female lay eggs within a few days
(Average eggs 200 per female)

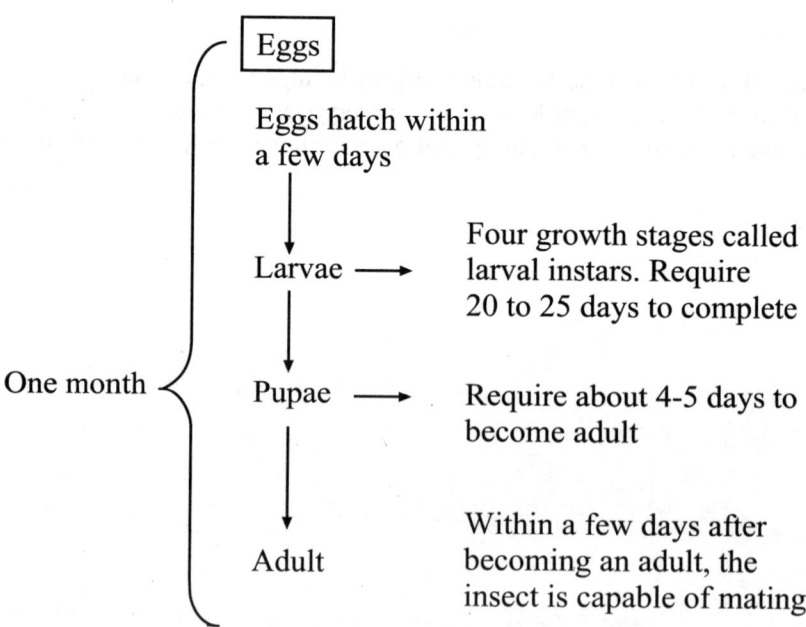

Eggs

Eggs hatch within
a few days

Larvae ⟶ Four growth stages called
larval instars. Require
20 to 25 days to complete

One month

Pupae ⟶ Require about 4-5 days to
become adult

Adult   Within a few days after
becoming an adult, the
insect is capable of mating.

There are a variety of pests to be managed or controlled in relationship to feed manufacturing. These pests are discussed with the concept in mind that the better the pest is understood, the more effectively the various control measures can be applied.

The primary pests of concern are the grain and cereal product insects, rodents that have adapted themselves to coexist in human environs, micro organisms (primarily fungi or mould) adapted to live in stored grains, birds and the human pest (J.R.Pedersen, 1985).

Insects

About 15 to 20 insects have adapted themselves to live and cause significant damage in the rather dry environment of grains and animal feeds. This relatively small group of insects includes both beetles (including weevils) and moths (butterfly-like insects). Recently A.D.Wales et al. (2010) reviewed the relationship between arthropods (flies, beetles and mites) that are commonly found in and around livestock premises and zoonotic bacteria. Salmonella is widely distributed in the flies of affected livestock units and is detectable to a lesser degree in beetles and mites. Persistent carriage appears to be common and there is some field and experimental evidence to support arthropod-mediated transmission between poultry flocks, particularly carry-over from one flock to the next. Campylobacter may readily be isolated from arthropods that are in contact with affected poultry flocks, although carriage is short-lived. The carriage of other zoonotic bacteria by arthropods has been documented. In view of this, sanitation and pest management has a greater role in preventing the spread of zoonotic pathogens such as Salmonella and Campylobacter.

Rodents

Feed plant operators and feed manufacturers are probably more aware of rodent problems than they are insect problems. Although rodents (rats and mice) consume sizeable quantities of grain, they are probably more important in feed plant operations from the standpoint of contamination of ingredients and finished products and the damage they do to plant facilities and product containers. Rodent contamination is particularly important because of the potential for disease transmission in urine and excrement (droppings).

Birds

Like rodents, birds are capable of consuming quantities of grains and feed products. Animal feed lots have reported substantial economic losses from starlings. However, birds at feed plants are a greater problem from the standpoint of product contamination and nuisance.

Pigeons and sparrows create the most problems. They tend to roost and/or nest on the plant structure where they find it convenient to feed on spillage in receiving and shipping areas. If the plant is not properly protected by screened windows, doors and other openings into the plant (or warehouse), birds will readily enter and be in the position to contaminate products with their droppings. Bird droppings create an undesirable appearance on plant exteriors and product containers and can potentially serve as sources of human and animal diseases. Bird nests can also be a source of Trogoderma insects that can infest grains and feed products.

Humans

Human beings do not like to be referred to as pests, though their actions (or inactions) often create sanitation problems more serious than those created by insects, rodents, micro organisms, and/or birds.

The attitudes and performance that employees show with respect to sanitation in the feed plant can be the result of many factors: lack of knowledge, lack of supervision, lack of management support, or other reasons. Management has the responsibility to see that good sanitation is maintained.

Sanitation and Pest Control: An integrated approach

Methods used in sanitation and pest control can be grouped broadly into four main categories:
1. Inspection
2. Housekeeping
3. Physical-mechanical methods
4. Chemical applications

Corrective steps need to be taken

Inspection

Inspections can be used to identify existing problems such as an active rodent population, grain which is infested, ingredients contaminated with mycotoxins, etc. Inspections can also be used to identify potential problems such as tall weeds and grass and spilled grains around the plant exterior that provide a habitat favourable for rodents, accumulations of stock in dead-spots in equipment that could provide a breeding place for insects, etc.

Housekeeping

Housekeeping involves cleanliness and orderliness. It includes maintaining the plant perimeter, exterior, and interior free of spilled grains and grain products that could provide attractants or breeding places for insect, rodent, microbial, and bird pests. Proper cleaning of interiors and exteriors of plant areas and equipment with frequency as needed and proper storage of equipment, ingredients, and finished products.

Housekeeping is considered the most effective preventive means of pest control and is accomplished primarily through good supervision and management. It is considered one of the primary means for preventing dust explosions. A properly maintained plant with good housekeeping is also a more productive plant.

Physical and Mechanical Methods

Physical means used in sanitation and pest control include temperature alteration, moisture control and pest exclusion. Reducing the temperature of stored grains below that favourable for insect development by use of aeration is a practical way of preventing losses due to insects. Heat treatment of plant interiors and equipment is being considered as a means for insect control, since chemicals for insect control are excluded (J.R.Pedersen, 1985). However, economics dictate what is to be done.

Mould growth in grains and feed products is controlled by maintaining the moisture content (or relative humidity) below that favourable for mould growth. Generally, grain in equilibrium with 70 percent relative humidity (13.5 to 14.5 percent) or less will not promote rapid mold growth. Conditions can be created within a feed plant or system that provides an environment favourable for mould development. Warm, moist conditions inside a grinder exposed to cool outside temperatures can result in condensation in the equipment and storage bins, thus encouraging mould development. This may be alleviated by suction on the system to remove the warm moist air, or it may be possible to reduce the potential for condensation by preventing the outside cooling effect.

Prevention of rodent and bird entry into feed plants is best accomplished by various physical barriers to exclude the pests. This can be as simple as keeping an existing door closed or providing special metal barriers on building exteriors to prevent rodent climbing of walls, conduit, or other structural elements. Screening of windows or other openings into a plant is another simple and effective way of excluding rodents and birds.

Some feed processing operations are considered effective in preventing insects from passing the system alive. The impact provided by hammermills or other grinders will destroy live insects. The temperature and pressures generated in pellet mills are probably sufficient to destroy insects and have been shown to reduce bacterial counts in contaminated ingredients.

There are a variety of mechanical traps available for rodent control and even simple glue boards have proven effective. Some other devices that are available for rodent and bird control include ultrasonic devices (rodents), rotating lights (birds), and electronic grids (flying insects).

Chemical Applications

Chemicals available for pest control are under scrutiny and are considered to be hazardous to use and subsequently removed from the market. The types of materials that have been available include **1. contact insecticides** used as grain protectants, surface sprays, fogs, or mists; 2. **fumigants**, materials which on exposure to the atmosphere form toxic vapours or gases; **3. rodenticides** in the form of acute or multiple dose positions; and **4. avicides**, including toxicants and repellants.

Coordinated effort

The various methods must be used in a coordinated manner to complement each other. This requires thorough planning and effective management. As an example, a contact insecticide is most effective as a surface spray when applied to a product free surface. One of the best times to spray would be shortly after sweeping in the area. The treatment can be made even more effective by cleaning and spraying just before plant shut down for a weekend. The clean, insecticide coated surface is then available for a longer period of time. In all situations, emphasis should be placed on the preventive aspects of the various methods of pest control and sanitation.

Rodent control checklist

- Identify primary areas of infestation by checking for rodent sings; gnawing marks, greasy smears along walls and rafters, rat droppings, burrows, etc.
- Measure extent of infestation by placing "control bait" (control bait is regular feed the rats have been eating in facilities) throughout building, and check frequently for rat consumption. The speed at which control bait is consumed should show extent of infestation.
- Remove rubbish, brush and weeds from around the facilities
- Seal off areas where trash and feed bags are stored, or store feed in tightly-covered containers.
- Close up access routes into buildings. Cement should be used to seal gaps around drains, pipes and foundations.
- Place small amounts of bait in most likely rodent dwellings. Pellets should be placed 6-10 feet apart along runways where rats travel, near burrows, and at entry points to buildings.
- Place water dishes near bait stations.
- Check bait station frequently, and refill immediately when empty.
- After 3-5 days of baiting, dead rats will start to appear. These should be discarded immediately.
- Once rodent problem seems under control, continue to re-fill bait stations and keep water available to year-round control.

Summary

It is evident from the preceding discussion that 'sanitation and pest management' at feed manufacturing plants is an important aspect of the total operation. Maintaining an effective and efficient sanitation programme requires considerable planning, supervision, and support from management. Greater emphasis needs to be given to sanitation and pest control at feed plants.

SECTION VII
Clinical Nutrition

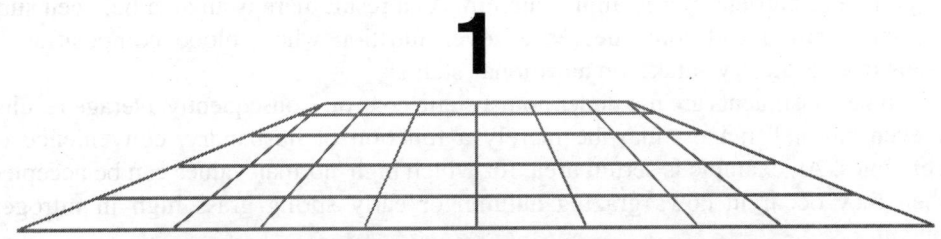

Relationship between *in vivo* Parameters and Nutritional Status of Dairy Animals

The concept of using blood, serum or plasma analysis as a means of assessing the metabolic status of an individual has been used for many years in the field of human medicine. In general terms, results outside the 'normal' range in human subjects are usually due to disease or physiological malfunction in the individual. Laboratory analyses can therefore be used as a means of identifying or confirming a medical diagnosis.

Metabolic profile system for animals

With animals, this use of blood analysis is a less common practice. Instead, a limited range of analyses has been used on selected animals within a herd to confirm (or help identify) suspected abnormalities of performance due to inadequate nutrition. Results of such analyses often lie partly within the 'normal' range, and for this reason it is necessary to test a number of animals (usually at least 6) to achieve a meaningful result. An example of this is the metabolic profile system for dairy cows devised and pioneered by Professor J M Payne, whereby a sufficient number of cows are selected out of a herd to allow the results to be analysed statistically.

Analysis of blood and animal tissues, including milk, are frequently carried out as a means of assessing the metabolic health of farm livestock, and as a diagnostic technique in the identification and treatment of certain disorders and diseases (Topps and Thomson, 1984). Further, it has been estimated that about 35% of the cows and buffaloes are culled from herds because of gynaecological complaints or failure of conception despite repeated inseminations. Fertility rates are especially affected with increasing milk yield. As a consequence, some of these analyses have become part of the work of veterinary investigation laboratories where use of the Compton profile, Blowey mini-profile and Edinburgh Dairy Herd Health & Productivity Scheme has been well established (Topps and Thompson, 1984).

General properties of blood characteristics

Many blood constituents are under some form of homeostatic control and for several nutrients the animal in a deprived state will improve its efficiency of utilization of the particular nutrient, for example calcium. As a result there is an area between sub-optimal nutrition and some degree of over-nutrition where blood composition is insensitive to dietary intake or nutritional status.

Some constituents are not under homeostatic control. Consequently average results, or even 'normal' ranges, may be merely a function of husbandry, convenience or economics. An example is serum urea, for which high 'normal' values can be accepted when they occur in cows grazing autumn or early spring grass high in nitrogen content.

Blood composition is affected by non-nutritional factors such as stage of lactation, age of the animal and time of year. Examples include packed cell volume (PCV), glucose and urea. Some blood constituents are noticeably affected by interaction with other elements, and may not always reflect the feed input/output relationship. Cows severely stressed at sampling may have very high values of glucose and NEFA.

Components such as serum urea and magnesium are subject to changes in level from hour to hour due to episodic feeding, whereas others do not show any pronounced diurnal variation.

The concentrations of certain constituents are seriously affected by disease. For example, liver damage caused by fluke parasites may change serum copper, and the nematode infestation of the gut may decrease serum albumin and inorganic phosphorus.

Constituents such as glucose and potassium may be affected by a delay in testing. Special anticoagulant, such as mixture of oxalate and fluoride salts, is used to prevent the loss of glucose due to oxidation.

Haematological measurements are made on blood to assess whether the animal is normal or deficient in relation to anaemia. The actual cause of the anaemia may be due to one or more of several factors.

Packed cell volume (PCV)

PCV and haemoglobin are closely correlated. PCV values fall in early lactation as milk yield rises, then tend to rise as lactation progresses. Values are highest in summer but in many circumstances high levels may be indicative of dehydration. Some times this can be due to a reduced water intake. The PCV value is not under full homeostatic control and time of sampling has little effect on it.

Haemoglobin

Haemoglobin reflects red cell function and status. At calving haemoglobin production ceases for a time, but synthesis increases again during the first four months of lactation. Anaemia can result from various infections and parasitic conditions as well as nutritional disorders. Copper, cobalt and iron are the chief minerals whose deficiency leads to anaemia, but iron deficiency is unlikely in normal farm practice.

Blood haemoglobin falls to a low level due to haemolysis on feeding certain forages, for example excess kale feeding. Deficiency of energy and protein over prolonged periods will reduce the total red cell mass, and it has been noted that in starved animals the hormone erythropoietin is markedly reduced.

Haemoglobin is not under close or rigid homeostatic control, and time of sampling has little effect on the value obtained.

Cell counts

Measurement of erythrocytes and leucocytes (lymphocytes, neutrophils, eosinophils) provides information on a nutritional problem. Total leucocytes often fall when feed intake is reduced, and a substantial reduction occurs with severe under-nutrition.

Characteristics associated with energy status (glucose, non-esterified fatty acids [NEFA], beta-hydroxy butyrate [BHB])

Blood metabolites such as glucose and NEFA, which are associated with the utilization of energy, are greatly influenced by hormones. In particular insulin and glucagon affect the metabolism of both glucose and NEFA. Insulin has a hypoglycaemic effect since it increases the movement of glucose into many peripheral tissues such as muscle and fat. It may also decrease lipolysis of adipose tissue. Glucagon is a hyperglycaemic hormone which promotes gluconeogenesis and to a small extent lipolysis. As a consequence, changes in hormone levels in blood may be the primary cause of variations in the concentrations of the metabolites that yield energy at tissue level.

Glucose: Glucose is normally determined in plasma, but either whole blood or serum can also be used. Glucose levels decline following under-feeding or fasting. Low glucose levels in dairy cows often occur when the milk produced has a low content of solids-not-fat (SNF). Conversely, high glucose values are sometimes found when the diet contains a high proportion of concentrate mixture. Concentrations of glucose tend to be lower in early lactation and occasionally in late pregnancy, which are broadly compatible with the negative energy balance (NEB). In high yielding animals the concentrations are lower than in those of average yield. High yielding cows with fatty livers tend to have low glucose values 1-2 weeks after calving.

Glucose is not as sensitive to changes in energy balance as BHB or NEFA because of homeostatic control. However, within the optimum range there is some evidence that plasma glucose can reflect weight change.

Non-esterified fatty acids (NEFA): When adipose tissue is mobilized to meet the energy needs of an animal, NEFA are released into blood plasma. High levels, therefore, reflect a degree of under-nutrition or negative energy balance. NEFA is a more direct measure of fat mobilization than BHB. However, it is not stable in transit. From 48 hours after collection it may start to rise. Cows severely upset at testing may show rises not relating to nutrition.

Beta-hydroxy butyrate (BHB): Measurement of this ketone, one of the four associated with ketoses in dairy cows, is regarded by some as an acceptable means (BHB is stable in blood and is more convenient to determine than total ketones) of assessing the dietary energy intake of dairy cows, particularly in early lactation. Beta-hydroxy butyrate (Fig.1) levels in dairy cows in early lactation are higher than

420

those in either dry cows or cows in mid-lactation, and that in general, high concentrations are directly related to the rate of mobilization of fat reserves. The concentration increases as the animal is under increasing energy stress.

Free glycerol: Free glycerol in the plasma of dairy cows has been found to show changes in concentrations which are similar to those of NEFA.

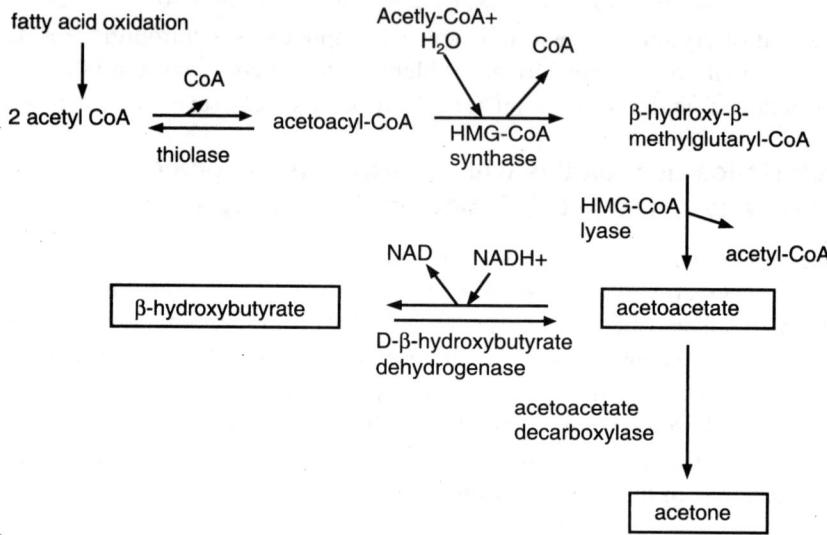

Figure 1. Formation of ketone bodies within mitochondria by condensation of acetyl-CoA. Metabolic conversions of acetoacetate, β-hydroxybutyrate, and acetone are shown. Enzymes that catalyze the different steps are indicated by arrows. CoA, coenzyme A; HMG-CoA, 3-hydroxy-3-methylglytaryl coenzyme A; NAD, nicotinamide adenine dinucleotide; NADH+, nicotinamide adenine dinucleotide (oxidized)

Urea: It is relevant to note that in circumstances where the intake of rumen degradable protein remains relatively constant, plasma urea may be inversely related to the intake of dietary energy.

Characteristics associated with protein status (urea, albumin, total protein, Hb and PCV)

Urea: 1.Concentrations of serum or plasma urea have been related to intake of protein, but other dietary factors can have a major effect on this fraction. In particular, the level of digestible energy in the diet controls the amount of ammonia produced in, and absorbed from, the rumen and this has an important effect on the concentration of urea in the blood. 2. The degradability of dietary protein is another factor.

In effect, the concentration of urea is a measure of the surplus supply ammonia arising from digestion and metabolism, which goes into the blood stream and is converted to urea by the liver. Blood urea nitrogen reflects very well the intake of effective rumen degradable protein (ERDP) and its balance with fermentable metabolizable energy (FME). Some of this urea is recycled to the gut via the saliva, but in most circumstances the major part of it is excreted in urine, via the kidneys.

Concentrations of urea fluctuate during the day and this reflects the amount of protein and non-protein nitrogen (NPN) fed and the rapidity of degradation in the rumen of different dietary proteins and sources of NPN. Normally serum urea reaches a peak 2-6 hours after a cow has eaten a quantity of high protein feed. The actual time lag and the extent of the peak depend on the rumen degradability of the protein and on the intake of digestible energy.

Serum albumin: Concentrations of serum albumin are in some ways a reflection of the animal's ability to synthesize and store protein, low values may indicate an insufficiency of protein and/or energy over an extended period. However, serum albumin is synthesized by the liver. Dysfunction of liver due to pathogens or parasites can result in less albumin being formed. In addition, certain gut parasites cause a loss of albumin into the gut and this will also show as a decrease in serum concentration. Serum albumin has a half life of about 30 days so that any decrease in synthesis is not usually seen for several weeks. An abrupt cessation of synthesis, which occurs at calving, however, may be seen sooner than this.

During lactation, generally low concentrations of albumin have been associated with lower yields and a low SNF content of milk. On the other hand, high yielding cows with fatty livers in early lactation have low concentrations of albumin, which may reflect changes in liver function.

There is no way of directly assessing through blood metabolites the adequacy of digestible undegradable protein (DUP) or metabolizable protein (MP) in a diet. Practically, however, if milk / milk protein performance is below expectation and if there is definitely no negative energy balance (normal BHB, NEFA and glucose in early lactation and body weight gain) and no shortage of ERDP (normal urea N), then additional DUP is worth trying.

Total protein and globulins: Globulin level is not measured itself. Globulins + albumin make up the total protein in serum and the concentration of globulins is obtained as the difference between laboratory determinations of total protein and of serum albumin. Globulins are antibodies of the type formed in response to chronic inflammation. The most common causes are things like mastitis, metritis or lameness. Infections such as Fasciola hepatica may be involved.

Haemoglobin and packed cell volume: Haemoglobin and PCV need to be mentioned again since intake of dietary protein can influence their concentration in blood. To confirm diagnosis of anaemia, Hb, PCV and plasma urea levels need to be measured and elicit whether prolonged feeding of kale to the animal has been a practice. When it is confirmed that low Hb and PCV values are associated with low plasma urea, the diet is likely to be seriously deficient in protein.

Characteristics indicating mineral or vitamin status

Calcium, phosphorus and magnesium: The concentrations of these elements in serum are controlled to varying degrees by endocrine factors. The mechanism for the control of calcium in blood is well established, whereas phosphorus and magnesium are not under any apparently strong homeostatic control. Even with calcium, a failure of homeostasis can occur in the dairy animal if there is a sudden demand for calcium when reserves from bone have not previously been required. Such a crisis is a common occurrence after calving, resulting in milk fever, and is more likely if a high calcium diet has been fed prior to calving.

The metabolites of vitamin D have an important role in calcium absorption and homeostasis, but sources in the diet or from sunlight are generally adequate. Serum calcium levels are depressed when diets are low in calcium or high in phosphorus, but the effect may be transient since calcium levels are maintained by mobilization of bone calcium. Starvation of progressive severity does not seem to affect serum calcium until feed intake becomes very low.

Low phosphorus diets generally result in a depression in serum phosphorus. Where intake of P is less than requirement, strong positive correlations have been demonstrated between P intake and serum or plasma P levels. However, blood P levels do not always reflect P intake. It has been observed that in cases of starvation or of inadequate energy or protein intake, or where weight loss is occurring, blood inorganic phosphorus levels increase. Low phosphorus diets tend to elevate serum calcium and urinary calcium excretion.

Extra magnesium in the diet lowers the level of serum phosphorus, and extra dietary phosphorus lowers serum magnesium level. Restriction of magnesium intake usually causes a drop in serum magnesium level, especially during pregnancy or lactation. Serum magnesium is also lowered by an excess of potassium in the diet following the application of a potassium-containing fertilizer to pasture. An increase in potassium intake results in a decrease in the absorption of magnesium and a reduction in its urinary excretion. However, the retention of magnesium may be unaltered and this may be why diets containing added magnesium do not necessarily increase serum magnesium levels.

In practice, dairy cows grazing young grass may succumb to grass tetany due to poor availability of the magnesium consumed, while a deficiency in milk-fed calves is likely to be due to a low intake of magnesium relative to requirements. Ruminants with low levels of serum or blood magnesium are at risk from 'grass staggers' but the incidence of clinical cases and death is comparatively low. This is because it is a low level of magnesium in the cerebrospinal fluid (CSF) which dictates the clinical condition. Magnesium level falls much more slowly in CSF than in blood and some cows seem able to maintain an adequate level in the CSF even when blood magnesium has been very low for some time. There is, however, a more rapid fall in CSF magnesium immediately prior to tetany and this explains the part played by stress factors in inducing 'staggers'. There is some indication that CSF magnesium is likely to be lower when both serum magnesium and serum calcium are low.

Sodium and potassium: Sodium concentrations are usually close to 140 m mol/litre and levels, which are 4 or more m mol lower, indicate an insufficiency of sodium. This may lead to the slow development of a depraved appetite as shown by hair licking, earth eating and urine drinking. Supplementation of common salt can prevent this situation. Dairy cows producing substantial amounts of milk secrete large amounts of sodium and a shortage of this element in the diet may reduce yield. High concentrations of serum sodium may indicate a partial deprivation of water. Low sodium levels have been found in herds with severe mastitis, which indicates that mastitis induces a fall in blood sodium.

Concentrations of potassium are usually close to 5.5 m mol/litre but higher values are often seen in animals grazing leafy or heavily fertilized pasture. High values have been reported when serum magnesium is low. Concentrations lower than normal are uncommon, and if they occur are probably not due to a dietary deficiency since most animal feeds contain adequate amounts of potassium.

Copper: Copper is usually determined in serum, but whole blood and plasma have been used in some laboratories. Grass is usually relatively low in copper content while concentrates are commonly high in copper level. Furthermore, molybdenum and sulphur in herbage reduce the availability of copper for ruminants because of interaction among them. Grasses and certain legumes contain elevated levels of molybdenum when grown on certain soils, especially after liming. Heavy metals such as iron, zinc and cadmium are also known to limit the availability of copper. Cows affected with liver fluke parasitsm often show low serum copper levels. Low blood copper has been associated in some instances with infertility problems.

Measurement of cobalt, selenium, iodine, vitamins E, A and B_{12}, and carotenoids are also important.

Examination of alternative materials

Blood samples are easily and conveniently obtained from animals and no serious attempt has been made to replace blood with any other tissue material as part of a screening system. However, it is important to remember that the use of blood is a practical expedient, and even in the best of circumstances changes in metabolite concentrations are not a true reflection of nutritional status. Measurements of plasma urea and serum vitamin B_{12} reflect to a significant extent changes, which occur in the gut or rumen of an animal. Storage and subsequent release of nutrients associated with bone and liver is not usually shown by changes in blood levels. Hence alternative materials such as saliva, urine, faeces, milk, hair, liver and rumen contents are helpful to assess the status of animals with respect to certain nutrients according to the situation.

Parotid saliva is most often used to assess sodium status and intake. The content of sodium and potassium responds rapidly to dietary insufficiency long before clinical signs appear. High content of potassium in parotid saliva from dairy cows gives an indication of very high intakes of potassium from heavily fertilized forage. These intakes have been associated with a greater incidence of infertility.

Liver biopsy samples can be used to assess the status of copper, vitamin B_{12} or vitamin A of animals. Rumen contents can be obtained by stomach tube and content of rumen ammonia, VFA, pH and vitamin B_{12} can be analysed.

The excretion of certain metabolites in urine tends to represent the final phase of a series of reactions, and many have a more consistent order of magnitude than the concentrations found in blood. It is well known that the milk of dairy animals may change in composition as a result of alterations to the diet. The most striking effects are lack of long roughage (which lowers milk fat content) and underfeeding of energy (which reduces protein and SNF content). Other major changes which affect lactose, sodium and chloride are usually due to mastitis.

Estimation of rumen microbial protein supply from PDC index

Daily excretion of purine derivatives (PD) in urine is accepted as procedure to estimate the supply of microbial protein in ruminant livestock. Quantitative relationships between urinary excretion of PD and intake of digestible organic matter and dry matter have been reported for ruminant animals. However, the use of this technique under field application is difficult because it requires total urine collection. Creatinine is excreted in urine in a fixed proportion relative to the metabolic body weight and is less affected by dietary factors. So when purine derivatives (PD=allantoin + uric acid) is expressed relative to creatinine excreted in urine corrected for metabolic body weight, it is called purine derivatives:creatinine (PDC) index.

Urinary purine derivatives to creatinine ratio (PDC index), obtained from spot urine sample, has been shown to be linearly correlated with daily PD excretion in sheep and buffaloes (M.T.Dipu, 2004) and in crossbred cattle (S.K.George, 2004) and thus it could provide a practical indicator of microbial protein supply under field conditions. The PDC index based on spot urine samples seems to be a powerful and handy technique for predicting the rumen microbial protein supply vis-à-vis nutritional status under farm conditions in cattle but not in buffaloes (Vijay Kumar Singh, 2007). The PDC index may be used as a practical indicator of microbial protein supply as well as nutritional status of animals under field conditions.

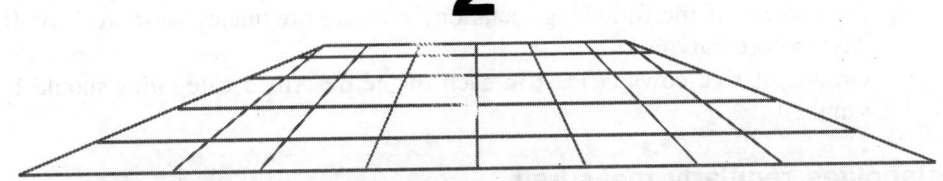

Metabolic Profile Tests; Use and Interpretation of Metabolic Profiles

INTRODUCTION

How well the animals are fed can be assessed by observation of daily milk yields, peak yields, lactation curves, body condition changes, fat and protein content of milk, strength of oestrous signs and conception rates. Metabolic profiles properly planned and organised will tell that something is wrong or about to go wrong, what it is and what is the best/most economic solution (David A.Whitakar, 2000).

Metabolic profile test

Metabolic profile test is intended to be a sequence of balance between 'nutrients absorbed' from gastrointestinal tract and 'nutrients furnished' for body functions (maintenance, pregnancy or lactation) as needed by the animal. If 'nutrients absorbed' are inadequate to match the 'demand of the body functions' levels of the metabolites in the blood and other body fluids may fall. The body's homeostatic mechanisms try to maintain the levels of different nutrients in the body initially. Hence, this fall may be slight and not manifested as a clinical abnormality. As the reduction in metabolite concentration progresses, it is reflected in clinical manifestation. The metabolic profile test can be used as both an early warning indicator of sub-clinical disease and as a diagnostic procedure.

Conduct of metabolic profile tests

- As there can be short term biochemical changes associated with feeding itself, cows should not be blood sampled soon after a larger concentrate feed. It is best to wait 1 hour after feeding, but 2 hours if cows receive more than 2 kg of concentrates at milking time.
- Cows should not be sampled within 2 weeks after a major diet change. This is to allow the rumen environment to become fully adapted to the new ration and so to utilise its potential.

- Tests should be planned to get the cows' opinion after any major diet change i.e. 2 weeks after the change and to know the metabolic status of cows in early lactation (10-20 days after calving), mid lactation group (around 100 days after calving) and dry cow group (the dry period is very important for the success of the following lactation) and late pregnancy (last week or 10 days before calving).
- Groups of five cows at least in each of the described categories should be sampled.

Metabolites regularly measured

- A wide range of metabolites can be measured in blood. But the number of such parameters as part of a nutritional advice programme needs to be kept to a minimum on the grounds of cost and to avoid over complication of results and interpretation.
- Practically the metabolite needs to be stable in an unseparated sample after collection for 2-3 days while in transit to a laboratory.
- The method of analysis needs to be rapid, accurate and not expensive.
- Metabolite values determined need to be compared with 'normal' or 'optimum' values (population mean ± 2 standard deviation). Nevertheless these values are guides only and should not be used too precisely.

I. Compton metabolic profile test: Thirteen metabolites were used by Payne et al. (1970) [PCV, haemoglobin, albumin, blood glucose, BUN, total protein, calcium, inorganic phosphorus, magnesium, potassium, sodium, copper and iron] while Kronfeld (1972) suggested twelve [Haemoglobin, blood glucose, albumin, total protein, Ca, P, Mg, FFA, acetoacetate, BHB, acetate dehydrogenase and lactate dehydrogenase] as alternative.

In this classical metabolic profile assessment, samples are obtained from animals which are representative of the stages in the production cycle namely, dry cows, cows in mid lactation and high yielding cows at their peak yield.

II. Mini metabolic profile test (Blowey et al., 1975): Three metabolites [glucose, albumin and urea nitrogen] are suggested. The animals are sampled at monthly interval

III. Individual preventive examination: Sommer (1975) suggested serum glutamic-oxaloacetic transaminase (SGOT) or aspartic transaminase (AST) or aspartate amino transferase and total cholesterol, Zepgi (1976) suggested SGOT, total cholesterol and blood glucose while Gnanaprakasam (1988) suggested SGOT, blood glucose, total cholesterol and rumen liquor.

In the individual preventive examination, the blood is sampled at 8 weeks prior to calving. It is considered that this procedure offered useful data concerning the susceptibility of each cow to several metabolic and nutritional disorders, because these parameters measure the stage of energy balance and the liver efficiency of each animal.

Energy Balance

- When cows-in-milk have high beta hydroxy butyrate (BHB) and/or high

- non- esterified fatty acids (NEFA), with normal or low glucose, this indicates a dietary energy problem but not necessarily a dietary deficiency.
- Cows-in-milk have high BHB, high NEFA and low glucose where there is no dietary energy problem, i.e. where milk yields are good and condition is not being lost.
- If milking cows have BHB, NEFA and glucose values within optimum ranges, this means cows are having their energy requirements met.
- In dry cows within the last 1-2 weeks of pregnancy, having BHB and/or NEFA above the optimum is a sign of negative energy balance. This can have important implications for production and fertility in the following lactation.

Protein

- If cows at any stage have low urea N values in their blood, this shows inadequate effective rumen degradable protein (ERDP) in the rumen and represents a situation inhibiting productivity. But it does not distinguish between a low dietary content and a low intake of a diet containing an adequate proportion of ERDP.
- A cow that does not eat properly during the previous 12-24 hours will have a low urea the next day.
- Where cows have high blood urea N there is an excess of ERDP in relation to fermentable metabolizable energy (FME) in the diet.

Minerals: Magnesium

- Plasma levels reflect current daily intake rather than reserves which are not quickly available.
- Low blood values are an early warning of the possibility of clinical problems. Subclinical deficiency can affect appetite and so milk yield.
- In dry cows, low plasma magnesium may be associated with a depressing effect on the calcium mobilisation system and consequently hypocalcaemia around calving. When this is happening blood magnesium levels may not drop until a day or two before calving.

Hypomagnesaemia/staggers: Low energy, high ammonia and high potassium in the rumen inhibit the absorption of dietary magnesium.

Inorganic phosphate

Plasma values reflect current dietary intake principally. Cows can tolerate low levels for some weeks while remaining productive and fertile.

Calcium

Variations in blood calcium are small except in the immediate periparturient period and have no relationship with dietary intake due to the strong homeostatic control mechanism.

Sodium and potassium

Homeostasis renders measurement of blood level of both sodium and potassium meaningless as a means of assessing dietary intake or content.

Thyroxine (T4)

Low values in milkers may be associated with poor production, but the main interest is low values in dry cows or pregnant heifers since such values are associated with abortions or the birth of dead calves.

Copper

Blood copper values are not an accurate guide to body and liver status, where most of it is found. If levels are low, productivity and health may be affected as copper is such an important part of many biochemical processes.

Glutathione peroxidase (GSHPx)

- Estimation of this selenium-containing enzyme allows a judgement to be made of selenium intake over the previous month or two.
- Direct measurement of selenium in blood can be done but is too expensive as a routine.

Deficiency conditions of selenium: Poor fertility in growing heifers, retained fetal membranes, still births and muscular dystrophy. Analysis of Vitamin E may also be done because of Se-Vitamin E interrelationship.

Measuring metabolites in milk: Urea

Urea N levels in milk mirrors accurately the blood level and so in individual cows these milk urea N levels can be used to assess in part the protein /energy dietary situation in cows.

- Very low bulk milk urea values would indicate a shortage of ERDP in the diet.
- 'Normal' or 'high' values reflect so many different situations, many of which are quite 'normal', that they can be hazardously misleading and should either be ignored or responded to by a metabolic profile blood test.

Faecal consistency of buffalo/cow

- The gross appearance of fresh faeces can provide valuable guidelines as to the nutritional status of the animal. The consistency of the faeces depends on water and fibre content of the feed it consumes.
- Normal faeces should have a medium porridge-like consistency and the pat should have a concave surface.
- A liquid or runny faeces with no real form suggests a diet low in fibre with too much degradable starch or protein in the diet. e.g. spring grass.

- Stiff or thick faeces are due to diets high in fibre and low in energy. Some diets low in ERDP will produce stiff faeces (David A.Whitakar, 2000).
- Slow rate of passage may result in a mucoid covering of the faeces.
- The presence of whole or partially digested grain may indicate incomplete digestion or accelerated rate of passage.

Use and interpretation of metabolic profiles

The results of metabolic profile (Table 1) tests need to be considered along with a whole range of supplementary data such as details of the animal (age, stage of lactation, yield), diet fed, condition of the animal, consistency of faeces, herd milk production and quality of milk, any clinical signs shown by the animal. Metabolic profiles are of maximum use when considered as an integral part of a planned preventive medicine programme. Full use and interpretation of metabolic profiles provides a major opportunity for the modern veterinary surgeon to exercise both the art and science of veterinary medicine to the positive benefit of productivity.

Production diseases

Metabolic diseases and secondary infections of uterus and udder occur immediately before or after calving. Rumen and liver play major role in the aetiology of 'production diseases'. The high producing dairy cow/buffalo can obtain the energy requirements through proper nutrition and gluconeogenesis, for which rumen and liver should be fully functioning. Hence it appears logical to conduct tests that indicate the health of rumen and liver. Symptoms of abnormality of rumen rarely produce dramatic effect as long as the liver is functioning normally. Hence, liver function deserves closest attention.

Importance of blood glucose and ketones in the evaluation of nutritional state of the ruminant

The concentrations of glucose and ketones (acetoacetate and ?-hydroxybutyrate) in the blood should be useful clinicochemical signs of the nutritional condition of the ruminant. Homeostasis of blood glucose level can be maintained by interactions between the forces to raise blood glucose (glucogan, epinephrime, glucocorticoid and growth hormone) and the forces to lower blood glucose (insulin).

Carbohydrate metabolism in ruminants-gluconeogenesis

The ingested feedstuffs are digested by microbial fermentation in the rumen (Fig. 1). The dietary carbohydrates are largely converted into VFA, so that little glucose is absorbed from the alimentary tract. But glucose is essential to meet certain obligatory requirements: for supply of milk sugar, lactose; for supply of energy to the fetus, for synthesis of triglycerides in adipose tissue and respiration of brain cells and working muscles. Hence, gluconeogenesis is a quantitatively more important process in the ruminant than in the nonruminant. Propionate and amino acids are the gluconeogenic materials.

430

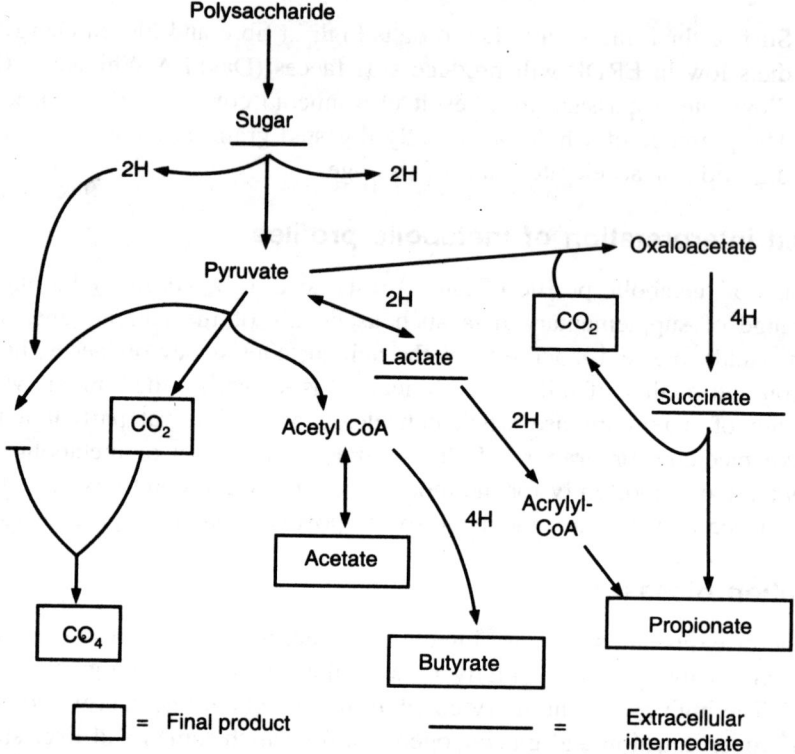

Figure 1. Carbohydrate fermentation in ruminants (Embden-Meyerhof glycolytic pathway for hexose catabolism, while majority pentose is metabolized by the pentose phosphate cycle coupled to glycolysis and some by the phosphoketolase pathway.

Ketogenesis

As glucose becomes less available in the blood, free fatty acids (FFA) and ketones become more important energy-supplying blood components, since most tissues can utilise ketones.

Ketones are synthesized in the liver and in the wall of the rumino-reticulum. The principal precursors of ketones are FFA derived from mobilised body fat and butyrate absorbed from the rumen contents. At low glucose levels ketogenesis increases, whether it be from rumen acids in the fed animal or FFA in the fasted animal.

Fatty liver syndrome

Fatty liver syndrome is a metabolic disorder which has been associated with decreased hepatic gluconeogenesis (due to inadequate oxaloacetate). Fatty liver has been associated with reduced production, reproductive performance and immune competence.

During periods of excessive fatty acid mobilisation from adipose tissue, ruminants are prone to the development of fatty liver. Hepatic uptake of fatty acids (NEFAs) is positively related to plasma concentration. When fatty acids are taken up by hepatocytes they are either oxidized to CO_2, partially oxidised to acetyl-coenzyme A and released as ketone bodies, or esterified mainly to triglycerides. Storage of triglycerides is increased as NEFA levels increase.

Fatty liver is commonly thought to develop postpartum, but it is likely that fat is often deposited from around day 17 prepartum to day 1 postpartum.

A major distinction between the metabolism of dietary fatty acids and those mobilized from adipose tissue is that dietary lipids do not have to enter the liver to be processed prior to use by other tissues. Thus, they are not likely to contribute to problems such as fatty livers and ketosis as do those mobilized from adipose tissue (Kronfeld et el., 1980).

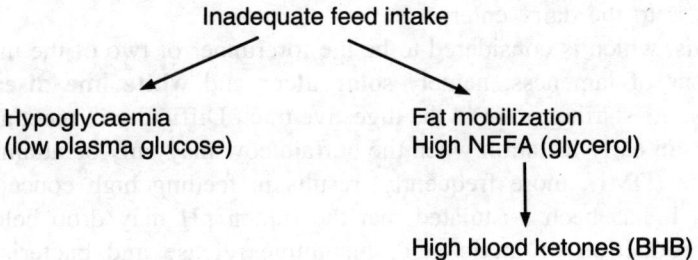

Liver fat levels can be determined using liver biopsy. An alternative method is to measure prepartum plasma NEFA, BHB and glucose levels. These parameters are strongly correlated with liver triglycerides levels at day 1.

Animals with over 35% hepatic lipid concentrations will be clinically ill and have a poor prognosis. At 25-35% levels there will often be clinical signs. At 15-25% there may be clinical signs but animals will be more susceptible to disease such as toxic mastitis.

Acetonaemia (Ketosis)

Acetonaemia or ketosis is a metabolic disorder of the periparturient period and is interrelated with fatty liver. Ketosis occurs due to insufficiency of carbohydrates. Excessive protein feeding may also lead into ketosis. Clinical signs include diminished appetite, decreased milk production, loss of weight, hypoglycaemia, hyperketonaemia and sometimes nervous signs. Blood glucose level is 28mg% against a normal level of 52. Ketone bodies are 41mg% against a normal level of 3.

Primary acetonaemia occurs when not enough food is consumed to meet requirements and body reserves are utilised, resulting in ketonaemia.

Secondary acetonaemia occurs when other diseases, e.g. mastitis or metritis, cause reduction in food intake and nutrient demands are not met.

Both fatty liver and ketosis are a result of fat infiltration into the liver and negative energy balance. When the dietary supply of glucose and that produced by gluconeogenesis are insufficient to meet requirements, fat is mobilised.

A decrease in the availability and concentration of oxaloacetate is a major causal factor in acetonaemia. Fat mobilisation may result in excessive fatty acid uptake by the liver and production of ketone bodies. Both conditions are characterized by elevated plasma NEFA and ketone levels. Excessive fat accumulation reduces glycogenesis.

Liver output of glucose is reduced, resulting in lowered insulin output with the vicious circle of further increase in fat mobilisation.

Bovine lactic acidosis and laminitis

Bovine lactic acidosis and laminitis are linked to imbalances in carbohydrate nutrition, mainly due to an excess of ruminally fermentable carbohydrate and inadequate fibre. Incidences of acidosis and therefore laminitis are more prevalent during the transition period in dairy cows. Laminitis is an aseptic inflammation of the dermal layers inside the foot, known otherwise as "Pododermatitis aseptic diffuse". Lameness has been highlighted as a major welfare problem for the dairy industry and it is a source of economic loss to the dairy enterprise.

Laminitis, which is considered to be the forerunner of two of the most common manifestations of lameness, namely **solar ulcer** and **white line disease**, is most likely to have its starting point in the digestive tract. Difficulty in meeting the energy requirements in early lactation when the buffalo/cow may only be attaining 75% dry matter intake (DMI), more frequently, results in feeding high concentrate/energy (grain) diet. It has been postulated that the rumen pH may drop below 5.5 with excessive production of lactic acid, histamine release and bacterial endotoxin production. These toxins may result in micro lesions in the laminae. However, the causes of laminitis can be manifold. These are nutritional, hormonal, infectious, managemental (hard surface of sheds, lack of bedding material) and miscellaneous causes.

Mineral imbalance resulting in rickets, copper deficiency causing developmental problems involving tendons and joints, and selenium deficiency associated with muscular dystrophy are all clear cut examples of cases where faulty nutrition undoubtedly results in lameness.

Bloat

The interaction of soluble proteins from excessively fed legumes, with rumen microbiota develops frothy bloat, as a result of which generated gases (CO_2, CH_4) are not eliminated from the rumen. Saponins and salivary mucoproteins also contribute towards foam formation. Bloat is characterized by a build up of pressure in the rumen. If timely intervention to release the pressure is not made, the affected animal dies.

Milk fever/hypocalcaemia/parturient paresis

It rarely occurs at first calving but commonly found in high milk yielders soon after calving. Low blood calcium and phosphorus are observed.

Metabolic disorders associated with excess nitrogen intake

In general, protein excess appears to produce more problems than protein deficiency in the feeding of dairy cows. Metabolic disorders associated with excess nitrogen intake are ammonia toxicity, disturbed intermediary metabolism and reduced fertility.

Table 1. Normal ranges of blood constituents for cattle
(J.H.Topps and J.K.Thompson, 1984)

Constituent	Older units mean	S.D.	S.I.units Mean	S.D.
Packed cell volume (blood)	33 %	3.9	0.33 l/l	0.039
Haemoglobin (blood)	11.3 g/100ml	1.0	11.3 g/dl	1.0
Glucose (plasma)	61.2 mg/100ml	5.4	3.4 m.mol/l	0.3
NEFA (plasma)	226 µeq/l	204	226 µ mol/l	204
BHB (blood)	5.0 mg/100 ml	2.10	0.48 m mol/1	0.20
Urea (plasma)	30.7 mg/100 ml	12.5	5.1 m mol /l	2.1
Albumin (serum)	3.5 g/100ml	0.41	35 g/l	4.1
Total protein (serum)	7.8 g/100ml	0.62	78 g/l	6.2
Globulin (serum)	4.3 g/100ml	0.81	43 g/l	8.1
Calcium (serum)	9.9 mg/100ml	0.44	2.48 m.mol/l	0.11
Phosphorus (serum)	6.0 mg/100ml	0.83	1.94 m.mol/	0.27
Magnesium (serum)	2.5 mg/100 ml	0.32	1.03 m mol/	0.13
Sodium (serum)	141 meq/l	1.01	41 m.mo/l	1.0
Potassium (serum)	5.6 meq/l	0.62	5.6 m.mol	0.62
Copper (serum)	0.70 mg/l	0.11	11.0	1.75
Vitamin B12 (serum)	Over 150 pg/ml	—	Over 110 p mol/l	—
Glutathione peroxidase (blood)	Over 19 iu/ml	—	—	—

High levels of ammonia can influence the normal functioning of the TCA cycle and thereby interfere with energy metabolism in the liver (Prior et al., 1970). Animals on a diet containing high levels of RDP or NPN absorb more ammonia so urea synthesis in the liver would be increased.

In studies on rats, Krebs et al. (1976) suggested that gluconeogenesis and urea synthesis are interconnected because they share a need for ATP and therefore compete for that source of energy particularly when the rates of glucose and urea synthesis are both very high.

A highly significant depression of the oxaloacetate concentration in the livers of affected animals has been reported.

It must be appreciated that the early lactating cow has an additional requirement for carbohydrate and ATP, namely, the synthesis of large volumes of milk.

Under these conditions attempts are made to meet the energy deficit by mobilizing depot fats with an accompanying increase in the blood NEFA levels.

Whatever the mechanisms involved, high protein intakes increase the susceptibility of dairy cattle to an induced ketosis. Feeding of large quantities of protein to cows in early lactation leads to an increase in the intake of potential ketone body precursors in the form of the ketogenic amino acids.

Haresign (1981) presented proof to show that excessive body weight loss in early lactation is detrimental to cow fertility. At this stage of lactation, high yielding dairy cows frequently have fatty livers. Excess protein feeding had been associated with reduced fertility since such cows showed high incidence of post-parturient endometritis and anoestrus.

Metabolic disorders associated with a low protein intake

One of the first effects of protein deficiency in the ruminant is a reduced feed consumption. There is a decrease in the feed intake and a decrease in the digestibility of the feed consumed. A protein deficient ration leads to a reduction in rumen microbial synthesis which in turn will reduce the protein supply to the animal. Cows under such regime show oestrus less regularly, they had decreased packed cell volumes, red cell counts and haemoglobin concentrations. Protein deficiency is known to affect wound healing, hair growth and the development of muscular tissue.

3

Disorders of Carbohydrate and Fat Metabolism

Hypoglycemic conditions

The genetic capacity to produce food for human consumption can challenge the metabolic capabilities of many of our farm animals. **Bovine Ketosis and ovine pregnancy toxemia** are hypoglycemic conditions of ruminants in which the ability to produce glucose is outpaced by the drain of glucose from the blood by the mammary gland or developing fetus. **Newborn animals also can develop hypoglycemia,** especially when they are chilled or they fail to nurse. The newborn pig is particularly susceptible to this syndrome as it has little body fat that it can use as an alternative source of fuel. Diabetes mellitus is increasingly diagnosed in our companion animals, just as it is in their owners (Goff, 2004). Overview of carbohydrate metabolism in animal cells is depicted in Figure 1.

Periparturient ketosis

In high-yielding milch animals, a more injurious form of ketosis appears. It develops in these animals during the first week after calving and seems to be associated with a rapid buildup of fat in the liver. These cows are often offered diets that are relatively high in starches, which should supply reasonable amounts of propionate to the cow. The syndrome seems to arise as a result of **inappetence in the cow during the immediate postpartum period.** The inappetence may be the result of the cow having dystocia, retained placenta, milk fever, or any other disorder. The dramatic reduction in feed intake at calving initiates a rapid increase in the mobilization of body fat, especially in fat cows carrying excess body condition. It appears that the rapid mobilization of body fat leads to a rapid buildup of triglyceride in the liver. Liver fat becomes a precipitating factor for ketosis.

Treatment options

These cows prove much more difficult to treat successfully. They often do not respond to a single injection of glucose intravenously. They are usually offered a diet

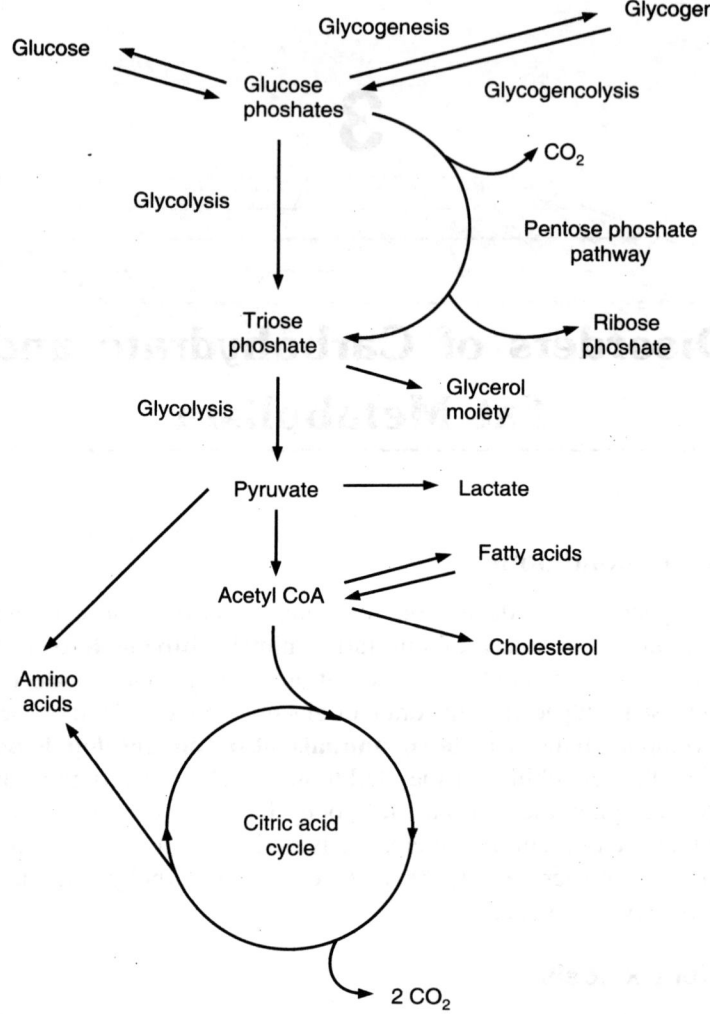

Figure 1. Overview of carbohydrate metabolism in animal cells

that would provide a good amount of propionate for gluconeogenesis, but they remain inappetent and so cannot take advantage of the diet. They also do not seem fully capable of utilizing the propionate to produce glucose. Ancillary treatments utilized by veterinarians include injection of synthetic glucocorticoids, presumably to stimulate gluconeogenesis by the liver. However, they also reduce milk production by the mammary gland. Both of these actions can be beneficial. Supplying gluconeogenic precursors in the form of drenches can often be helpful as well. Propylene glycol, glycerol, and sodium or calcium salts of propionate can be used for this purpose. Propylene glycol is converted in the liver to phosphoenol pyruvate and then to glucose. Glycerol is converted to diacyl-glycerol and then to glucose. Propionate is converted to succinate and enters the TCA cycle, where it is eventually converted to glucose as well.

Pregnancy Toxemia

Pregnancy toxemia is a hypoglycemic condition commonly observed in ewes and does. The disorder usually occurs in late gestation and is associated with the presence of multiple fetuses. In most cases, the plane of nutrition the animals are on in late gestation is not adequate to support the development of more than one fetus. In sheep, the amount of glucose that must be made each day to maintain the body of the ewe is about 100 g/day. In late gestation, the amount of glucose increases by about 80 g/day in ewes carrying a single fetus. This is complicated by the reduced rumen volume, reducing feed intake in late gestation as the fetuses demand more space within the abdomen. Fat ewes suddenly experiencing a period of poor nutrition seem to be at increased risk because they will mobilize large amounts of triglycerides of adipose origin and overwhelm the liver's capacity to metabolize or export the fatty acids. The disease is also often complicated by concurrent hypocalcemia, hypomagnesemia, and hypophosphatemia.

Fatty liver

Excessive mobilization of body fat can cause a buildup of triglycerides within the parenchyma of the liver. Fatty liver is a clinically important finding in dairy cattle and laying hens. The etiology of the fatty liver syndrome of these two species is quite different (Goff, 2004).

Limitations on ability of the liver to oxidize fatty acids

The oxidation of fatty acids requires that they enter the TCA cycle. In order to enter the TCA cycle, acetyl coenzyme A must be combined with a molecule of oxaloacetate (OAA) to form citrate. One theory suggests that the demand for OAA during gluconeogenesis is so great that the liver cells are depleted of OAA. Without OAA the oxidation of acetyl coenzyme A cannot proceed, and it instead is converted to ketone bodies. Fatty acids build up within the hepatocytes and the formation of triglycerides is stimulated, resulting in fatty liver. Unfortunately, recent studies have been unable to demonstrate a reduced level of OAA in the hepatocytes of cows with ketosis, suggesting that the cause of the defective catabolism of fatty acids lies elsewhere.

Fatty liver syndrome in poultry

Fatty liver syndrome is most common in laying hens. The liver and abdomen become infiltrated with fat. The liver becomes friable, and a common cause of death is rupture and hemorrhage of the liver. The disease is associated with excessive calorie intake. The typical hen has a very high calorie requirement while she is laying eggs. However, at the time of molting she quits laying eggs and no longer requires the high energy diet. The liver and adipose tissue accumulate the extra energy and deposit it as triglyceride. Caged layers seem to be at higher risk-perhaps because they do not exercise as much as floor-housed birds and thus have an even lower calorie requirement. In some cases, mycotoxins (aflatoxins) interfere with lipid metabolism and cause excessive body fat accumulation.

4

Negative Energy Balance and its Impact on Fertility of the Dairy Animals

Optimum reproductive efficiency of dairy buffalo and cow leads to profitable dairy animal production. Buffalo and cattle rearing is one of the livelihood supporting enterprises for many a landless cattle owners and rural farmers in India. Nutritional intervention is imperative to improve the reproductive efficiency of their dairy animals. Cows are expected to rebreed within 2-3 months of calving for optimum economic return. Poor fertility is a serious economic consideration in the dairy enterprise and is strongly linked to the animal's health around calving.

Though negative energy balance in early lactation is a common feature in milk yielders, the intensity and length of period of negative energy affects the fertility of the animals. However, improper feeding of heifers/cows and buffaloes such as feeding oilseed cakes and energy supplements inappropriately leads to elevated serum urea levels and thus affect their conception rates.

Negative energy balance (NEB)

High yielding dairy cows are under considerable metabolic stress in early lactation, as they cannot meet the energetic demands for milk production entirely from feed intake (Bauman and Currie, 1980). Immediately after calving high rates of mobilization of body energy resources are associated with a negative energy balance (NEB) status. Analyzing data published by Nielsen et al. (2003) of 400 cow lactations, Friggens and Newbold (2007) reported that the cows were in substantial negative energy balance at 14 days postcalving and feed intake on that day was only 80% of the maximum intake attained. It was concluded that the observed body lipid mobilization in early lactation was largely genetically driven.

Nutrient partitioning

Despite consuming equal quantities of the same diet, two heifers at their first calving (Table 1) exhibited marked differences in nutrient partitioning during the first 67 days of lactation. Cow 1, yielded 12.3 kg milk and gained 39.1 kg of body weight while cow 2, yielded 26.3 kg milk and lost 51.8 kg body weight. Similar differences in partitioning of absorbed nutrients were observed in the comparison of genetically diverse groups of cows. High milk yields in dairy cows are related to the ability to mobilize body energy reserves. Animals of high genetic merit produce more milk, have greater voluntary intakes and use more of their body reserves in early lactation than those of low merit.

Table 1: Example of animal differences in nutrient partitioning*

Variable	Cow 1	Cow 2
Initial body weight, kg	517	519
Intake of diet	equal	
Live weight change, kg	+39.1	-51.8
Average daily milk yield, kg 3.5% FCM	12.3	26.3

*Adapted from Swan (1976)

Nutrient partitioning is the major component of productive efficiency that differs among the cows. A sustained, high level of milk yield is dependent on the adaptation of many tissues of the body. A coordinated approach of metabolism of body tissues in support of lactation is important. One adaptation of major importance is the use of body fat reserves in the first portion of lactation. Marked mobilization of body reserves during early lactation, and replacement of these reserves in late lactation, is an important component of the increased productive efficiency that genetically superior cows achieve by dilution of maintenance.

Postpartum uterine microbial contamination

Following calving, the uterus must undergo extensive remodeling to reduce in size, remove cellular debris, and restore normal architecture (Sheldon and Dobson, 2004). Most dairy cows suffer uterine microbial contamination postpartum. The most common recognized pathogens are *Arcobacterium pyogenes, Escherichia coli, Fusobacterium necrophorum, Prevotella melaninogenicus,* and *Proteus* spp. Uterine defenses rely initially on classical innate immunity and mucosal defense systems rather than adaptive immunity (Sheldon et al., 2006). Failure in this defense system results in uterine disease. Metritis is present in some (40%) of the cows within 2nd week of calving, and some cows (15%) have a persistent endometritis in the 3-6 week postpartum period. Subclinical endometritis may be observed from 6 week postpartum onward and is characterized by an extensive leukocytic infiltration of the endometrium and chronic inflammation (Sheldon et al., 2006). Subclinical endometritis is associated with longer intervals to conception.

Impact of negative energy balance on fertility of animals

The negative energy balance is reflected by alterations in blood metabolite and hormone profiles. Both nonesterified fatty acids (NEFAs) and ?-hydroxybutyrate (BHB) concentrations are elevated, which are indicative of lipid mobilization and fatty acid oxidation. The liver coordinates the extensive biochemical and morphological modifications required via upregulation of genes involved in fatty acid oxidation and gluconeogenesis, and down-regulation of triacylglycerol synthesis (Loor et al., 2005). However, excessive fat mobilization (accumulation) postpartum impairs liver function, compromising glucose production and increasing inflammatory responses. Production of insulin and insulin-like growth factor I (IGF-I) are also reduced at this time (Drackley et al., 1999; Fenwick et al., 2008).

Excessive lipid mobilization is associated with metabolic and reproductive disorders (Roche, 2006). Cows with a low nadir in IGF-I in the first 2 week postpartum take longer to resume estrous cyclicity and are less likely to conceive when the breeding period is reached (Taylor et al., 2004). Immune function is also suppressed over the periparturient period, and poor energy balance (EB) status and fatty liver can impair peripheral blood neutrophil function (Hamman et al., 2006).

Wathes et al. (2009) tested the hypothesis that metabolic changes in postpartum cows can delay uterine repair mechanisms and promote a state of chronic inflammation, resulting in an unfavourable uterine environment that is likely to contribute to reduced fertility. They studied the effect of mild and severe NEB in early lactation.

- Circulating concentrations of IGF-I remained lower in the severe NEB group, whereas blood nonesterified fatty acid and ?-hydroxybutyrate concentrations were raised.
- White blood cell count and lymphocyte number were reduced in severe NEB cows.
- Cows in severe NEB were still undergoing an active uterine inflammatory response 2 week postpartum, whereas mild NEB cows had more fully recovered from their energy deficit, with their endometrium reaching a more advanced stage of repair.
- The severe NEB cows had clear evidence of liver damage, associated with lipid infiltration, high circulating NEFAs and BHB, and reduced glucose and IGF-I (Fenwick et al., 2008). In late pregnancy falling insulin and elevated placental lactogen stimulate adipose mobilization, providing nutrients for fetal growth (Bell, 1995).
- Cows are also under oxidative stress around calving, as indicated by an increase in reactive oxygen metabolites, decreased CuZn-superoxide dismutase (SOD), and raised plasma Se-glutathione peroxidase (GSH-Px) (Bernabucci et al., 2005).
- Uterine involution and elimination of contaminant bacteria will be delayed in animals in NEB postcalving (Lewis, 1997; Wathes et al., 2009). An increased rate of uterine involution is associated with earlier resumption of ovarian activity (Mateus et al., 2002). Conversely, endometrial damage associated with subclinical endometritis delays cervical involution, disrupts the preovulatory LH surge, and perturbs embryo survival, leading to prolonged intervals to conception with many cows failing to conceive at all (Sheldon and Dobson, 2004).
- Therefore, severe negative energy balance may prevent cows from mounting an effective immune response to the microbial challenge experienced after calving, prolonging the time required for uterine recovery and compromising subsequent fertility.

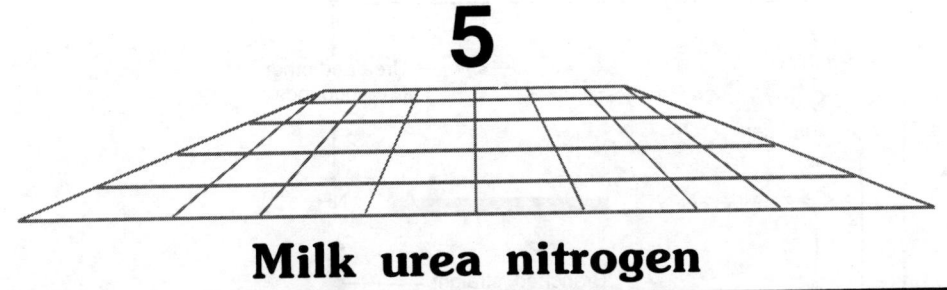

5

Milk urea nitrogen

Milk urea nitrogen (MUN) is considered a normal nonprotein nitrogen (NPN) component in milk. Urea concentration in milk results as a byproduct of protein metabolism. Ruminant growth and milk production are possible with urea as the sole source of dietary nitrogen, which agree with the concept that ammonia has a central role in ruminal nitrogen metabolism (Fig 1). Digestion of dietary protein results in the production of ammonia. Ammonia is converted to urea primarily in the liver. Urea is (recycled into rumen then) excreted from the body primarily through urine, but is also found in blood and milk. Milk urea nitrogen levels have been used to evaluate herd nutritional status, as well as assess nitrogen excretion to the environment. Elevated MUN concentrations have been documented to adversely affect fertility.

Evaluation of milk urea nitrogen (MUN) as a diagnostic of protein feeding

The basic function of milk producing ruminants is to convert low-quality noncompetitive feed sources into high quality protein for human consumption. Often the amount and quality of protein absorbed from the small intestine can limit milk production. However, feeding excess protein in relation to requirements increase environmental N emissions and can impair reproductive performance. There is, therefore, an urgent need for on-farm diagnostic to monitor the adequacy of protein feeding offering the opportunity to optimize the efficiency of N utilization with respect to both milk protein production and N emissions into the environment.

Blood urea nitrogen (BUN) is the major end product of N metabolism in ruminants, and high concentrations of it are indicative of an inefficient utilization of dietary N. However, BUN cannot be measured routinely due to difficulties in obtaining regular and reliable samples. It is well established that urea equilibrates rapidly with body fluids, including milk, and thus there is a close relationship between MUN and BUN. Milk urea nitrogen can be determined accurately by enzymatic or physical methods. Milk urea is also derived from arginine catabolism in the mammary glands, but this does not appear to be quantitatively important. It is, therefore suggested that MUN in the pooled milk tank could be used as a diagnostic of on-farm efficiency of N utilization.

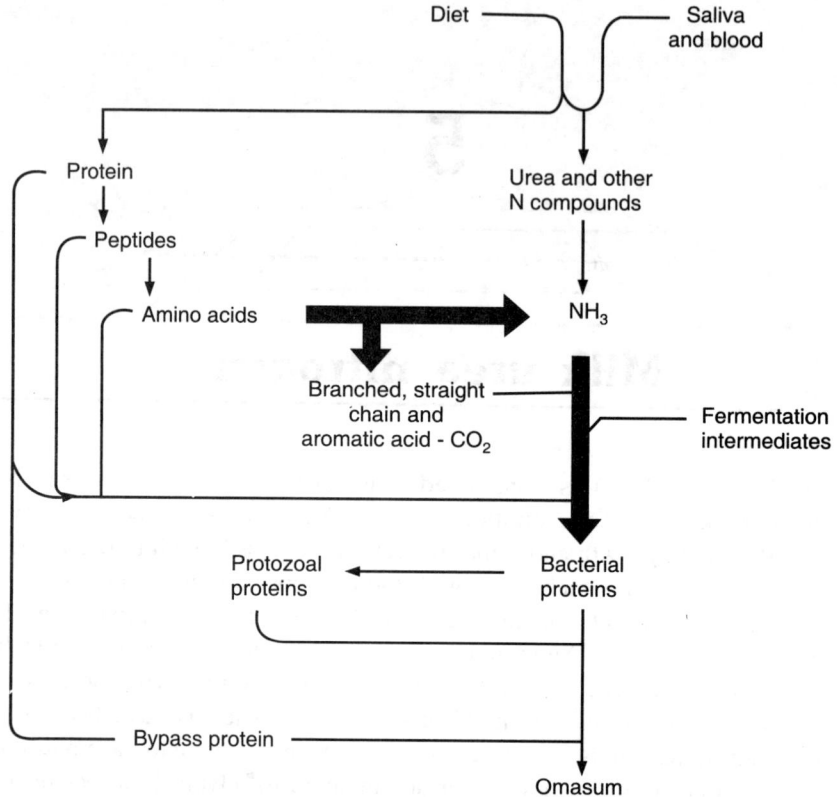

Figure 1. Transformations of nitrogenous substances in the rumen

Levels of MUN: The normal/target values for MUN are considered to be within the range from 10 to 15 mg/dl (Moore and Varga, 1996). Thus, MUN concentrations can be used as a practical tool to monitor dietary CP and energy intake relative to requirements. This type of monitoring can play an important role in dairy herd management, because 1) excess protein intake may impair reproductive performance, 2) consumption of excess CP increases energy requirements, 3) protein supplements are costly feed ingredients and 4) excess N excretion has a negative environmental impact (Broderick and Clayton, 1997).

Mean MUN concentrations in some of the high producing herds were between 10 to 11 mg/dl. Using MUN to monitor and adjust ration energy-protein balance might provide an opportunity to reduce feed costs and to improve profitability of the herd (Rajala-Schultz and Saville, 2003).

Sources of variation in milk urea nitrogen

Several studies have shown that milk urea nitrogen concentration is related to dietary CP intake, the percentage of rumen degradable and undegradable protein as well as protein-energy ratio in the diet (Baker et al., 1995).

Nousiainen el el. (2004) confirmed that dietary crude protein (CP) content is the most important nutritional factor influencing MUN, and that measurements of MUN can be utilized as a diagnostic of protein feeding in the dairy cow and used to predict urea N excretion. Based on experimental studies, a number of other factors in addition to feed intake and dietary composition, are also known to be related to MUN concentrations. Such factors are sampling time, method of analysis, days in milk (DIM), BW, parity, and milk yield of a cow (Rajala-Schultz and Saville, 2003).

The results of 15-month research study conducted on 9 buffalo herds in Italy (Francia et al., 2003) suggested that high milk production was achieved using rations with high protein content, which led to increased milk urea concentrations. However, milk urea was not associated with milk fat and protein content or somatic cell count. Milk urea was related to milk yield, crude protein index, excess of nitrogen intake and nitrogen efficiency. The findings indicate that milk urea measured at group level can offer a useful indication to monitor the efficiency of N utilization in commercial buffalo herds.

MUN as a reproduction performance indicator in dairy herds

Seven dairy herds in Sao Paulo State, Brazil were selected for sampling monthly during 12 months (Peixoto Jr, 2003). Urea levels were analysed in milk samples and CP was determined in feed samples.

- Milk production presented linear effect on MUN levels.
- Dietary CP evaluated in the conception month had a significant linear effect on service period and conception rate and a quadratic effect on the time between parturition and first service, although the number of services per pregnancy was not affected.
- Dietary protein in the month before the conception showed significant linear effect on service period and on the conception rate, while protein in the month after the conception service only affected the pregnancy rate.
- MUN levels in the month of conception did not cause changes on the reproductive parameters, but MUN levels in the month before the conception affected the service period, number of services, interval between parturition and first service and pregnancy rates in the herds evaluated.

MUN levels evaluated in dairy cows on the month of conception are not indicative of reproductive performance. The study showed that MUN levels estimated in the month before the conception can be used as indicators of reproductive performance. Hence, continuous monitoring of MUN levels certainly helps in tracking the reproductive performance and productivity of buffaloes and cows. BUN or MUN concentrations above 19 to 20 mg/dl may be useful to associate with decreased conception rates in cows (Butler et al., 1998).

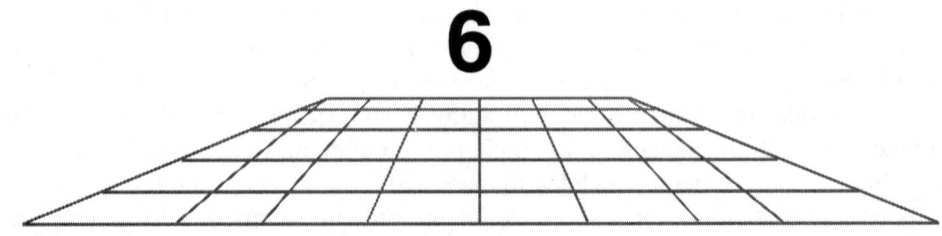

6

Nutritional and Metabolic Infertility in Buffaloes and Cows

In general it has been observed there is reduced fertility in high yielding dairy animals. But in India reduced conception rate in dairy animals may also be due to improper / imbalanced feeding.

Effect of nutrition on fertility

Malnutrition or nutritional diseases result from the ingestion or absorption of insufficient quantities of nutrients required by the animal. Malnutrition (nutrient imbalances and nutrient deficiencies) affects growth, production and reproduction. Many times animals continue to produce milk, albeit in less amount. But such cows and buffaloes will not conceive. That is reproduction can be affected by acute or subacute nutrient deficiencies, which could not be compensated by the body's homeostatic mechanisms. This infertility caused by malnutrition is called nutritional infertility. T.J.McClure (1968) adopted the generic term 'metabolic infertility' for this kind of acute-nutrient-imbalance-induced causes of fertility since it differs little from the recognized metabolic diseases of cattle such as ketosis, milk fever/hypocalcaemia and hypomagnesaemia.

Most chronic nutritional deficiencies cause first the slowing of the growth rate, then the loss of body condition (muscle and subcutaneous fat) and weight, become infertile, and, in extreme cases, become emaciated and die.

Energy and protein status and infertility

Energy is the first limiting dietary component to optimal dairy cow performance in early lactation because feed intake cannot match nutritional needs. As energy output (through milk production) exceeds the energy intake, the cow will mobilise her own body resources. This is perhaps inevitable, but it is the magnitude of the deficit that may influence subsequent fertility. The extent and duration of negative energy status of the cow is one of the most important factors influencing when the cow will return to normal ovarian function after calving. The degree of energy deficit in the first 20 days post calving can have a very significant effect on the time of first ovulation.

Effect of protein on the health of dairy animals

The effect of high crude protein intakes on reproduction of the dairy cow is controversial. The results of experimental work have been equivocal and research is continuing. If more rumen degradable protein (RDP) is fed than the animal can utilize, urea levels in body tissues can rise. Raised blood urea levels have been related to delay of first ovulation, to lowered conception rates, increased embryonic death and general reproductive inefficiency. Hibbit (1984) reviewed the literature on effect of protein on the health of dairy cows. Deviation from the optimum in the feeding of high yielding dairy cows can produce changes in the animal's metabolism affecting production, fertility and the general body condition.

Nutritional and metabolic infertility can occur in the following circumstances:

T.J.McClure (1994), an Australian veterinarian described the events based on his research experience since 1960.

1. When the amount of feed available is restricted during critical stages of growth of heifers from weaning to puberty, during late pregnancy and during the early lactation period. The fertility of heifers is most affected compared to cows/buffaloes since heifers are still growing.
2. Cattle grazing dry mature grass: Dry mature grass is poorly digestible and is deficient in protein, carotene and minerals including phosphorus.
3. When lactating cows are fed lush young pasture or young forage crops: These feeds provide sufficient crude protein but insufficient energy and possibly undegraded dietary protein (UDP) to meet the requirements for maintenance plus milk production. This type of feeding does not appear to be associated with infertility when cows are also fed sufficient grain-based concentrate rations (McClure 1970)
4. When a large part of the diet consists of one species of plant (or product manufactured from that plant) and the plant contains toxic substances or is deficient in essential nutrients. Examples include
    *   Lucerne and clovers containing phytoestrogens
    *   Kale (*Brassica oleracea*), which sometimes contains goitrogens and tends to be deficient in copper, phosphorus and manganese
    *   Maize silage, which contains little carotene and often insufficient methionine and other essential amino acids and little selenium
    *   Sugar beet (*Beta vulgaris*) tops and pulp which often contain insufficient phosphorus and manganese.
5. When cows are fed on compounded feeds which are not nutritionally balanced
6. When cows are fed on crops or pastures, which are grown on soil containing high concentrations of molybdenum or are contaminated by industrial pollution or when cows drink water containing high concentrations of fluorine.
7. When cows calve in fat condition
8. When cows are fed excess rumen degradable protein (RDP)
9. When minerals such as cobalt, copper, manganese, phosphorus and selenium, which are considered to be essential for reproduction, are insufficient in feeds

Reproductive physiology

The physiology of reproduction relevant to nutritional and metabolic infertility is briefly described here. **During pregnancy,** oestrogen and progesterone are secreted by the placenta and circulate in the maternal blood, inhibiting the secretion of gonadotrophin-releasing hormone (GnRH) by the hypothalamus.

The gonadotroph cells of the adenohypophysis are then deprived of sufficient stimulation to maintain the synthesis of follicle-stimulating hormone (FSH) and luteinizing hormone (LH). These must be restored **after parturition** before normal cycles can commence. Restoration is completed by day 10 in cows, episodic release of LH normally commences on day 13, and reaches a peak mean concentration and frequency two weeks before the first post-partum oestrum (between day 17 and day 42).

The function of the reproductive endocrine system is modulated by nervous signals from other hypothalamic nuclei and higher centres, the ovarian hormones oestradiol, progesterone and inhibin and the endogenous opioid peptides.

In the 21-day cyclic cow, the concentration of progesterone falls from its peak of 6-8 ng/ml to less than 1ng/ml 16-19 days after oestrus. The plasma oestradiol-17β concentration rises from its minimum of less than 10pg/ml to a peak of 15-25 pg/ml on the day before next oestrus and falls within two to five hours after the beginning of oestrus to its basal level. The concentration of LH in the plasma rapidly increases from its basal level of 2-3 ng/ml to higher than 10-15 ng/ml for six to eight hours with a peak of 10-65 ng/ml corresponding to the onset of oestrus. Progesterone appears in the blood in appreciable quantities five days after oestrus and continues to increase until the 16th or 17th day by which time it has reached its peak of 6-8ng/ml (Stabenfeldt et al., 1969).

Reproductive failure

Reproductive failure can occur at three stages: 1. pituitary synthesis/release of luteinizing hormone, 2. ovarian function, or 3. ovulation, fertilization and development of the ovum, embryo and fetus. The evidence from cattle, sheep and laboratory rodent experiments indicates that energy deficiency can inhibit reproduction at all three stages. The failure may be due to energy deficiency, protein deficiency and excess NPN /RDP, mineral and vitamin deficiencies.

Reproductive performance of cows is often associated with body weight, body weight change and condition. Body weight as appropriate for the breed is often taken as an important criterion to breed the heifers. Severe body weight loss is usually accompanied by anoestrus. Loss of body weight after parturition seems to delay the recurrence of oestrus. It was reported a delay of 19 days for every 10% loss of body weight.

Cows which calve in fat condition eat less during early lactation, mobilize more body tissue and lose more weight after calving than those calving in moderate condition. There is some evidence suggesting that these cows are less fertile and more susceptible to metabolic diseases (Treacher et al., 1986). Genetic merit plays some part in the live weight and condition changes which can occur during lactation, with superior cows producing more milk while losing more body weight (Holmes and Macmillan, 1982).

Nutritional inappropriateness/deficiencies
Energy

Negative energy balance during early lactation is the major nutritional link to low fertility in lactating dairy animals. Negative energy balance delays recovery of postpartum reproductive function and exerts carryover effects that reduce fertility. The most common and most important nutritional cause of reproductive failure in the buffalo and cow is the failure of the digestive and hepatic systems to provide sufficient energy for maintenance, growth, pregnancy and lactation.

- The substrates for energy, which are absorbed from the alimentary tract, are the volatile fatty acids, mainly acetate, butyrate and propionate, amino acids and a little glucose.
- Feeding cows on diets deficient in energy causes plasma glucose, insulin, growth hormone, luteinizing (LH), oestrogen and progesterone concentrations to fall, and NEFA and β-hydroxibutyrate concentrations to rise (Donaldson et al., 1970).

Plane of nutrition

Effect of underfeeding: Underfeeding during growth delays puberty; during late pregnancy delays the recurrence of oestrous cycles after parturition; during the post-partum period reduces pregnancy rates. During underfeeding blood glucose concentration, pool-size and the rate of entry of glucose into cells are reduced and the pulsatile release of LH by the pituitary is suppressed (McClure, 1994).

In making efforts to achieve higher profits, least cost rations are formulated and the animals are fed the minimal quantity of feed, where there is always some risk that the amount of feed made available will fall below the optimum to such an extent that fertility suffers. However, restricting the intake of balanced feedstuffs within reasonable limits, even though cause appreciable losses in body weight, did not affect either the blood glucose concentration or fertility.

Shortage of feed: If feed availability is in short supply and the animals must be underfed, animals can be safely underfed between the time of implantation and the end of the seventh month of pregnancy without any effect on their fertility provided that they are well-fed subsequently.

Effect of monensin: Feeding cows on monensin increases the molar proportion of propionate at the expense of acetate, increases the blood glucose concentration, hastens the ability of the hypothalamus and pituitary to respond to oestrogens early in the post-partum period, reduces the age of heifers at puberty, and reduces the calving-to-conception interval (Randel, 1990).

Feedstuffs

Feedstuffs should be utilized appropriately in feeding the buffaloes and cows so that their rumens function efficiently. Feedstuffs should also supply all the required nutrients post-ruminally complementing the ruminal synthetic products for optimum production of milk and meat. When byproducts are included in the ration, care should be taken to ensure that they are free from contaminants such as heavy metals, insecticides and other chemical poisons, mycotoxins and bacterial toxins.

Chemical composition of the feed: The critical components are the available carbohydrate content, the protein content and its quality in terms of RDP and UDP and the mineral content. The chemical composition of the feed influences the quantity of energy which is absorbed and also the nature of the energy substrates, whether they are glucogenic or ketogenic.

Available carbohydrate: Pastures and crops contain low concentrations of available carbohydrate when very young and again when approaching maturity.

- Lactating cows fed on either immature or overmature forage were found to have lower blood glucose concentrations and to be less fertile since such forage has lesser soluble carbohydrate plus starch.
- Concentrate feeds should provide an adequate ruminal propionate: acetate ratio.

Forages are to be fed at the optimal stage of growth, i.e. just before the flower stems emerge, when the yield of digestible organic matter (DOM) is at its peak. Very immature grass is deficient mainly in readily available carbohydrate, DM and UDP. Very immature grass (high in RDP) and grass-dominant pastures can be fed, if supplemented by green legumes, hay or preferably grain-based concentrates containing a source of UDP. These allow a higher intake of DOM and, in particular readily fermentable carbohydrate and protein yielding more VFA and non-ammonia nitrogen to enter the duodenum.

In mature grasses and crops, the vegetative parts at the flowering and later stages of growth contain an increasing proportion of fibre and a decreasing proportion of available carbohydrate, protein, minerals and ultimately carotene. Fibrous roughages can be improved by addition of urea alone only to a small extent. It becomes difficult to prepare balanced rations with such mature grasses/straws. Supplementation strategy can be used in such instances with poultry droppings, molasses, bran, highly digestible young plants, and/or, protein supplements such as fishmeal, cottonseed meal which slowly releases nitrogen and energy into the rumen. This combination of protein-, non-protein nitrogen- and energy-supplements is a good strategy to meet the requirements of rumen microorganisms and the host animals.

Protein and non-protein nitrogen: Insufficient dietary NPN and RDP reduce the digestibility of the feed. In turn, this causes a dietary energy deficiency and reduces the flow of microbial protein (Orskov, 1982), slows the growth rate of the heifer, delays or inhibits puberty and the commencement of oestrous cycles after calving, and reduces the pregnancy rate to first and subsequent services (Nolan et al., 1988).

Crude protein concentrations in the diets of cows in the range of 13-20% can sustain normal reproduction. Feeding cows from late pregnancy through to early lactation on diets containing insufficient RDP and NPN reduces appetite and food intake and has the same effect as underfeeding. Pituitary LH and FSH contents are reduced (Nolan et al., 1988), the recommencement of post-partum oestrous cycles is delayed or suppressed, ovulation may fall, and pregnancy rates are reduced and calving-to-conception intervals increased.

High crude protein concentrations in the diets of cows have been associated with infertility. The effect may be due to

1. A depression in the total soluble sugar and water soluble carbohydrate content of the grass, which is induced by heavy application of nitrogenous fertilizer to the pasture or lack of sunlight (Bryant and Ulyatt, 1965).

2. An effect of NO_3 on the carbohydrate fermentation by the ruminal flora encouraging the production of acetate at the expense of the glucogenic fatty acids. The addition of urea to the feedstuffs has been observed to cause blood glucose concentration to fall.

3. The magnitude of the UDP component: The depression of fertility in lactating cows may be due to insufficient UDP, since high-producing cows may not absorb sufficient amino acids for both tissue metabolism and milk secretion (Ferguson and Chalupa, 1989). In these circumstances the main limiting amino acids are likely to be methionine and /or lysine.

4. High CP diets containing high RDP: low UDP ratios with insufficient readily available carbohydrate for the rumen microorganisms may not fully utilize the free nitrogen from the RDP (McClure, 1970).

Relation between serum urea nitrogen and conception rate

It is known that serum urea nitrogen concentration is found to be negatively associated with conception rate in dairy cows (Ferguson et al., 1993). Diets high in CP (17 to 19%) are typically fed during early lactation to both stimulate and support high milk production. However, feeding higher protein diets have been associated with reduced reproductive performance (Butler, 1998). As a result of feeding high protein, the increased blood/plasma urea concentrations (BUN or PUN) may interfere with the normal inductive actions of progesterone on the microenvironment of the uterus and, thereby cause suboptimal conditions for support of embryo development (Butler, 2001). The concentration of BUN depends upon the dietary CP intake, the balance of dietary protein fractions (RDP and RUP), the availability of fermentable carbohydrates and protein-energy ratio in the diet. Consumption of excess CP increases energy requirements. This exacerbates the energy deficiency, which is a major problem in animal feeding.

As part of the progression of events involved in establishing pregnancy, high dietary RDP seems not to impact follicle development or ovulation, but results in reduced concentrations of plasma progesterone in lactating cows, which appears to be linked to the effects of exacerbated negative energy balance. The effects of RDP on energy status may also impair embryo development. Embryo survival and growth depend upon the quality of the uterine luminal environment, and the intake of high dietary protein alters uterine secretions.

Detrimental effects of high plasma urea nitrogen levels on viability of embryos

Rhoads et al. (2006) evaluated the quality of embryos flushed from superovulated lactating cows having moderate or high PUN concentrations. Subsequent embryo survival was determined after transfer to recipient heifers with either low or high PUN. Lactating Holstein dairy cows (n=23; 50-120 days in milk) were randomly assigned to one of two diets designed to result in moderate or high PUN concentrations (15.5±0.7 and 24.4±1.0mg/dl, respectively) and were fed for 30 days before embryo flushing and recovery. Embryos (n=94) were evaluated morphologically, frozen and subsequently transferred into synchronized virgin heifers that were fed one of two diets designed to result in either low or high PUN concentrations (7.7±0.9 and 25.2±1.5mg/dl, respectively). The number, quality and stage of development of recovered embryos were similar for cows with moderate or high PUN.

Transfer of embryos from moderate PUN donor cows resulted in a higher pregnancy rate (35%; P<0.02) than the transfer of embryos from high PUN donor cows (11%). Pregnancy rate was not affected by either recipient diet or the interaction of donor and recipient diets (P>0.05). These results indicate that high PUN concentrations in lactating dairy cows decrease embryo viability through effects exerted on the oocyte or embryo before recovery from the uterus 7 days after insemination (M. Rhoads et al., 2006).

In conclusion, the poor fertility of high producing dairy cows reflects the combined effects of a uterine environment that is dependent on progesterone, but has been rendered suboptimal by antecedent effects of negative energy balance or postpartum health problems and has been further compromised by the effects of urea resulting from intake of high dietary protein. Possible effects on gametes, hypophyseal-pituitary-ovarian axis, embryonic viability or its implantation have all been suggested as the cause of infertility. It could be argued that the effects attributed to excess protein in the diet are in actual fact ultimately due to energy deficiency.

Minerals and Vitamins

Minerals: Most of the minerals required by buffaloes and cattle for growth and metabolism are also required by the ruminal microbiota for the fermentation of the plant cell-walls and the release of the cell contents. Thus they play an essential role in digestion and thus influence appetite and feed intake. Diets containing insufficient concentrations of essential minerals (these include P, S, cobalt) for microbial metabolism have the same effects as those containing insufficient NPN and RDP. Fermentation rate, appetite and intake are low and an energy deficiency may ensue.

Importance of minerals in the metabolism

1. Diets which contain low concentrations of cobalt, copper, iodine, manganese, phosphorus and selenium or high concentration of molybdenum, have been reported to cause infertility in cows
2. Cobalt deficiency prevents the formation of vitamin B12, which is required for conversion of propionate to succinate. This reduces gluconeogenesis and the activity of TCA cycle (cobalt deficiency may also reduce the amount of adenosyl-cobalamine (Adocbl) coenzyme which is necessary for the incorporation of deaminated glucogenic amino acids into the TCA cycle), and results in hypoglycaemia.

3. Copper is widely distributed in the body in the enzyme cytochrome oxidase, copper-superoxide dismutase, dopamine-?-hydroxylase, monoamine oxidase, ceruloplasmin and lysyloxidase. Copper deficiency may cause infertility because of its effect on the integrity of the small intestine (i.e. cellular damage to the small intestine affects absorption) which would lead to a general nutrient deficiency, and its role in energy metabolism and as an antioxidant.

4. Iodine deficiency occurs as the result of feeding pasture or crops grown on iodine-deficient soils containing <2mg I/kg dry matter or excessive quantities of goitrogens such as thiocyanates in the feedstuffs. It prevents thyroid hyperplasia and it forms part of the thyroxine molecule which stimulates mitochondrial ATP production. Deficiency of iodine reduces the oxygen uptake by cells indicating a reduction in the rate of energy metabolism.

5. Manganese deficiency has been reported in cows fed on diets containing <22mg Mn/kg dry matter and appears to cause anoestrus or suboestrus, delayed ovulation, low first-service pregnancy rates and the birth of deformed calves. This infertility occurs mainly in cattle grazing pasture grown on manganese-deficient or heavily limed soils or fed supplements containing excessive amounts of calcium. Manganese has a key role in gluconeogenesis, since it is a cofactor for, or a component of, the enzymes phosphoglucomutase, pyruvate carboxylase (PC) and phosphoenolpyruvate carboxykinase (PEPCK).

6. The ions Na^+, Ca^{2+}, and Mg^{2+} play critical roles in regulation of cellular function.

Approaches to provide minerals to the animals

There are several approaches to provide the minerals to the animals.

1. Mineral content of pastures can be improved by addition of minerals such as P, Co, Mn, Se, Cu to fertilizers and applied to the soil. Copper and phosphorus, being essential for plant growth, are best applied as fertilizers where pasture production is sufficient to make this method economic.

2. Supplementation of mineral mixture to the diet offered to the animals

3. Supplementation minerals in the form of licks or trace minerals (copper, cobalt and selenium) incorporated in slow-release capsules or pellets administered per os. Cobalt and selenium are required by animals but not by plants. Hence this is considered as the most appropriate.

4. Mineral deficiencies in pasture or crops caused by excessive soil acidity or alkalinity are best controlled and prevented by correcting soil pH by applying or withholding lime, dolomite or sulfate fertilizers. Examples include manganese deficiency caused by excessive liming and selenium deficiency in pasture grown in very acid soils which responds to fertilization with dolomite or lime.

Antioxidants

Deficiencies of antioxidants are reported to be potential causes of reproductive failure. Reproductive failure due to deficiencies of these antioxidant nutrients may be due to their effect on ovum, embryo or fetus.

Importance of antioxidants in the metabolism

Antioxidant role of copper (copper-superoxide dismutase), selenium (a component of glutathione peroxidase), β-carotene and α-tocopherol: Of these, α-tocopherol and glutathione peroxidase scavenge free radicals that initiate the oxygenation of unsaturated phospholipids and critical sulfhydryl groups and help to inhibit lipid peroxidation and maintain the integrity of cell membranes (Putnam and Comben, 1987). α-tocopherol is required particularly during fetal development. Rammel (1983) concluded that the ruminant requires tocopherol only to overcome the toxic effect of PUFA in the diet, or to prevent lipid peroxidation and membrane (both cellular and subcellular) damage in the absence of the far more efficient glutathione peroxidase.

β-carotene has a vital role in reproduction in buffaloes and cows that is unrelated to vitamin A. Goto et al. (1989) found the superovulated cows with high plasma β-carotene concentrations had higher embryonic survival rates (50%) than those with low concentrations (27%).

1. Selenium deficiency can occur where cattle are fed on pasture, crops or grain from crops grown on soils containing <0.5 mg Se per kg DM, and feedstuffs containing <0.05 mg Se per kg DM.
2. α-tocopherol deficiency can occur in cattle when they are fed on:
   - Dry mature pasture, straws, hay, containing <0.7 mg α-tocopherol per kg DM (normal values for immature pasture are ≥20).
   - Stored hay, silage, rootcrops, acid-preserved grain which may contain no vitamin E
   - Diets supplemented with polyunsaturated fatty acids or rancid fats, e.g., oilseeds and fish liver oil.
3. Dietary PUFA could be the precipitating cause of the infertility in cows fed on pasture grown on selenium-deficient soils and the response to selenium may depend upon the amount of PUFA, and the other antioxidants (α-tocopherol, β- carotene) and possibly copper and molybdenum in the body.

REFERENCES

Bauman, D.E. 2000. Regulation of nutrient partitioning during lactation: homeostasis and homeorhesis revisitied. In Ruminant physiology: digestion, metabolism, growth and reproduction (ed. PB Cronje), pp. 311-328. CAB International, Wallingford, UK.

Bauman, D.E. and Currie, W.B. 1980. Partitioning of nutrients during pregnancy and lactation: A review of mechanisms involving homeostasis and homeorhesis. J Dairy Sci 63: 1514.

Bell, A.W. 1995. Regulation of organic nutrient metabolism during transition from late pregnancy to early lactation. J Anim Sci 73: 2804.

Bernabucci, U., Ronchi, B., Lacetera, N., and Nardone, A. 2005. Influence of body condition score on relationships between metabolic status and oxidative stress in periparturient dairy cows. J Dairy Sci 88: 2017.

Fenwick, M.A., Fitzpatrick, R., Kenny, D.A., Diskin, M.G., Patton, J., Murphy, J.J. and Wathes, D.C. 2008. Interrelationships between negative EB (NEB) and IGF regulation in liver of lactating dairy cows. Domest Anim Endocrinol 34: 31.

Friggens, N.C. and Newbold, J.R. 2007. Towards a biological basis for predicting nutrient partitioning: the dairy cow as an example. Animal 1: 87.

Hammon, D.S., Evjen, I.M., Dhiman, T.R., Goff, J.P. and Walters, J.L. 2006. Neutrophil function and energy status in Holstein cows with uterine health disorders. Vet Immunol Immunopathol 113: 21.

Haresign, W. 1981. In: Recent Developments in Ruminant Nutrition. Pp. 1-16. Eds Haresign, W and Cole, D.J.A., Butterworths, London.

Hibbit, K.G. 1984. Effect of protein on the health of dairy cows In: Recent advances in animal nutrition1984 eds by William Haresign and DJA Cole, Butterworth Publications.

Krebs, H.A., Lund, P. and Stubbs,. M.1976. In: Gluconeogenesis: Its Regulation in Mammalian Species. Pp.261-291. Eds Hanson, R.W. and Mehlman, M.A. John Wiley, New York.

Lewis, G.S. 1997. Uterine health and disorders. J Dairy Sci 80: 984.

Loor, J.J., Dann, H.M., Guretzky, N.A., Everts, R.E., Oliveira, R., Green, C.A., Litherland, N.B., Rodriguez-Zas, S.L., Lewin, H.A. and Drackley, J.K. 2005. Plane of nutrition prepartum alters hepatic gene expression and function in dairy cows as assessed by longitudinal transcript and metabolic profiling. Physiol Genomics 27: 29.

Nielsen, H.M., Friggens, N.C., Lovendahl, P.L. Jensen, J. and Ingvartsen, K. L. 2003. The influence of breed, parity and stage of lactation on lactational performance and the relationship between body fatness and live weight. Livestock Production Sci 79: 119.

Prior, R.L., Clifford, A.J., Hogue, D.E. and Visetz, W.J. 1970. J Nutr. 100, 438-444.

Sheldon, I.M. and Dobson, H. 2004. Postpartum uterine health in cattle. Anim Reprod Sci 82-83: 295.

Sheldon, I.M., Lewis, G.S., Leblanc, S., Gilbert, R.O. 2006. Defining postpartum uterine disease in cattle. Theriogenology 65: 1516.

Swan, H. 1976. The physiological interrelationship of reproduction, lactation and nutrition in the cow. In: H Swan and W H Broster (ed) Principles of Cattle Production. Pp 85 -102. Butterworths, Kent, England.

Topps, J.H. and Thompson, J.K. 1984. Blood characteristics and the nutrition of ruminants An appraisal of the relationships between blood characteristics (and other in vivo parameters) and the nutritional status of farm ruminants Published by Her Majesty's Stationery Office 1984

Wathes, D. C., Cheng, Z., Chowdhury, W., Fenwick, M.A., Fitzpatrick, R., Morris, D.G., Patton, J and Murphy,J.J. 2009. Negative energy balance alters global gene expression and immune responses in the uterus of postpartum dairy cows, Physiological Genomics 39:1- 13.

SECTION VIII
Quality Control of Feed

1

Feed Quality Control

Importance of quality control of feeds

Quality control of feedstuffs (Reddy, 2001) can play a vital role in the development of feed manufacturing industry and also for maximum exploitation of the production efficiency of animals. The overall mission of feed formulation and manufacturing is to provide customers with efficiently manufactured feeds which are correctly delivered to their facilities and consistently contain the available nutrients required by animals for body maintenance, growth, production or reproduction (Jones, 1996). The feed manufacturers who implement a quality assurance programme will have a competitive edge over others and remain in the business.

Individual feed ingredients - Variation in nutrient content

Feeds for livestock and poultry contain cereal grains, oilseed cakes, animal protein supplements, cereal byproducts or certain agroindustrial byproducts, minerals, vitamins and other feed additives in different proportions to supply a balanced ration. Quality begins with formulation of a balanced ration for a particular species of animal at a certain physiological stage of life. Therefore, it is obviously necessary to assess the suitability of various feed ingredients. Procurement of the feed ingredients is the crucial part of the feed production and plays a key role in determining the feed quality because good quality feed ingredients only can get good quality finished feed.

There is a constant pressure to reduce the cost of feed to produce animal products at a competitive price and ensure their availability at affordable cost to majority of the population. Hence many byproducts and unusual feedstuffs (for example soya hulls, tapioca waste powder, groundnut shell powder), where due attention may not be given for their quality, are often integrated into a feeding programme. Variations in nutrient content of finished feeds may occur. Large portion of the variation in the nutrient content of finished feeds can be traced to feed ingredients due to variation in ingredients from batch to batch. Poor mixing of ingredients or segregation of ingredients after mixing and improper weighing of individual ingredients also contributes. Such variations in nutrient content of finished feed affect either the credibility of the supplier if it contains lower nutrients than specified or the business profits if it contains excess nutrients. Ingredients alone can account for 70 - 90% of the cost of producing feeds for livestock and poultry. Ingredient quality and cost, therefore, need considerable attention in the production of good quality economic complete feed/concentrate mixture.

Procurement of feed ingredients

Feed ingredients are to be procured keeping a focus on quality as well as cost. Low quality feed ingredients are generally characterized by the presence of adulterants such as hulls in groundnut cake, scales and silica in fish meal, bones and horns in meat meals, husk in rice bran and rice polish, etc. Good quality feed ingredients can be purchased by following few simple "field methods of feed quality control" (Narahari, 2004).

Physical inspection and sensory evaluation

Physical inspection and sensory evaluation of the feed ingredient forms one of the important phases of the quality control to identify the gross adulteration. Well dried feeds and feedstuffs are free flowing. The cereal grains must be free from dust, stones, extraneous materials, insect infestations and fungus growth. Damaged food grains from warehouses, sometimes, are available for animal feeding. Such materials have to be ascertained for the extent of damage due to insects. Materials with high infestation would contain more number of holes in the grain and also weigh less.

Byproducts such as wheat bran, rice bran, rice polish, deoiled rice bran, maize gluten, maize bran, gram husk, broken gram, etc. are used in animal feeding. All these byproducts must be free from musty or stale odour, lumps, dirt, extraneous material, fungus growth or insect infestations. Rice polish must be fresh with fine aroma and taste, soft to touch and free from rancidity. A good quality rice polish shows the finger impressions whereas the adulterated one crumbles on pressing a handful of it in the fist. Take a pinch of rice bran/ DORB and rub between fingers to know adulteration of it with rice husk, which would be coarse and rough.

Oilseed cakes and meals (soybean meal, full fat soya, groundnut cake, sesame cake, sunflower cake, etc.) should have original texture and should be free from rancidity, insect or fungus infestation, musty or other objectionable odours. Animal byproducts such as fish meal and meat meal should have the characteristic odour and should be free from any off-smell indicative of spoilage, free from adulterants, insect or mite infestation and also free from visible fungal growth.

Collection of samples for laboratory analysis of feeds

Various feed ingredients are available for animal feeding in the shopping complexes of Pondicherry region. Samples of feed ingredients were collected from such shops located in rural, periurban and urban regions of Pondicherry. A total of 102 samples of feed ingredients (cereals and millets, pulses, oil cakes and byproducts of food industry) were analysed.

Sampling of feeds

The preparation of sample for analysis is just as important as the analytical procedure and hence it should be done with the same attention. Great care must be taken to obtain truly representative samples. The sample must always be taken at random so that the opinion of the operator may in no way influence the selection [look for details in appendix 1: Sampling of compounded feeds for cattle (IS: 2053 -1979)].

- Take representative samples from different parts of each bag
- If the feed to be sampled is present in the form of a pile, take small quantities of sample from as many parts of the pile as are accessible so that the proportion of coarse and fine particles in each small amount will be the same as in the total amount of feed being sampled.
- In shoveling a feed to be sampled, every fifth shovelful or every tenth shovelful, etc. may be taken depending upon the amount of total feed and the size of the sample desired.
- Sampling of materials-in-process: Materials-in-process can be sampled more conveniently from a stream than by probing a deep bag. Greater accuracy in sampling can be obtained while material drops from a chute of a grinder/ mixer/pelletiser. When taking the samples, use a pail or a receptacle which can be swung completely across the flowing stream, in a brief interval of time so as to take "all of the stream, part of the time". Under no circumstances should the sampling receptacle be allowed to overflow.

Preparation of sample for analysis

The sample received for analysis is poured into a dry enamel/plastic tray. The feed sample is mixed thoroughly and a representative sample (100g) is taken for lab analysis. The remaining sample is deposited back into the cover and kept in safe custody.

Laboratory analysis of feeds

Samples of feed ingredients and finished feeds were analysed for proximate principles and acid insoluble ash (AIA).

After taking a sample for moisture analysis, the representative feed sample is ground in a Wiley mill through 1mm screen and the ground sample is used for laboratory analysis. After allowing the ground material to equilibrate with air it is stored in prelabelled wide-mouthed containers (up to 80% of their capacity) fitted with tight lids. The container is rolled thoroughly to obtain uniform mixing, before taking sample for analysis. Crude protein is estimated with fresh samples, while total ash is estimated either on fresh or oven-dried sample (at 100° C) and ether extract and crude fibre with oven-dried samples. Proximate analyses of feeds were estimated as per the methods described by Association of Official Analytical Chemists (AOAC, 1995).

Moisture was estimated by keeping about 5-10g feed sample in aluminium/ porcelain moisture cup in hot air oven at 100±1° C for overnight (a minimum of 8 hours) and recording the loss of weight.

Nitrogen was estimated by Kjeldahl method by either manual Kjeldahl digestion and distillation apparatus or autoanalyser Kjeltek apparatus using boric acid and standard sulpuric acid method/ standard sulphuric acid and standard sodium hydroxide method. Crude protein was calculated by multiplying N with 6.25.

Dried sample was placed in a thimble (closed by absorbent cotton) for **ether extract** (EE) estimation in Soxhlet extraction apparatus for 6-8 hours of extraction period using petroleum ether (60-80° C) as solvent and a condensation rate of 4-6 drops per second; dry the receiver flask in hot air oven at 100±1° C overnight and the increase in weight of receiver flask was recorded as EE.

Dried and fat free sample was used to estimate **crude fibre** in a refluxing apparatus (tall form one litre spoutless beaker and round bottom flask) for 30 min. each with 200ml of 1.25% sulphuric acid and 1.25% sodium hydroxide, successively, and filtering through a cloth (free from starch and contain 18-22 threads per centimeter of cloth) by repeated hot water washings with the aid of filter pump to make it acid and alkali free; difference in weight of residue on the filter cloth between drying and ashing gave the crude fibre of the sample.

Total ash content of the sample (5-10g) was estimated in muffle furnace at 600° C for 2 hours after charring it in silica basin and the increase in weight of the basin was the ash content. Nitrogen free extract was calculated by deducting the sum of CP, EE, CF and total ash in DM from 100.

Acid insoluble ash (AIA) was estimated by dissolving the ash in hydrochloric acid (with a few drops of nitric acid) and igniting the dried residue on filter paper in muffle furnace at 600° C for 1 hour and recording the increase in weight as the AIA. Calcium and phosphorus were estimated as per the methods described by Talapatra et al. (1940).

Results and discussion of the feed analysis

Proximate analysis of the feed ingredients gives some idea about their adulteration. Moisture is the single most important factor that affects the quality of feeds (refer appendix 2). Lower crude protein (CP) and higher crude fibre (CF) content of an oilseed cake than its specifications indicate the presence of some fibrous feed such as hulls/husk. If the fibre remains higher than the specified level and CP within normal range, it may be inferred that the cake is adulterated with urea and/or some inferior quality oil cake, like mahua cake, castor cake, karanj cake, etc. Rice bran/ deoiled rice bran may have high CF and acid insoluble ash (AIA). The main adulterants are rice husk, tapioca waste powder, sand, zeolite, limestone, etc.

Proximate composition and AIA of feed ingredients

Proximate composition and AIA of feed ingredients are presented in Table 1. Minimum of three samples were analysed for each ingredient. Feed ingredients are categorized into cereals & millets, pulses, oilseed cakes and byproducts from food industry. The cereals & millets group includes rice broken, wheat broken, barley, maize, sorghum, bajra desi variety, bajra improved and ragi. Average moisture was 10.94%. Crude protein (CP) ranged from 7.27 % in case of bajra improved variety to 11.36% for bajra *desi* variety (*pottu cumbu*). Ether extract (EE) ranged from 0.46% for barley to 4.48% in case of bajra desi variety. Crude fibre (CF) ranged from 0.45% in barley to 4.49% in ragi and total ash ranged from 0.90% for barley grain to 8.6% for ragi grain.

The pulses analysed were bengalgram, cowpea, soyabean, friedgram broken and redgram dhal, some of which are frequently used in animal feeding. The CP content of bengalgram, friedgram broken, redgram dhal and cowpea ranged from 23.01 to 28.17, the EE from 0.46 to 4.27, the CF from 1.54 to 9.75 and total ash from 3.82 to 6.84%. Soyabeans contained 36.36% CP, 16.53% EE, 4.93% CF, 6.18% total ash, 36.00% NFE and 0.45% of AIA.

Oilseed cakes analysed were groundnut cake, gingelly cake, sunflower cake, coconut cake, soybean meal and mahuaseed cake. Among the oilseed cakes/meals analysed, soybean meal contained 46.64% CP, groundnut cake 44.06%, gingelly cake 35.95%, sunflower cake 26.72%, coconut cake 22.10% and mahuaseed cake 20.95%. The crude fibre percentages are sunflower cake 29.21, coconut cake 9.44, soybean meal 7.59, groundnut cake 7.56, gingelly cake 7.21 and mahuaseed cake 6.56. The total ash contents are gingelly cake 11.09%, soybean meal 9.58%, groundnut cake 8.78%, coconut cake 8.54%, mahuaseed cake 8.21% and sunflower cake 8.15%. The AIA ranged from 1.5% to 2.0% in the oil cakes tested.

Bengalgram husk, blackgram husk, greengram husk, redgram husk, brewers' dried grain, roasted bengalgram meal, tapioca chips and tapioca thippi, seaweed meal, rice brans and wheat bran, the valuable byproducts of food industry for animal feeding, were also analysed. The range (%) of CP observed is 12.73-16.32, CF 27.45-42.46 and AIA 2.43-4.08 in the gram husks. Brewers' dried grain and seaweed meal, respectively, contained 19.93 and 18.90% CF, 16.82 and 9.95% CP, 6.71 and 32.17% total ash and 2.58 and 9.29% AIA. Roasted bengalgram meal has 20.26% CP, 7.45% EE, 1.80% CF, 2.57% ash and 0.22% AIA. Tapioca chips and thippi contained CP of 5.19% and 6.89%, CF 5.22 and 16.66, ash 7.43 and 10.34 and AIA 1.31 and 3.95%. The CP 12.61 and 15.34%, CF 16.68 and 8.58% and AIA 10.27 and 0.20%, respectively, were present in DORB and wheat bran.

It is important to specify the quality standards because "you cannot improve what you do not control; you cannot control what you do not measure; you cannot measure what you do not define". Bureau of Indian Standards (BIS) specified the standards for cattle feeds (IS: 2052, 1979 and reaffirmed 1990), chicken feeds (IS: 1374, 1992) and pig feeds (IS: 7472, 1986). Compound Livestock Feed Manufacturers' Association (CLFMA) also developed specifications for compound feeds for dairy cattle and buffaloes as per the level of production of our animals.

Variability in chemical composition of some common feed ingredients

Variability in protein, fibre and AIA levels of some common feed ingredients are presented in Table 2. The CP of rice broken varies from 8.13 to 8.94 with a mean of 8.61%, CF from 0.24 to 3.45 with a mean of 1.70% while the AIA is minimum of 0.03 and maximum of 0.86 with average of 0.35%. The range of crude protein (%) are 9.19-11.38 for wheat broken, 9.94-10.62 for maize, 9.88-11.06 for *jowar*, 7.31-

11.59 for bajra and 9.13-10.80 for ragi. Among the oil cakes, gingelly cake has wide variation in crude protein and the range is 28.53-41.5%; CF ranges from 3.62 to 9.68 while AIA ranges from 0.86% to 2.56%. The CF content is widely variable in groundnut cake samples and the range is 3.89-10.27. In case of sunflower cake, range (%) of CP, CF and AIA, respectively, are 22.63-29.77, 26.08-31.92 and 0.86-2.56. Similar is the case with coconut cake, where the CP range is 19.15-25.0, CF range is 8.56-11.24 and AIA ranges from 0.11 to 3.26%. The variation among the soybean meal samples tested is less, the ranges (%) being 44.81-47.56 for CP, 6.28-9.29 for CF and 1.47-2.10 for AIA.

Work done at Feed Analytical and Quality Control Laboratory, Namakkal, Tamil Nadu (Krishna Reddy, 2003) also revealed high variability of groundnut meal, sunflower meal and soybean meal. The protein content of groundnut meal varied from 30.15 to 47.05 and the mean was 40.81 while the CF varied from 6.07 to 27.74 with a mean of 13.58%. In case of soybean meal, the CP range was 33.07 - 52.17 (mean=45.18%) and the CF range was 2.63 - 9.68 (mean=6.66%). The protein content ranged from 22.14 to 34.90 (mean = 26.77%) and the fibre varied from 19.65 to 34.25 (mean = 27.56%) for sunflower meal.

Feed analysis done during Nov 2003-Oct 2004 at the R.R.Labs, Hyderabad (Souvenir, 2004) revealed much variability in nutrient levels among the feed ingredients. For example among the 340 samples of soybean meal, the CP ranged between 35.42 and 50.32 with an average of 43.68%. Sand content observed ranges from 0.60 to 9.51 with an average of 3.54% for a sample size of 25. The CP (n = 270) content of deoiled groundnut cake ranges from 35.7 to 49.0 with a mean of 42.81% and the oil content (n = 12) range was 0.64–1.02 with a mean of 0.83% while in case of groundnut cake (expeller) the CP (n = 6) range was 39.8–47.26 with an average of 44.01% and the oil content varied from 5.12 to 7.51%. Sunflower cake (deoiled) contained a minimum of 20.35% and a maximum of 31.40 with a mean of 28.3% CP (n = 117) and the fibre (n = 6) ranged from 18.28 to 27.16 with a mean of 24.13%.

Among the byproducts (Table 2), husks showed wide variation in crude fibre and crude protein, tapioca thippi in crude protein and DORB in crude fibre, acid insoluble ash and crude protein. The crude protein in DORB ranged from 8.93 to 14.5, CF ranged from 3.31 to 29.13 and AIA ranged from 2.68 % to 18.05%. The R.R.Labs, Hyderabad (Souvenir, 2004) also reported similar findings: Crude protein (n = 54) of deoiled rice bran (DORB) ranged from 9.62 to 18.15 and the average was 12.91%. The CF (n = 11) content range was 15.59–20.67 and the mean was 19.86%.

Conclusions

1. The soybean meal contained 46.64% CP, groundnut cake 44.06%, gingelly cake 35.95% and sunflower cake had 26.72% and the CF values are sunflower cake 29.21, coconut cake 9.44, soybean meal 7.59, groundnut cake 7.56 and gingelly cake 7.21.

2. Considerable variation was observed in CP, CF and AIA of gingelly cake and CF content of groundnut cake. In case of sunflower cake, range (%) of CP, CF and AIA, respectively, are 22.63-29.77, 26.08-31.92 and 0.86-2.56.

3. Gram husks and brewers' dried grain can be used as valuable roughage sources. Roasted bengalgram meal may be considered as a protein supplement with 20.26% CP and 7.45% EE.

4. Brans are popular feeds among the animal farmers though there is a wide variation in the protein, fibre and silica content in the rice bran.

Table1. Proximate composition and AIA of feed ingredients [% on dry matter (DM) basis except for DM]*

Feed Ingredients**	DM	CP	EE	CF	TA	NFE	AIA
Cereals/Millets							
Rice broken	89.83±0.60	8.61±0.24	1.15±0.70	1.70±0.94	2.88±1.99	85.67±3.35	0.35±0.26
Wheat broken	89.90±0.40	10.32±0.63	2.94±0.19	3.90±0.63	8.40±2.72	74.44±3.69	1.31±0.44
Barley grain	88.61±0.19	9.05±0.30	0.46±0.03	0.45±0.03	0.90±0.02	89.15±0.33	0.013±0.003
Maize grain (n=4)	88.70±0.25	10.24±0.15	4.14±0.08	3.13±0.12	6.91±1.78	75.59±1.52	1.05±0.30
Jowar grain	88.69±0.45	10.36±0.36	3.13±0.10	4.26±0	8.08±0.12	74.18±0.51	0.96±0.15
Bajra grain (Desi)	87.88±0.11	11.36±0.51	4.48±0.12	2.24±0.14	3.79±0.06	79.11±0.52	1.27±0.04
Bajra grain (Improved)	90.20±0.01	7.27±0.14	3.46±0.07	1.55±0.07	2.28±0.14	85.44±0.41	0.32±0.07
Bajra grain	88.92±0.48	9.82±0.91	3.57±0.29	3.65±1.05	6.05±1.81	76.93±3.24	0.95±0.22
Ragi grain	88.77±0.45	9.77±0.52	2.88±0.69	4.49±0.29	8.60±2.52	74.25±2.96	1.01±0.61
Pulses Bengalgram	91.28±0.34	23.01±1.16	4.27±0.78	9.75±0.68	4.50±0.95	58.47±2.45	0.49±0.23
Cowpea	92.25±2.11	24.40±0.74	4.56±1.71	7.05±1.10	5.45±0.87	58.55±0.78	0.29±0.12
Soyabean	90.67±0.57	36.36±0.61	16.53±2.34	4.93±0.25	6.18±0.69	3.01±2.00	0.45±0.17
Friedgram, broken	88.43±0.19	28.17±3.09	0.46±0.02	2.80±0.14	6.84±0.25	61.73±3.08	0.42±0.03
Redgram dhal	89.49±0.25	23.41±0.80	1.75±0.09	1.54±0.20	3.82±0.08	69.48±1.26	0.06±0.01
Oil cakes							
Groundnut cake	90.75±0.31	44.06±0.20	7.24±0.59	7.56±1.90	8.78±1.78	32.36±2.83	2.04±0.10
Gingelly cake (n=4)	90.23±0.53	35.95±2.84	9.13±1.29	7.21±1.33	11.09±0.90	36.62±4.35	2.01±0.39
Sunflower cake	91.0±0.76	26.72±2.12	0.50±0.20	29.21±1.70	8.15±1.06	35.42±1.76	1.50±0.53
Coconut cake (n=4)	90.85±0.52	22.10±1.22	4.25±2.18	9.44±0.61	8.54±0.92	55.67±0.63	2.04±0.68
Soybean meal	91.13±0.47	46.64±0.92	1.07±0.18	7.59±0.89	9.58±1.45	35.11±1.52	1.71±0.20
Mahuaseed cake	90.01±0.03	20.95±0.32	1.35±0.03	6.56±0.02	8.21±0.12	62.94±0.42	1.63±0.08

Table1. Proximate composition and AIA of feed ingredients [% on dry matter (DM) basis except for DM]* (contd.)

Feed Ingredients**	DM	CP	EE	CF	TA	NFE	AIA
Byproducts from food industry							
Bengalgram husk	90.79±0.42	12.73±0.53	1.60±0.65	42.56±6.63	9.31±2.45	33.80±3.46	2.43±1.13
Blackgram husk	89.91±0.35	12.73±1.97	1.38±0.28	30.96±5.16	9.48±0.92	45.45±5.06	3.31±0.30
Greengram husk	90.02±0.19	13.84±1.91	1.81±0.40	27.45±2.82	11.17±0.85	45.73±0.66	4.08±1.46
Redgram husk	89.09±1.50	16.32±1.84	1.65±0.65	31.43±4.10	8.36±1.15	42.24±2.95	2.97±0.17
Brewers' Dried grain	92.54±0.85	16.82±0.20	1.76±0.16	19.93±0.64	6.71±1.52	54.78±1.10	2.58±1.11
Roasted bengalgram meal	90.34±0.08	20.26±0.07	7.45±0.03	1.80±0.07	2.57±0.10	67.93±0.16	0.22±0.02
Seaweed meal	93.90±0.06	9.95±0.06	0.74±0.05	18.90±0.12	32.17±0.09	38.24±0.16	9.29±0.07
Tapioca chips (including skin)	93.30±3.06	5.19±0.38	0.83±0.47	5.22±0.77	7.43±0.74	81.34±0.65	1.31±0.52
Tapioca thippi	90.25±0.74	6.89±3.26	1.03±0.47	16.66±0.21	10.34±0.80	65.08±2.39	3.95±0.21
Brans Deoiled Rice bran (n=5)	89.85±0.42	12.61±0.97	2.07±0.81	16.68±4.09	17.89±1.27	50.75±4.07	10.27±2.98
Rice polish	89.59±0.01	12.50±0.16	11.94±0.66	12.68±0.56	12.42±1.40	50.46±1.48	3.49±0.22
Wheat bran (n=4)	88.22±0.71	15.34±1.20	3.83±0.48	8.58±0.66	4.83±0.27	67.43±2.38	0.20±0.07

* Mean ±Standard Error

**Average of 3 samples analyzed unless otherwise stated

Table 2. Variability in protein, fibre and AIA levels of some common feed ingredients

Feed Ingredients	CP %			CF %			AIA %		
	Min	Max	Mean	Min	Max	Mean	Min	Max	Mean
Rice broken	8.13	8.94	8.61	0.24	3.45	1.70	0.03	0.86	0.35
Wheat broken	9.19	11.38	10.32	2.71	4.87	3.90	0.65	2.15	1.31
Maize grain	9.94	10.62	10.24	2.96	3.47	3.13	0.21	1.59	1.05
Jowar grain	9.88	11.06	10.36	4.26	4.26	4.26	0.69	1.21	0.96
Bajra grain	7.31	11.59	9.82	1.46	5.63	3.65	0.32	1.27	0.95
Ragi grain	9.13	10.80	9.77	3.92	4.88	4.49	0.06	2.14	1.01
Groundnut cake	43.75	44.42	44.04	3.89	10.27	8.24	1.84	2.15	2.07
Gingelly cake	28.53	41.50	35.95	3.62	9.68	7.21	0.86	2.56	2.01
Sunflower cake	22.63	29.77	26.72	26.08	31.92	29.21	0.86	2.56	1.50
Coconut cake	19.15	25.0	22.10	8.56	11.24	9.44	0.11	3.26	2.04
Soybean meal	44.81	47.56	46.64	6.28	9.29	7.59	1.47	2.10	1.71
Bengalgram husk	11.88	13.69	12.73	35.31	55.79	42.56	0.20	3.89	2.43
Blackgram husk	10.25	16.63	12.73	25.30	41.26	30.96	2.89	3.90	3.31
Greengram husk	11.69	17.65	13.84	21.95	31.26	27.45	2.55	7.01	4.08
Redgram husk	13.00	19.37	16.32	24.24	38.45	31.43	2.74	3.29	2.97
Tapioca thippi	3.63	13.41	6.21	16.24	16.91	16.66	3.54	4.18	3.95
Deoiled Rice bran	8.93	14.5	12.61	3.31	29.13	16.68	2.68	18.05	10.27
Wheat bran	12.18	18.03	15.34	7.41	10.44	8.58	0.10	0.41	0.20

APPENDIX-1

Sampling of compounded feeds for cattle (IS: 2053 -1979)
General requirements of sampling

In drawing, preparing, storing and handling samples, care should be taken that the properties of the material are not affected. The following precautions and directions shall be observed.

- Samples shall be taken in a place not exposed to damp air, dust or soot.
- The sampling instrument shall be clean and dry when used.
- Precautions shall be taken to protect the samples, the material being sampled, the sampling instrument and the containers for samples from adventitious contamination.
- The samples shall be placed in clean and dry glass containers. The sample containers shall be of such a size that they are almost completely filled by the sample.
- Each container shall be sealed air-tight with a stopper or a suitable closure after filling in such a way that it is not possible to open and reseal it without detection, and marked with full details of sampling, date of sampling, batch or code number, name of the manufacturer and other important particulars of the consignment.
- Samples shall be stored in such a manner that there is no deterioration of the material.
- Sampling shall be done by a person agreed to between the purchaser and the vendor and if desired by any of them, in the presence of the purchaser (or his representative) and the vendor (or his representative).

Scale of sampling

1. **Lot** -The quantity of cattle feed of a particular type, produced under relatively similar conditions in a day shall constitute a lot (Note: Relatively similar conditions would mean the use of raw material having insignificant variations and similar conditions of manufacture).
   Samples shall be tested for each lot for ascertaining conformity of the material to the requirements of this standard.
2. The number of bags to be selected from the lot shall depend on the size of the lot and shall be in accordance with col.1 and col. 2 (Table -1)
3. The bags shall be chosen at random as per the following procedure: "Starting from any bag count 1, 2, 3... etc, up to r and so on in a systematic manner and withdraw the rth bag; r being the integral part of the N/n; where N is the total number of bags in the lot, and n the number of bags to be selected according to Table 1"

Table 1. Number of bags to be selected for sampling

Lot size (N)	Number of bags to be selected (n)
(1)	(2)
Up to 50	1
51 to 100	3
101 to 300	4
301 to 500	5
501 and above	7

Test samples and Referee samples

(a) **Preparation of individual samples:** Draw with an appropriate sampling instrument, equal quantities of the material from the top, bottom and the sides of each bag selected according to the Table 1. The total quantity of the material drawn from each bag shall be not less than 1.5kg. Mix all the portions of the material drawn from the same bag thoroughly. Take about 0.75kg of the material and divide it into three equal parts. Each portion, thus obtained, shall constitute the test sample representing that particular bag and shall be transferred immediately to clean and dry sample containers and sealed air-tight. These shall be labelled with particulars as mentioned in general requirements of sampling. The individual samples thus obtained shall be formed into three sets in such a way that each set has a test sample representing each bag selected. One of the sets shall be for the purchaser, another for the vendor and the third for the referee.

(b) **Preparation of composite samples:** From the mixed material from each selected bag remaining after the individual samples have been taken, equal quantities of the material from each bag shall be taken and mixed together so as to form a composite sample weighing not less than 0.75kg. This composite sample shall be divided into three equal parts and transferred to clean and dry containers and labelled with particulars as mentioned earlier and sealed air-tight. One of these samples shall for the purchaser, another for the vendor and the third for the referee.

(c) **Referee samples:** Referee samples shall consist of a set of test samples and a composite sample and shall bear the seal of the purchaser and the vendor and shall be kept at a place agreed to between the two.

APPENDIX-2

Storage of feeds

Ingredients as well as finished feed should be stored properly since high temperature and relative humidity increase the probability of deterioration in their nutritive value.

They should be stored in dry and cool places separately. Moisture content of feeds is the single most important factor in maintaining the keeping quality of feeds. However, in our climatic conditions, it is better to avoid storage of finished feeds for longer periods. The feed bags are stored on pallets away from walls in the sanitized and rodent-proof godowns.

Moisture level-Feed quality

Moisture, temperature, relative humidity are the important physical factors that affect the food value and deterioration during storage. The lower the temperature, higher is the level of permissible moisture for safe storage. Bureau of Indian Standards specified 11% moisture as the maximum level for safe storage of feeds. Moisture content of feed is an important factor in the activity of insects and moulds. At low moisture contents (below 9%) most of the destructive insects become inactive e.g., rice weevils and maize weevils. Flour beetles (e.g., Tribolium spp) on the other hand can produce progeny in brans that are extremely dry. During larval development and growth, an insect produces metabolic water and heat. It has been reported that when the density of *Sitophilus oryzae* (weevil) rose from 15 adults to 2100 in a closed container of wheat the moisture content increased from 15 to 35%.

Mould growth can readily develop in stored materials if the moisture content in any one area rises above 11%. Thus insect activity is usually beneficial to mould growth. The increase in moisture content and temperature due to growth of insects, frequently, is followed by rapid growth of moulds. More over, insects - weevils and beetles may also be carriers of moulds such as Aspergillus and Penicillium spp. in their intestinal flora. The interaction of moisture content, moulds and insects can rapidly lead to spoilage of stored materials. Insect infestation enhances the moisture content of stored feeds due to their metabolism and can result in temperature increase up to 42° C. Increased moisture and temperature are conducive for the growth of moulds.

2

Genetically Modified Feedstuffs—Issues Related to Food Safety

Genetically Modified crops

The development and use of genetically modified (GM) crops could offer considerable potential to ensure a satisfactory diet for an ever-increasing number of people in the context of decreasing crop lands due to urbanization. As a result of consistent and substantial benefits during the first dozen years of commercialization from 1996 to 2007, farmers have continued to plant more biotech crops every single year (James Clive, 2007). In 2007, the USA, followed by Argentina (19.1 million ha), Brazil (15.0 million ha), Canada (7 million ha), India (6.2 million ha) and China (3.2 million ha) continued to be the principal adopters of biotech crops (principal crops being **soybean, maize, cotton, canola**) globally, with the USA retaining its top world ranking with 57.7 million hectares. Notably, 63% of biotech maize, 78% of biotech cotton, and 37% of all biotech crops in the USA in 2007 were stacked products containing two or three traits that delivered multiple benefits. Stacked products are a very important feature and future trend, which meets the multiple needs of farmers and consumers.

Deliverables from Crop Biotechnology (James Clive, 2007)
1. **Increase global crop productivity to improve food, feed and fibre security in sustainable crop production systems that also conserve biodiversity:** Biotech crops are more tolerant to the biotic stresses caused by pests, weeds and diseases.
2. **Contribute to the alleviation of poverty and hunger:** Fifty percent of the world's poorest people are small and resource-poor farmers, and another 20% are the rural landless dependent on agriculture for their livelihoods. Thus, increasing income of small and resource-poor farmers contribute directly to the poverty alleviation of a large majority of the world's poorest people.
3. **Reduce the environmental footprint of agriculture:** Conventional agriculture has impacted significantly on the environment. Biotechnology can be used to reduce the environmental footprint of agriculture. Significant

reductions in pesticides, saving on fossil fuels and decreasing CO_2 emissions through no/less ploughing are already visible.

4. **Mitigate climate change and reduce greenhouse gases:** Biotech crops are already contributing to reducing CO_2 emissions by precluding the need for ploughing a significant portion of cropped land, conserving soil and moisture, reducing pesticide spraying as well as sequestering CO_2.

5. **Contribute to the cost-effective production of biofuels:** Biotechnology can be used to cost effectively optimize the productivity of biomass per hectare of first generation food/feed and fibre crops and also second generation energy crops. This can be achieved by developing crops tolerant to abiotic stresses (drought and salinity) and biotic stresses (pest, weeds, diseases) and also to raise the ceiling of potential yield per hectare through modifying plant metabolism. There is also an opportunity to utilize biotechnology to develop more effective enzymes for the downstream processing of biofuels.

Impact of Agricultural Biotechnology on Consumers

The consumer benefits that could be developed through agricultural biotechnology include enhanced nutritional and nutraceutical composition, prolonged shelf-life, resistance to spoilage, improved flavor and appearance, and the elimination of naturally occurring toxicants including allergens.

Questions in the mind of consumer

There is growing concern however within the United Kingdom and Europe regarding safety issues over the introduction of genes into plant genomes using recombinant DNA technology. What is the fate of DNA and resultant proteins derived from introduced traits? This has led to several important questions; (1) could the DNA of inserted or modified genes, or their products, if transferred to animals, cause adverse health effects in these animals; (2) could these DNA fragments or proteins be transferred to and accumulate in the products (milk, meat, eggs) of animals fed GM crops and (3) will consumption of agricultural crop materials or animal products derived from GM crops lead to adverse health effects in humans (Beever and Kemp, 2000).

Concept of substantial equivalence

The concept of substantial equivalence has been a key, though sometimes misunderstood, feature of the safety assessment of genetically modified foods from the outset of international deliberations (FAO/WHO, 1996). The concept of substantial equivalence arose from the goal that the genetically modified food should be as safe as its traditional counterpart. In practice, the currently approved genetically modified varieties of traditional crops, such as maize and soybeans, are altered very little from their traditional counterparts. In the concept of substantial equivalence, the safety evaluation would then focus on those differences while assuming that the unaltered components are just as safe as the same components in the traditional counterpart varieties (Taylor, 2003).

In the concept of substantial equivalence, the genetically modified food (or food ingredient) is compared with its traditional counterpart for such attributes as the origin of the novel genes, agronomic parameters, composition including key nutrients, anti-nutrients and allergens, and consumption patterns. Three possible outcomes can arise from the comparisons made through the concept of substantial equivalence (FAO/WHO, 1996):

1. The genetically modified food would be considered substantially equivalent to its traditional counterpart;
2. The genetically modified food would be considered substantially equivalent to its traditional counterpart except for one or more defined differences; or
3. The genetically modified food would not be considered to be substantially equivalent to its traditional counterpart

In the first scenario, the genetically modified food could be judged to be substantially equivalent to its conventional counterpart. In this case, no further safety testing would be required. In reality, this possibility would occur only on rare occasions. This situation might occur if a gene is removed or silenced but no novel genes are introduced. This situation might also occur with ingredients such as cottonseed oil where the plant would have some defined differences from the expression of specific novel proteins but the oil fraction would not contain these novel proteins and would be equivalent in composition to cottonseed oil derived from traditional varieties of cottonseed. Some of the confusion surrounding the adequacy of the safety assessment of genetically modified foods is based on the incorrect assumption that most genetically modified foods are considered to be substantially equivalent to their traditional counterparts and, therefore, that no safety studies are conducted. In fact, the vast majority of genetically modified foods are not considered to be completely equivalent to their traditional counterparts, and regulatory agencies have required safety studies on those features of the genetically modified food that are distinct and different from the traditional counterpart.

With most of the current genetically modified crops, the foods for food ingredients derived from these crops could be judged to be substantially equivalent to their conventional counterpart except for the defined differences associated with the introduced traits. In this situation, the safety testing would focus upon the safety of the introduced trait or gene product, usually a novel protein. Even in the cases where several genes are introduced, the product could be considered to be substantially equivalent to its conventional counterpart except for the various gene products derived from the specific introduced and novel genes.

Finally, the genetically modified food could be judged to be not substantially equivalent to the conventional food for food ingredient. More extensive safety assessments would probably be required for such products. Since no products have yet been released to the commercial marketplace or approved by worldwide regulatory agencies, the nature of the requirements for safety assessment of such products has not been delineated specifically. Certainly, the safety assessments would need to be conducted in a flexible manner depending upon the nature of such novel food products. More rigorous nutritional and toxicological evaluation would be likely to be desired with any products of this type that are developed. Although no such products have yet been released into the commercial marketplace, agricultural biotechnology offers the promise of many such products in the future.

Extensive compositional analyses are conducted on genetically modified foods to compare them with their conventional counterparts. Of course, the composition of the conventional counterpart can vary significantly as a result of varietal differences, climatic conditions and agronomic conditions. The choice of the conventional counterpart for comparative purposes is extremely important. In such comparisons, the crops and the foods or food components produced therefrom are compared for protein, carbohydrate, fat, fatty acid composition, starch, amino acid composition, fibre, ash, minerals, vitamins and other factors. If known anti-nutrients are present in either the source material for the novel gene or the host plant, the comparative levels of these anti-nutrients are determined. Similarly, if the biological sources of the novel gene or the host plant are known to be allergenic, the presence and levels of the allergens are determined in the transgenic variety and compared with the traditional counterpart. The allergenicity of the host plant is a lesser concern because, for example, consumers with soybean allergy will probably avoid all soybeans whether genetically modified or not.

Safety for animal feeding purposes

Maize, soybeans, canola and cottonseed are among the genetically modified crops that are important in the feeding of domestic animals. Feed safety assessment typically involves feeding studies with the appropriate target animal species and comparisons for typical performance parameters such as growth rate.

Genes, genomes, DNA and bioengineering

Deoxyribonucleic acid (DNA) provides the genetic coding for all plants, animals, bacteria and many viruses. In plants and animals it exists as a long molecule, basically one per chromosome, comprising of many ($>10^6$) small molecular units or nucleotides. Each nucleotide contains a pentose sugar, a phosphate group and one nitrogen-containing base (adenine, cytosine, guanine or thymine). Nucleotides are arranged in specific sequences, and matched by complimentary nucleotides on the opposite strand of the anti-parallel double helical molecule, held together by hydrogen bonds. Linear groups of 1000 or more nucleotides act together as a functional unit known as genes. Each gene provides the blueprint for the production of specific proteins, whilst some genes contain regulatory sequence segments which do not code for proteins, but control specific functions including the spatial, temporal and quantitative expression patterns of genes throughout the lifetime of the organism. An average plant species contains between 20 and 50×106 different genes.

Many plants are diploid, having one homologous copy of each chromosome from each parent. Equally crop plants can be multiploid, containing four (eg soyabean; autotetraploid) or six (eg wheat; allohexaploid) haploid genomes. Polyploidy in cultivated crops is associated with agronomic vigour leading to increased yields. The haploid sequence of soyabeans was estimated by Clark (1997) to contain 1.1×10^9 bp, equivalent to the DNA content of the pollen or the primary nucleus of the ovule.

The maize haploid genome is approximately 2.5×10^6 bp (base pairs) whilst the human genome is slightly larger (3×10^6 bp). In addition to the nuclear genome, two subcellular organelles (mitochrondia and chloroplasts) contain small plasmid-like chromosomes with additional genes.

Bioengineering involves extracting or manipulating the DNA, which makes up the genes of all living things. Scientists cut a desired gene out of a string of genes, called a chromosome, of a particular plant, animal or bacteria and put the gene into another plant cell. Success depends upon the introduced DNA becoming stably integrated into one of the chromosomes, with this DNA being passed to new plant generations through conventional breeding procedures. Once integrated and duplicated, the molecular characteristics of the transferred DNA segment will be identical to the original plant DNA. Genetically modified foods are agricultural foods grown from seeds that have had the chromosomes re-engineered with genes spliced from viruses, bacteria and even animals.

Genomic sizes

The size or length of DNA inserted into the genome of an alternative organism will vary, but is usually of the order of 2 to 14×10^6 bp, examples being 4×10^6 for insect-resistant maize and 2.5×10^6 for herbicide-tolerant soyabean. The haploid genome size of these crops is approximately 1×10^9 bp, with the inserted DNA constituting less than 0.00016 to 0.00066% of the genomic DNA in the modified plant.

Consumption of DNA

Both the World Health Organisation (1993) and the US Food and Drug Administration (1992) have previously concluded that there is no inherent risk in consuming DNA, including that derived from GM crops. The basis of their conclusion was that mammals have always consumed significant quantities of DNA from a wide variety of sources, including plants, animals, bacteria, parasites and viruses.

Dietary exposure to foreign DNA

The obvious route for human and animal exposure to foreign DNA is by oral consumption. Most foodstuffs contain a complex mixture of proteins, lipids, carbohydrates, nucleic acids, minerals and vitamins. The relative proportions of these may vary widely, but the quantity of DNA in most food crops is generally less than 0.02% (dry matter basis), with Watson and Thompson (1988) reporting values of 0.005% in some crops.

DNA in the diet, regardless of sources, is not considered to be toxicologically significant (Beever and Kemp, 2000). Virtually all foods contain DNA, and DNA is ingested in significant quantities. Human dietary intakes of RNA and DNA are estimated to range from 0.1 to 1.0 g per day (Doerfler and Schubbert, 1997). Ingestion of novel DNA from genetically modified foods is insignificant by comparison and would probably represent <1/250,000 of the total amount of DNA consumed (FAO/WHO, 2000). DNA is also highly digestible (FAO/WHO, 2000). Thus, the novel

DNA contained in genetically modified foods is extremely unlikely to pose any safety concerns.

Two examples are presented here to have awareness on the amount of ingestion of recombinant DNA from GM crops in relation to total DNA intake.

Example 1: Consider the impact of GM maize fed to dairy cows either as forage maize silage or as maize grain (Beever and Kemp, 2000). Based on maize silage and maize grain accounting for 40% and 20% respectively of total DM intake (i.e. 60% of the complete diet), transgene DNA consumption would amount to 2.3 µg/day in a 600kg dairy cow. It is assumed that no degradation of DNA occurred in the gut following ingestion. This permits estimation of the maximum possible intake of recombinant DNA from GM crops in relation to total DNA intake, taking into account the proportion of total DNA to total feed intake, and the proportion of each commodity in the diet.

$$\frac{4000 \text{ bp insert DNA}}{2.5 \times 10^9 \text{ bp genomic DNA}} \times 0.0001 \text{ g DNA/g DM} \times 0.60 \text{ g maize/g DM} \times 24000 \text{ g feed/day}$$

This compares with a total diet DNA intake of 608 mg/day, equating to a GM DNA to normal plant DNA ratio of 1:264,000 or 0.00038% of total dietary DNA. On this basis it appears that exposure to introduced DNA of GM crop material will be negligible compared with normal exposure to non-GM crop DNA.

Example 2: In mid lactation, a cow may consume up to 600 mg of maize DNA per day. The maize diploid genome is approximately 5×10^9 bp; the length of DNA inserted in GM maize is 4000 bp (one copy per diploid genome); the relative amount of transgenic DNA fed to the cow is $(4000 \div 5 \times 10^9) \times 600 \text{ mg} = 0.48 \text{ µg}$.

In vivo fate of DNA

Comprehensive data relating to DNA exposure and possible fate can be derived from studies involving the analysis of human and animal milk, designed to estimate the dietary requirements of nucleotides (as phosphate esters of nucleosides; adenosine, guanosine, thymidine, cytidine, uridine; as free molecules and as components of DNA and RNA) for suckling neonates (Gil and Uauy, 1995). As nucleotides are generally abundant in food relative to dietary requirements, little attention has been paid to the occurrence of DNA and RNA in food (Jackson et al., 1997; Yu, 1998).

Ingested DNA is rapidly cleaved into small fragments by the mechanical processes of mastication along with buccal and gastro-intestinal enzymatic digestion and acid hydrolysis. Few studies have attempted to measure in vivo DNA degradation and published evaluations occurred prior to the development of analytical methods that could distinguish the source of DNA (plant, digestive tract microbes, epithelial cells etc). In particular the methods could not determine the length of the DNA fragments but were able to establish the catabolism of DNA to nitrogenous bases, free bases and secondary metabolites (McAllan, 1980).

The enzymes involved in DNA hydrolysis include high concentrations of DNase I, an endonuclease that disrupts the double stranded DNA and is produced and secreted by the salivary glands, as well as the pancreas, the liver and the Paneth cells of the small intestine. DNase I has optimal activity at neutral pH. DNase II has a pH optima of between 4.6 and 5.5. This enzyme is also secreted but its primary function is in lysosomes within phagocytes, involved in the catabolism of DNA as well as the fragmentation of genomic DNA during apoptosis.

McAllan, (1982) estimated that more than 85% of the plant DNA consumed by ruminants is reduced to nucleotides or smaller constituents before entering the duodenum, with most of the larger nucleic acid fragments in small intestinal contents arising from rumen microbes.

In addition to enzymatic digestion, low pH conditions in stomach (monogastrics) or abomasal (ruminants) contents should remove most adenine and guanine bases from naked DNA fragments. This process will destroy the genetic information in long strands of DNA.

DNA transfer

A small proportion of plant or microbial DNA fragments remaining in intestinal digesta could potentially be absorbed through the intestinal mucosa either directly by epithelial cells or by antigen presenting cells of the immune system. If the intestinal epithelial surface has been damaged, DNA and other macromolecules may also diffuse into the lamina propria. It is suggested, however, that most of this DNA would be phagocytised by tissue macrophages, dendritic cells or other terminally differentiated phagocytes of the immune system.

The possibility of the transfer of genes from genetically modified foods to mammalian cells has also been examined, and the probability of such occurrence is considered very low. The transfer of DNA from genetically modified plants into mammalian cells under normal conditions of dietary exposure would require that all of the following conditions be met (FAO/WHO, 2000):

1. The relevant gene in the plant DNA would have to be released probably as a linear fragment.
2. The gene would have to survive nucleases in the plant and in the gastrointestinal tract.
3. The gene would have to compete for uptake with dietary DNA from traditional sources.
4. The recipient mammalian cells would have to be competent for transformation and the gene would have to survive their restriction enzymes.
5. The gene would have to be inserted into the host DNA by rare repair and recombination events.

Detection of a plant DNA fragment

Klotz and Einspanier (1998) reported the detection of a plant DNA fragment in tissues taken from a cow. The fragment was from the abundant soyabean chloroplast gene (ribulose-1, 5-biphosphate carboxylase/oxygenase (Rubisco) large subunit) and was detected in white blood cells of a cow fed a diet containing GM soyabean meal. The reported assay used the highly sensitive polymerase chain reaction (PCR) method followed by Southern blotting to detect the amplified DNA fragment. In the same experiment, attempts to detect the presence of DNA from the GM transgene CP4 5-enolpyruvylshikimate-3-phosphate synthase (EPSP synthase) in cows blood were unsuccessful, despite being detectable in the soyabean meal. Equally they could not detect fragments of Rubisco or EPSP synthase DNA in milk collected from that cow.

In another study, microbial DNA was fed directly into the gastrointestinal lumen and tissues of mice and fragments of this DNA were detected in some mouse white blood cells (leukocytes) at 24 hours or more after initial exposure (Schubbert et al., 1994, 1997, 1998; Doerfler et al., 1997; Doerfler and Schubbert, 1998). However, this observation has been seriously questioned (Beever and Kemp, 2000). FAO/WHO (2000) concluded that no data exist to demonstrate that plant DNA can be transferred to and stably maintained in mammalian cells. Additionally, FAO/Who (2000) concluded that no evidence exists that intact genes from plants can be transferred to and be expressed in mammalian cells.

The possibility of the transfer of genes from genetically modified foods to gastrointestinal bacteria has also been examined. No evidence exists to suggest that such transfer has occurred in humans ingesting genetically modified foods. The likelihood of such transfer is considered to be quite low (FAO/WHO, 2000). The transfer of genes from plant cells into microbial cells is considered very unlikely except in circumstances where the gene from the genetically modified plant shows homology with prokaryotic genes (FAO/WHO, 2000). Gene transfer has been observed under laboratory conditions, but only in situations where homologous recombination is possible (Nielsen *et al.*, 1998). Gene transfer has not been demonstrated to occur from plant cells to microbes in experiments conducted in the gastrointestinal tracts of animals.

Effect of feed processing DNA integrity

Cells contain DNA in large fragments (hundreds of thousands of base pairs) protected by a nuclear membrane. It is recognized that certain processes involved in animal feed preparation will cause significant fragmentation of the DNA, whilst other processes appear to have little or no effect. Forbes *et al.* (1998) studied the effect of feed processing conditions on DNA fragmentation. The study provided data on DNA fragment size from various processed feed fractions of wheat, maize, soyabean, linseed, rape seed, sugar beet and rye grass. Treatments involved in the preparation of feed material including variations in mechanical processing, heating in dry air or with steam at different pressures and possible cubing / extrusion of the final product. Results indicated grinding and milling to have little effect on DNA fragment size, whilst mechanical expulsion of oil from seeds, or chemical extraction caused extensive DNA fragmentation. Dry heat applied to plant material at 90°C appeared to have no effect, while 95°C for 5 minutes caused considerable fragmentation of the plant DNA. Equally steam heat at low to moderate pressures effected substantial DNA fragmentation, whilst ensiling of forage had no detectable effect.

Antibiotic resistance marker DNA

In a recent publication Forbes (1998) suggested that feeding GM plants containing genomic antibiotic resistant marker genes could lead to the development of new antibiotic resistant microbes. Transmission of antibiotic resistance among bacterial strains is well documented, and occurs by transfer of plasmids, small circular extra-chromosomal pieces of DNA or in some bacterial species by insertion of intact antibiotic resistant genes from genomic DNA of one bacterium to that of another. Additionally, the extensive use of powerful antibiotics as often occurs in intensive animal farming, has resulted in multiple resistance microbes. This must be a far greater cause for concern than the potential for resistance to the antibiotics commonly used for selection during the genetic modification process.

Labelling

Labelling of GM food products to provide consumer choice is required in Europe, and already occurs under the present regulations relating to herbicide tolerant soyabean and maize. Suitable methods are available to test for the presence of the protein product or the inserted DNA of the GM crop. It has also been recommended that threshold limits are established that would be set to designate the limits of which products would require labelling as GM commodities, with those foods containing less than the threshold level of GM product not requiring to be labelled.

When the question raised by consumers becomes one of choice regarding the consumption of meat, dairy or poultry products from animals that may or may not have consumed GM crop material, the relevance and the practicality of implementing and enforcing any labeling policy would be challenging. When livestock consume plant DNA and proteins, nearly, if not all of the protein and DNA from the plant will be digested and the identifiable characteristics of the GM material would be destroyed. Once that plant material passes the stomach or abomasum, it is unlikely that any of the transgenic protein products would be detectable. Because most of the GM transgenic proteins are expressed at low concentrations, it is often difficult to detect them when the concentration of the plant is less than one percent of the test matrix, included in the feed or processed food.

A thorough literature search (Beever and Kemp, 2000) has not identified any studies describing the detection of plant proteins which are expressed at levels comparable to current GM products, in products including meat, milk and eggs derived from animals consuming the plant. Furthermore, as indicated in the discussion above, there are no examples of the detection of the DNA from single copy plant genes in animal products even when highly sensitive PCR assays were employed. Therefore, any suggestion to label food products derived from animals fed GM plant material could be impractical or difficult to enforce. One solution would be to allow the marketing of food products derived from animals that were not fed GM feed to be labelled as such, as long as proof of appropriate assurance schemes established that they were fed GM crop free feed.

Safety of food products derived from animals fed GM crops

Two key questions confront the animal producers and feed manufacturers when they try to cope with looming GM issues. Can traces of GM material find their way into meat, milk or eggs? Will GM-derived food products be acceptable to the consumer?

On the first question, it seems that the likelihood is extremely small, certainly no higher than 1 in 10,000 or 0.01%. Regarding the consumer acceptability, survey of European consumers revealed that there is a great reluctance to contemplate eating such foods, despite the assurances that GM foods are safe. Elsewhere it is not like that. Probably, it may be difficult to get a food / feed product in USA totally free from GM material.

Conclusion

In the USA and other countries, genetically modified foods pass through numerous regulatory hurdles between the early gene discovery phase and product commercialization. Accordingly, the products of biotech crops currently sold for food /feed purposes around the world have been subjected to intensive safety evaluations. The safety assessment of genetically modified feeds usually begins with a comparison of the novel food with its traditional counterpart. In most cases currently, the novel food is comparable with its conventional counterpart except for a few defined differences resulting from the introduction of the particular gene(s) of interest. As a result, the safety assessment is then focused upon the safety of the introduced gene and especially the novel protein produced from the gene. Current genetically modified foods are well documented to be safe for their intended uses under the anticipated conditions of consumption because they have been subjected to such safety evaluations.

3

PCR-based Methods for Detection of Animal-derived materials in Feedstuffs

INTRODUCTION

Proliferation of bovine spongiform encephalopathy (BSE) in the British cattle is thought to have emerged originally from initial interspecies transmission of the Scrapie - agent into cattle by the feeding of Scrapie - infected sheep meal, plus bone meal products to cattle. BSE or mad cow disease is one of the neurodegenerative and prion-transmitted zoonotic terminal diseases of many animal species, incubation period of which being 3 to 9 years (Marsh, 1991). BSE and other strains of BSE - like transmissible encephalopathies have been encountered in human beings, cats, sheep, mink, hamsters, mice, ostrichs and zoological animal (wild elk). Prion - type diseases include sheep Scrapie; BSE in cattle; Cruetzfeldt - Jacob disease (CJD), Gerstmann straussler - Scheinker disease (GSS), and fatal familial insomnia (FFI) of humans, and transmissible mink encephalopathy of mink (TME). Swine have also been infected with spongiform encephalopathy (Bradley, 1996).

In view of the possible link between BSE and human's CJD, World Health Organization recommended certain things to be followed to lessen the risk of BSE. These include ban on the use of ruminant tissues in ruminant feed, slaughter and safe disposal of TSE affected animals so that TSE infectivity cannot enter any food chain and all countries should review their rendering procedure to ensure that they effectively inactivate TSE agents. In the wake of the devasting BSE crisis in the UK, there is a continuing crisis of confidence among consumers of beef and beef products in particular.

Rendering systems: European renderers along with the European Commission conducted research on rendering systems capable of destroying the BSE and Scrapie disease agents. Based on these results, EC permitted from April 1997, only rendering systems operating at a minimum of 133°C with 3 bar pressure for 20 min for the manufacture of mammalian animal protein for use in farm animal feeds. However, this was contradicted later in July 1997 conference and the specified conditions may not be sufficient to totally inactivate the BSE agent. Macerated bovine brain with the BSE agent and rodent brain infected with scrapie agent were autoclaved at 134°C to 138°C for 60 min without complete inactivation. The BSE-infective agent is resistant to formaline fixative and cremation at 360°C is inadequate to destroy the infectiveness.

Feed manufacturers and animal nutritionists have to protect the animals from various forms of zoonotic prion diseases. Since normal transmission of prion - associated diseases is through food and feed intake and the disease is always lethal, the prevention of BSE in food animals (cattle, buffaloes, sheep, goats) and companion animals (cats, dogs) should be relatively straightforward. Hence the ban on feeding of meat and bone meal derived from ruminants to ruminants came into force from July 1988 in UK. Later the ban was extended throughout the Europe in 1994, and it prohibited the feeding of mammalian protein to ruminants.

In the United States, regulation 21 CFR 589.2000 of the US FDA prohibited the use of proteins derived ruminant tissue in feed for ruminant animals to prevent the spread and amplification of BSE in the United States.

Consequent upon the reports of clinical diseases caused by Transmissible Spongiform Encephalopathy (TSE) group of agents occurring in different countries, Government of India in its order No. 2-4/99-AHT/FF dated 21st June 1999, reiterated the prohibition on the use of meat meal, bone meal and blood meal in the manufacture of ruminant feeds as a matter of abundant caution. It cautions the State Governments to enhance the surveillance to prevent cross contamination of feeds during the handling, manufacture, storage and transportation of animal feeds.

Animal byproducts such as meat meal, blood meal, meat and bone meal, fish meal, etc. have a high content of good quality protein and a high energy value. They are rich sources of lysine and the sulphur containing amino acids and biologically available sources of minerals. In view of the ban of meat and bone meal in ruminant feeds, there is a potential to adulterate fish meal with these banned terrestrial animal products.

There is a need to develop cost-effective analytical methods to detect the presence of ruminant animal protein in animal feeds.

Methods for detection: Rapid identification of bovine and other animal materials in animal feedstuffs is essential for effective control of a potential source of BSE. Several methods for the detection and identification of animal materials in feed have been developed ever since BSE was recognized. Species identification of animal products is possible by three major methods.

1. Enzyme-linked immunosorbent assay (ELISA): ELISA is simple and convenient, but not sensitive enough to detect heat-treated proteins produced during the rendering process.

2. Feed microscopy: It is based on microscopic structure identification. It is tissue-specific and mostly unaffected by heat treatment of the samples. But feed microscopy is reliable only when the operator is expert.

3. DNA analysis: In DNA analysis, use of the PCR has improved feed analysis for traceability of foods of animal origin because of its simplicity, species specificity and sensitivity for detecting feed components. With species-specific primers (Tartaglia et al., 1998; Wang et al., 2000; Lahiff et al., 2001;

Matsunaga et al., 1999) and analysis of restriction fragment length polymorphism (Bellagamba et al., 2001), material from cattle, sheep, goats, pigs and chickens can be detected and identified.

PCR-based methods for rapid detection of animal-derived materials in feedstuffs

Tartaglia has first proposed the polymerase chain reaction (PCR)-based approach in 1998 to detect bovine mitochondrial DNA as marker for bovine-derived proteins in ruminant feeds. In this context, species-specific mitochondrial DNA sequences have been investigated, for a possible application for the traceability of foods of animal origin. Primers for PCR have been based on mitochondrial DNA (Tartaglia et al., 1998; Lahiff et al., 2001; Matsunaga et al., 1999) because there are some 2500 copies of the mitochondrial genome in each cell.

The PCR method developed by Tartaglia et el. (1998) for the detection of bovine materials present in animal feedstuffs requires 24 h to complete and is a tedious multi-step purification process. This method can detect a concentration of 0.125 % bovine-derived meat and bone meal (MBM) with a bovine specific primer. Further, guanidine thiocyanate (GuSCN) buffer used for extraction process can produce a toxic gas and thus associated with hazardous waste (Boom et al., 1999). Boom et al. (1999) reported that PCR inhibitors in the feed samples may interfere with assay performance. The species-specific PCR method of Lahiff et al. (2001) has a detection limit in MBM of a contamination by single species is5 %, 1 %, and 5 % for sheep, pigs and chickens, respectively. Matsunaga et al. (1999) reported that 0.25 ng of genomic DNA from cattle, sheep, goats, pigs and chickens is the limit for detection with multiplex PCR.

In view of the drawbacks of Tartaglia method and findings of Boom et al., an alternative sample preparation procedure to enhance the speed, simplicity and reproducibility of the PCR method was developed (Wang et al., 2000). Animal feed samples were prepared by a Chelex-100 treatment method, then subjected to PCR detection. The assay can be completed in 2 h including 30 min for sample preparation, 35-65 min for PCR cycling and 30 min for gel electrophoresis. This method is not only rapid, simple and consistent, but also avoids a hazardous waste disposal issue associated with a previously described GuSCN extraction-PCR method.

PCR Detection of DNAs of animal origin by primers based on sequences of short and long interspersed repetitive elements

The repetitive sequences in genomes can be markers for DNA-based species identification. Among the highly repetitive sequences, short and long interspersed nucleotide elements (SINEs and LINEs) are transposable. The primers (for PCR) designed on the basis of these sequences are present in more copies than mitochondrial DNA. SINEs are from 80 to 500 bp long and they often are present in 105 copies per mammalian genome. LINEs are 3 to 7 kb long. The chicken genome contains 105 copies of the chicken repeat1 (CR1) LINE. Such interspersed repetitive elements have been found in various animals. If PCR primers are designed on the basis of sequences of SINEs or LINEs from a particular animal, sensitivity for detection of materials of animal origin in feed might be improved.

Keeping this in mind Tajima et al. (2002) undertook the design of new PCR primers for the detection of materials from ruminants, pigs and chickens, using sequences of Art 2 SINE, PRE-1 SINE and CR1 LINE, respectively. Total DNA isolated from cattle, sheep, goats, chickens was used as a control template. Test feeds were prepared with commercial meat and bone meal (MBM) added to final concentrations of zero, 0.001, 0.01, 0.1 and 1.0 % to the MBM-free feed. Total DNAs from animals and feeds were extracted with the QIAamp DNA stool mini kit (Qiagen, Tokyo, Japan) and measured at 260 nm with a Bio-Rad Smartspec 3000 (Bio-Rad, Tokyo, Japan).

The designed primers amplified the SINE or LINE from total DNA extracted from the target animals and from test feed containing commercial MBM. PCR was done with Takara Ex Taq Hot Start version Kit (Takara Bio Inc., Shiga, Japan). With these primers, detection of Art 2, PRE-1, or CR1 in test feed at concentrations of 0.01 % MBM or less was possible. These primers are advantageous over primers of Tartaglia et al. (1998). The Art 2 detect not only bovine material, but also that from sheep and goats; the use of this primer allow us to check for ruminant materials in feed. Another advantage is the improved sensitivity of detection.

PCR detection of multiple animal-derived materials in animal feed

In the United States, Myers et al. (2001) validated the PCR-based assay of Tartaglia et al. (1998) which is specific only for bovine-derived materials in animal feed. But animal feed may contain rendered feed ingredients from many species of animals. Hence Myers et al. (2003) studied the characterization of a PCR primer set capable of amplifying a mitochondrial DNA segment of multiple species (cattle, sheep, goats, deer and elk) whose rendered products are prohibited from being fed to ruminants. The primer set also amplifies DNA derived from the rendered remains of pigs and horses.

Test feeds used were feeds with either 2 % bovine MBM or 10 % pig blood meal and dry dog feeds labeled as containing either lamb, chicken, chicken and fish, or turkey. DNA from the blood of exempt species (dog, cats, rabbits, turkeys, poultry, horses and pigs) and prohibited species (cattle, deer, elk, sheep and goats) was isolated from heparinized blood with the Promega Wizard Genomic DNA Purification Kit. This method isolates both genomic and mitochondrial DNA. The experimental procedure followed for PCR amplification of DNA extracted from animal feed or dog food were of Myers et al. (2001) and Tartaglia et al. (1998). Five microliters of the DNA-containing solution was used for the PCR reaction.

The results of this study provide a practical approach for the simultaneous detection of materials derived from several species banned from ruminant feed. The principal drawback of this approach is that it also detects DNA derived from equine and swine species. Rendered materials from both of these species are exempt under the US FDA's current feed ban. A positive PCR result could be due to the presence or absence of one or more of these species.

484

PCR-based analysis to detect terrestrial animal protein in fish meal: Meat meal-based feedstuffs are banned in animal feeding to avoid the risk of the diffusion of mad cow disease. Bellagamba et al. (2003) conducted a study to describe a DNA monitoring method to examine fish meal for contamination with mammalian and poultry products. They have developed and evaluated a PCR method based on the nucleotide sequence variation in the 12 S ribosomal RNA gene of mitochondrial DNA. Three species-specific primer pairs were designed for the identification of ruminant, pig and poultry DNA. The specificity of the primers used in the PCR was tested by comparison with DNA samples for several vertebrate species and confirmed. The PCR specifically detected mammalian and poultry adulteration in fish meals containing 0.125% beef, 0.125% sheep, 0.125% pig, 0.125% chicken and 0.5% goat. A multiplex PCR assay for ruminant and pig adulteration was optimized and had a detection limit of 0.25%.

REFERENCES TO THE LITERATURE (PARTIAL LIST)

Anonymous, 2005. "A survey on feed quality control in Pondicherry" conducted by Department of Animal Nutrition, RAGACOVAS, Pondicherry.

AOAC 1995. Official methods of analysis. 16th ed. Association of Official Analytical Chemists, Washington, D.C. 2044.

Beever, D.E. and Kemp, C.F. Safety issues associated with the DNA in animal feed derived from genetically modified crops. University of Reading, U.K.

Bellagamba, F., Moretti, V.M., Comincini, S. and Valfe, F. 2001. Identification of species in animal feedstuffs by polymerase chain reaction: restriction fragment length polymorphism analysis of mitochondrial DNA. J Agric Food Chem 49: 3775-3781.

Bellagamba, F., Valfre, F., Panseri, S., Moretti, V.M. 2003. Polymerase chain reaction-based analysis to detect terrestrial animal protein in fish meal. J Food Prot 66 (4) 682-685.

Boom, R., Sol, C. J. A., Beld, M., Weel, J., Goudsmit, J. and Wertheim-van Dillen, P.W., 1999. Improved silica-guanidiniumthiocyanate DNA isolation procedure based on selective binding of bovine alpha-casein to silica particles. J Clin Micro 37:615-619.

Bradley, R.1996. The research programme on Transmissible Spongiform Encephalopathies in Britain with special reference to Bovine Spongiflrm Encephalopathy. Dev. Biol. Stand. 80:157-170\

Jones, F.T. 1996. Quality control in feed manufacturing. Feedstuffs, July17, pp135-138.

Krishna Reddy, T. 2003. Quality control of feed ingredients. In: Feed Processing Technology (Reddy, G.V.N., Krishna, N., Prasad, V.L.K., Reddy, K.J. and Reddy, Y.R. eds.) Compendium of short term training programme organized by TOE on Feed Technology and Quality Assurance (NATP), Department of Veterinary Biochemistry, College of Veterinary Science, ANGRAU, Hyderabad pp285-289.

Lahiff, S., Glennon, M., O'Brien, L., Lyng, J., Smith, T., Maher, M. and Shilton, and., 2001. Species-specific PCR for the identification of ovine, porcine and chicken species in meat and bone meal (MBM). Mol.Cell. Probes 15:27-35.

Marsh, R.F. 1991. Symposium BSE and Scrapie:Pathobiology and Public Health Policy. University of Illinois, March 14.

Matsunaga, T., Chikuni, K., Tanabe, R., Muroya, S., Shibata, K., Yamada, J. and Shinmura, Y., 1999. A quick and simple method for the identification of meat species and meat products by PCR assay. Meat Sci., 51: 143-148.

Myers, M. J., Friedman,S. L., Farrell,D. E., Dove-Pettit, D. A., Bucker, M. F., Kelly, S.,

Madzo, S., Campbell, W., Wang, R-F., Paine, D and Cerniglia, C.E. 2001. Validation of a polymerase chain reaction method for the detection of rendered bovine-derived materials in feedstuffs. J Food Prot 64: 564-566.

Myers, M. J., Yancy, H. F. and Farrell, D. E., 2003. Characterization of a polymerase chain reaction-based approach for the simultaneous detection of multiple animal-derived materials in animal feed. J Food Prot 66: 1085-1089.

Narahari, D. 2004. Feeds and Feedstuffs. Published by Pixie Publications India (P) Ltd, Karnal.

Prusiner, S.B. 1994. Annal Review Microbiol 43:655-686.

Reddy, D.V. 2001. Principles of Animal Nutrition and Feed Technology. Published by Oxford and IBH Publishing Co. Pvt. Ltd., New Delhi. pp. 337-345.

Souvenir 2004. R.R. Labs, First Anniversary Celebrations 2004, Ravinder Reddy, S., Krishna Kumar, C. V. R. and Rao, M.N. (eds), Hyderabad, pp 28-29.

Tajima, K., Enishi, O., Amari, M., Mitsumori, M., Kajikawa, H., Kurihara, M., Yanai, S., Matsui, H., Yasue, H., Mitsuhashi, T., Kawashima, T and Matsumoto, M., 2002. PCR detection of DNAs of animal origin in feed by primers based on sequences of short and long interspersed repetitive elements. Biosci. Biotechnol. Biochem., 66:2247-2250.

Talapatra, S.K., Roy, S.C. and Sen, K.C. 1940. Estimation of phosphorus, chlorine, calcium, magnesium, sodium and potassium in foodstuffs. Indian Journal of Veterinary Science and Animal Husbandry, 10: 243-258.

Tartaglia, M., Saulle, E., Pestalozza, S., Morelli,L., Antonucci, G. and Battaglia, P.A., 1998. Detection of bovine mitochondrial DNA in ruminant feeds: a molecular approach to test for the presence of bovine-derived materials. J Food Prot 61:513-518.

Wang, R-F., Myers, M.J., Campbell, W., Cao, W-W., Paine, D. and Cerniglia, C. E., 2000. A rapid method for PCR detection of bovine materials in animal feedstuffs. Mol. Cel. Probes 14:1-5.

SECTION IX
Appendix

APPENDIX

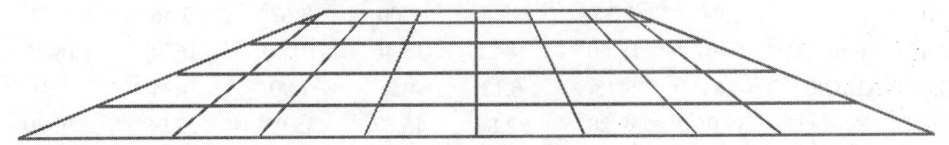

1. ANALYSIS OF CELL WALL FRACTIONS ON ASH FREE BASIS IN TREE LEAVES: METHODOLOGY AND DATA

Carbohydrates are defined as fibre carbohydrates [equal to neutral detergent fibre (NDF)] and non-fibre carbohydrates. Rumen microbes and animals utilize the different fractions of protein, non-fibre carbohydrate and structural (fibre) carbohydrate fractions differently and their estimation in the feedstuffs elucidates more information about their availability (Sniffen et al 1992). Inadequacies in the nitrogen free extract of the Weende analysis have been addressed by development of methods to quantify the nonstructural carbohydrates (NSC), which are mainly starches and sugars. The NSC and non-fibre carbohydrates (NFC) or neutral detergent soluble carbohydrates (NDSC), which are calculated by difference, are distinct fractions (NRC 2001). NDSC include some fibre carbohydrates such as pectins, β-glucans and fructans.

Table 1. Cell wall fractions and protein bound to cell wall fractions (%) of certain tree leaves on dry matter basis* D.V.Reddy and N.Elanchezhian, LRRD, 20, 5, 2008.

Tree leaves / Constituents	Acacia auric- uliformis	Cashew nut	Gliricidia	Jack	Sesbania grandi- flora	Subabul	Yellow gold mohur
Neutral detergent fibre (NDF)	36.94	45.79	38.38	30.09	18.99	40.37	49.02
NDF excluding ash (NDFom)	34.01	43.31	37.17	28.06	17.86	38.84	47.66
Acid detergent fibre (ADF)	30.08	39.08	27.11	25.22	15.82	28.33	30.39
ADF excluding ash (ADFom)	28.25	36.81	25.38	23.75	14.35	26.23	28.56
Acid detergent lignin	14.13	15.25	7.86	7.30	4.31	5.19	13.47
Silica	1.84	2.27	1.73	1.46	1.47	2.11	1.83

Hemicellulose (NDF-ADF)	5.76	6.50	11.79	4.31	3.51 ·	12.61	19.10
Cellulose (ADF-ADL)	14.12	21.58	17.52	16.45	10.04	21.04	15.09
NDICP	7.75	4.88	10.56	6.56	11.53	8.50	7.03
NDICP, % of CP	50.00	51.81	43.31	50.70	33.06	38.64	57.81
ADICP	2.94	1.75	4.44	2.00	3.63	3.56	2.22
ADICP, % of CP	18.97	18.60	18.21	15.46	10.40	16.18	18.26
NDICP-ADICP	4.81	3.13	6.12	4.56	7.90	4.94	4.81
NFC*	39.05	39.28	22.84	46.87	35.95	22.06	30.80
NFC**	46.80	44.16	33.40	53.43	47.48	33.11	37.83
NFC: NDF ratio	1.38	1.02	0.90	1.90	2.66	0.85	0.79

*NDICP, Neutral detergent insoluble crude protein; ADICP, Acid detergent insoluble crude protein; *NFC= .non-fibre carbohydrate calculated by difference 100 - (% CP + %NDF + %ether extract + % total ash); **NFC = 100 - [% CP + (%NDF - %NDICP) + % ether extract + % total ash)*

Tree leaves were analysed for neutral detergent fibre (NDF) without using α-amylase and sodium sulphite (Van Soest et al 1991) and acid detergent fibre (ADF), acid detergent lignin (ADL) and silica (Goering and Van Soest 1970). The NDF was expressed exclusive of residual ash (referred henceforth as NDFom) and ADF was corrected by the ash content of the ADL residue (ADFom), as recommended by Van Soest (2006), because of varying soil contamination in forages and feeds. The neutral detergent insoluble crude protein (NDICP) was derived by determining CP of the insoluble residue of the NDF extraction. The acid detergent insoluble crude protein (ADICP) was determined as the CP associated with the insoluble residue of an ADF extraction. Nitrogen free extract (NFE) and non-fibre carbohydrate (NFC) fraction that is soluble in neutral detergent (Neutral detergent soluble carbohydrates, NDSC) were calculated (Table 1).

2. Analysis of polyphenolic compounds in tree leaves: Methodology and data

Extraction and determination of total phenolics and tannins

Fresh tree leaves were hand plucked in the month of April 2007 and brought to the laboratory. The tree leaves were sun-dried with due care separately and ground to fine mesh. Sun drying was preferred because oven drying of feeds that contain proanthocyanidins, even at temperatures below 60°C, increased NDF, fibre bound nitrogen and lignin.

Leaf samples (200 mg) were extracted with ultrasonicator (Cell Disrupter Ultrasonic Probe, Model 1000L) at 4°C in 10 ml aqueous acetone solution (acetone/water: 7/3 v/v). After centrifugation (3000 x g at 4°C for 20 min), the supernatants (total phenolics extract) were analysed for phenolic components (total phenolics, non-tannin phenolics, total tannin phenolics and condensed tannins) as described by Makkar (2003b) using Spectronic[R] Genesys 2 Spectrophotometer. The facilities available at molecular biology lab of Department of Veterinary Biochemistry with the courtesy of Prof K.V.S.Reddy and Dr J.Thanislass were utilized and their assistance is gratefully acknowledged.

Contents of total phenolics was analysed using the Folin – Ciocalteu's reagent (Sisco Research Laboratories Pvt Ltd, Mumbai, India) based on tannic acid standard (Qualigens fine chemicals, GlaxoSmithKline Pharmaceuticals Ltd, Mumbai, India). Total phenolics consist of simple phenolic compounds or non-tannin phenolics and pure tannins or total tannin phenolics. Polyvinyl polypyrrolidone (PVPP; Sigma – Aldrich) has the property to bind tannins but not the simple phenolics. Two ml distilled (triple glass) water and 2 ml total phenolics extract were added to the test tube containing 200 mg PVPP and vortexed twice and filtered through Whatman No 1 filter paper. The filtrate was used to estimate non-tannin phenolics, which was subtracted from total phenolics to obtain total tannins. The concentration of total phenolics and total tannins were expressed as tannic acid equivalent.

Condensed tannin

Three ml n-butanol – HCl (95:5 v/v) and 0.1 ml ferric ammonium sulphate (1%) were added to the test tube containing 0.5 ml phenolics extract. The test tube was closed with a glass marble and heated in a boiling water bath for 60 min. The absorbance of the red anthocyanidin products (i.e., condensed tannin) was measured at 550 nm and condensed tannin was expressed as leucocyanidin equivalent (Table 2).

3. Protein and carbohydrate fractions in feedstuffs

The nitrogen (N) content of the ruminant feedstuffs continues to be one of the most commonly used index in feed evaluation. N solubility in mineral solvents and detergent solutions such as bicarbonate phosphate buffer (BCP), burrough's mineral mixture diluted to 10% with distilled water (BMM), McDougall's artificial saliva, 0.15% M NaCl and borate phosphate buffer (BF) has been tested for several feeds. Pichard and Van Soest (1977) and Krishnamoorthy et al. (1982, 1983) fractionated feeds into various categories based on chemical constituents as well as protein degradation rates.

The Cornell Net Carbohydrate and Protein System (CNCPS)

The Cornell Net Carbohydrate and Protein System (CNCPS) is a mathematical model to evaluate diet and animal performance. It was developed from basic principles of rumen function, microbial growth, feed digestion and passage and animal physiology. **The CNCPS partitions CP into 5 fractions using 3 solvents and a protein-precipitating agent.** The protein fractionation scheme used in the CNCPS is the most widely used and sophisticated multi-chemical approach for quantifying N fractions in feedstuffs (Sniffen et al., 1992; Fox et al., 2000). The 5 fractions are: A (NPN; soluble in borate-phosphate buffer but not precipitated with tungstic acid), B1 (rapidly degraded true protein; soluble in borate-phosphate buffer and precipitated with tungstic acid), B2 (moderately degraded true protein and large peptides; calculated as the difference between total CP and the sum of the other 4 CP fractions), B3

Table 2. Polyphenolic compounds (%) of certain tree leaves on dry matter basis*

Tree leaves / Constituents	Acacia auric- uliformis	Cashew nut	Gliricidia	Jack	Sesbania grandi- flora	Subabul	Yellow gold mohur
Total phenolics[1]	13.44	20.31	5.63	15.63	9.38	11.25	12.50
Non-tannin phenolics[1]	0.48	0.86	0.35	0.94	0.74	0.48	0.53
Total tannin phenolics[1]	12.96	19.45	5.28	14.69	8.64	10.78	11.98
Condensed tannins[2]	12.29	16.43	3.44	13.23	5.71	7.28	11.03

[1]*as tannic acid equivalent;*   [2]*as leucocyanidine equivalent*

* D.V.Reddy and N.Elanchezhian, LRRD, 20, 5, 2008.

(slowly degraded true protein; calculated as the difference between neutral detergent insoluble CP [NDICP] and acid detergent insoluble CP [ADICP]), and C (undegraded true protein; measured as ADICP).

In situ and multi-chemical derived protein fractions are used in NRC (2001) and CNCPS, respectively, to predict ruminal degradation of feed CP. A comparison of the two methods for predicting RDP/RUP and RUP digestibility indicated remarkable similarity. Both models appropriately recognize the fact that the proportional concentrations of RDP and RUP in feedstuffs are not static values and provide similar estimates of RUP and RUP digestibility by combining ruminal degradation of CP with rates of degradation and passage. Moreover, both models are sensitive to protein inputs, and both provide a good framework for the industry.

Cornell Net Carbohydrate and Protein System

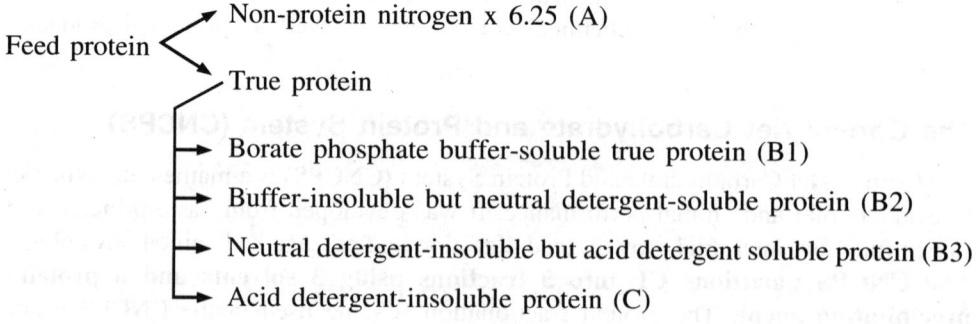

Feed protein
- Non-protein nitrogen x 6.25 (A)
- True protein
  - Borate phosphate buffer-soluble true protein (B1)
  - Buffer-insoluble but neutral detergent-soluble protein (B2)
  - Neutral detergent-insoluble but acid detergent soluble protein (B3)
  - Acid detergent-insoluble protein (C)

According to CNCPS, Sniffen et al. (1992) and NRC (2001), protein fractionation based on their solubility in borate phosphate buffer and detergent solution along with the rumen fermentation characteristics are useful to predict rumen degradability, microbial biomass synthesis and digestible amino acid flow to the duodenum.

Borate phosphate buffer soluble nitrogen, PBSN

Borate phosphate buffer insoluble nitrogen, PBIN = 100 − PBSN

Neutral detergent insoluble nitrogen, NDIN

Acid detergent insoluble nitrogen, ADIN

Borate phosphate buffer insoluble nitrogen (PBIN) estimation

Take 0.5 g sample into a 100 ml beaker.

Add 5 ml of 10% t-butyl alcohol (wetting agent) and 5 ml borate phosphate buffer.

Pichard's method: The sample is soaked at room temperature with stirring every 10 min for 1 hour and filter on Whatman No. 54 filter paper. Residue was washed with 50 ml buffer and 250 ml distilled water. Residual nitrogen is estimated by micro-kjeldahl.

(Borate phosphate is prepared by adding 12.2 g of $NaH_2PO_4.H_2O$ and 8.91 g of $Na_2B_4O_7.10H_2O$ per litre of distilled water). Borate phosphate is preferred since it is more stable compared to other solvents such as bicarbonate phosphate buffer, burrough's mineral mixture, McDougall's artificial saliva, 0.15% M NaCl.

NDIN & ADIN: NDF and ADF are isolated with Whatmen No 54 filter paper substituted for Gooch Crucibles. Nitrogen content is determined. The respective N contents are NDIN and ADIN.

A + B1 = Soluble protein

PBIN − NDIN = B2

NDIN − ADIN = B3

ADIN = C

Protein fractions as a percentage of C.P.

- Protein fraction of A of CP is NPN that enters the ruminal ammonia pool directly.
- B1 is true protein that has a rapid Kd and is nearly completely degraded in the rumen.
- C is ADICP and is assumed to be unavailable.
- B3 or slowly degraded protein fraction.
- B2 fraction, which is partly degraded in the rumen, is estimated as the difference between CP and the sum of soluble, B3 and C, where soluble protein equals A + B1.

Intestinal digestibility of the amino acids is assumed to be 100% for B1 and B2 and 80% for B3 protein pools.

Carbohydrates are categorized into A, B1, B2 and C fractions (Table 3).

1. A fraction: It is very rapidly fermented, water soluble, pool that is largely composed of sugars, although it also contains organic acids and short oligosaccharides.
2. B1 fraction is primarily starch and pectin.
3. B2 pool is composed of available NDF.
4. C pool is an indigestible fraction and it is computed as NDF × Lignin × 2.4% DM.

Table 3. Protein and Carbohydrate fractionation relative to ruminal availability

Fraction	Protein	Carbohydrate	Rumen availability
A	Ammonia N, soluble amino acids, proteins	Sugars, some starch, fructans	Soluble (generally highly available, 4% per min to 2% per hour
B1	Very rapid degrading proteins, oligopeptides	Fast degrading starch, pectin, oligosaccharides	Insoluble potentially digestible (1-30% per hour)
B2	Fast degrading protein	Slow degrading starch	——
B3	Medium degrading proteins	——	——
C	ADF bound proteins	Lignin	Nondigestible (0% per hour)

4. Limitations of Goering and Van Soest (1970)

P.J.Van Soest, J.B.Raobertson and B.A.Lewis (1991, Methods for Dietary Fiber, Neutral Detergent Fiber, and Nonstarch Polysaccharides in Relation to Animal Nutrition J. Dairy Science, 74: 3583) published the recommended procedures.

The pH of neutral detergent solution should be checked and adjusted to pH 7.0 using either HCl or NaOH. Solution should be discarded if it is not between 6.0 and 8.0, initially.

The original **NDF** method was applied to forages, and its subsequent application to starchy foods and feeds revealed interference by starch, thus presenting difficulties for the original neutral detergent **(ND)** method.

In the original ND method, starch removal was facilitated by using 2-ethoxyethanol. However, 2-ethoxyethanol (ethyleneglycol monoethyl ether) now is recognized as health risk. Its use appears necessary for optimal removal of starch. Therefore, 2-ethoxyethanol should be replaced by a safer reagent. Use of triethylene glycol at the same concentration gives equivalent values and is on safe list. Thus, even with the use of efficient amylases, addition of either 2-ethoxyethanol or triethylene glycol seems necessary for concentrate feeds. However, triethylene glycol does not have the antifoaming activity of 2-ethoxyethanol.

Use of sulfite

The use of sodium sulfite in the NDF procedure remains optional. Hence, addition of sulphite or otherwise needs to be indicated accordingly. Its purpose is to lower the protein level and remove keratinaceous residues of animal origin. Sulfite cleaves disulfide bonds and thus dissolves many cross-linked proteins. Its general use for ruminant feeds is discouraged, especially if the residues are to be used as an assay for ND insoluble protein, because the sulfite reaction is nonbiological. The ND and acid detergent (AD) insoluble proteins from animal products tend to be indigestible.

Sodium sulphite should be included in routine NDF analysis to remove nitrogen contamination, especially if feeds have been heated (maillard or nonenzymatic products).

Lipid Interferences

Lipid contents above 10% are a problem for both ND and AD if a separate oil layer forms in the solution because the detergents are more soluble in the lipid phase than in water. High values of ADF and NDF result. Simple removal of lipid may be done by brief heating in ethanol and filtering on the pretared crucible to be used subsequently for NDF or ADF. Contents and crucible are boiled in the NDF or ADF reagent as required.

Acid-Insoluble Ash

Neutral detergent reagent dissolves pectin and biogenic silica but not silicaceous soil minerals. On the other hand, Acid detergent solution precipitates pectic acid as the quaternary detergent salt and quantitatively recovers all silica. Acid-insoluble ash is conveniently measured as the residue from ADF after ashing at 525°C. The insoluble ash after lignin determination by either KMnO4 or Klason procedures is identical to that of the original ADF, provided that asbestos or other filter aids are not used.

5. Feed efficiency for milk production in purebred Holstein cows, crossbred cows and buffaloes

Variation between animals in feed conversion efficiency (FCE) may have genetic components, allowing selection for animals with greater efficiency and reduced environmental impact. A major source of variation in FCE is feed digestibility, and thus approaches that improve digestibility should improve FCE if rumen function is not disrupted. Methane represents a substantial loss of digestible energy from rations. Major determinants of methane emission are the amount of feed consumed and the proportions of forage and concentrates fed. In addition, feeding fat has long been known to reduce methane emission. A myriad of other supplements and additives are currently being investigated as mitigators of methane emission.

Dairy efficiency is defined as yield of milk per unit of dietary dry matter (DM) consumed. It is not commonly measured in dairy herds as is feed conversion to weight gain in swine, beef, and poultry. Feed efficiency for milk production depends on diet and other environmental factors and on the genetic ability of the cow to utilize these inputs to produce milk. Greater daily milk yield, high quality forages and improved feed digestibility increases dairy efficiency. Animals in early lactation have higher dairy efficiency. Inclement environmental / weather conditions, animals in late lactation, animals of first lactation have low dairy efficiency. See the data in the following table.

6. Comparison among pseudo ruminants, true ruminants, herbivores and monogastric animals

Rumen microorganisms

Bacteria can be cultured easily compared to protozoa. Clostridia can be distinguished from bacilli by anaerobic growth. Bacilli are aerobic spore-formers. The highest total counts of bacteria have been recorded with diets largely composed of concentrates.

All cellulose digesters need ammonia strictly. Ammonia is essential and they use it in preference to amino acids. The branched and straight-chain fatty acids required for many rumen bacteria arise through fermentation of the amino acids. Cellulose digestion is stimulated. Valine, proline, leucine and isoleucine are fermented to isobutyrate, valerate, 3-methyl butyrate and 2-methyl butyrate, respectively. These amino acids are synthesized from the same fatty acids by cellulolytic bacteria e.g. *Ruminococcus flavefaciens.*

Purebred Holstein cows, USA, UK

S.No	Feed dry matter per kg milk yield	Source
1	0.54 to 0.87	T R Dhiman et al., 1993, J Dairy Sci, 76, 1945
2	0.55 to 0.91	T R Dhiman and L D Satter 1993, J Dairy Sci, 76, 1960
3	0.65 to 0.73	T R Dhiman et al., 2001, Anim Feed Sci Technol, 90, 169
4	Early lactation = 0.53 to 0.56 Mid lactation = 0.71 to 0.75 Late lactation = 0.94 to 1.09	R M Kirkland and F J Gordon, 2001, Livest Prod Sci 72, 213.

Crossbred cows, India

S.No	Feed dry matter per kg milk yield	Source
1	0.95 to 1.04	S K Chouraba et al., 2003, Indian J Anim Sci73, 1353.
2	0.85 to 0.87	Puranik et al., 1997, Indian J Anim Sci 67, 146.
3	2.03 to 2.07	S Radotra and V S Upadhay, 2002, Indian J Anim Sci72, 815.
4.	1.94 to 2.15	R C Saha et al., 2002, Anim Nutr Feed Tech., 2, 83.
5	2.42 to 2.84	K S Rao et al., 1999, Indian J Anim Nutr., 16, 155.

Buffaloes, India

S.No	Feed dry matter per kg milk yield	Source
1	3.44 to 3.85	D P Tiwari and B R Patle, 1997, Indian J Anim Nutr., 14, 98.
2	2.80 to 3.22	D Nagalakshmi et al., 2004, Anim Nutr Feed Tech., 4, 23.
3.	1.60 to 1.82	A K Mishra et al., 2007, Indian J Anim Sci 77, 405.

Acetic acid is produced by more rumen species. Propionate and butyrate are formed by only a fourth of the species. *Selenomonas ruminantium, Megasphaera elsdenii* produce propionate. *Butyrivibrio fibrisolvens, Clostridium polysaccharolyticum, Clostridium lochheadii* produce butyrate. Butyrivibrio may use hydrogen in the reduction of acetate, but otherwise the only species known to utilize hydrogen is Methanobacterium.

Products of carbohydrate fermentation

Proportion of VFA in the rumen liquor in a sheep

Complete diet Hay: Concentrate	TVFA m.moles/litre	Molar proportions, % Acetic	Propionic	Butyric	Others
100 : 0	97	66	22	9	3
80 : 20	80	61	25	11	3
60 : 40	87	61	23	13	2
40 : 60	76	52	34	12	3
20 : 80	70	40	40	15	5

Proportion of VFA in blood (peripheral blood, cattle)

Acetic acid	93.3%
Propionic acid	2.4%
Butyric acid	2.5%
Higher fatty acids	1.8%

Pyruvate, hydroxypyruvate, glyoxylate, α-ketoisovalerate, α-ketoisocaproate, α-keto-β-methylvalerate, oxaloacetate, and α-ketoglutarate are detected in rumen fluid 30 min after the animal was fed.

Nutrient needs of ruminant versus monogastric species

The dietary needs of ruminants are simpler and often cheaper than for non-ruminants. Ruminants derive much of their energy from fibrous roughages. Ruminants don't have dietary amino acid requirement, only a nitrogen or crude protein requirement. Ruminants don't have a dietary requirement for the B-complex vitamins. Non-ruminants can utilize only limited amounts of fibrous material (Table 4). These differences are due to the microorganisms in the rumen. As a result of ruminal fermentation, ruminants are able to convert poor quality feed sources, which are unusable or poorly usable by non-ruminants, to high quality meat and milk which can be used by man and other non-ruminants.

Table 4. Differences in fibre digestion between ruminants and hindgut digesters

Attributes	Horses	Ruminants
1. Total stomach capacity	Less than 20 L	About 250 L for cow
2. Fermentative digestion	Postgastric	Pregastric
3. Feed passage time through GIT	24 h less time for hindgut fermentation; so less complete fibre digestion	72 h

4. Microbial activity	Less	More
	Limited amount of protein, B-vitamins and vitamin K are synthesized. The smaller capacity and less fermentation means a horse can't handle as much forage as ruminants. Fibre must be of higher quality. Little or no NPN should be fed. B-vitamin supplementation may be necessary.	
5. Efficiency of absorption of fermentation products	Less	More
	Small intestine with its immense absorptive surface never gets a chance at the ingesta from the caecum and colon. Most microbial production in the hindgut is excreted in the faeces.	Rumen microbial cells are digested in abomasum and small intestine.

Rumen microbial fermentation cause less efficient use of high quality proteins and energy utilization is lowered by methane production. Ruminants can't use as much dietary fat as non-ruminants because of adverse effects of fat on rumen microbial fermentation and of limited pancreatic lipase activity. Ruminants can't digest as much starch, maltose and sucrose in the gastrointestinal tract as non-ruminants can, but these nutrients are usually be fermented in the rumen which eliminates the need for extensive intestinal digestion of these nutrients.

Pseudoruminant llamas (*Lama glama*) versus pecoran ruminants

There have been many questions regarding the relative digestion efficiencies of pseudoruminant llamas (three compartment stomach) and pecoran ruminants (true ruminants; four compartment stomach). It has been suggested that llamas and their close relative, the alpaca, have superior digestive capabilities compared to pecoran ruminants. However, some research workers have found no differences between these taxa, especially on high crude protein diets. Llamas are more efficient on low-quality feeds because they lose less urinary N than do ruminants. Under confined laboratory conditions camelids have been reported to have a higher efficiency in extracting energy and protein from forages than pecoran ruminants.

7. Bioavailability of Minerals from Pulses

The mineral content of legumes is generally high, but the availability is poor due to the presence of phytate, which is a main inhibitor of iron (Fe) and zinc (Zn) absorption. The negative influence on iron absorption is nutritionally the most important because in many developing countries the diet is based on cereals and legumes. Deficiency of iron, and perhaps zinc, is highly prevalent in developing countries. All the more, it is more crucial in a vegetarian diet.

Mineral content (mg/100 g) of legumes

legume	Fe	Zn	Ca	Mg
Phaseolus vulgaris	7.0	3.0	197	250
Peas (Pisum sativum)	7.36	3.01	96	132
Chickpeas/Bengalgram	6.96	3.54	124	155
Lentils	7.50	3.73	71	129
Soybeans	6.64	4.18	201	220

Legumes contain varying amounts of polyphenols and generally the amounts are considered higher in coloured seeds. Beans of species *Phaseolus vulgaris* are found to contain high amounts of polyphenols whereas the content of polyphenols in peas (*Pisum sativum*) is very low. These Fe-binding polyphenols inhibit Fe absorption. Further, soya protein per se has an inhibiting effect on Fe absorption. A certain amount of oxalic acid occurs in Phaseolus beans and oxalic acid is known to decrease calcium absorption in monogastric animals.

How to increase the bioavailability of minerals?

Efficient removal of phytate, and polyphenols can be obtained by enzymatic degradation during food processing, either by increasing the activity of the naturally occurring plant phytases and polyphenol degrading enzymes, or by addition of enzyme preparations. Degradation of phytate can occur both during food processing and in the gastrointestinal tract. Efforts have been made to reduce the amount of phytate in foods by means of phytate-degrading enzymes, phytases, present naturally in the plant foods or present in yeasts or other microorganisms used in food processing. In case of oxalic acid, both cooking and dehulling reduced it.

Ascorbic acid is a potent enhancer of iron absorption and it can counteract the inhibitory effect of phytate. Increasing the ascorbic acid concentration is a good means of improving iron absorption. Certain organic acids formed during fermentation may also improve iron absorption.

Practical means to enhance the bioavailability of minerals

Biological food-processing techniques such as soaking, germination, fermentation, etc., increase the activity of native enzymes of cereals and legumes. During germination, phytase enzymes are synthesized or activated; ascorbic acid content is generated and enhanced. Lactic fermentation leads to lowering of pH as a consequence of bacterial production of lactic acid and other organic acids, which is favourable for cereal phytase activity. Germination of lentils reduced the amount of phenolic compounds.

Strictly vegetarian diets based on unrefined cereals and legumes will result in low absorption of iron and zinc. Otherwise in a balanced diet containing animal protein, a high intake of legumes does not imply a risk of inadequate mineral supply. The absorption of minerals depends on the total composition of the meal rather than a particular foodstuff.

8. Dietary Phytoestrogens

Evidence is emerging that dietary phytoestrogens play a beneficial role in obesity and diabetes. Phytoestrogens are shown to have antioxidative, antiproliferative and antiangiogenic activities. Hence higher consumption of phytoestrogens might be protective against certain chronic diseases. Epidemiological studies suggest that consumption of a phytoestrogen-rich diet is associated with a lower risk of coronary heart disease, osteoporosis, menopausal symptoms and cancers of prostate, breast and colon.

What are phytoestrogens?

Phytoestrogens are a group of biologically active plant substances (Table 5). Phytoestrogens are classified into three main classes: isoflavones, lignans and coumestans. Structurally, coumestans and isoflavones resemble endogenous steroid estrogen, estradiol.

Phytoestrogens are found in various foodstuffs consumed by humans. Their biochemistry, absorption and metabolism are described briefly in the following lines.

Isoflavones

The major bioactive isoflavones are genistein and daidzein. They are both present in plants and may also be metabolized from other isoflavonoid plant precursors, biochanin

Table 5. Prominent Food Sources of Phytoestrogens

Food Source Phytoestrogen content	Phytoestrogen present µg/g
Roasted soybeans	
Isoflavones: Total	2661
Genistein	1426
Diadzein	941
Glycitein	294
Flaxseed	
Lignans: Secoisolariciresinol	3699
Matairesinol	10.9
Soybean	
Lignans: Secoisolariciresinol	2.73
Matairesinol	Trace
Peanuts	
Lignans: Secoisolariciresinol	3.33
Matairesinol	Trace

A and formononetin, respectively. The most abundant food sources of isoflavones are soybean and soybean products. Other beans, lentil, peas, nuts and clover contain a very small quantity of isoflavones. In soybean, the isofavones are tightly associated with protein. Roasted soybeans and commercially available soy products (soy flour and textured protein) contain 0.1- 5 mg isoflavones/ g protein.

Isoflavones exist primarily in plants as glycosides in their inactive form. Once ingested, isoflavone glycosides (genistin and daidzin) are hydrolyzed in the intestines by bacterial β-glucosidases and are converted to corresponding bioactive aglycones (genistein and daidzein) while further fermentation proceeds in the distal intestine.

The aglycones are then absorbed from the intestinal tract and conjugated mainly in the liver to glucuronides, which are either reexcreted through the bile, and reabsorbed by enterohepatic recycling or excreted unchanged in the urine. Daidzein may be further metabolized (by gut bacterial flora) to equol, dihydrodaidzein, or O-demethylangolensin(O-Dma), whereas genistein may be metabolized to p-ethylphenol in the colon. Daidzein, genistein, equol, and 0-demethylangolensin are the major isoflavones that have been detected in the blood and urine of animals and humans. Dihydrodaidzein, p-ethylphenol, and glycetin have also been detected in human plasma.

Lignans

Lignans are constituents of many plants and form the building blocks for the formation of lignin in the plant cell wall. They are more predominant in the plant kingdom compared to isoflavones. The two major mammalian lignans, enterolactone and enterodiol, are produced from matairesinol and secoisolariciresinol, respectively, and possibly from other plant precursors, by gut microflora.

Common food sources include whole oil seeds, whole grain cereals, nuts, fruits, vegetables and coffee and tea. The highest concentrations of lignans are found in flaxseed while other foods have very small quantities. Modern processing techniques tend to deplete grains of their lignan content because they remove the outer fibre layer that has highest concentration of lignan precursors.

Plant lignans also undergo intestinal hydrolysis by bacterial β-glucosidases. The lignan glycosides matairesinol and secoisolariciresinol are converted to their corresponding metabolites, enterolactone and enterodiol, by the action of colonic bacteria; further enterodiol is readily oxidized to enterolactone. These metabolites are then absorbed in the colon and conjugated with glucuronic acid or sulfate in the liver. Some of the metabolites may also undergo enterohepatic circulation. Lignans are excreted in bile and urine as conjugated glucuronides and in faeces in the unconjugated form. The major metabolites, enterolactone and enterodiol, are excreted in the urine.

Coumestans

Coumestans occur predominantly during germination. Coumesterol is the most important form of coumestan consumed by humans. The major food sources of coumesterol are alfalfa sprouts, clover sprouts, dry round split peas and other legume sprouts.

How do they act?

Phytoestrogens, especially the isoflavones and coumestans, have certain hormonally mediated influences because of their structural resemblance to endogenous steroid estrogen. Isoflavones and coumestans are able to bind to the estrogen receptor; their plasma concentration is several fold lower than that of endogenous estradiol. It is also suggested that isoflavones and coumestans act as anti-estrogens by competing with the more potent endogenous estrogen on the estrogen receptor. Lignans hardly show binding affinity to the estrogen receptor. In addition, phytoestrogens have beneficial effects through several other mechanisms.

Concentration of phytoestrogens in plasma and urine

Plasma isoflavone concentrations increase markedly in the micromolar range (1-4 ?mol/L) after ingestion of soy diets while the corresponding figures are in the nanomolecular range (< 40 nmol/L) for healthy humans consuming diets without soy. Similarly urinary excretion of isoflavones increases markedly after ingestion of isoflavone-rich diets.

In healthy young women consuming diets supplemented with flaxseed, plasma lignan concentrations increased from 29 to 52 nmol/L after ingestion of flaxseed. Urinary lignan excretion also increased with increasing dietary intake of lignan precursors.

Biomarkers, such as plasma or urinary excretions, usually represent only a short period (up to 48h) of phytoestrogen intake, and are influenced by the bioavailability of phytoestrogens consumed. Bioavailability of phytoestrogens varies among individuals and depends on many factors, such as habitual diet, duration of soy consumption, presence of gut microflora, use of antibiotics, gender, differences in individual metabolism patterns that might be due to genetic factors.

Effect of soybeans on glucose and lipid metabolism

Studies in healthy human beings showed that soy polysaccharides reduce postprandial glucose and triacylglycerol concentrations. Studies in obese subjects with type 2 diabetes, also revealed that the soy polysaccharide (10 g fibre) reduced the postprandial hyperglycemia and triacylglycerol concentrations. Beneficial effect of feeding soy hull (26-52 g fibre/day for 2-4 weeks) to type 2 diabetics on glucose tolerance, lipid indexes and glycated/glycosylated haemoglobin has also been reported. This effect may have been due to the effect of nongelforming fibre of soy polysaccharide.

Soy proteins are rich in arginine and glycine, which are involved in insulin and glucagon secretion from the pancreas; soy proteins induced a lower postprandial insulin-glucagon ratio in healthy and hypercholesterolemic subjects; decreased plasma insulin by soy protein may be due to decreased release from the pancreas or increased hepatic removal; decreased postprandial insulin and glucose is associated with a significant reduction in serum total cholesterol, LDL-cholesterol and triacylglycerol concentrations; higher glucose disposal rates were also observed indicating an improvement in peripheral insulin sensitivity. All these findings emphasize that soybean diets provide potential benefits in conditions associated with impaired glucose tolerance, hyperlipidemia, and reduced insulin sensitivity.

Effect of flaxseed on obesity and diabetes

It has been reported that 50 g carbohydrates from flaxseed or 25 g flaxseed mucilage (soluble fibre) lowered postprandial glucose by 27% in healthy women. In healthy and hyperlipidemic subjects, ingestion of whole flaxseed lowers serum total cholesterol and LDL-cholesterol. These beneficial effects may be due to n-3 α-linolenic acid and lignans.

Like soy isoflavones, lignans have antioxidant activity. The antioxidant activity of secoisolariciresinol and enterodiol is higher than that of vitamin E or the parent glucoside present in flaxseed.

Common Food Sources of Phytoestrogens

Isoflavones	Coumestans	Lignans
Soybeans/Soy foods	Groundnuts	Broccoli, Brussels sprouts, Mushrooms, Cabbage,
(e.g. Tofu)		Cauliflower, Beans, Garlic, Onion
Peas and beans		Carrots, Beetroots, Tomato, Pears, Orange,
		Groundnuts Grapes, Coffee & tea
		Groundnuts, Almonds, Cashew nuts, Walnuts

9. Whole Pulses are Functional Foods

Pulses are commonly defined as 'the edible seeds of leguminous plants cultivated for food, as peas, beans, lentils, etc.' In India popular pulses include greengram (mung bean), blackgram, redgram (*tur/arhar*), bengalgram (chick pea), lentil, cowpea, field bean, *rajma*, soybean. Of these, greengram, bengalgram, cowpea, pea, soybean, field bean, *rajma* are used as whole gram. Protein of pulses is deficient in methionine while redgram is deficient in methionine and tryptophan. Pulses when used as whole such as bengalgram, cowpea, field bean, soybean, rajma can contribute maximum benefits. Greengram sprouts are excellent; whole gram *dhals* e.g., greengram, blackgram, are excellent.

Grain legumes are considered to be good for health due to their mutual compatibility with cereals. It has long been recognized that legumes are functional foods that promote good health and have therapeutic properties. Pulses contain a wide range of nutrients and non-nutrient bioactive microconstituents. Nutrients include vegetable protein, resistant starch, nonstarch polysaccharides (soluble and insoluble dietary fibre), oligosaccharides, folates, selenium, zinc while non-nutrients include enzyme inhibitors (protease and amylase inhibitors), lectins, phytates, oxalates, phenolic compounds, saponins, alkaloids. Legumes are considered as low glycaemic index foods and the resistant starch seems to confer protection against colorectal cancer.

Increased intake of pulses, preferably in their whole form, have beneficial effect on blood pressure, provide better control over blood glucose levels and thus reduce the risk of diabetes, protect from development of obesity and be useful in weight management and possibly, colon cancer. Pulses are excellent food choices because of their nutritional values and their cardioprotective effects. Several of these beneficial effects attributable to pulses result from a synergism between the nutrient and non-nutrient bioactive microconstituents, which are integrated in pulses.

Mechanisms for the hypocholesterolaemic effects of pulses

The hypocholesterolaemic effects of pulses appear related to the following factors: soluble dietary fibre, vegetable protein, oligosaccharides, isoflavones, phospholipids and fatty acids, phytosterols, saponins and other factors.

Soluble or viscous fibres

Psyllium, guar gum and other fibres from pulses, in the same order, reduce serum cholesterol and LDL-cholesterol levels. The major effects of these soluble fibres on serum lipoproteins appear related in bile acid binding and decreased reabsorption of bile acids. Fermentation of soluble fibres in the colon with production of short-chain fatty acids appears to contribute to decreased hepatic cholesterol synthesis. Changes in serum insulin concentrations might also contribute to a lower serum cholesterol levels (Pulses are low-glycaemic index foods).

Isoflavones, phytosterols, saponins and phospholipids in pulses could contribute to hypocholesterolaemic effects.

Effects of pulses on hypertension, diabetes and obesity

Generous intake of dietary fibre (fruits, vegetables, wholegrain cereals and pulses) decreases blood pressure. That is why, in general, vegetarians have lower blood pressures than nonvegetarians, though dietary differences and life-style differences between these groups also matters.

Increasing dietary fibre intake is usually associated with a decrease in blood pressure. Pulses are a good source of starch, dietary fibre, protein and minerals such as calcium, iron, potassium, magnesium and zinc. They are also lower in sodium and contain no cholesterol. A low sodium intake has been reported to decrease systolic blood pressure by 9mmHg and diastolic blood pressure by 4.5mmHg.

Pulses being low glycaemic index foods can offer an important benefit for blood glucose control for diabetic individuals.

Pulses in their whole form are excellent sources of dietary fibre. Extensive epidemiological data supported a role for dietary fibre in the management of obesity. Experimental studies in men suggest that high fibre intakes are associated with the following attributes: longer eating times because of the lower energy density of high-fibre diets; delayed gastric emptying, leading to earlier sense of fullness; earlier satiety because of the gastric and intestinal effects of fibre; decreased absorption of nutrients.

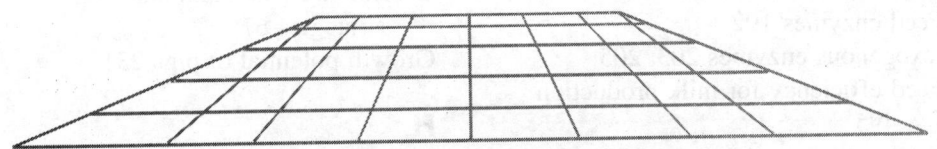

SUBJECT INDEX